Lasers and Energy Devices for the Skin

Lasers and Energy Devices for the Skin

Second Edition

Edited by

Mitchel P. Goldman, MD
Volunteer Clinical Professor of Dermatology/Medicine, University of California, San Diego, California, USA
Goldman, Butterwick, Fitzpatrick, Groff, and Fabi Cosmetic Laser Dermatology, San Diego, California, USA

Richard E. Fitzpatrick, MD
Volunteer Associate Clinical Professor of Dermatology/Medicine, University of California, San Diego, California, USA
Goldman, Butterwick, Fitzpatrick, Groff, and Fabi Cosmetic Laser Dermatology, San Diego, California, USA

E. Victor Ross, MD
Scripps Clinic Laser and Cosmetic Dermatology Center, San Diego, California, USA

Suzanne L. Kilmer, MD
Laser & Skin Surgery Center of Northern California, Sacramento, California, USA

Robert A. Weiss, MD, FAAD, FACPH
Associate Professor, Johns Hopkins University School of Medicine, Baltimore, Maryland, USA
Director, Maryland Laser, Skin, and Vein Institute, Baltimore, Maryland, USA

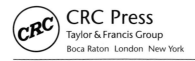

CRC Press
Taylor & Francis Group
Boca Raton London New York

CRC Press is an imprint of the
Taylor & Francis Group, an **informa** business

CRC Press
Taylor & Francis Group
6000 Broken Sound Parkway NW, Suite 300
Boca Raton, FL 33487-2742

© 2013 by Taylor & Francis Group, LLC
CRC Press is an imprint of Taylor & Francis Group, an Informa business

No claim to original U.S. Government works

Printed on acid-free paper
Version Date: 20130208

Printed and bound in India by Replika Press Pvt. Ltd.

International Standard Book Number-13: 978-1-84184-933-1 (Hardback)

Visit the Taylor & Francis Web site at
http://www.taylorandfrancis.com

and the CRC Press Web site at
http://www.crcpress.com

Contents

v

List of Contributors

R. Rox Anderson
Department of Dermatology
Wellman Center for Photomedicine
Massachusetts General Hospital
Boston, Massachusetts, USA

Mathew M. Avram
Department of Dermatology
Massachusetts General Hospital
Harvard Medical School
Boston, Massachusetts, USA

Karen L. Beasley
Department of Dermatology
The University of Maryland School of Medicine and
The Maryland Laser, Skin, and Vein Institute
Hunt Valley, Maryland, USA

Sabrina G. Fabi
Goldman, Butterwick, Fitzpatrick, Groff, and
Fabi Cosmetic Laser Dermatology
San Diego, California, USA

Richard E. Fitzpatrick
University of California and Goldman, Butterwick,
Fitzpatrick, Groff, and Fabi Cosmetic Laser Dermatology
San Diego, California, USA

Lilit Garibyan
Laser, Cosmetic Center and
Wellman Center for Photomedicine Massachusetts
General Hospital and Department of Dermatology
Harvard Medical School Boston,
Massachusetts, USA

Mitchel P. Goldman
University of California and Goldman, Butterwick, Fitzpatrick,
Groff, and Fabi Cosmetic Laser Dermatology
San Diego, California, USA

Omar A. Ibrahimi
Connecticut Skin Institute, Stamford, Connecticut, USA
Wellman Center for Photomedicine, Massachusetts General
Hospital and Harvard Medical School,
Boston, Massachussets, USA

H. Ray Jalian
Laser and Cosmetic Center and Wellman Center for
Photomedicine, Massachusetts General Hospital and
Department of Dermatology, Harvard Medical School
Boston, Massachusetts, USA

Suzanne L. Kilmer
Laser & Skin Surgery Center of Northern California,
Sacramento, California, USA

William T. Kirby
Laser Tattoo Removal and Laser Hair Removal, Beverly Hills,
California, USA

Andrew C. Krakowski
Pediatric Dermatology, University of California and
Rady Children's Hospital, San Diego, California, USA

Woraphong Manuskiatti
Department of Dermatology, Faculty of Medicine Siriraj
Hospital, Mahidol University, Bangkok, Thailand

Ane B.M. Niwa Massaki
Former fellow at Goldman, Butterwick, Fitzpatrick, Groff and
Fabi Cosmetic Laser Dermatology,
San Diego, California, USA

Melanie D. Palm
Art of Skin MD, Solana Beach, and Laser Skin Care Center,
Long Beach, California, USA

Jennifer D. Peterson
Dermatology and Laser Surgery Center, Houston, Texas, USA

E. Victor Ross
Laser and Cosmetic Dermatology Center, Scripps Clinic,
San Diego, California, USA

Penny J. Smalley
Technology Concepts International, Chicago, Illinois, USA

Robert A. Weiss
Johns Hopkins University School of Medicine and The Maryland
Laser, Skin, and Vein Institute, Baltimore, Maryland, USA

Douglas A. Winstanley
Laser and Cosmetic Dermatology Center, Scripps Clinic,
San Diego, California, USA

Jennifer G. Wojtczak
Weiss Memorial Hospital, Chicago, Illinois, USA

1 Laser–tissue interactions*

E. Victor Ross and R. Rox Anderson

INTRODUCTION

When using a light source, many physicians dial in "suggested" settings and proceed, using identifiable endpoints to determine if the parameters are appropriate. For example, when treating a port-wine stain (PWS) with the pulsed dye laser (PDL), the physician looks for immediate purpura and is vigilant to ensure that no surface whitening occurs. Although this is a good way, perhaps the best, to ensure that a favorable outcome is secured, it is instructive for the operator to know from first principles how the clinical endpoint was achieved. This will allow the physician to expand his laser repertoire and optimize the use of this very expensive equipment. For example, armed with an education in laser–tissue interactions (LTIs), one can cajole the PDL to treat pigmented lesions without purpura by compressing the lesions with a clear plastic piece (Fig. 1.1). This removes blood as a chromophore and increases the ratio of melanin to vascular heating (1). There are many other creative ways to use light-based technologies, but without a basic understanding of LTIs, one is reduced to treating skin ailments like one microwaves popcorn (according only to the instructions with no license to do it better). In short, an understanding of light–tissue and electrical–tissue interactions optimizes clinical outcomes in cutaneous laser surgery.

MACROSCOPIC BASIS OF LTI

Light demonstrates both wave and particle properties. Normally, wave behavior accurately describes light's behavior in space and at large interfaces (i.e., skin and air) (2). However, the particle properties (and quantum physics) are more useful in characterizing electromagnetic radiation (EMR)–tissue interactions on a molecular level (vide infra) (3). On a macroscopic level, light behavior conforms to various laws and equations that are consistent with our "eyeball" observations in nature. For example, we are familiar with refraction and reflection (4). Normally, the percentage of incident light reflected from the skin surface is determined by the index of refraction mismatch between the skin surface (stratum corneum, $n = 1.55$) and air ($n = 1$) (2). The Fresnel equations can be used to describe how much light will be reflected from the

skin (4). Depending on the angle between the light beam and the skin, this value varies considerably. More light is reflected as the angle of incidence between the beam and the surface approaches zero. It follows that, in most laser applications, we want to maintain a perpendicular angle to minimize reflective losses (5,6). This regular reflectance is about 4–7% for light incident at right angles to the skin (Fig. 1.2). One can reduce interface losses by applying an alcohol solution ($n = 1.4$) or even water ($n = 1.33$). This allows for optical coupling (vide infra). On the other hand, because of multiple index of refraction mismatches (keratin–air–keratin–air, etc.), dry skin reflects a great deal of light (hence the white appearance of a psoriasis plaque). Light not reflected at the skin surface penetrates into the epidermis. At this point, further light propagation in skin is determined by wavelength-dependent localized absorption and scattering (vide infra) (4). Overall, because of scattering, much incident light is remitted (remittance refers to the total light returned to the environment due to multiple scattering in the epidermis and dermis, as well as the regular reflection from the surface; Fig. 1.2). The amount of light "wasted" because of remittance varies from 15% to as much as 70% depending on wavelength and skin type. For example, for 1064 nm, 60% of an incident laser beam may be remitted. One can easily verify this by holding a finger just adjacent to the beam near the skin surface. Considerable warmth will be felt with higher fluences, all of which is due to a remitted portion of the beam. For our purposes, light can be divided into the ultraviolet (UV; 200–400 nm), visible (VIS; 400–760 nm), near-infrared (NIR; 760–1400 nm), mid-infrared (MIR; 1.4–3 μm), and far-infrared (FIR; 3 μm and beyond). These are the wavelength ranges that are important in laser dermatology (2).

TYPES OF LASERS AND PROPERTIES OF LASERS

Lasers as light sources are useful because they can, depending on parameters, allow for exquisite control of where and how much one heats. However, most reactions with biological systems are nonspecific to radiation from laser sources and at least in principle could be induced by thermal sources as well (3). What are the advantages of laser? For the most part, properties of laser light (i.e., coherence) are irrelevant insofar as the way light interacts with skin in therapeutic applications. This contention is supported by the increasing use of filtered flashlamps in dermatology. There are four properties that are common to all laser types: (*i*) beam directionality, (*ii*) narrow beam divergence, (*iii*) spatial and temporal coherence of the beam, and (*iv*) high intensity of the beam (7).

---

* The reader should note that although the title of this chapter is "Laser–tissue interactions", the introduction of many new and diverse technologies makes the term somewhat obsolete. We will continue to use the term, but a more appropriate is "electromagnetic radiation (EMR)–tissue interactions." Both terms are used interchangeably in the remainder of the text.

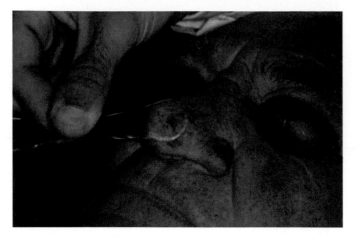

Figure 1.1 Example of compression technique. The plastic piece is used to "remove" blood so that lentigo can be treated with 1.5-ms pulsed dye laser without purpura.

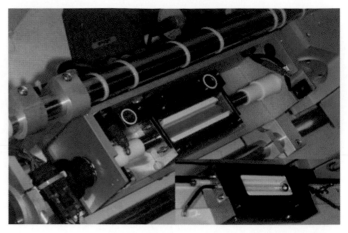

Figure 1.3 Ruby rod attached to high-power voltage. Flashlamp assembly is adjacent to rod. Normally the lamp is attached atop the rod assembly. Mirror allows the rod to be excited circumferentially.

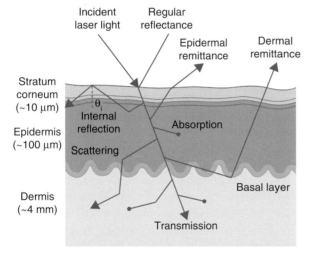

Figure 1.2 The behavior of light at skin surface.

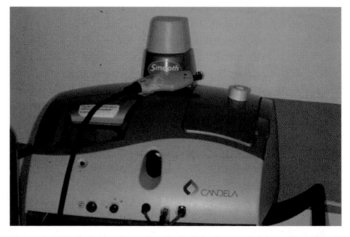

Figure 1.4 Diode laser where the diode light is coupled into fiber that is attached to the handpiece.

The greatest advantages of laser light are the intensity and the monochromaticity—this allows a degree of precision that is hard to reproduce with nonlaser sources. The beam of the laser is easy to manipulate. The beam can, for example, be expanded, or focused, quite easily. On the other hand, with nonlaser sources, such as flashlamps, one cannot exceed the brightness of the source lamp. It follows that the intensity of the beam can only be attenuated once emitted from the lamp surface. Lasers can create very high intensity light because of the property of stimulated emission. With laser, a lamp similar to the intense pulsed light (IPL) flashlamp pumps the laser cavity. The amplification of the light within the cavity sets laser light apart from other sources. Laser is really a fancy way to convert lamplight to a more powerful monochromatic form (8). The high power of the light (especially peak power with pulsed lasers) is not attainable outside of laser sources. The ability to focus the laser beam is an important contributor to the peak power density of the laser. Very small beam angles can be obtained that are not possible with intrinsically divergent nonlaser light sources (i.e., IPL) (9).

With respect to lasing media, there are diode lasers, solid-state lasers, and gas lasers. An example of a solid-state laser is the neodymium (Nd) laser. These lasers have a rod that is pumped by a flashlamp (Fig. 1.3). Miniaturized diode lasers have become more powerful and popular. Some diode lasers are housed separate from the handpiece (Fig. 1.4). Others are configured with the laser diodes in the handpiece (Fig. 1.5). Modern diode lasers are capable of much higher powers than in the past years, but their peak powers are still limited compared with most pulsed solid-state lasers (10).

IPL devices are becoming increasingly popular (11–17). Because the absorption spectra of skin chromophores are not monochromatic, a broadband light source is a logical approach for cosmetic applications. Rather than using a lamp to pump a laser, these devices use the lamp directly. Appropriate filtration creates the optimal output spectrum for a particular application. Much like a slide projector with a specific color slide, these bright lamps produce spectra that can mirror the absorption spectrum of melanin, hemoglobin, and even water. The advantages of these devices are their flexibility, but one disadvantage is that one must hold the lamp, cooling, and the high-voltage source in the hand. This creates a larger "umbilical cord" compared with the fibers and articulated arms used by most laser devices. Also, the beam diverges quickly, and nonlaser beams are not optically as easily manipulated as true laser beams. Very short pulses (e.g., Q-switched nanosecond (ns)

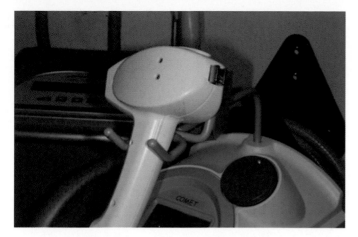

Figure 1.5 Another diode laser; in this case, the diodes are in the handpiece. This configuration allows for more direct application of laser light. However, placement of diodes in the handpiece requires that "high voltage" and laser cooling be attached to the handpiece by larger "umbilical" cord.

pulses) are not possible with these sources alone; they can, however, be used to pump a Q-switched laser, and newer IPLs have featured a Q-switched attachment (Fig. 1.6).

Basic parameters for any EMR procedure are power, time, and spot size for continuous wave (CW) lasers, and for pulsed lasers, the energy per pulse, pulse duration, spot size, fluence, repetition rate, and the total number of pulses (18). Energy is measured in joules (J). The amount of energy delivered per unit area is the fluence, sometimes called the dose or radiant exposure, is given in J/cm^2. The rate of energy delivery is called power, measured in watts (W). One watt is 1 joule per second (W = J/s). The power delivered per unit area is called the irradiance or power density, usually given in W/cm^2. Laser exposure duration [called pulse width (pw) for pulsed lasers] is the time over which energy is delivered. Dermatology uses EMR exposures ranging from many seconds to nanoseconds. The fluence is equal to the irradiance times the exposure duration (19). Power density is one of the most important parameters, for it often determines the action mechanism in cutaneous applications (Fig. 1.7). For example, a very low irradiance (typical range of 2–10 mW/cm^2) does not markedly increase tissue temperature and is associated with diagnostic applications, photochemical processes, and biostimulation. On the other extreme, a very short ns pulse can generate high peak power densities associated with photomechanical injury and even plasma formation (20). Other important factors are the laser exposure spot size (which greatly affects intensity inside the skin), whether the incident light is convergent, divergent, or diffuse, and the uniformity of irradiance over the exposure area (spatial beam profile). The pulse profile, that is, the character of the pulse shape in time (instantaneous power vs. time) is another feature that can impact the tissue response (18).

When we train residents, one of the greatest challenges is understanding all of these above terms within the context of a specific EMR device. When a novice confronts a laser instrument panel, there is often a grimace born of confusion. The staggering array of options on some user interfaces can be overwhelming (Fig. 1.8). Many physicians would prefer to have fewer options and a simpler display, especially early on in their use of a particular laser. However, like the driver who feels confined by an automatic transmission, the experienced

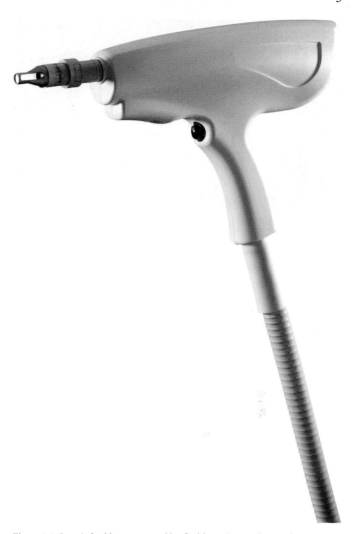

Figure 1.6 Q-switched laser pumped by flashlamp in IPL device (from ALMA Laser website). The laser rod is in the handpiece.

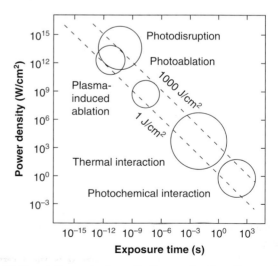

Figure 1.7 The relative mechanisms of action as a function of power density ranges. *Source*: Modified from Ref. 157.

laser surgeon usually wants the flexibility in tweaking parameters. Many manufacturers have accommodated both types of users, providing preset parameter sets (and "go-bys") while still allowing for experienced physicians to choose parameter configurations of their liking.

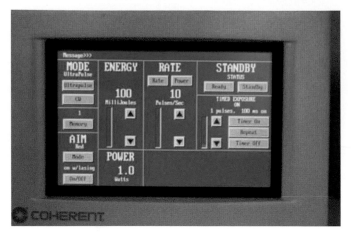

Figure 1.8 Instrument panel of a common carbon dioxide laser. The panel is intuitive once the operator is experienced.

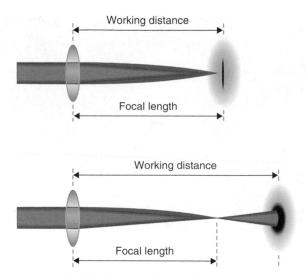

Figure 1.9 A focusing handpiece like that typically used with continuous wave carbon dioxide laser. Operator can vary spot size and therefore power density "on the fly" simply by moving the handpiece away and toward the skin surface.

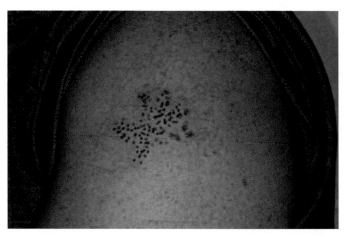

Figure 1.10 Immediate postoperative result on tattoo on shoulder. In this case, the operator inadvertently moved the toggle "spot size" switch from 4 to 2 mm. Fluence in 532 Q-switched mode increased from 3 to 12 J/cm² (fourfold increase). This resulted in loud snap and punctate bleeding.

Most lasers in modern skin surgery are pulsed, and the "instrument" panel fields are given in terms of pulse duration and fluence. Also, the spot size is often displayed. However, some carbon dioxide (CO_2) lasers, for example, provide only the pulse energy on the panel, or in CW mode, the number of watts. Likewise, our photodynamic therapy (PDT) system (a KTP-pumped 630-nm dye laser) gives the display in "watts." In these cases, one must know the spot size and time (in CW applications) to calculate the total light dose (fluence). It is helpful in these cases to attach a sheet of paper on the side of the laser with different fluences for the various spots and times.

In CW mode, the user must know the spot size, exposure time, and power density to determine the fluence. In many CW applications (e.g., wart treatment with CO_2 laser), the fluence is not too helpful in characterizing the overall tissue effect. One normally observes the tissue responses in real time and suspends the procedure when an appropriate endpoint is reached. On the other hand, in PDT applications with CW light, the total fluence and power density are very important in predicting the tissue response.

For CW mode, the CO_2 laser is typically used with a noncollimated handpiece. This allows one to control the spot size, as the operator can vary the power density or fluence simply by moving the handpiece tip toward or away from the skin (Fig. 1.9). For the accomplished laser surgeon, particularly in ablative applications for small lesions, this configuration offers "on-the-fly" flexibility and control not available with more modern locked-in spot sizes and fluences.

The "enlightened" laser practitioner should have an *intimate* knowledge of his particular devices. For example, some lasers "know" what spot size is being used (e.g., insertion of the handpiece into the calibration port can signal the spot size to the laser), whereas with others, you select the spotsize on the display, and the laser calculates the fluence accordingly. For example, one of our Q-switched lasers has a toggle that allows us to choose 2-, 4-, or 6-mm spots. However, the handpiece does not communicate the spot size to the laser control system. The user "tells" the laser what spot is to be used, and the laser calculates the fluence based on this user input. In this case, if one inadvertently changes the spot size (e.g., by inadvertently moving the toggle to the 2-mm from the 4-mm spot), the laser still "thinks" the 4-mm spot is being used, so that the actual surface fluence is now 4× fluence on the panel. The resulting small spot, which impacts the skin with a loud snap and punctate bleeding, should alert the savvy operator that something is amiss (Fig. 1.10). The operator then can examine the device and ensure that all the knobs are in the proper position before proceeding. The reader should note well that if tissue response looks unusual, most likely there is a problem and the physician should do a laser "walk around" before proceeding (akin to the pilot who dutifully checks the exterior of his plane before taking off). Most newer lasers allow for calibration through the end of the handpiece. This configuration allows for interrogation of the entire system, from the lamps to the fiber to the handpiece optics. This setup ensures that any problem is identified before patient care. For example, if a fiber is damaged, the laser will be unable to "make" calibration, and a failure message appears on the panel.

There are some quick and dirty, but not infallible, ways to check for system integrity. One can examine the aiming beam as it illuminates a piece of white paper, checking that the beam edges are sharp (usually the aiming beam and treatment

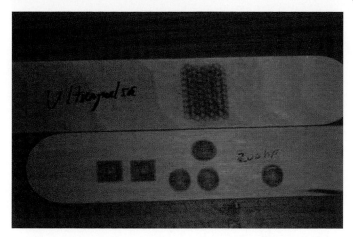

Figure 1.11 Scan pattern with two carbon dioxide lasers. Both patterns show uniform coverage. Scanners appear to be working properly.

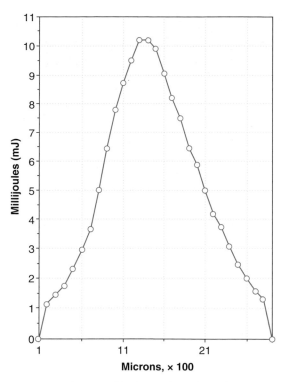

Figure 1.12 Gaussian beam profile of a popular carbon dioxide laser, as measured by author.

beam are following the same optical path). This suggests that the treatment beam is also sharp and the profile is according to the manufacturer's specifications. Also, burn paper can be used—here the laser is used with a low energy and the spot is checked for uniformity from beam edge to edge. With FIR lasers [erbium (Er):yttrium-aluminum-garnet (YAG) and CO_2], a tongue depressor can be used. This is especially useful for Er:YAG and CO_2 lasers, where calibration is typically carried out only internally. It follows that by checking the impact pattern on wood, one can uncover damaged mirrors in the knuckle of the articulated arm, or a bad focusing lens that renders the laser unstable or unsafe. Likewise, for scanners, it is wise to check the tongue depressor with FIR lasers to ensure that skin coverage will be uniform (Fig. 1.11).

Beam Profiles—Top Hat vs. Gaussian

Laser beam profiles can be of various shapes. A common profile is the Gaussian profile. This has the shape of a bell curve and is the fundamental mode of most lasers (Fig. 1.12). One often sees this shape when the beam has been delivered through an articulated arm (with mirrors at the knuckles). For some wavelengths, this is still the most effective way to deliver energy (CO_2 and Er). The disadvantage of the arm is the limited motion and the counterweight of the arm pulling against the surgeon's hand (10). The Gaussian profile is often disparaged as an inferior profile for lasers. In many applications, the criticism is well founded. For example, in treating a lentigo with a typical Q-switched ruby laser, one will often observe complete ablation of the epidermis at the center of the "spot," but only whitening at the periphery. On the other hand, sometimes a bell-shaped profile is desirable, for example, when applying a small spot FIR beam with a scanner. In this scenario, the wings of the beam allows for some overlap without delivering "too much" energy at points of overlap (see Fig. 1.11, note scan at the top of tongue depressor).

In most applications, a flat top profile is desirable, and with many fiber delivery systems, this is the case, as the beam is mixed by the multiple internal reflections within the fiber. Fibers have become increasingly popular with VIS light lasers, NIR lasers, and MIR lasers. Some high peak power Q-switched lasers exceed fiber damage thresholds, such that articulated arms are still required.

Pulse Profiles: Square vs. Spiky

The pulse profile is the temporal shape of the laser pulse (21). Many laser physicians assume that, for example, a 10-ms pulse with a pulse dye laser comprises a single burst of energy. In fact, in many pulsed laser applications, particularly the pulse dye laser, the "macropulse" comprises several smaller pulses (Fig. 1.13) (22). Depending on the application, the temporal pulse profile may impact the tissue effect. For example, we evaluated various pulse durations in the treatment of leg veins with a Nd:YAG laser. We found, for example, that in applying a 40-ms macropulse, where the micropulses were delivered in four "installments" versus 14 installments, the purpura threshold did not change. On the other hand, a very different response was observed in the application of green–yellow (GY) light. In this wavelength range, purpura thresholds are much lower, making the tissue response more susceptible to subtle changes in the pulse structure. For example, in our own experience and that of others (23), even with longer pulse PDLs, purpura (both inside the vessel and extending throughout the spot) is more likely after PDL than KTP lasers. Although both lasers generate pulse trains, the PDL delivers the energy in very energetic narrow spikes, whereas the long-pulse KTP laser delivers a smoother temporal pulse profile (21). The spiky pulse profile is more likely to cause immediate thrombosis and vessel rupture versus the smooth pulse profile, which is more likely to contract the vessel wall. We have observed that even by extension of the macropulse duration with the PDL (125-μs micropulse width) up to 20 ms, fluences sufficient to achieve vessel contraction or persistent bluing (two typical endpoints for effective vessel reduction), there is still a risk for immediate or delayed purpura. On the other hand, the IPL, even when configured with pulse trains, the micropulses are usually over 2-ms long (macropulse width about 20–30 ms),

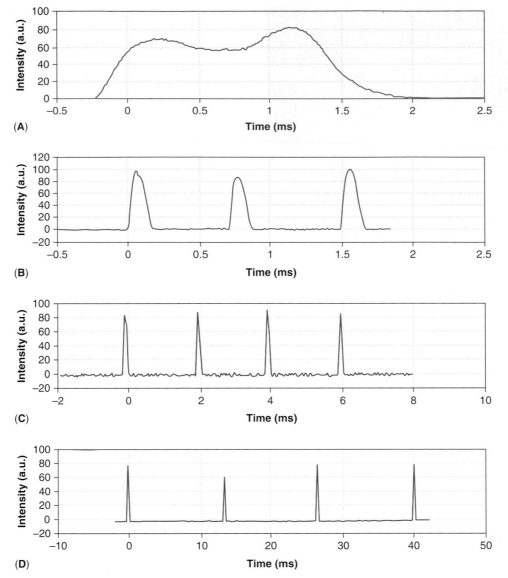

Figure 1.13 Various pulse profiles for pulsed dye laser. (**A**) Scleropus 1.5 ms; (**B**) V-Beam 1.5 ms; (**C**) V-Beam 6 ms; (**D**) V-Beam 40 ms. *Abbreviation:* a.u., arbitrary units.

and is not normally associated with purpura. This suggests that there is a critical difference in purpura threshold for this wavelength range (500–600 nm) between 125- and 2000-μs micropulse durations, regardless of the total macropulse length.

MOLECULAR BASIS OF LTI

Most devices *developed* for cosmetic rejuvenation are based on photothermal or "electrothermal" mechanisms, that is, the conversion of light or electrical energy to heat. Two fundamental processes govern all interactions of light with matter: absorption and scattering. Besides scattering and absorption, photons can be totally internally reflected at a tissue–air interface, or they can be remitted out of the tissue (Fig. 1.14) (4,18). Absorption and excitation are necessary for all photobiologic effects and laser–tissue interactions. Plank's law describes how much energy is invested in one photon as a function of wavelength. Energy is proportional to frequency and inversely proportional to wavelength. Thus, a 532-nm photon (532 nm is the distance between two of the transverse waves in a stream of

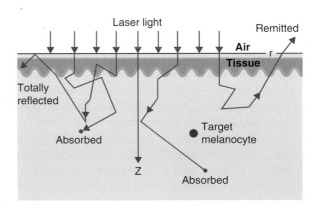

Figure 1.14 The behavior of light at and just below the skin surface.

light) is twice as energetic as a 1064-nm photon (5,24,25). When absorption occurs, the photon loses its energy to an atom or molecule, known as a chromophore. Upon absorption, the photon ceases to exist, and the chromophore becomes excited; it may undergo photochemistry or may dissipate the energy as either heat or reemission of light (e.g., fluorescence).

The probability that absorption will occur depends on specific transitions between allowed electron orbitals and molecular vibration modes. Thus chromophore molecules exhibit characteristic bands of absorption around certain wavelengths (19).

The molecular basis of LTIs is based on electronic transitions for the UV and VIS wavelengths. However, NIR wavelengths and beyond are absorbed via rotational and vibrational excitations in biomolecules (all of which are hydrocarbons with the exception of pigments). The reactions can be considered a two-step process. In the first, the molecule is excited to an excited state. Then, through a process known as nonradiative decay, there are inelastic collisions with nearby molecules, giving rise to an increase in kinetic energy and therefore temperature. The temperature rise results from the transfer of photon energy to kinetic energy. In most biological systems, tissue constituents show broad absorption bands with only a few distinct absorption peaks. Goldman and Rockwell (26) noted years ago that the biggest difference between tissue necrosis with laser and nonlaser devices, such as high-frequency electrical current, was the specificity of the reaction for color. For example, unlike the electric needle, only the darkly pigmented areas strongly absorb laser radiation in the VIS and NIR range. Thus the heterogeneity of the skin (in this case, melanin in small concentrations in tissue water) allows for selective heating with chromophore-specific wavelengths (27).

From 200 to 290 nm (UVC), light is absorbed by all cellular constituents (2) and all biological objects (cells and tissue) absorb energy very strongly. From 290 to 320 (UVB) nm, only a limited number of biomolecules show absorption (aromatic amino acids and nucleic acids). For UVA (near-UV) 320–400, light is weakly absorbed by colorless skin parts. From 400 to 1000 nm, only very few biomolecules absorb (mainly pigments such as bilirubin, blood, melanin). But it is over this wavelength range that the heterogeneity of the skin allows for discrete heating and therefore most of the magical properties of laser. For >1100 nm, all biomolecules have specific strong vibrational absorption bands. The principal absorber is tissue water, and all processes are guided by absorption of tissue water.

The absorption spectra of major skin chromophores dominate laser–tissue interactions in dermatology. The absorption coefficient (μ_a) is the probability per unit path length that a photon at a particular wavelength will be absorbed. It is therefore measured in units of 1/distance and is typically designated μ_a, given as cm^{-1}. The absorption coefficient depends on the concentration of chromophores present. Skin contains pigments and distinct microscopic structures that have different absorption spectra (Fig. 1.15) (4).

If tissues were clear, only absorption would be required to characterize light propagation in skin. However, the dermis is white because of light scatter. Scattering is responsible for much of the light's behavior in the skin (beam dispersion, spot size effects, etc.). The main scattering wavelengths are between 400 and 1200 nm, where the average distance a photon travels between two scattering events is between 0.05 and 0.2 mm. Although absorption occurs where the frequencies of the wavelength equal the natural frequency of the free vibrations of the particles (absorption is associated with resonance) (4), scattering takes place at frequencies not corresponding to those natural frequencies of particles (4). The resulting oscillation is determined by forced vibration. Scattering is decreased

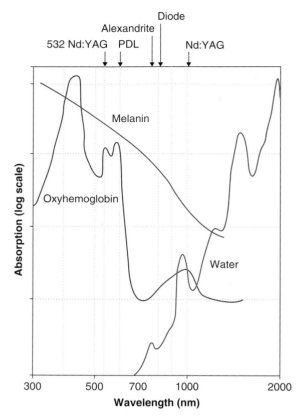

Figure 1.15 Absorption spectra of three major skin chromophores. *Abbreviations*: Nd:YAG; neodynium:yttrium-aluminum-garnet; PDL, pulsed dye laser.

as wavelength increases. In most biological tissues, it has been found that photons are preferably scattered in the forward direction.

There are three chromophores of interest (water, blood, and melanin). Water makes up about 65% of the dermis and lower epidermis. There is some water absorption in the UV. Between 400 and 800 nm, water absorption is quite small (which is consistent with our real-world experience that light propagates quite readily through a glass of water). Beyond 800 nm, there is a small peak at 980 nm, followed by larger peaks at 1480 and 10,600 nm. The water maximum is 2940 nm (Er:YAG).

Hemoglobin

There is a large oxyhemoglobin (HbO$_2$) peak at 415 nm, followed by smaller peaks at 540 and 577 nm. An even smaller peak is found at 940 nm. For deoxyhemoglobin (deoxyHb), the peaks are at 430 and 555 nm. Because of the discrete peaks of hemoglobin absorption, the laser physician can optimize heating of the vessel with excellent protection of the surrounding structures. If one examines Figure 1.15, there are multiple opportunities for selective heating blood vessels. Conjugated double bonds in their structure are responsible for the absorption of deoxyHb and HbO$_2$ by VIS light (3).

Melanin

Most pigmented lesions result from "too" much melanin in the epidermis. By choosing almost any wavelength (<800 nm), one can preferentially heat epidermal melanin (Fig. 1.16). Shorter wavelengths will tend to create very high superficial epidermal temperatures, whereas longer wavelengths tend to bypass epidermal melanin (i.e., 1064 nm).

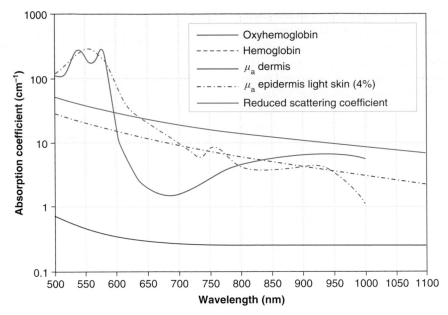

Figure 1.16 Hb absorption versus bloodless dermis. Note that Hb absorption always exceeds bloodless dermis. *Abbreviations*: μ_a, absorption coefficient; Hb, hemoglobin.

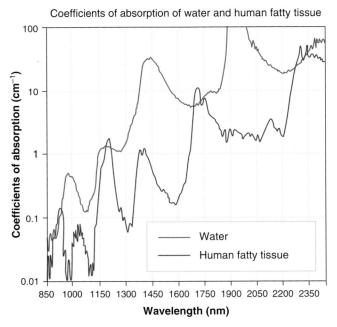

Figure 1.17 Water and fat absorption curves.

Fat

Fat shows strong absorption at 1200 and 1700 nm (Fig. 1.17). Although the ratios of fat-to-water absorption are small, the small differences could be exploited with the proper choice of parameters (or possibly through interstitial therapy).

Carbon

Carbon is not per se a chromophore but rather a product of prolonged skin heating. Once carbon is formed at the skin surface, the skin becomes "opaque" to most laser wavelengths (i.e., most energy will be absorbed very superficially). It follows that the dynamics of surface heating changes immediately once carbon is formed. This can be used creatively as an advantage. For example, one could use a layer of carbon paper to convert a deeply penetrating laser to one that would only

affect the surface. If the pulse were short enough, a 694-nm laser, for example, could optically act as a CO_2 laser (28)!

Collagen

Dry collagen shows absorption peaks near 6 and 7 μm. With a free electron laser, these peaks can be exploited for selective molecular targeting. In this manner, collagen is directly heated rather than relying on heat conduction due to its close bonds to tissue water (where Er:YAG and CO_2 lasers work). Ellis et al. found that this approach provided more efficient resurfacing and might allow for less tissue irradiation and less thermal damage than CO_2 laser (29).

SELECTIVE PHOTOTHERMOLYSIS

With the exception of water, heating in the skin is based on discrete heating by chromophores of relatively low concentration (i.e., melanin, hemoglobin). Anderson described the concept of selective photothermolysis (SPT) more than 30 years ago (24). Although Goldman argued for color as a means to selectively damage dermal targets as early as 1963, SPT offered an elegant and mathematically rigorous rationale for developing different tissue-selective lasers. As described by Anderson, extreme *localized heating* achieved with SPT relies on the following: (*i*) a wavelength that reaches and is preferentially absorbed by the desired target structures, (*ii*) an exposure duration less than or equal to the time necessary for cooling of the target structures, and (*iii*) sufficient energy to damage the target. The heterogeneity of the skin allows for very selective injury in thousands of microscopic targets. Unlike tracing out blood vessels with an electric needle (or using a CO_2 laser on a wart), the physician can apply a large light beam without the need to aim at the target. The effect is like the legendary "magic bullet," which seeks only the desired target. In contrast to gross thermal injury, SPT (with discrete targets, i.e., melanin and Hb) allows for focal heating with large volumes of undamaged skin between chromophores. The focal nature of the heating decreases the likelihood of catastrophic pancutaneous thermal damage. Because temperature elevations are localized, there is often less pain than with devices targeting tissue water.

Thermal Relaxation Time

In simple terms, the thermal relaxation time (τ) is the time taken for a target to cool to a certain percentage of its peak temperature (24). We know from experience that larger volumes require longer time than smaller volumes to cool. For example, a tubful of warm bathwater requires about 1 hour to cool to room temperature, whereas a thimbleful requires only a few minutes. In laser scenarios, we assume instantaneous heating of the target, so that τ is usually thought of as the time for cooling after the pulse. However, if the pulse is long, the target can cool during the pulse, akin to one pouring water into a leaky bucket. If the water represents heat, one observes that the bucket never fills (akin to a target never becoming very hot). If one wants to spatially confine heating, one chooses a short pulse that coincides roughly with the τ of the chromophore. For the same volume, a sphere will cool faster than a cylinder, which will cool faster than a slab. When defining thermal relaxation time, one should consider the immediate target and the boundaries of the target. Normally, it is defined by

$$\delta^2/g\kappa \qquad (1)$$

where δ is the optical penetration depth for homogeneously absorbing layers (such as tissue water for IR applications). For discrete absorbers, that is, the melanosome, τ is defined in terms of the particle size, and δ represents the diameter of the particle. κ is the thermal diffusivity, a quantity based on the thermal conductivity and specific heat of the medium, and "g" is a constant based on the geometry of the target (slab, cylinder, or sphere) (30). The optical penetration depth of laser irradiation is wavelength dependent and defined as the depth where fluence is attenuated to 37% of its incident value. The often-used term "thermal relaxation time of the skin" is meaningful only when used for specific wavelengths (or specific skin structures, i.e., the epidermis). For example, with a ubiquitous absorber such as tissue water, τ should be considered within the context of δ, not the dimensions of the skin constituents. For example, if one uses the 1540-nm laser, the entire epidermis and large portions of the dermis are heated, and τ is on the order of seconds, because δ is several hundred micrometers. So even though τ of the epidermis is about 10 ms on a dimensional basis, because a thick slab of skin is heated at 1540 nm, the number is somewhat irrelevant. In this case, the epidermis will take several seconds to cool because there is no real gradient between its temperature and the dermis.

On the other hand, when establishing τ of the epidermis with the melanosome as the immediate chromophore, one can consider either the entire epidermis as the target (thickness of 80–100 μm) or the dermal–epidermal (DE) junction (10 μm) or, finally, the melanosome itself when using melanin as chromophore. Each skin "unit" will have its own respective τ. A Q-switched laser pulse will confine high temperatures to the melanosome. The upper epidermis is heated only after postpulse heat conduction away from the DE junction. On the other hand, in treating with a 10-ms 532-nm pulse, heat will diffuse freely from the melanosome during the pulse, resulting in more uniform epidermal heating. This diffuse and gentle epidermal heating may be desirable or undesirable depending

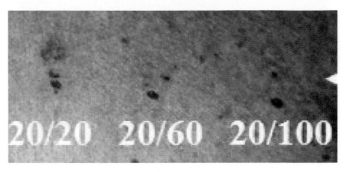

Figure 1.18 The impact of pulse duration on epidermis. The fluence was 20 J/cm² for all sites with an intense pulsed light. The second number at each site represents the pulse width in milliseconds. Note the decrease in epidermal damage as pulse duration increases.

on the specific clinical indication. Most importantly, the physician can titrate the degree of epidermal heating by manipulation of the pulse duration (Fig. 1.18).

With a too short pw, pulses "violently" vaporize targets, leading to substantial immediate or delayed vessel wall damage and hemorrhage in the treatment of vascular lesions (25). With longer pulses, one can gently heat targets without causing rupture of the vessels. On the other hand, the shortcoming with a long-pulsed ruby laser for nevus of Ota is that the pigmented nevus cells cool off too fast during the delivery of the pulses; also, the very high fluence can damage the pigmented epidermis (8).

For most tissue targets, a simple rule of thumb can be used: the thermal relaxation time in seconds is about equal to the square of the target dimension in millimeters. Thus a 0.5-μm melanosome (5×10^{-4} mm) should cool in about 25×10^{-8} seconds, or 250 ns, whereas a 0.1-mm PWS vessel should cool in about 10^{-2} seconds, or 10 ms. The natural variation of target sizes in tissue leads to an even greater variation in thermal relaxation times, such that much more precise calculations, although certainly possible, are probably unnecessary (24). This is a feature that should be noted well by the reader. The τ is derived from a solution of the general heat equation. It follows that these values are not absolute cooling times, but rather provide ballpark figures of pulse durations that achieve varying degrees of thermal confinement. Also remember that perfect thermal confinement is not always desirable, as gentle heating sometimes is a preferred method in cutaneous laser applications.

Two "offshoots" of SPT are the concepts of thermal damage time and thermokinetic selectivity (TKS).

Thermal Damage Time

In some applications, the immediate chromophore and the final target are not collocated (i.e., hair shaft and hair bulb/bulge). In this case, thermal damage time is defined as the time required for irreversible target damage with sparing of the surrounding tissue. For a nonuniformly absorbing target structure, the thermal damage time is the time when the outermost part of the target reaches the target damage temperature through heat diffusion from the heater. In this case, the eventual target and the heater (e.g., hair shaft) are different and at a considerable distance from each other (31). Using this model, the thermal damage time can be many times longer than the thermal relaxation time.

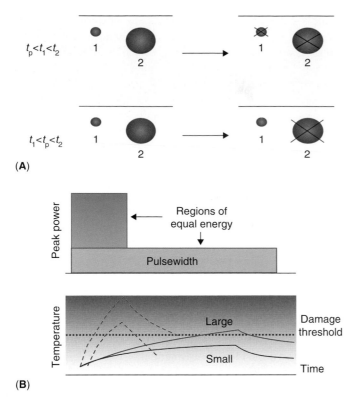

(A)

(B)

Figure 1.19 (**A**) Target-size selectivity by choice of pulse width. (**B**) Relationship between size of target and pulse duration to peak temperature. The longer pulse favors heating of the larger target (blood vessel) versus the smaller melanosome.

Thermokinetic Selectivity

Along the same lines is the concept of thermokinetic selectivity (TKS). In this model, one selects larger or smaller targets based on pulse duration (Fig. 1.19A,B). For example, if one wants to heat larger targets while sparing relatively smaller ones, the pulse duration is extended beyond the thermal relaxation time of the smaller target. In this manner, that is, a melanosome will be heated to a lower temperature than the subjacent vessel.

REACTION TYPES

Photothermal

Most laser applications in dermatology rely on heating. Temperature is directly related to the average kinetic energy of molecules. As temperature is raised, tissue coagulates (19). A familiar example of denaturation and coagulation is the cooking of an egg white. Thermal denaturation is both temperature and time dependent, yet it often shows an all or none like behavior. For a given heating time, there is usually a narrow temperature region above which complete denaturation occurs. This is readily evident in Figure 1.20. As a rule, for denaturation of most proteins, one must increase the temperature by about 10°C for every decade of decrease in the heating time to achieve the same amount of thermal coagulation (19).

Photothermal processes depend on type and degree of heating, from coagulation to vaporization. A mild to moderate temperature increase results in breakage of hydrogen bonds and van der Waal bonds leading to denaturation of enzymes and function. If the heating is very fast, a phase change occurs (27). Depending on the rate of energy delivery, photovaporization occurs with or without inertial confinement (vide infra), where

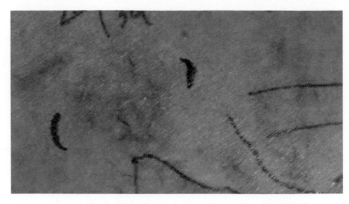

Figure 1.20 The effect of pulse stacking on skin overlying leg vein. Two previous pulses caused no effect, then immediate whitening was noted. Biopsy would show full-thickness necrosis (treatment was with neodynium:yttrium-aluminum-garnet laser).

time is short compared with the time for pressure relaxation. Here the laser-induced pressure causes compressive stresses in tissue. Microcracks in the tissue are the result of these large stress gradients (27).

Thermal Injury to Cells

There is a range of measurable effects on skin based on temperature. Below 43°C, the skin remains unharmed, even for very long exposures (4). Thus one can exceed body temperature by about 5°C without a measurable change in the skin. The first change is a conformational change in the molecular structure. These typically occur at temperatures from 42°C to 50°C. After several minutes, there will be tissue necrosis as described by the Arrhenius equation (an equation that quantitatively describes conversion of tissue from a native to denatured state). Thermal denaturation is a rate process: heat increases the rate at which molecules denature, depending on the specific molecule. For example, at 45°C, cultured human fibroblasts die after about 20 minutes. However, the same cells can withstand over 100°C for 10^{-3} seconds (32). In general, a temperature of >60°C lasting for at least 6 seconds leads to irreversible damage (4).

Coagulation

This is normally the first heating step that is identifiable on routine light microscopy. An absolute temperature for coagulation–denaturation does not exist. It appears that for very short times, higher temperatures than the often-quoted "62–65°C" would be required. It is not known to what extent the Arrhenius formulation holds for very short heating times (less than 1 second) (33). In most scenarios of light–tissue interaction, tissues and cells may be reversibly or irreversibly damaged. Normally, pathologists examine tissue for changes such as vacuolization, hyperchromasia, and protein denaturation (birefringence loss). Moderate temperature-induced damage phenomena in tissue have been difficult to assess with conventional methods of detection, such as light microscopy. However, particularly in light of newer large volume low-intensity heating devices for rejuvenation, more sensitive tools might be required to characterize subtle thermal effects. Beckham et al. (33) found that over a narrow temperature range, heat shock protein (HSP) expression correlated with laser-induced heat stress, and that the HSP production followed the Arrhenius integral. Thus HSP expression [(in addition to tissue ultrastructure, i.e., electromagnetic (EM)] might be an excellent tool to examine low-intensity high-volume heat injury.

Vaporization

At a certain threshold power density, coagulation gives way to vaporization. Often, this process is referred to as ablation and is an important component of laser skin resurfacing (LSR). At this higher power density (and higher fluence), water expands as it is converted to steam. Vaporization is beneficial in that much of the heat is carried away from the skin during the process (4). The vaporization energy for water is approximately 2.4 kJ/cm^3. When there is vaporization, there is also increasing pressure as the water tries to expand in volume. The expansion leads to localized microexplosions. At temperatures beyond 100°C (without further vaporization), carbonization takes place, which is obvious by blackening of adjacent tissue and the escape of smoke. Carbon is the ultimate end product of all living tissues being heated and carbon temperatures often reach up to 300°C (34). Normally, this should be avoided, because the depth of tissue injury will extend well beyond the blackened skin surface. This is particularly true, for example, when treating something like a rhinophyma or performing LSR.

Photomechanical

With even more rapid heating, there is insufficient time for pressure relaxation. In this scenario, there will be disassembly and microcracks in the tissue. On the other hand, with slow energy deposition, there will be no pressure increase. Mechanical damage plays an important role in SPT with high-energy, submicrosecond lasers for tattoo and pigmented lesion removal. Inertially confined ablation occurs when there is high pressure at constant volume. In a very short pulse, the energy is invested so quickly one that there is no time for the pressure to be relieved. Under these conditions of inertial confinement, there is not enough time for material to move—this can lead to the generation of tremendous pressures. New studies support a role for femtosecond ablation of skin where beam can be focused from the surface to create small "holes" 300–500 µm below the stratum corneum. In this scenario, the overlying skin is undamaged (35).

Photochemical

Photochemical reactions are governed by specific reaction pathways and are becoming increasingly important in dermatology (4). The most common type of photodynamic action in dermatology is one where singlet oxygen is created. In the reaction, a photosensitizer is excited by a certain wavelength of light. In the presence of oxygen, oxygen is transformed from its triplet state, which is its normal ground state, to an excited singlet state. The excited singlet state oxygen reacts with biological molecules and often attacks plasma and intracellular membranes. The most common photosensitizer (PS) in dermatology is PpIX. This PS is formed by skin cells by the prodrug, aminolevulinic acid (ALA). The proper combination of wavelength and power density will achieve the best results. Overall, most photochemical reactions proceed more efficiently with lower power densities, such that, for example, the Blu-U light (DUSA, Vahalla, New York, USA) will normally outperform a pulsed source (IPL, KTP, or PDL) for actinic

keratoses (AKs) with one treatment (36). However, pulse light sources can theoretically also be used and have proved to be useful in a range of skin disorders (37,38). There is little *endogenous* photochemistry beyond 319 nm. Some exceptions are photoisomerization of bilirubin (450 nm) and singlet O$_2$ production by *Propionibacterium acnes* porphyrins (similar absorption peaks as PpIX). Beyond 800 nm, photochemistry, even with exogenous photosensitizers or prodrugs, is unlikely.

Pulsed Light Sources and PDT

It has been shown that lower irradiances demonstrate a more marked PDT effect for equivalent total light doses (39). Although pulsed light sources have been shown to be as effective as CW sources in some experiments, the PDT effect was only equivalent *if the light doses and average irradiances were similar*. Most pulsed light sources in dermatology do not meet the theoretical PDT saturation threshold (4×10^8 W/m^2) (40). All of this suggests that an optimal pulsed light PDT configuration might require multiple passes with blue, green, yellow, or red light. The interval between passes should be designed, such that the average irradiance is similar to that of CW devices with similar emission spectra.

Excimer Laser (308 nm)

The mechanism of action for the excimer laser (XeCl) is thought to be the same as narrow band UV therapy. There is an erythema action spectrum determined by plotting a reciprocal of the minimal erythema dose against wavelength. It appears a reduction in cellular proliferation and most likely plays a part in UV radiation shorter than 320 nm. This range has a profound influence on epidermal cellular DNA synthesis and mitosis. In the original study of Parrish in 1981, he showed that wavelengths between 300 and 313 nm were most effective (41). It appears that the excimer laser works through in an immunomodulatory way much like UVB. The precise chromophore is unknown. There may be a thermal component as well at fluences >800 mJ/cm^2.

Biostimulation

Biostimulation is thought to belong to the group of photochemical interactions. However, the term biostimulation has not been scientifically very well defined. Most biostimulation studies involve low-power lasers and have been a subject of controversy for decades. Typical fluences are in the range of 1–10 J/cm^2, and normally there is no acute temperature elevation. Some scientists define biostimulation by the absence of any thermal mechanism (4). The most vexing problem about many biostimulation studies is the difficulty in assessing what is occurring at a clinical level (beyond the cell culture model). It is unknown if any features of laser light, coherence, monochromaticity, polarization, are really relevant for biostimulation (4). One example of a "biostimulation" device in dermatology is the Gentlewaves LED Photomodulation unit (Light BioScience, LLC, Virginia Beach, Virginia, USA). This device uses 590-nm light in a high repetition rate and low-power density to purportedly increase collagen synthesis and enhance facial tone. Cell culture work supports this concept (42). However, more work clearly needs to be done in this arena of biostimulation. Is it really plausible to unlock the code for subcellular processes through low-level irradiation?

Plasma-Induced Ablation

With very high power densities exceeding 10^8 W/cm^2, a phenomenon called optical breakdown occurs. With plasma-induced ablation, very clean and well-defined removal of tissue without evidence of mechanical or thermal damage can be achieved when choosing appropriate parameters. Plasmas are sometimes produced by laser tattoo removal, where one can observe a spark (19,27). Also, there is a new resurfacing system that uses this fourth state of matter to target the skin surface. The plasma is created by a radio frequency (RF) excited N$_2$ gas, which is directed toward the skin. The plasma is above the surface, creating very high but superficially confined temperatures. The goal is to achieve damage to the skin surface with minimal residual thermal damage (RTD). RF pixilated devices can now create microplasmas on the skin surface to correct acne scars and striae.

SKIN OPTICS

The optical properties of human skin determine the penetration, absorption, and internal dosimetry of laser light in skin. The cosmetic surgeon can divide the skin into two main components: (*i*) the epidermis (primarily an absorber of VIS light due to melanin) and (*ii*) the dermis (which can be envisioned as a carton of milk with red dots in it). When one uses a laser, one should envision where the photons and/or electrical energy is going and where the primary heating is. The laser surgeon should memorize the absorption spectra of the main chromophores in planning the procedure. He should remember that the optical properties of the skin are not static. For example, just a positional change in the arm will change the dermal blood fraction. Also, just a few minutes in the sun will increase the pigmentation index. Light–tissue interactions can be broken down into (*i*) the transport of light in tissue, (*ii*) absorption of light and heat generation in tissue, (*iii*) localized temperature elevation in the target tissue (and denaturation of proteins), and (*iv*) heat diffusion away from the target (Fig. 1.21).

The optical properties of the skin mimic those of a turbid medium intermixed with focal discrete VIS and IR light absorbers (blood, melanin, bilirubin, and dry collagen). There is absorption by proteins, nucleic acids, and other compounds in the UV spectrum, but outside of photochemistry, possibly with a blue light source, these light–tissue interactions are probably irrelevant for skin rejuvenation. In any light–tissue interaction, the thermal or photochemical effects depend on the *local* energy density at the target. Surface fluence represents the energy per unit area incident on the skin. Once the light penetrates the surface, it undergoes a complex series of absorbing and scattering events. Characterization of the light pathways is best understood by thinking of the incident beam in terms of its constituent photons, where the photons statistically are either scattered or absorbed in a wavelength-dependent fashion (43). The probabilities of absorption or scattering (Table 1.1), designated μ_a and μ_s, respectively, are determined by experiment. For a path length, L, the probability of photon will not be absorbed or scattered is

$$e^{-\mu_a L} \tag{2}$$

Jacques notes that a typical bloodless tissue value for μ_a in the VIS range is 1 cm^{-1} and the mean free path of a photon is therefore 1 cm (44). For most VIS light, there are typically 100 scattering events before a photon is absorbed. As it turns out, the photon scatters roughly 10 times before it loses its orientation with respect to the initial direction as it migrates in a random walk. With scattering, there is *backscattered* light that augments the delivered irradiance to yield a higher fluence beneath the tissue than at the tissue surface (Fig. 1.22) (44). An often-used term is the penetration depth (δ), which describes the path length that causes 1/e attenuation of light. For a clear solution, δ accurately conveys the depth-dependent fluence

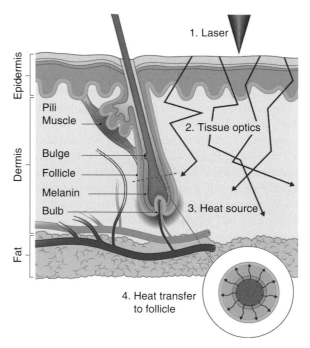

Figure 1.21 The cascade of events in typical laser–tissue interaction with discrete chromophore (in this case the hair follicle).

Table 1.1 Absorption Coefficients (cm^{-1}) for Various Chromophores

Wavelength (nm)	410	532	595	694	755	810	940	1064
OxyHb (40% Hct)	1990	187	35	1.2	2.3	3.6	5.2	2.2
DeoxyHb	1296	138	96	6.6	5.2	2.7	3.0	0.6
Melanin[a]	140	56	38	23	17	13	7	5.7
Water	6.7×10^{-5}	0.00044	0.0017	0.005	0.03	0.02	0.27	0.15
Bloodless dermis	10	3	2	1.2	0.8	0.6	0.5	0.4
OPD in skin (μm)	100	350	550	750	1000	1200	1500	1700

[a]Net epidermis for moderately pigmented adult: 10% melanin volume fraction in epidermis (46,141).
Abbreviations: DeoxyHb, deoxyhemoglobin; Hct, hematocrit; OPD, optical penetration depth; OxyHb, oxyhemoglobin.

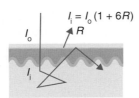

λ (nm)	R	I_i/I_o
585	0.3	2.8
694	0.6	4.6
1064	0.7	5.2

Figure 1.22 How backscattered light can result in subsurface fluence exceeding incident fluence. I_o is the surface fluence. R is the total light reflected from the skin for the respective wavelength. Note that ratio increases with wavelength over this range.

attenuation. However, for turbid tissue such as the dermis, where backscattering can be considerable, the "real" penetration depth can be $>\delta$. This value may be 2–3× δ, for example, with 1064 nm (43–45). One will see different charts showing different penetration depths in different bodies of literature. For example, in an article by Reinisch (10), the optical penetration depths are somewhat larger than those in another article by Anderson (5). The trends are the same in both articles, and neither chart is "wrong." The δ can change based on how it is defined. Therefore one will see a wide range of different values for similar wavelengths.

One should consider the choice of laser within the context of the application and the respective absorption and scattering coefficients. If the absorption coefficient is greater than 200 cm^{-1}, one typically is looking at a "what you see is what you get laser" (examples are Er:YAG and CO_2). Between 1 and 200 cm^{-1}, one sees a wavelength range where lasers that can sometimes be useful (i.e., PDL, KTP, alexandrite). Finally, when one considers μ_a less than 1 cm^{-1}, we are typically dealing with deeply penetrating light sources where one can injure the skin without obvious surface changes [a "what you don't see can hurt you laser"; an example being the neodynium:yttrium-aluminum-garnet (Nd:YAG)] (20).

Beyond 600 nm, the increase in penetration and a brisk cut-off in Hb absorption make for a therapeutic window between 600 and 1200 nm. In this range, radiation penetrates biological tissues at a lower loss, thus enabling treatment of deeper tissue structures (19). At times, the various skin pigments can play optical "tricks" on the cutaneous surgeon. For example, poikiloderma appears to be a mix of hyperpigmentation and hypervascularity. In fact, although there is some melanin influence—the red-brown appearance—the dyschromia is by far more a disorder of matted telangiectasia. This is confirmed by the response of the condition to the PDL, even with surface cooling. Additionally, with diascopy, often skin appears no browner than the surrounding apparently normal skin. The explanation is that deoxyHb contributes to a "pigmented skin appearance." This finding follows from the absorption spectrum of deoxyHb in the 630–700 nm range, which is very similar to the absorption spectrum of epidermal melanin. The size of the vessels in the superficial venous plexus is such that the transmitted light through these vessels is approximately 50% lower than the incident intensity. These vessels therefore appear dark (Fig. 1.23) (46).

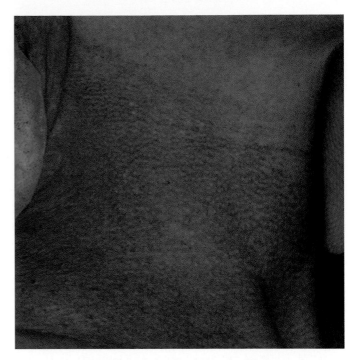

Figure 1.23 Note dark red neck skin of poikiloderma.

Heat Generation

All laser–tissue interactions are guided by the same energy balance rules that guide all of physics. Heat generation can occur in one of the two ways. In one scenario, it occurs at discrete chromophore sites. In this case, there is very precise localized heating consistent with the theory of SPT. These hot spots under the skin allow for only the bad guys to be damaged. The good guys (normal skin), so long as the ratio of absorption coefficients (i.e., blood vs. bloodless dermis) is high enough (optimally >10), remain unharmed. The primary areas where SPT is helpful in dermatology are in the treatment of vascular lesions, tattoos, and pigmented lesions. However, even in applications where water is the chromophore, the principles of SPT are useful (24). When treating by heating tissue water, the injury is typically from "top to bottom," the exception being deeper penetrating NIR and MIR wavelengths coupled with surface cooling. In this scenario, one can coordinate heating and cooling to damage specific slices of subsurface skin.

Once the local subsurface energy density has been determined using models, heat generation can be predicted by energy balance (conservation of energy) and the wavelength-specific absorption for that target. Depending on the amount of thermal diffusion during the pulse, the local peak temperature can be determined. The temperature increase of a desired target can be roughly calculated by knowing the absorption and scattering coefficients, surface light dose, size of the target, and the length of the pulse, as follows:

$$\Delta T = \frac{F_z \mu_a}{\rho c} \left(\frac{\tau_r}{\tau_r + \tau_p} \right)^{g/2} \qquad (3)$$

where F_z is the local subsurface fluence, ρ is the density, c is the specific heat, "g" is a geometric factor ("1" for planes, "2" for cylinders, and "3" for spheres), τ_p is the laser pulse duration, and τ_r is the thermal relaxation time of the

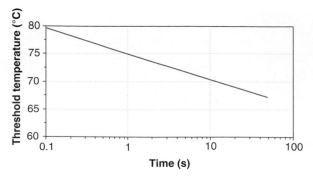

Figure 1.24 Denaturation as a function of *t* and *T*. *Abbreviations*: *t*, time; *T*, temperature.

target (time for target to cool to 37% of peak temperature), defined by

$$\tau_r = \frac{D^2}{g\kappa} \qquad (4)$$

where *D* is the thickness or diameter of the target. Thus one can perform some quick algebraic calculations to estimate the peak temperatures of local targets in the skin.

Spatially selective temperature elevation is possible when (*i*) the absorption coefficient of the target exceeds that of collateral tissue (SPT) or (*ii*) when the "innocent bystander" tissues are cooled so their peak temperatures do not exceed some damage threshold. Localized heating, for example, in telangiectasia and lentigines, follows from the concentrations of blood and melanin there, respectively, such that μ_a is focally increased.

Coagulation

As noted above, denaturation depends on time and temperature, and at least over times greater than 1 second, appears to conform to a rate process as described by the Arrhenius equation (Fig. 1.24). The characteristic behavior of the Arrhenius-type kinetic damage model is that, below a threshold temperature, the rate of damage accumulation is negligible; it increases precipitously when this value is exceeded. This behavior is to be expected from the exponential nature of the function. Pearce and Thomsen define a critical temperature, T_{crit}, as the temperature at which there is roughly 100% damage in 1 second. A range of values for T_{crit} from 60°C to 85°C have been reported for various human tissues (47).

Heat Conduction Away from the Chromophore

Once heat is generated, heat losses are based on heat conduction, heat convection, or radiation. Radiation can be neglected in most types of laser applications. A good example of heat convection is transfer from blood flow. Heat conduction is a considerable heat lost term and is the primary mechanism by which heat is transferred to unexposed tissue structures.

WAVELENGTH RANGES USEFUL FOR CUTANEOUS SURGERY

In this section, wavelength ranges useful for cutaneous surgery are examined briefly:

1. *UV laser and light sources*: they have been used primarily for the treatment of inflammatory skin diseases

and/or vitiligo, as well as striae. The presumed action is immunomodulatory. The XeCl excimer laser emits at 308 nm, near the peak action spectrum for psoriasis. Other UV nonlaser sources have also been used for hypopigmentation, striae, and various inflammatory diseases (48,49).

2. *Violet IPL spectra and low-power 410-nm LED and fluorescent lamps*: both are used either alone or with ALA. Alone, the devices take advantage of endogenous porphyrins and kill *P. acnes* (50–53). After application of ALA, this wavelength range is highly effective in creating singlet O_2 after absorption by PpIX. Uses include treatment of AKs, actinic cheilitis, and basal cell carcinomas (BCCs) (54).

3. *VIS (GY)*: these wavelengths are highly absorbed by Hb and melanin and are especially useful in treating epidermal pigmented lesions and superficial vessels (11,12,23,55–59). The relatively poor penetration in skin (and the even poorer penetration in blood, Table 1.2) makes them poor choices for treatment of *deeper* pigmented lesions or *deeper larger* vessels. The effective portions of many IPL spectra include the GY range. There are absorption peaks for PpIX in the GY range, making these wavelengths useful for PDT (i.e., sodium lamp, IPL, or PDL) (52,60).

4. *Near-IR(A) (755–810 nm)*: these two popular wavelengths are used primarily in hair reduction but have also been used to treat blood vessels and hyperpigmented lesions. They are positioned in the absorption spectrum for blood and melanin between the GY wavelengths and 1064 nm. They will penetrate deeply enough in blood to coagulate vessels up to 2 mm (61,62); also, they are reasonably tolerant of epidermal pigment in hair reduction (with surface cooling) so long as *very* dark skin is not treated (63).

5. *Near-IR(B) 940 and Nd:YAG*: these two wavelengths have been used extensively for various sized vessels on the legs and face (64–66). They occupy a unique place in the absorption spectrum of our "big 3" chromophores (i.e., *blood, melanin, and water*). Because of the depth of penetration (on the order of millimeters), they are especially useful for hair reduction and coagulation of deeper blood vessels. On the other hand, they are not well suited for epidermal-pigmented lesions. Also, although water absorption is poor, it exceeds that of the VIS and near-VIS wavelengths. The result is that 940 and 1064 nm can cause large volume mild temperature

Table 1.2 Thermal Relaxation Time of Some Potential Targets

Target	Thermal Relaxation Time
Erythrocyte	2 μs
200-μm hair follicle	40 ms
0.5-μm melanosome	0.25 μs
10-μm nevus call	0.1 ms
0.1-mm diameter vessel	10 ms
0.4-mm diameter vessel	80 ms
0.8-mm diameter vessel	300 ms

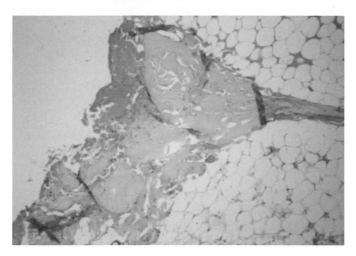

Figure 1.25 Full-thickness necrosis in ex vivo sample after multiple pulses of a neodynium:yttrium-aluminum-garnet laser.

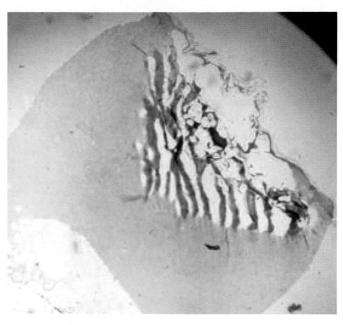

Figure 1.26 Effect in pigskin of a 1540-nm laser with a 2.5-mm spot without cooling and fluence of ~15 J/cm².

elevation in the skin, and with repeated laser impacts, because of the slow cooling of this volume (large τ), catastrophic pancutaneous thermal damage is possible. We observed this phenomenon when treating a piece of discarded tissue after Mohs surgery. After exposing the tissue to one, three, and six repeated exposures of Nd:YAG laser at 1 Hz, we noted widespread coagulation that occurred as an "all-or-none" phenomenon between the third and sixth pulses, consistent with the threshold behavior of protein denaturation (Fig. 1.25). This wavelength (1064 nm) represents the extreme example of a "what you don't see can hurt you laser" (20). They are extremely useful, but the user must develop an understanding of where this energy is going to effectively harness it and benefit his patients. One can appreciate firsthand that the Nd laser penetrates deeply by taking a fingertip on one side of the ear and applying the laser to the opposite side of the lobe. The author promises a hot finger!

6. *MIR lasers and deeply penetrating lamps:* these lasers and lamps heat tissue water. Depending on where we want to heat, we can "choreograph" our laser and/or cooling settings to maximize the skin temperature in certain bands. In general, with more deeply penetrating wavelengths, larger volumes are heated. On the other hand, achieving temperature elevations in the volume will require higher fluences than with highly absorbing wavelengths. With more highly absorbing wavelengths, one will heat a tighter band of dermis. This is referred to as selective dermal heating. Accordingly, without surface cooling, unless very small fluences are applied, a top to bottom thermal injury occurs (Fig. 1.26). The absorption coefficients for the 1320, 1450, and 1540 nm systems are ~3, 20, and 8 cm⁻¹, respectively (67,68), whereas the effective scattering coefficients are about 14, 12, and 11 cm⁻¹. The corresponding penetration depths are ~1500, 300, and 700 µm. It follows that for equal surface cooling and equal fluences, the most superficial heating will occur with

the 1450-nm laser, followed by the 1540- and 1320-nm lasers. The advantage of deeper penetration (i.e., less absorption) is that surface cooling does not need to be as aggressive. On the other hand, higher fluences must be applied and the peak temperature elevation will tend to be slightly deeper. Newer deeply penetrating lamps have been introduced (Titan, Cutera, Brisbane, California, USA). They emit light over a 1- to 2-µm band with relatively low power densities and long exposures (several seconds). In a typical scenario, the irradiation begins after a roughly 2-second period of cooling. At this point, a band of tissue from roughly 700-µm deep to 1.5-mm deep in the skin is heated. By varying the fluence, this relatively large volume can be heated to different peak temperatures (Fig. 1.27). As part of each iteration, post-pulse cooling is included. This is because such a large volume of skin is heated that a "thermal wake" of several seconds is created. It follows, that if one removes the handpiece too quickly, there is a tendency for heat to build up near the skin surface with the possibility of pain, dermal thermal injury, and scarring. One can make various arguments for large-volume deep subsurface heating versus heating a precise band of dermis more superficially (i.e., the deep papillary or superficial reticular dermis). As one attempts to confine heat superficially, a more highly water absorbing MIR laser is optimal, but the counterpoint is that the cooling must also be confined superficially. It follows that, as one tries to heat superficially and spare the epidermis, the heating–cooling tandem must become ever more synchronized, lest one overheat the epidermis or overcool the dermis. On the other hand, with more penetrating wavelengths, heating will occur in the deeper dermis, often below the level of solar elastosis, the very pathology we presumably are trying to reverse.

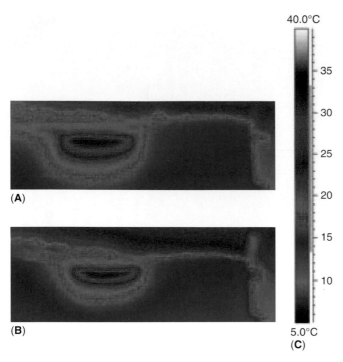

Figure 1.27 Heating bands with a mid-infrared heat lamp (Titan, Cutera, California, USA). By filtering out water, the depth and the thickness of the heated slab increase.

Despite the various modalities used in selective dermal heating, the degree of rhytid improvement typically seen after Er:YAG and CO_2 LSR has not been observed (69) Even where fibroplasia is observed histologically, clinical improvement is often modest (70). Several reasons for this apparent discrepancy are suggested: (*i*) Although selective dermal heating can be achieved with deeply penetratingMIR lasers combined with topical cooling, the zone of heating in the dermis will always be broader and deeper than the fine band of basophilic staining denaturation observed with Er:YAG and FIR lasers. The wounds are quite dissimilar, and if one creates a subepidermal zone of injury with the complete denaturation characteristics of the CO_2 laser, pitted scarring will be most likely. Thus in MIR-based NSR, one is substituting a larger volume of gentler heating for the precise and complete denaturation observed after typical short-pulsed CO_2 LSR.

7. *FIR systems*: the major lasers are the CO_2 and Er:YAG lasers. Using models, as well as experiments, one can determine the relative rates of ablation and heating (30,71,72). Overall, the ratio of ablation to heating is much higher with the Er:YAG laser. However, one can extend the thermal field of the Er:YAG laser by extending the pulse or increasing the repetition rate, and likewise one can decrease the thermal field of CO_2 laser by decreasing pw or increasing fluence (73,74). It follows that for applications where precision is required in ablation, Er:YAG is preferred. On the other hand, depending on settings, the CO_2 laser combines an enviable blend of ablation and heating. The depth of RTD is typically more uniform with CO_2 than the depth of *ablation* with Er:YAG,

such that the CO_2 laser is more useful for global skin improvement (fine or moderate wrinkle without severe contour defects) on the face. The thresholds for ablation for CO_2 and Er lasers vary inversely with their optical penetration depths in tissue (20 and 1 μm, respectively). This assumes thermal confinement. It follows that less surface fluence is required for ablation with the Er laser. With the CO_2 laser, we are operating *at ablation threshold* in typical resurfacing applications, so a large fraction of energy is invested in tissue heating. This results in low ablation efficiency, and only a small mass of dermal tissue is ablated. In contrast, the Er laser operates well above threshold (approximately 8–10× for a fluence of 5 J/cm²), resulting in greater ablation and less thermal denaturation. The CO_2 laser at typical operating parameters performs self-limited controlled heating of the skin, whereas the Er laser operates in an almost purely ablative regime.

Radio Frequency Technology

RF–skin interactions are fundamentally different from the optical ones. Rather than "optical" fluence and absorption coefficients, local heat generation depends on the local resistance and local current density. With most RF systems, there is a rapidly alternating current which, given the impedance of the skin, generates heat. The distribution of the current density is determined by the configuration of the electrodes relative to the skin anatomy. Depending on the type of surface cooling, one can create various zones of heating under the skin. There are two types of electrode deployments. In one scenario, bipolar electrodes are combined with either a diode laser or an IPL device (Fig. 1.28). In this configuration, there is so-called synergy between the two applications (75). With the bipolar electrode configuration, electrical field density is intrinsically confined fairly superficially (the field intensity reaches about as deep as one-half the distance between the electrodes).

In monopolar configurations, the dispersive electrode is located at a distant point on the body. Monopolar skin rejuvenation systems tend to create large volumes of heating. They disperse the electrical energy over the breadth of the electrode through a concept known as capacitive coupling. This type of coupling helps to prevent the natural accumulation of electrical energy at the electrode edge (76). The first nonablative RF device (Therma Cool TC, Thermage, Hayward, California, USA) uses cryogen spray cooling (CSC), where the spray is started before the RF current. With a large monopolar electrode (>1 × 1 cm), for example, current is deposited diffusely in the dermis and the effects tend to be deep; that is, large volume of skin is heated. The goal is uniform heating of the deep dermis and fat. Depending on the dose, electrode configuration, time, and local skin structure, one observes various immediate ultrastructural changes (76).

On the other hand, if both positive and negative electrodes are placed in the contact tip (bipolar electrode), current density tends to flow superficially (path of least resistance from electrode to electrode, and therefore temperature elevation is confined to superficial skin). By placing the electrodes further apart, the current density depth will increase. Otherwise, control of

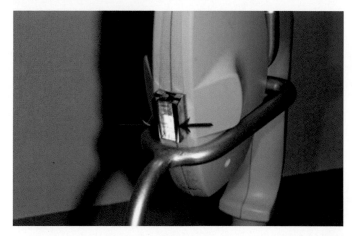

Figure 1.28 Tip of diode-radiofrequency device (metal rails (*arrows*) are the electrodes in bipolar configuration; Comet, Syneron, Canada).

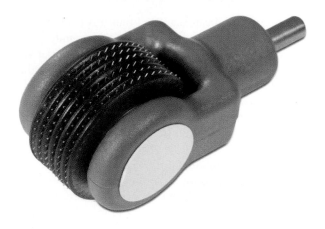

Figure 1.29 Radio frequency fractional handpiece; the small electrodes create plasma on skin as device rolls over surface.

the tissue heating is determined by variations in electrode type, power, and cooling times (75). If one uses "rail" metal-type electrodes placed next to a flashlamp crystal, EM field theory predicts that there will be a hot spot near the edge of the electrode. These hot spots can be reduced by electrically coupling the energy into the skin (e.g., ensuring that the dry stratum corneum, with high intrinsic impedance, is wetted with an electrolyte solution).

One device (Aurora SR, Syneron, Richmond Hill, Ontario, Canada) combines RF energy and a flashlamp. The near-simultaneous application of electrical and optical fields is proposed to optimize efficacy and safety. In this configuration, the local optical energy (fluence) increases the discrete chromophore temperature (i.e., hair, vessel). This localized heating reduces impedance (skin is treated as an electrolyte with decreasing impedance as a function of increasing temperature) and therefore in higher localized current densities. Thus, there is "synergy" between the optical and electrical parts of the device (75). A purported advantage of the treatment is that lower optical energies can be used to selectively heat subsurface targets than if a light source were used alone (thus enhancing epidermal preservation). There is some evidence that white hairs could be reduced with this technology. The working theory is that although there is little melanin in white hairs, there is higher current density around the follicle (as the current navigates around the high-resistance shaft) (75,77,78) The current density in the tissue adjacent to the hair shaft is roughly twice the current density and other parts of the skin; this is because the electrical current streams around the hair shaft concentrating in a layer just around the hair. Although certainly promising in principle and based on sound scientific principles, no study has clearly shown at the time of this writing that the "synergy," at least in its present configurations, is clinically relevant. That is, for example, no peer-reviewed study has shown that hair removal without RF is more effective than that with RF (with all other parameters held constant). Many studies that may or may not support the role of RF energy and optical energy as good dance partners are pending.

More recently fractional RF devices have been introduced for skin rejuvenation. Both bipolar and monopolar designs have been applied to create microwounds at and just below the skin surface (Fig. 1.29) (79–82).

A BRIEF OVERVIEW OF APPLICATIONS
Psoriasis
In psoriasis, one can target the microvasculature with vascular-specific lasers or, alternatively, vaporize plaques with resurfacing lasers. Owing to the size of the vessels, the PDL with its shorter pulse is the most logical choice among vascular lasers (83–85). Laser resurfacing has also been used to remove lesions (86). The excimer laser has been used. Here photochemistry is the primary mechanism (87). PDT configurations have also been applied with varying degrees of plaque clearing (88–90).

Hypopigmentation
The excimer laser and UV lamp sources have been used to restore pigment through photochemical pathways (48,91).

Postinflammatory Hyperpigmentation
This is typically very resistant to laser therapy. Some exceptions are Q-switched laser therapy for long-standing hyperpigmented areas on the extremities. Also, the PDL, in treating certain hyperpigmented hypertrophic scars, can reduce both the pigmentation and vascular aspects of the scar. Finally, long-pulsed KTP lasers and IPLs can sometimes reduce postinflammatory hyperpigmentation.

Wrinkle and Scar Reduction
They are typically achieved via ablative mechanisms. The CO_2 and Er:YAG lasers are ideally suited for LSR. The CO_2 laser functions more as a heating tool with typical parameters (5–10 J/cm^2 in pulsed mode), whereas the Er:YAG laser acts more as a purely ablative tool. A summary of the mechanisms follows. In brief, when energy deposition occurs rapidly, water does not vaporize at 100°C because the pressure is higher than 1 atm. Energy is deposited isovolumetrically and the temperature may reach 300°C with pressures up to 1000 atm (19). These high-pressure gradients can assist tissue removal because, depending on the mechanical properties of the tissue, the explosive removal process can be more energetically efficient than the 2500 J/cm^3 latent heat of vaporization for water. For example, the heat of ablation for epidermis is small, and portions of the friable cellular epidermis can be observed in the plume. Thus not all of the tissue is actually vaporized but rather forcibly ejected from the surface. For dermis, about 4.3 kJ/cm^3 are required for ablation by many CO_2 lasers—almost twice that needed for water

vaporization. It has been suggested that this is related to the high tensile strength of collagen fibers. A large induced pressure is necessary to disrupt the tissue (92). The Er laser vaporizes tissue more explosively than with CO_2 LSR, so that at fluences of only 5–10 J/cm², there is violent ablation, and particles are ejected at supersonic velocities. There is recoil at the tissue surface—the skin actually appears to be "pushed down" in real time. Momentum transfer produces stress waves, which combined with the small level of RTD may contribute to the tendency for bleeding after Er:YAG LSR. In general, in any laser resurfacing procedure, by confining energy both spatially and temporally, more efficient vaporization occurs with less thermal decomposition of proteins and less chance of charring. Nonablative skin remodeling has also been used with water as a chromophore (1320, 1450, and 1540 nm) and is intended to heat a subsurface "slab" of tissue (without epidermal damage). Both wrinkles and scars have improved with these approaches, but results are normally modest compared with properly applied ablative approaches. PDLs and other VIS light modalities have proved effective in scars (67,93–96). Although there is an indirect effect of VIS light technologies on wrinkles in some cases, no VIS light modality has achieved the same improvement in fine wrinkling as ablative modalities with traditional fluences. Fractional lasers have expanded greatly since the last edition of this book. Both ablative and nonablative approaches have played an ever-increasing role in wrinkle reduction (97–99).

Acne

There are many EMR-based approaches to acne treatment, which are limited only by our understanding of the pathophysiology of acne. Mechanisms for improving acne include suppression of *P. acnes* (PDT with endogenous and exogenous PS), normalization of the keratinization process through infundibular heating (some MIR lasers), and possible sebaceous gland damage through deep heating with IR lamp, deep MIR, and RF technologies (100). Of all the techniques, the only one that shows long-term acne reduction with *microscopic* evidence of marked sebaceous gland damage is *red light ALA-PDT*. This histologic picture has only been observed with long ALA incubation times (>4 hours) coupled with low power density light sources (101). A new system undergoing studies uses gold nanoshells that are targeted by 755- and 810-nm lasers to disrupt and damage the infundibulum and sebaceous glands. Delivery of the shells to the target relies on a transfolllicular route (102).

Pigmented Lesions

Melanosome heating conforms well with the basic theory of SPT (19). With very short pulses (nanoseconds), one observes immediate frost whitening at the surface (Fig. 1.30) added. Although the exact cause is unknown, it is most certainly related to the formation of gas bubbles that intensely scatter light (19). Over several minutes, these bubbles dissolve, causing the skin color to return to nearly normal. As the pulse duration increases, melanosome heating becomes more gentle, and there tends to be focal DE junction heating but with considerable diffusion outside the melanosome. Pigmented lesions can be divided into superficial and deep. Static epidermal pigmented lesions such as lentigos tend to be straightforward to

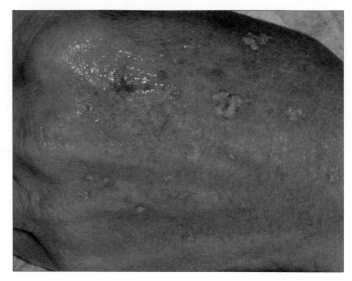

Figure 1.30 Note whitening response of lentigo on hand after Q-switched alexandrite laser.

treat. In most cases, the most complete removal (with only one treatment session) is achieved via Q-switched technologies. On the other hand, the least invasive and gentlest removal is via long pulse (milliseconds) technologies in the VIS light spectrum, such as IPL devices as well as KTP lasers. Long-pulse alexandrite lasers have also been employed as well as long-pulsed diode lasers to gently heat epidermal static pigmented lesions. "Dermal" static pigmented lesions such as nevus of Ota respond best to Q-switched lasers (103). This is consistent with the theory of SPT. With longer pulses (millisecond-domain), the dermal melanocytes, which are of relatively low concentration (compared with melanocytic nests in compound nevi or highly pigmented basal cell layers in lentigos), simply do not become hot enough to achieve pigment reduction (8). For light lentigos, the contrast between the skin's background color and the lesions may become too small for effective reduction by long-pulsed GY sources. In these cases, the shorter pulses of Q-switched lasers are required for selective heating of pigmented lesions. Melasma is a challenging condition to treat via lasers, most likely due to its dynamic and inflammatory nature (compared with the static nature of lentigos) (104). Ablative lasers can sometimes result in improvement; however, the ablation normally has to be carried out deeply, or postinflammatory hyperpigmentation may outweigh any achievement gains. Q-switched lasers typically result in only temporary improvement (followed by PIPA that worsens the appearance!) (104). On the other hand, longer pulsed VIS light laser technologies can sometimes achieve gradual improvement in melasma so long as the settings are not too high (105,106).

Vascular Lesions

Selective microvascular injury can be achieved well into the penetrating red visible wavelengths. The absorption coefficient of bloodless dermis is only 0.1–0.3 cm⁻¹ throughout the red wavelength region, and Hb absorption exceeds bloodless dermis throughout the red and NIR spectrum. It follows that even lasers with relatively poor Hb absorption, such as the ruby laser, have been used for PWS treatment. Despite competition from melanin, GY wavelength (532–595 nm) laser pulses appear to work well for treating larger vessel (0.1- to 1-mm diameter) PWSs or telangiectasia, and at the longer pulses appropriate to PWS treatment, pigment cell injury is minimized. By adding a second pass to vascular lesions, the dermal blood fraction will have increased from the first pass, and the blood absorption can increase manyfold. This has been shown to result in more comprehensive vessel heating within a volume of treated tissue (107). Part of the improvement may also stem from methemoglobin production (108,109). With GY lasers and IPLs, longer pulses (or pulse sequences) allow for some epidermal cooling between vascular events. The rationale is that the vessel will have a longer τ than the DE junction. It follows that longer pulses should allow for a greater ratio of vascular to epidermal heating (Fig. 1.19). This is supported by our work, which shows that longer IPL pulses allowed for greater epidermal sparing (Fig. 1.18). Recently, an enhanced role for PDT in vascular lesions has been reported. In these cases, vascular-specific photosensitizers, such as hematoporphyrin monomethyl ether, have been applied to PWS (110,111).

Hair

In this application, the target is either the bulge or the bulb, and the innocent bystander is the DE junction. The goal is to maximize the ratio of bulb to epidermal heating. The melanin density of the bulb normally exceeds the DE junction (most people have darker hair than skin). The challenge in laser hair reduction (LHR) is that the bulb lies deep in the skin (about 1–3 mm), such that the local fluence at the DE junction will exceed the bulb fluence. However, we can maximize the bulb-to-epidermal temperature ratio by (*i*) extending the pulse, (*ii*) using longer wavelengths, (*iii*) applying epidermal cooling, and (*iv*) compressing the skin (which decreases the bulb-to-surface distance) (112). In LHR, the heater (shaft) and the target (bulb or bulge) are not collocated. It follows that pws should be designed that exceed the τ of the shaft but not be so long that the dermis is overheated beyond the bulb (113). Too short pulses provide only temporary hair reduction and for the same reasons, very short pulses are ineffective in treating vascular lesions–heating is too confined to the immediate chromophore and does not extend to the intended target. Nanosecond pulses result in vaporization, but with or without a carbon suspension, hair reduction is akin to that of laser waxing. Very short nanosecond pulses expel the melanosomes outside the shaft but do not allow for significant heat conduction, and an immediate leukotrichia may be observed (the pulses are so short that the skeleton of the hair shaft remains) (114). With longer pulses (1–3 ms) and high power densities, the entire shaft is often coagulated, and it tends to coil up on the surface. Thus, like the blood vessel, one observes a continuum in the immediate laser light–hair response as a function of pulse duration. What about immediate endpoints and their relationship to the laser–tissue interaction? We normally think of perifollicular edema (PFE) as a necessary (and possibly) sufficient condition for semi- or permanent hair reduction. However, PFE can be a deceptive endpoint. Most likely it represents peribulbar damage. However, no one has characterized an association between the level of damage and the PFE severity. The failure of PDL, for example, to cause PFE despite obvious hair vaporization at the surface, suggests that deeper heating is required for PFE. Shorter

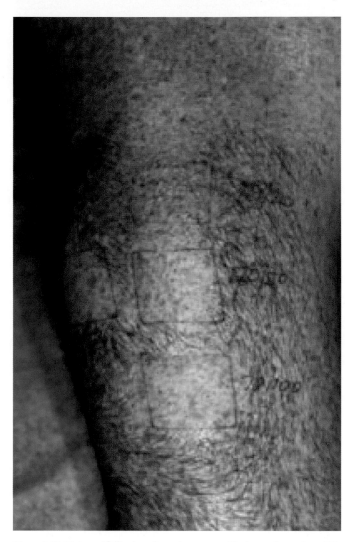

Figure 1.31 Note perifollicular edema increases with decreasing pulse width for same fluence with 1064-nm laser.

pulses, at least in a range from 3 to 100 ms) cause more PFE than longer ones with other parameters held constant, most likely due to more "intense" short-term damage to the follicle (Fig. 1.31). It follows that there is no reliable endpoint for permanent reduction. The presence of PFE always signals short-term reduction, but its absence does not preclude delayed LHR. For example, with a very long pulse (200–400 ms) 810-nm diode laser (Super Long Pulse, Palomar, Burlington, Massachusetts, USA), we have observed permanent LHR without PFE. What is the optimal wavelength for LHR? Theory suggests that longer wavelengths (e.g., 1064 vs. 755 nm) will always achieve a greater ratio of dermal-to-epidermal heating (112). But studies have not confirmed that longer wavelengths are necessarily more effective in LHR (115–119). Overall, the greatest limitation in using longer wavelengths is the absolute decrease in melanin absorption. For example, let us take the typical case of a young type II patient with dark coarse hair on the neck. If one compares the 810-nm diode laser with the 1064-nm laser, for example, treating one side with a 10-mm spot at 810 nm and 44 J/cm² and 21 ms and the other side with identical parameters with the YAG laser, although both lasers will achieve marked hair reduction, LHR will be better on the 810-nm side. We can use arguments from the skin optics and heat generation sections (vide supra) to support this result. We can also use those same arguments to optimize our parameters to enhance 1064-nm LHR. 810-nm light is absorbed roughly 2.5× that of 1064 nm. It follows that scattering and penetration issues aside, 2.5× the fluence should be required for identical bulb heating for the two wavelengths. However, more 1064-nm light will penetrate 3-mm deep into the skin, such that there are about 25% more photons at this depth versus 810 nm (120). It follows that to achieve identical bulb heating, assuming all other parameters are held constant, simple algebra suggests that about 2× more fluence must be delivered at the surface for similar bulb heating. Most YAG lasers, however, do not routinely allow for fluences above 80 J/cm^2 with big spots. Also, with larger spots and high fluences, although the epidermis is preserved, the YAG laser poses a risk for generalized dermal heating with multiple pulses. It follows that YAG lasers are ideal when the skin is very dark or the hair is very thick and black (Fig. 1.32). In these scenarios, the bulb-to-epidermal heating ratio is greater than 1, and even with lower fluences, μ_a of the follicle is so large (~75 cm^{-1} for a thick dark hair vs. 10 cm^{-1} for a fine brown hair at 1064 nm) that sufficient heat is generated (the hair is "saturated" with heat). With lighter finer hairs, one can use very high fluences and shorter pulses and still achieve some degree of permanent LHR with 1064 nm. We were able to see this in sandy brown haired patient, where a biopsy showed that a combination of 150 J/cm^2 and a 5-mm spot was necessary to see the earliest clearly identifiable heat changes in the bulb. Still, this heating was far less than that seen with a very thick black hair at 50 J/cm^2. For the author's own fine black arm hair, 120 J/cm^2 with 1064 nm achieved the same degree of PFE as 50 J/cm^2 with 810 nm. Hair reduction is a good example of why studies must be carefully examined before proclaiming victory for one laser over another (or at least one wavelength over another!). Often a study will compare lasers in their *commonly deployed* parameters (and not the optimal parameters) and then score the results. In the investigators' defense, often the optimal parameters are not available with a particular device. Unfortunately, some YAG lasers compromise too low fluences, and shorter wavelength lasers usually prevail in head-to-head studies unless the studied hairs are very thick and/or very black. Although the alexandrite and diode lasers can be used in most skin types (so long as effective surface cooling is applied), the one exception is very dark skin (i.e., darkest African-American) (115,121). In this case, we have found that no matter how long the pulse and how exquisite the cooling, 1064 nm offers the *greatest* ratio of efficacy to safety. This finding is consistent with our pigment readings with reflectance spectrophotometers, which show that a dark-skinned African-American is about 1.8× a dark as a light-skinned African American, but that the light-skinned African-American is only about 1.2× as dark as a tanned medium complexion Caucasian. PDT is another potential means for LHR. The major advantage is its nondependence on pigment. At this time, no system is readily available for ALA-assisted hair reduction, and several obstacles (pain, incubation time of ALA) remain before such a system can be deployed over large areas. A device that combines RF and light has been proposed to work in whitish hairs (vide supra).

Sebum and Fat

Laser lipolysis has been examined; however, no device has truly exploited the fat/sebum absorption maxima (relative to water) at 915, 1200, 1700, and 2200 nm (122). An RF device selectively heats fat in some applications at some threshold power.

Tattoo Removal by SPT

Tattoos consist of mainly intracellular, submicrometer size insoluble ink particles that have been ingested by phagocytic skin cells after intradermal injection. The stability and longevity of most tattoos show that many phagocytic skin cells do not traffic or migrate widely, although tattoos do become less distinct over decades (19). A great variety of inks are used in professional tattoos, which consist mainly of insoluble metal salts, oxides, or organic complexes (123). Amateur tattoos are almost always carbon in some form—India ink (amorphous carbon), graphite, or ash. Goldman first noted that tattoos were responsive to pulsed laser treatment, using normal mode ruby laser pulses (8). A dose–response and histologic study of Q-switched ruby laser pulses was subsequently performed, which led to widespread interest in Q-switched ruby lasers in the United States, followed by further ultrastructural studies of response (124). It is now apparent that the Q-switched ruby laser is generally effective and relatively well tolerated in the treatment of black, blue-black, and green tattoos. Multiple treatments are required at fluences ranging from 4 to 10 J/cm^2. Typically, four to six treatments given 1-month interval are needed for amateur tattoos, and six to eight for professional tattoos, although individual response is extremely variable. The risk of scarring is about 5–10% for the series of treatments, although over one-fourth of patients have transient textural changes. The Q-switched ruby laser causes blistering and hypopigmentation in most patients and permanent depigmentation in about 1–3%. The mechanisms involved in tattoo removal are largely unknown (123). It is clear that much of the ink, although apparently removed from the skin, is not removed from the body. All persons with tattoos have tattoo ink pigmentation of the lymph nodes draining the tattooed skin, and it is likely that this is the fate of most of the ink after laser treatment. Lightening of the tattoo occurs gradually about 1 week after each treatment and may go on for months. Occasionally, it is clear that ink is present in the scale crust that forms following epidermal injury and sheds 1–2 weeks after treatment, but it is equally apparent that tattoos are removed in cases where no scale crust is formed. Before treatment, ink particles are

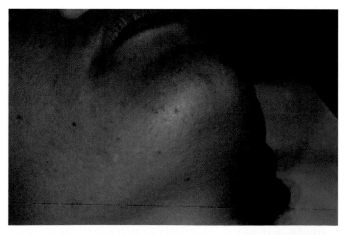

Figure 1.32 Selective heating of thicker black hairs with 1064 nm. The thinner hairs were unchanged on the surface after treatment with 1064-nm laser at 80 J/cm^2 and 40 ms with a 5-mm spot.

contained in phagolysosomes in fibroblasts, macrophages, and mast cells. After treatment by Q-switched ruby laser, electron microscopy suggests that some ink particles are fractured into 10–100 smaller fragments, which are extracellular, presumably released by rupture of the phagocytic cells (125). A study comparing nanosecond and picosecond 1064-nm pulses showed that carbon black particles became more electron-lucent after irradiation both in vivo and in vitro (126). The threshold fluences for these changes were less for the shorter pulses. Also, a cuvette of a carbon black suspension was lightened by simply irradiating its contents. The gradual reduction in absorbance has been shown to be due to a well-known steam carbon reaction; this reaction occurs when particles are heated sufficiently to cause a chemical reaction between carbon and surrounding water. The products are H_2 and carbon monoxide gases (69). This suggests that changes in optical properties of the particles may play a role in the tattoo-lightening process. Observations strongly suggest but do not prove that the primary effects of Q-switched lasers are (i) fragmentation of ink particles, (ii) laser-induced optical property changes, (iii) release into the extracellular dermal space, (iv) partial elimination of ink in a scale crust if present, (v) probably greater elimination into lymphatics, and (vi) rephagocytosis of laser-altered residual tattoo ink particles. Irreversible changes can occur in tattoo inks, especially those used in cosmetic skin-colored tattoos. Photochemical changes may conceivably affect tattoo ink removal for some kinds of ink. This appears to be especially true for tattoos containing red (ferric oxide) and titanium dioxide (vide infra) (127,128). All of the pulsed lasers used for tattoo removal occasionally cause irreversible immediate darkening of these tattoos, which may be temporarily obscured in part by the immediate whitening reaction, discussed above. It is therefore prudent to perform a small test exposure of cosmetic red, flesh-colored, or white tattoos to see whether immediate darkening occurs. In some cases, the darkened ink cannot be removed by subsequent laser treatments and adds to the disfigurement. The mechanism of red tattoo ink darkening is not known but probably involves reduction of ferric oxide (rust color) to ferrous oxide (black). Pure ferric oxide is easily converted in this manner by Q-switched laser pulses in vitro and is present in many cosmetic tattoos (127). During tattoo treatment, there is surface whitening (as in epidermal pigmented lesions, vide supra). This is accentuated where there is the highest pigment concentration. The proposed causes have already been discussed. In treating black tattoos with 1064 nm (where there is little epidermal effect), one can also see a subsurface transient bright light. This probably represents laser-induced incandescence with maximum temperatures around 2000 K. At 4000 K carbon particles vaporize (123). There are a few controlled studies to understand and optimize tattoo removal. The study cited above addressed the role of pulse duration (nanosecond vs. picosecond domain pulses) in tattoo removal (126). One of the study goals was to examine the role of inertial confinement in laser–tattoo reactions. Somewhat analogous to the concept of thermal confinement, inertial confinement can be achieved when the laser pulse is delivered within the time for which pressure can be relieved from the ink particles. The inertial confinement time is simply the particle diameter divided by the speed of sound, which for tattoo ink particles equals about 1 ns. Because of the

high pressures, shock waves (bulk disruption of the material) can occur, which should increase the probability of mechanical fracture. It may therefore be that all of the laser pulses being used now are too long. Ross et al. (126) showed that the picosecond domain pulses were more effective than nanosecond pulses in black tattoo removal for the same radiant exposures, suggesting that tattoo removal is very sensitive to power density. A theoretical model predicts that the nanosecond pulses would only generate peak temperatures about 3% that of the nanosecond pulses, so that photothermal effects alone could explain the more efficient tattoo resolution with shorter pulses. It is unclear if shock waves were generated with the picosecond pulse. Significant details of wavelength-dependent effects are unknown. One study has examined the spectra for most colors and showed absorption peaks for all known colors; however, many tattoos are resistant to multiple treatments, especially green tattoos (129). In a study of tattoos at our laboratory, TiO_2 was detected by X-ray diffraction in 4/5 resistant green tattoos, and the Q-switched alexandrite laser produced an immediate blue-black discoloration of TiO_2 ink; the ink is often used as a brightener for green and other colors. Paradoxically, with additional treatments, some laser-darkened tattoos can be lightened (128). It may be that once all the photochemistry has taken place that the newly formed products are also capable of absorbing VIS or IR radiation. The chemical identity of most tattoo inks and how they are affected by high-intensity laser pulses are unknown and, most importantly, have never been linked to clinical response. In the previous edition of this text, several unresolved issues were listed in tattoo removal, only a few of which have been answered: (i) Is a laser-induced plasma involved? Possibly, if the generation of surface plasma facilitates ink removal through generation of shock waves. (ii) Must the ink particles be fractured? Ink particles need not be fractured for clinical resolution. This has been shown for carbon black, where particles may actually increase in size yet lighten through a change in chemistry. It appears that more crystalline particles are more likely to fracture than relatively amorphous organic substances (130). (iii) Is it the ink or the cells containing it are the targets? It appears that the ink is the target but that cell death is associated with clearing, since this allows ink release from the cell. (iv) How is the ink removed, and where does it go? The ink is removed by the mechanisms cited above; in addition, optical property changes in the ink itself may contribute to clearing for some inks. (v) What role might phagocytosis by different cell types play in the retention of ink following treatment, and how can this be optimized? Attempts have been made to modulate the immune response in tattoo removal. Recently, imiquimod cream has been used in the interval between laser treatment sessions to augment ink removal. Also, at least one study showed that repeated laser treatment in the same office visit at 20-minute intervals could accelerate tattoo clearing. Presumably, the delay allows the whitening response to resolve and permits enhanced transmission of the subsequent set of laser impacts (131).

Cooling

Before the availability of surface cooling, fluence thresholds for efficacy and epidermal damage were often close. VIS light technologies (especially GY light sources such as IPL, KTP laser, and PDL) are popular in cutaneous laser surgery. They are also the wavelength ranges where epidermal damage is most likely. The epidermis is an innocent bystander in cutaneous laser applications where the intended targets, such as hair follicles or blood vessels, are located in the dermis. Specifically, absorption of light by epidermal melanin causes epidermal heating. Melanin is distributed throughout the epidermis but is especially concentrated in the basal cell layer. Melanin absorption of VIS light causes heating of melanosomes and through thermal diffusion, subsequent damage to the entire epidermis. This is especially true for GY light, but the risk of selective DE junction–derived epidermal injury extends to wavelengths as long as 1064 nm. Overall, shorter wavelengths pose a greater risk to the skin surface, because the ratio of epidermal-to-dermal heating is higher. This ratio derives from (*i*) a higher absorption of melanin by shorter wavelengths and (*ii*) a tendency for photon scatter to limit penetration of shorter wavelengths. This leads to an accumulation of energy near the DE junction (58,132–134).

Beyond VIS light (green, yellow, and red) sources, surface cooling has also been employed in NIR and MIR lasers. With NIR lasers, surface cooling is important, but not only because of DE junction–derived epidermal heating. In addition, deep beam penetration may cause catastrophic bulk heating. With MIR lasers (1.32, 1.45, and 1.54 μm), the chromophore is water. It follows that with even very low fluences, surface cooling is imperative. Without cooling, water's ubiquitous nature in the skin causes laser-induced top-to-bottom injury. There is no discrete heating. All of the techniques are susceptible to operator error and device failure. It follows that as physicians rely more heavily on cooling devices, any lack of their proper deployment unveils the *dark* side of cooling.

The first goal of surface cooling is preservation of the epidermis. Unintentional heating of the basal cell layer can lead to vesiculation, crusting, and, at times, scarring. The second and related goal of surface cooling is to allow for delivery of higher fluences to the intended target (i.e., the hair bulb and/or bulge or a subsurface blood vessel). Often, the highest fluence that can be used in targeting hair and/or subsurface vessels is limited by heating of the epidermis. By cooling the epidermis, higher fluences and therefore higher temperature elevations are possible in the targeted structures in the dermis. Another benefit of surface cooling is analgesia, as almost all cooling strategies will provide some pain relief (135–141).

The timing of the cooling relative to the laser pulse is important. Cooling can be before the pulse (pre), during the pulse (parallel), or after the pulse (post) (134). All three cooling periods are important. For example, postcooling may prevent retrograde heating (i.e., from the vessel back to the epidermis) from damaging the skin surface. A cooling protection factor (CPF) has been proposed by Anderson, who likens it to the sun protection factor concept used in sunscreen assessments. The cooling protection factor is the ratio of fluence, with and without surface cooling, that spares the epidermis. It can be evaluated from the following equation:

$$CPF = \frac{T_c - T_{ic}}{T_c - T_i} \qquad (5)$$

In the above equation, T_{ic} and T_i are basal layer temperatures before laser irradiation with and without cooling, respectively. T_{crit} is the critical temperature at which thermal injury occurs. The detailed calculations described later indicate that if the initial skin temperature is 30°C, contact cooling reduces the temperature of the basal layer to about 20°C. If T_{crit} is assumed to be 60°C (it is actually somewhat higher for the brief laser exposure times in this analysis), this would give the CPF as (60–20)/(60–30) or 1.33. Similarly, cryogen cooling reduces the temperature to about 0°C, thus giving a CPF value as (60–0)/(60–30) or 2.0. In summary, the CPF values provided by CSC and contact cooling are predicted as 2.0 and 1.33, respectively. Finally, there is convective air cooling, where cold air is commonly used in skin chilling. The Zimmer (Cyro5, Zimmer MedizinSysteme, Ulm, Germany) directs −10°C air at the skin at a rapid rate (1000 L/min). This system proves for good bulk cooling but spatial localization of the cooling is poor. The CPF, depending on the air temperature and nozzle velocity, is near that of contact cooling (142).

Besides protection of the DE junction from pigment "unfriendly" wavelengths, sometimes bulk cooling is required because the volume heated is large and there is a risk for large volume overheating and catastrophic scarring (i.e., with 1064 nm). There are some scenarios where cooling is unlikely to prove beneficial: (*i*) when the absorption of the wavelength is very strong by water (i.e., Er:YAG and CO_2), here the cooling and heating zone are collocated so that preservation of epidermal *viability* is unfeasible; also (*ii*) when using Q-switched lasers in the range from 532 to 1064 nm, cooling achieves pain reduction but will only modestly reduce the high peak temperatures generated by these ultrashort pulses in melanin and exogenous inks (tattoos).

SOME INTERESTING CONCEPTS AND IDEAS IN LASER–TISSUE INTERACTIONS
Focusing the Laser Beam
A trick to increase the dermal-to-epidermal damage ratio is use of a convergent lens. This tool increases the local photon density in the dermis (targeting the hair bulb, a blood vessel, or dermal water). Theoretically, one should be able to use smaller incident fluences, therefore achieving some protection of the epidermis (143). Because of scattering and subsequent beam broadening, the increased subsurface photon densities that would be predicted in a transparent medium are not realized. Still, there should be a relative increase in deeper photon density versus using a more collimated beam.

Vacuuming the Target in the Laser Beam
A company (Aesthera, Livermore, California, USA) has proposed a pneumatic device whereby the skin is vacuumed into the light path, such that the light penetration into skin is enhanced (Fig. 1.33). In this way more energetic high-frequency photons can be delivered, for example, to the hair follicle, with relative epidermal sparing.

Pixilated Injury (Also Known As Fractional Photothermolysis)
One can use a "pixilated" injury with water as a chromophore in what is called fractional photothermolysis. Roughly

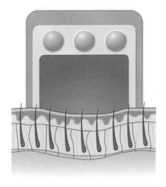
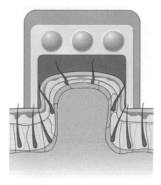
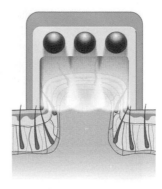
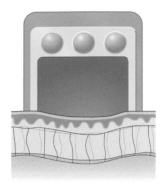

(**A**) Handpiece is placed on treatment area

(**B**) Targets elevated closer to skin's surface
Blood concentration reduced
Melanin concentration reduced

(**C**) Light applied to treatment area

(**D**) Targets are safely and painlessly destroyed

Figure 1.33 (**A–D**) Device that "vacuums" skin into the light path; skin is stretched and thinned, providing enhanced "relative" penetration of the beam.

100- to 430-μm spots have been used with 250- to 500-μm spacing (144). The tissue can recover from this fractional injury without the widespread epidermal loss observed after traditional resurfacing applications.

Optical Damping

Optically, replacing air ($n = 1.0$) with a higher-index medium at the skin surface such as glass ($n = 1.5$) or sapphire ($n = 1.7$) tends to spare the epidermis. This effect has nothing to do with heat transfer, but rather is a consequence of optical scattering behavior. At wavelengths from about 600 to 1200 nm, the majority of light in Caucasian epidermis is actually back- and multiple-scattered light. Indeed, the contribution of scattered light can be almost an order of magnitude higher than that of the laser beam itself! By providing a closer match to the skin's refractive index, internal reflection of the back-scattered light is greatly reduced, decreasing the natural convergence of photons at the skin surface. This version of optical epidermal sparing requires a physically thick external medium such as a thick layer of gel.

Compacting the Dermis

One can decrease the depth photons must propagate by applying pressure over the treated area. This maneuver may, for example, decrease the relative depth of the bulb and bulge up to 30% relative to the skin surface. Disadvantages might include variability in the amount of pressure, such that adjacent treatment areas are exposed to different subsurface fluences. Also, it is unclear if compacting the dermis might alter its scattering properties. In theory, compression should decrease water content and improve dermal transmission (19). Most recently fractional lasers have been configured with compression optics to enhance penetration of the microbeams. The pressure displaces tissue water and creates a tubular light guide to decrease scattering losses (Fig. 1.34A,B) (145,146).

Spot Diameter

In general, the spot size should be $3–4\times > \delta$, as larger spots make it more likely that photons will be scattered back into the incident collimated beam (112). Photons that are scattered out of the beam are essentially wasted. Traveling "alone," they carry insufficient energy to cause macroscopic thermal responses in tissue. The consequences of spot size are explained as follows. Basically, for small beams (narrow) scattered photons are carried out of the beam path after only a few scattering events. A good analogy is a highway with exits. With a narrow highway, any movement obliges the auto to "take" the exit, and the car does not return to the road. On the other hand, on a superhighway with many lanes, cars can move about and stay within the original boundary of the thoroughfare. Only cars on the extreme left and right are likely to "get" off the road. Large spots increase the dermal-to-epidermal damage ratio as well as the relative penetration depth. However, *absolute* epidermal damage will be greater with the larger spot with the same fluence as the smaller spot. It follows that it is prudent to reduce the fluence by 20%, for example, if one increases the spot size between treatment sessions in care of a PWS. Also, one should note that for any turbid medium, even if the spot is "top hat," there will be an accumulation of photons near the center of the beam, such that a greater clinical effect will often be noted at the center of the spot. As a clinical example of the effect of spot size, we have found for 3- versus 6-mm spots with the YAG laser that roughly half the fluence is required with the larger spot for leg vein clearance. For shallow-penetrating lasers such as CO_2 and Er where the $\delta \ll$ spotsize, the diameter of the beam does not intrinsically affect the tissue response. That is why equivalent results can be obtained for skin resurfacing, using pulsed CO_2 lasers versus scanned, tightly focused CW CO_2 lasers (147).

Changing Optical Properties in Real Time

One should always be aware of the changing chromophore concentrations as a function of time during a treatment session. One should never consider each laser–tissue interaction as an independent event, but rather a cumulative process where visual endpoints are the most important ally for the physician. Optical properties of the skin are like the weather (5), and one must accommodate the changes in real time. For example, the dermal blood fraction increases after one pass of the PDL, such that for a second pass, the skin temperature will increase due to the higher μ_a (148). A failure to

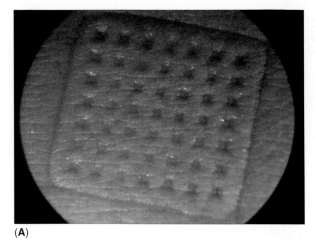

(A)

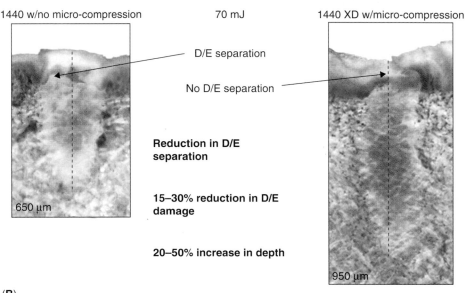

(B)

Figure 1.34 (**A**) Note microindentations after application of compression optic; (**B**) histology correlate—the pressure enhances transmission of beam. *Abbreviation*: D/E, dermal/epidermal.

respond to these real-time changes accounts for many laser complications.

Optical Clearing with Hyperosmolar Solutions

One can increase the transparency of the dermis by topical application or intradermal injection of solutions such as glycerin (149). The working theory is that water and collagen become less bound, such that the effective scattering coefficient of the dermis is reduced. Already this concept has been applied to increase the visibility of blood vessels from the surface. Possible applications include tattoo removal, where particles often are found several millimeters deep in tissue.

"Carbonization" at the Surface

Carbon will cause all wavelengths to increase absorption, such that one can convert a deeply penetrating laser to a more superficially penetrating laser by having a fine carbon layer at the surface. For example, one can "convert" a 694-nm ruby laser into a laser with CO_2 laser-like effects by applying a fine layer of graphite from a copy machine to the skin surface. In this way, the 694-nm laser energy is confined to the surface by the almost 100% absorption by carbon. This fine layer of

Table 1.3 μ_a for Fine Layer of Carbon on Surface

Laser	Wavelength (nm)	μ_a (cm^{-1})
Argon ion	488	504
Argon ion	514	463
HeNe	633	317
Diode	805	183
Nd:YAG	1064	80

Abbreviations: HeNe, helium neon; Nd:YAG, neodynium:yttrium-aluminum-garnet; μ_a, absorption coefficient.

heated material then cools much like a superficial layer of tissue heated by a CO_2 laser alone (Table 1.3).

Photon Recycling

The remittance of human skin is wavelength dependent and ranges from 15% to 70% through the VIS and NIR regions of the EM spectrum. These reflected photons are scattered into the environment and essentially "wasted" in surgical laser applications. One can (and we did) design a simple hemispherical reflector to return reflected light to the incident spot on the skin (Fig. 1.35). In theory, the gain in total energy available to

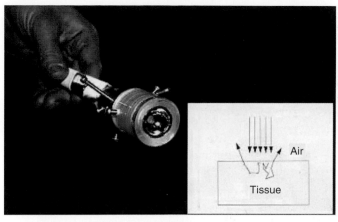

Figure 1.35 Hemispheric mirror that "sits" over the skin and reflects remitted photons back to the skin surface (so-called photon recycling).

skin is a factor of $\dfrac{1}{(1 - R_S R_M)}$, where R_S is the skin reflectance and R_M is that of a hemispherical mirror. For example, if R_S is 0.7 and R_M is 0.9, a gain of $\dfrac{1}{(1 - 0.63)}$, or almost threefold, can be achieved.

Plasma for Skin Regeneration

Gas plasmas have been used in surgical devices for many years. Typically, ionized gas acts as a conducting pathway to deliver RF energy to achieve superficial tissue coagulation. The plasma energy is relatively small, as the tissue effect is achieved primarily by RF energy. In contrast, the Portrait PSR (plasma skin resurfacing), (Rhytec, UK) uses ultrahigh-frequency (UHF) RF energy to ionize a flow of nitrogen gas producing millisecond pulses of plasma (3). The plasma, characterized by a lilac glow transitioning to a yellowish light called a Lewis–Rayleigh Afterglow as it flows out of the nozzle of the handpiece, produces short-lived rapid elevations in the temperature of the skin's surface. The disruptive effect of energy conversion through an intermediate chromophore found with high-energy lasers is avoided. The important clinical reason for selecting nitrogen is that it purges oxygen from the skin's surface so that oxidative carbonization is minimized, eliminating unpredictable "hot spots" and charring that can produce scarring. A new pixilated RF plasma system (RF Pixel, Alma Lasers, Buffalo Grove, IL, USA) uses a rolling set of electrode tips to create microwounds in the skin (Fig. 1.29).

Pigment/Erythema Meters to Assist in Guiding Parameters

Many laser complications stem from a failure of the operator to consider subtle pigmentary differences between patients and the transitory nature of pigmentary status in the same patient. For example, a tanned Caucasian patient may appear to be equally dark as an Asian-American patient who is untanned. However, in LHR, the patient with the higher constitutive coloration will normally show a greater epidermal tolerance. Tanned skin is injured skin, and newly introduced spectrophotometers can allow the operator to distinguish between levels of coloration within the context of erythema and time. Proper use of these handheld devices allows the astute operator to adjust settings based on absolute pigment levels as well as ratios of pigment to erythema. Also, step-off

regions between tanned and untanned areas can be accounted for (150). One newer device integrated into an IPL system is the Skintel™, a built-in pigment meter that sends a Bluetooth signal from the skin surface to the base device and suggests safe start settings to the operator for that local anatomic region.

Using a Polarizing Lamp to Enhance Illumination

One can optimize laser treatment by using a polarizing lamp during procedures to enhance the appearance of blood and pigment dyschromias (Fig. 1.36A,B) (151).

Selective Cell Targeting

A process called selected cell targeting has been examined as a way to destroy selected cells. This precise energy deposition is achieved by using laser pulses and light absorbing immunoconjugates tagged to the respective cells. The investigators in one study showed, for example, that lymphocytes could be selectively damaged by attaching iron oxide microparticles absorbing 565-nm radiation at those sites (152). One can imagine, in the future, using this type of modality to treat T-cell-mediated diseases, such as atopic dermatitis or psoriasis. In this way, one makes the "bad guy" more noticeable to the laser.

Scatter-Limited Therapy Using Small Microbeams

Reinisch (153) proposed the use of variously sized beams to limit penetration into the dermis. By using the aforementioned spot size arguments, one can exploit the properties of small spots to change the way particular wavelengths behave in the skin. For example, one can tailor a 1064-nm laser to heat progressively larger depths of skin by increasing the spot size (Fig. 1.37).

Two-Photon Excitation

We often are limited in dermatology by using VIS light laser technologies with which are intrinsically nonpenetrating. By using very high power density sources, there is a concept known as "two-photon excitation" (154). This concept allows for optimal beam penetration while still preserving tissue target selectivity for shorter wavelengths. If, for example, one wants to target a red tattoo deep in the skin with 532-nm light, high-fluence 1064-nm light can be applied to the surface. By chance some photons will arrive simultaneously at the target, creating one higher energy photon. Although presently only used in diagnostic applications in the future, this sort of technology might overcome some obstacles in our present approaches.

Enhanced Drug Delivery Through Microchannels

Investigators have examined the role for fractional lasers in drug delivery through the skin. Already, enhanced delivery of ALA has been reported (155,156). Another potential role for fractional lasers is sequential firing whereby the first pulse creates a gateway for the second pulse. For example, a CO_2 laser vertical channel could create a hole for a subsequent beam. The second beam would have a "head start" and travels deeper into the skin (157).

Finally, the reader should note that most of this chapter has dealt with the physical portion of the skin's reaction to light and electricity. However, oftentimes a characterization of the reaction between the tissue and the energy source is not as difficult as the subsequent biological sequelae. For example, as Dr. Martin van Gemert remarked, why do DE junction-derived blisters (after KTP laser) often cause scars but CO_2 laser, even

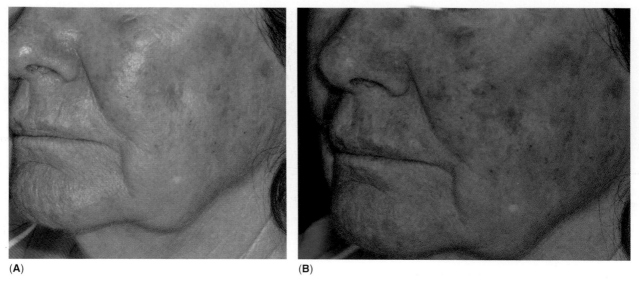

Figure 1.36 Blood vessels (**A**) with and (**B**) without cross-polarization.

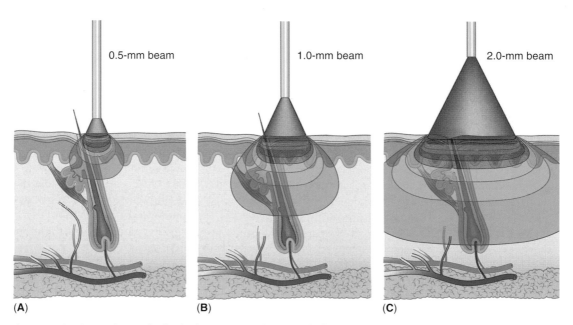

Figure 1.37 Note how spot size changes impact the depth of penetration. Shown are the fluence patterns for 1064-nm light with beams (**A**) 0.5 mm, (**B**) 1.0 mm, and (**C**) 2.0 mm in diameter on the skin surface.

after obvious removal of the epidermis, does not? Obviously, much of the work in the future for scientists will involve a more complete "mapping" of these complex responses.

Laser, nonlaser light sources, and other physical modalities will undoubtedly play different roles than the traditionally destructive ones that they have played to date. As we further harness and understand EMR, the role of light will expand into real-time bedside diagnostic tools. One day the dermatologist could well diagnose a BCC noninvasively, prepare the patient for PDT, and months later "re-biopsy" the patient with optical coherence tomography for test of cure! All of this would occur without disruption of even the stratum corneum! The future is indeed exciting.

REFERENCES

1. Kono T, Isago T, Honda T, Nozaki M. Treatment of facial lentigines with the long pulsed dye laser by compression method. Lasers Surg Med 2004; 34(Suppl 16): (abstract): 33.
2. Grossweiner L. The Science of Phototherapy. Boca Raton: CRC, 1994.
3. Hillenkamp F. Interaction between laser radiation and biological systems. In: Hillenkamp FRP, Sacchi C, eds. Lasers in Medicine and Biology. Vol Series A New York: Plenum, 1980: 37–68.
4. Welch A, van Gemert MJ, Starr JC, Wilson BC. Definitions and overview of tissue optics. In: Welch AJ, van Gemert MJ, eds. Optical-Thermal Response of Laser-Iradiated Tissue. New York: Plenum, 1995: 15–46.
5. Anderson RR, Parrish JA. The optics of human skin. J Invest Dermatol 1981; 77: 13–19.
6. van Gemert MJ, Jacques SL, Sterenborg HJ, Star WM. Skin optics. IEEE Trans Biomed Eng 1989; 36: 1146–54.

7. Goldman L, Rockwell R. Laser systems and their applications in medicine and biology. In: Levine S, ed. Advances in Biomedical Engineering and Medical Physics. New York: Interscience, 1968: 317.

8. Anderson RR. Dermatologic history of the ruby laser: the long story of short pulses. Arch Dermatol 2003; 139: 70–4.

9. Knappe V, Frank F, Rohde E. Principles of lasers and biophotonic effects. Photomed Laser Surg 2004; 22: 411–17.

10. Reinisch L. Laser physics and tissue interactions. Otolaryngol Clin North Am 1996; 29: 893–914.

11. Angermeier MC. Treatment of facial vascular lesions with intense pulsed light. J Cutan Laser Ther 1999; 1: 95–100.

12. Bitter PH. Noninvasive rejuvenation of photodamaged skin using serial, full-face intense pulsed light treatments. Dermatol Surg 2000; 26: 835–42; discussion 843.

13. Cliff S, Misch K. Treatment of mature port wine stains with the PhotoDerm VL. J Cutan Laser Ther 1999; 1: 101–4.

14. Goldberg DJ, Cutler KB. Nonablative treatment of rhytids with intense pulsed light. Lasers Surg Med 2000; 26: 196–200.

15. Raulin C, Greve B, Grema H. IPL technology: a review. Lasers Surg Med 2003; 32: 78–87.

16. Sadick NS, Weiss R. Intense pulsed-light photorejuvenation. Semin Cutan Med Surg 2002; 21: 280–7.

17. Weiss RA, Goldman MP, Weiss MA. Treatment of poikiloderma of Civatte with an intense pulsed light source. Dermatol Surg 2000; 26: 823–7; discussion 828.

18. Welch AJ, van Gemert MJ. Overview of optical and thermal interaction and nomenclature. In: Welch AJ, van Gemert MJ, eds. Optical Thermal Response of Laser- Irradiated Tissue. New York: Plenum, 1995: 1–14.

19. Anderson R, Ross E. Laser-tissue interactions. In: Fitzpatrick R, Goldman M, eds. Cosmetic Laser Surgery. St. Louis: Mosby, 2000: 1–30.

20. Fisher JC. Basic biophysical principles of resurfacing of human skin by means of the carbon dioxide laser. J Clin Laser Med Surg 1996; 14: 193–210.

21. Kimel S, Svaasand LO, Cao D, Hammer-Wilson MJ, Nelson JS. Vascular response to laser photothermolysis as a function of pulse duration, vessel type, and diameter: Implications for port wine stain laser therapy. Lasers Surg Med 2002; 30: 160–9.

22. Tanghetti E, Sierra RA, Sherr EA, Mirkov M. Evaluation of pulse-duration on purpuric threshold using extended pulse pulsed dye laser (cynosure V-star). Lasers Surg Med 2002; 31: 363–6.

23. West TB, Alster TS. Comparison of the long-pulse dye (590-595 nm) and KTP (532 nm) lasers in the treatment of facial and leg telangiectasias. Dermatol Surg 1998; 24: 221–6.

24. Anderson RR, Parrish JA. Selective photothermolysis: precise microsurgery by selective absorption of pulsed radiation. Science 1983; 220: 524–7.

25. Anderson RR, Parrish JA. Microvasculature can be selectively damaged using dye lasers: a basic theory and experimental evidence in human skin. Lasers Surg Med 1981; 1: 263–76.

26. Goldman L, Rockwell RJ Jr. Laser systems and their applications in medicine and biology. Adv Biomed Eng Med Phys 1968; 1: 317–82.

27. Itzkan I, Izatt J. Medical Use of Lasers. Encyclopedia of Applied Physics. Washington, D.C.: VCH Publishers, Inc. & American Institute of Physics, 1994: 33–59.

28. Jacques SL. Spectrum of carbonized tissue. 1998. [Available from: http://omlc.bme.ogi.edu/spectra/carbonizedtissue/index.html]

29. Ellis DL, Weisberg NK, Chen JS, Stricklin GP, Reinisch L. Free electron laser infrared wavelength specificity for cutaneous contraction. Lasers Surg Med 1999; 25: 1–7.

30. Walsh JT Jr, Flotte TJ, Anderson RR, Deutsch TF. Pulsed CO_2 laser tissue ablation: effect of tissue type and pulse duration on thermal damage. Lasers Surg Med 1988; 8: 108–18.

31. Altshuler GB, Anderson RR, Manstein D, Zenzie HH, Smirnov MZ. Extended theory of selective photothermolysis. Lasers Surg Med 2001; 29: 416–32.

32. Polla BS, Anderson RR. Thermal injury by laser pulses: protection by heat shock despite failure to induce heat-shock response. Lasers Surg Med 1987; 7: 398–404.

33. Beckham JT, Mackanos MA, Crooke C, et al. Assessment of cellular response to thermal laser injury through bioluminescence imaging of heat shock protein 70. Photochem Photobiol 2004; 79: 76–85.

34. Verdaasdonk RM, Borst C, van Gemert MJ. Explosive onset of continuous wave laser tissue ablation. Phys Med Biol 1990; 35: 1129–44.

35. Chung SH, Mazur E. Surgical applications of femtosecond lasers. J Biophotonics 2009; 2: 557–72.

36. Smith S, Piacquadio D, Morhenn V, Atkin D, Fitzpatrick R. Short incubation PDT versus 5-FU in treating actinic keratoses. J Drugs Dermatol 2003; 2: 629–35.

37. Alexiades-Armenakas MR, Geronemus RG. Laser-mediated photodynamic therapy of actinic cheilitis. J Drugs Dermatol 2004; 3: 548–51.

38. Karrer S, Baumler W, Abels C, et al. Long-pulse dye laser for photodynamic therapy: investigations in vitro and in vivo. Lasers Surg Med 1999; 25: 51–9.

39. Finlay JC, Conover DL, Hull EL, Foster TH. Porphyrin bleaching and PDT-induced spectral changes are irradiance dependent in ALA-sensitized normal rat skin in vivo. Photochem Photobiol 2001; 73: 54–63.

40. Sterenborg HJ, van Gemert MJ. Photodynamic therapy with pulsed light sources: a theoretical analysis. Phys Med Biol 1996; 41: 835–49.

41. Parrish JA, Jaenicke KF. Action spectrum for phototherapy of psoriasis. J Invest Dermatol 1981; 76: 359–62.

42. Weiss RA, McDaniel DH, Geronemus RG, Weiss MA. Clinical trial of a novel non-thermal LED array for reversal of photoaging: Clinical, histologic, and surface profilometric results. Lasers Surg Med 2005; 36: 85–91.

43. Jacques SL. Laser-tissue interactions. Photochemical, photothermal, and photomechanical. Surg Clin North Am 1992; 72: 531–58.

44. Jacques S. Simple optical theory for light dosimetry during PDT. In: Tuchin V, ed. Selected Papers on Tissue Optics. Vol MS 102 Bellingham: SPIE- International Society for Optical Engineering, 1992: 655.

45. Jacques S. Skin optics summary. 1998. [Available from: http://www.omlc.ogi.edu/news/jan98/skinoptics.html]

46. Stamatas GN, Kollias N. Blood stasis contributions to the perception of skin pigmentation. J Biomed Opt 2004; 9: 315–22.

47. Pearce J, Thomsen SL. Rate process analysis of thermal damage. In: Welch AJ, van Gemert MJ, eds. Optical Thermal Response of Laser-irradiated Tissue. New York: Plenum, 1995: 561–608.

48. Alexiades-Armenakas MR, Bernstein LJ, Friedman PM, Geronemus RG. The safety and efficacy of the 308-nm excimer laser for pigment correction of hypopigmented scars and striae alba. Arch Dermatol 2004; 140: 955–60.

49. Raulin C, Greve B, Warncke SH, Gundogan C. Excimer laser. Treatment of iatrogenic hypopigmentation following skin resurfacing. Hautarzt 2004; 55: 746–8.

50. Gold MH, Rao J, Goldman MP, et al. A multicenter clinical evaluation of the treatment of mild to moderate inflammatory acne vulgaris of the face with visible blue light in comparison to topical 1% clindamycin antibiotic solution. J Drugs Dermatol 2005; 4: 64–70.

51. Omi T, Bjerring P, Sato S, et al. 420 nm intense continuous light therapy for acne. J Cosmet Laser Ther 2004; 6: 156–62.

52. Gold MH, Bradshaw VL, Boring MM, et al. The use of a novel intense pulsed light and heat source and ALA-PDT in the treatment of moderate to severe inflammatory acne vulgaris. J Drugs Dermatol 2004; 3: S15–19.

53. Tzung TY, Wu KH, Huang ML. Blue light phototherapy in the treatment of acne. Photodermatol Photoimmunol Photomed 2004; 20: 266–9.

54. Itkin A, Gilchrest BA. delta-Aminolevulinic acid and blue light photodynamic therapy for treatment of multiple basal cell carcinomas in two patients with nevoid basal cell carcinoma syndrome. Dermatol Surg 2004; 30: 1054–61.

55. Bjerring P, Christiansen K. Intense pulsed light source for treatment of small melanocytic nevi and solar lentigines. J Cutan Laser Ther 2000; 2: 177–81.

56. Bjerring P, Christiansen K, Troilius A. Intense pulsed light source for treatment of facial telangiectasias. J Cosmet Laser Ther 2001; 3: 169–73.

57. Chan H. The use of lasers and intense pulsed light sources for the treatment of acquired pigmentary lesions in Asians. J Cosmet Laser Ther 2003; 5: 198–200.

58. Kauvar AN, Frew KE, Friedman PM, Geronemus RG. Cooling gel improves pulsed KTP laser treatment of facial telangiectasia. Lasers Surg Med 2002; 30: 149–53.

59. Lee MW. Combination 532-nm and 1064-nm lasers for noninvasive skin rejuvenation and toning. Arch Dermatol 2003; 139: 1265–76.

60. Avram DK, Goldman MP. Effectiveness and safety of ALA-IPL in treating actinic keratoses and photodamage. J Drugs Dermatol 2004; 3: S36–9.

61. McDaniel DH, Ash K, Lord J, et al. Laser therapy of spider leg veins: clinical evaluation of a new long pulsed alexandrite laser. Dermatol Surg 1999; 25: 52–8.

62. Dover JS. New approaches to the laser treatment of vascular lesions. Australas J Dermatol 2000; 41: 14–18.

63. Eremia S, Li C, Umar SH. A side-by-side comparative study of 1064 nm Nd:YAG, 810 nm diode and 755 nm alexandrite lasers for treatment of 0.3-3 mm leg veins. Dermatol Surg 2002; 28: 224–30.

64. Passeron T, Olivier V, Duteil L, et al. The new 940-nanometer diode laser: an effective treatment for leg venulectasia. J Am Acad Dermatol 2003; 48: 768–74.

65. Kaudewitz P, Klovekorn W, Rother W. Effective treatment of leg vein telangiectasia with a new 940 nm diode laser. Dermatol Surg 2001; 27: 101–6.

66. Major A, Brazzini B, Campolmi P, et al. Nd:YAG 1064 nm laser in the treatment of facial and leg telangiectasias. J Eur Acad Dermatol Venereol 2001; 15: 559–65.

67. Trelles MA, Allones I, Levy JL, Calderhead RG, Moreno-Arias GA. Combined nonablative skin rejuvenation with the 595- and 1450-nm lasers. Dermatol Surg 2004; 30: 1292–8.

68. Paithankar DY, Clifford JM, Saleh BA, et al. Subsurface skin renewal by treatment with a 1450-nm laser in combination with dynamic cooling. J Biomed Opt 2003; 8: 545–51.

69. Chen H, Diebold G. Chemical generation of acoustic waves: a giant photo-acoustic effect. Science 1995; 270: 963–6.

70. Kopera D, Smolle J, Kaddu S, Kerl H. Nonablative laser treatment of wrinkles: meeting the objective? Assessment by 25 dermatologists. Br J Dermatol 2004; 150: 936–9.

71. Ross EV, Domankevitz Y, Skrobal M, Anderson RR. Effects of CO_2 laser pulse duration in ablation and residual thermal damage: implications for skin resurfacing. Lasers Surg Med 1996; 19: 123–9.

72. Walsh JT Jr, Flotte TJ, Deutsch TF. Er:YAG laser ablation of tissue: effect of pulse duration and tissue type on thermal damage. Lasers Surg Med 1989; 9: 314–26.

73. Smith KJ, Skelton HG, Graham JS, et al. Depth of morphologic skin damage and viability after one, two, and three passes of a high-energy, short-pulse CO_2 laser (Tru-Pulse) in pig skin. J Am Acad Dermatol 1997; 37: 204–10.

74. Majaron B, Verkruysse W, Kelly KM, Nelson JS. Er:YAG laser skin resurfacing using repetitive long-pulse exposure and cryogen spray cooling: II. Theoretical analysis. Lasers Surg Med 2001; 28: 131–8.

75. Sadick NS, Makino Y. Selective electro-thermolysis in aesthetic medicine: a review. Lasers Surg Med 2004; 34: 91–7.

76. Zelickson BD, Kist D, Bernstein E, et al. Histological and ultrastructural evaluation of the effects of a radiofrequency-based nonablative dermal remodeling device: a pilot study. Arch Dermatol 2004; 140: 204–9.

77. Sadick NS, Laughlin SA. Effective epilation of white and blond hair using combined radiofrequency and optical energy. J Cosmet Laser Ther 2004; 6: 27–31.

78. Sadick N, Sorhaindo L. The radiofrequency frontier: a review of radiofrequency and combined radiofrequency pulsed-light technology in aesthetic medicine. Facial Plast Surg 2005; 21: 131–8.

79. Gold MH, Biron JA. Treatment of acne scars by fractional bipolar radiofrequency energy. J Cosmet Laser Ther 2012; 14: 172–8.

80. Cho SI, Chung BY, Choi MG, et al. Evaluation of the clinical efficacy of fractional radiofrequency microneedle treatment in acne scars and large facial pores. Dermatol Surg 2012; 38: 1017–24.

81. Lee HS, Lee DH, Won CH, et al. Fractional rejuvenation using a novel bipolar radiofrequency system in Asian skin. Dermatol Surg 2011; 37: 1611–19.

82. Taub AF, Garretson CB. Treatment of acne scars of skin types II to V by sublative fractional bipolar radiofrequency and bipolar radiofrequency combined with diode laser. J Clin Aesthet Dermatol 2011; 4: 18–27.

83. Bjerring P, Zachariae H, Sogaard H. The flashlamp-pumped dye laser and dermabrasion in psoriasis—further studies on the reversed Kobner phenomenon. Acta Derm Venereol 1997; 77: 59–61.

84. Hern S, Allen MH, Sousa AR, et al. Immunohistochemical evaluation of psoriatic plaques following selective photothermolysis of the superficial capillaries. Br J Dermatol 2001; 145: 45–53.

85. Zelickson BD, Mehregan DA, Wendelschfer-Crabb G, et al. Clinical and histologic evaluation of psoriatic plaques treated with a flashlamp pulsed dye laser. J Am Acad Dermatol 1996; 35: 64–8.

86. Alora MB, Anderson RR, Quinn TR, Taylor CR. CO_2 laser resurfacing of psoriatic plaques: a pilot study. Lasers Surg Med 1998; 22: 165–70.

87. Taylor CR, Racette AL. A 308-nm excimer laser for the treatment of scalp psoriasis. Lasers Surg Med 2004; 34: 136–40.

88. Cather JC, Abramovits W. Investigational therapies for psoriasis. J Am Acad Dermatol 2003; 49: S133–8.

89. Ibbotson SH. Topical 5-aminolaevulinic acid photodynamic therapy for the treatment of skin conditions other than non-melanoma skin cancer. Br J Dermatol 2002; 146: 178–88.

90. Szeimies RM, Landthaler M, Karrer S. Non-oncologic indications for ALA-PDT. J Dermatolog Treat 2002; 13: S13–18.

91. Hartmann A, Brocker EB, Becker JC. Hypopigmentary skin disorders: current treatment options and future directions. Drugs 2004; 64: 89–107.

92. Walsh J. Pulsed laser angioplasty: a paradigm for tissue ablation. In: Welch AJ, van Gemert MJ, eds. Optical thermal Response of Laser-Irradiated Tissue. New York: Plenum, 1995: 925.

93. Friedman PM, Jih MH, Skover GR, et al. Treatment of atrophic facial acne scars with the 1064-nm Q-switched Nd:YAG laser: six-month follow-up study. Arch Dermatol 2004; 140: 1337–41.

94. Fulchiero GJ Jr, Parham-Vetter PC, Obagi S. Subcision and 1320-nm Nd:YAG nonablative laser resurfacing for the treatment of acne scars: a simultaneous split-face single patient trial. Dermatol Surg 2004; 30: 1356–9.

95. Hirsch RJ, Dayan SH. Nonablative resurfacing. Facial Plast Surg 2004; 20: 57–61.

96. Bowes LE, Alster TS. Treatment of facial scarring and ulceration resulting from acne excoriee with 585-nm pulsed dye laser irradiation and cognitive psychotherapy. Dermatol Surg 2004; 30: 934–8.

97. Wind BS, Meesters AA, Kroon MW, et al. Formation of fibrosis after nonablative and ablative fractional laser therapy. Dermatol Surg 2012; 38: 437–42.

98. Smith KC, Schachter GD. Technical characteristics of fractional light devices. Facial Plast Surg Clin North Am 2011; 19: 235–40.

99. Munavalli GS, Turley A, Silapunt S, Biesman B. Combining confluent and fractionally ablative modalities of a novel 2790 nm YSGG laser for facial resurfacing. Lasers Surg Med 2011; 43: 273–82.

100. Elman M, Lebzelter J. Light therapy in the treatment of acne vulgaris. Dermatol Surg 2004; 30: 139–46.

101. Hongcharu W, Taylor CR, Chang Y, et al. Topical ALA-photodynamic therapy for the treatment of acne vulgaris. J Invest Dermatol 2000; 115: 183–92.

102. Kauvar A, Lloyd J. Wang Cheung, et al. Selective photothermolysis of the sebaceous follicle with gold-coated nanoshells for treatment of acne. Lasers Surg Med (abstract) 2012; 44: 351.

103. Kang W, Lee E, Choi GS. Treatment of Ota's nevus by Q-switched alexandrite laser: therapeutic outcome in relation to clinical and histopathological findings. Eur J Dermatol 1999; 9: 639–43.

104. Taylor CR, Anderson RR. Ineffective treatment of refractory melasma and postinflammatory hyperpigmentation by Q-switched ruby laser. J Dermatol Surg Oncol 1994; 20: 592–7.

105. Chan HH, Kono T. The use of lasers and intense pulsed light sources for the treatment of pigmentary lesions. Skin Therapy Lett 2004; 9: 5–7.

106. Negishi K, Kushikata N, Tezuka Y, et al. Study of the incidence and nature of "very subtle epidermal melasma" in relation to intense pulsed light treatment. Dermatol Surg 2004; 30: 881–6.

107. Koster PH, van der Horst CM, van Gemert MJ, van der Wal AC. Histologic evaluation of skin damage after overlapping and nonoverlapping flashlamp pumped pulsed dye laser pulses: A study on normal human skin as a model for port wine stains. Lasers Surg Med 2001; 28: 176–81.

108. Fournier N, Brisot D, Mordon S. Treatment of leg telangectasias with a 1,064 nm Nd YAG laser in multipulse mode emission and contact cooling (abstract). Paper presented at: World Congress of Dermatology, 2002.

109. Fournier N, Brisot D, Mordon S. Treatment of leg telangiectases with a 532 nm KTP laser in multipulse mode. Dermatol Surg 2002; 28: 564–71.

110. Huang N, Cheng G, Li X, et al. Influence of drug-light-interval on photodynamic therapy of port wine stains—simulation and validation of mathematic models. Photodiagnosis Photodyn Ther 2008; 5: 120–6.

111. Qiu H, Gu Y, Wang Y, Huang N. Twenty years of clinical experience with a new modality of vascular-targeted photodynamic therapy for port wine stains. Dermatol Surg 2011; 37: 1603–10.

112. Ross EV, Ladin Z, Kreindel M, Dierickx C. Theoretical considerations in laser hair removal. Dermatol Clin 1999; 17: 333–55; viii.

113. Kelly KM, Kimel S, Smith T, et al. Combined photodynamic and photo-thermal induced injury enhances damage to in vivo model blood vessels. Lasers Surg Med 2004; 34: 407–13.

114. Dover JS, Margolis RJ, Polla LL, et al. Pigmented guinea pig skin irradiated with Q-switched ruby laser pulses. Morphologic and histologic findings. Arch Dermatol 1989; 125: 43–9.

115. Bouzari N, Tabatabai H, Abbasi Z, Firooz A, Dowlati Y. Laser hair removal: comparison of long-pulsed Nd:YAG, long-pulsed alexandrite, and long-pulsed diode lasers. Dermatol Surg 2004; 30: 498–502.

116. Goh CL. Comparative study on a single treatment response to long pulse Nd:YAG lasers and intense pulse light therapy for hair removal on skin type IV to VI—is longer wavelengths lasers preferred over shorter wavelengths lights for assisted hair removal. J Dermatolog Treat 2003; 14: 243–7.

117. Goldberg DJ, Silapunt S. Hair removal using a long-pulsed Nd:YAG Laser: comparison at fluences of 50, 80, and 100 J/cm. Dermatol Surg 2001; 27: 434–6.

118. Goldberg DJ, Silapunt S. Histologic evaluation of a millisecond Nd:YAG laser for hair removal. Lasers Surg Med 2001; 28: 159–61.

119. Gold MH, Bell MW, Foster TD, Street S. One-year follow-up using an intense pulsed light source for long-term hair removal. J Cutan Laser Ther 1999; 1: 167–71.

120. Zhao Z, Fairchild P. Dependence of light transmission through human skin on incident beam diameter at different wavelengths. Proc SPIE 1998; 2681: 468–77.

121. Greppi I. Diode laser hair removal of the black patient. Lasers Surg Med 2001; 28: 150–5.

122. Jalian HR, Avram MM. Body contouring: the skinny on noninvasive fat removal. Semin Cutan Med Surg 2012; 31: 121–5.

123. Anderson RR. Shedding some light on tattoos? Photochem Photobiol 2004; 80: 155–6.

124. Taylor CR, Gange RW, Dover JS, et al. Treatment of tattoos by Q-switched ruby laser. A dose-response study. Arch Dermatol 1990; 126: 893–9.

125. Taylor CR, Anderson RR, Gange RW, Michaud NA, Flotte TJ. Light and electron microscopic analysis of tattoos treated by Q-switched ruby laser. J Invest Dermatol 1991; 97: 131–6.

126. Ross V, Naseef G, Lin G, et al. Comparison of responses of tattoos to picosecond and nanosecond Q-switched neodymium: YAG lasers. Arch Dermatol 1998; 134: 167–71.

127. Anderson RR, Geronemus R, Kilmer SL, Farinelli W, Fitzpatrick RE. Cosmetic tattoo ink darkening. A complication of Q-switched and pulsed-laser treatment. Arch Dermatol 1993; 129: 1010–14.

128. Ross EV, Yashar S, Michaud N, et al. Tattoo darkening and nonresponse after laser treatment: a possible role for titanium dioxide. Arch Dermatol 2001; 137: 33–7.

129. Haedersdal M, Bech-Thomsen N, Wulf HC. Skin reflectance-guided laser selections for treatment of decorative tattoos. [erratum appears in Arch Dermatol. 1996 July;132(7):818. Note: Hodersdal M [corrected to Haedersdal M]]. Arch Dermatol 1996; 132: 403–7.

130. Zelickson BD, Mehregan DA, Zarrin AA, et al. Clinical, histologic, and ultrastructural evaluation of tattoos treated with three laser systems. Lasers Surg Med 1994; 15: 364–72.

131. Kossida T, Rigopoulos D, Katsambas A, Anderson RR. Optimal tattoo removal in a single laser session based on the method of repeated exposures. J Am Acad Dermatol 2012; 66: 271–7.

132. Aguilar G, Majaron B, Karapetian E, Lavernia EJ, Nelson JS. Experimental study of cryogen spray properties for application in dermatologic laser surgery. IEEE Trans Biomed Eng 2003; 50: 863–9.

133. Choi B, Pearce JA, Welch AJ. Modelling infrared temperature measurements: implications for laser irradiation and cryogen cooling studies. Phys Med Biol 2000; 45: 541–57.

134. Zenzie HH, Altshuler GB, Smirnov MZ, Anderson RR. Evaluation of cooling methods for laser dermatology. Lasers Surg Med 2000; 26: 130–44.

135. Hohenleutner U, Walther T, Wenig M, Baumler W, Landthaler M. Leg telangiectasia treatment with a 1.5 ms pulsed dye laser, ice cube cooling of the skin and 595 vs 600 nm: preliminary results. Lasers Surg Med 1998; 23: 72–8.

136. Greve B, Hammes S, Raulin C. The effect of cold air cooling on 585 nm pulsed dye laser treatment of port-wine stains. Dermatol Surg 2001; 27: 633–6.

137. Chan HH, Lam LK, Wong DS, Wei WI. Role of skin cooling in improving patient tolerability of Q-switched Alexandrite (QS Alex) laser in nevus of Ota treatment. Lasers Surg Med 2003; 32: 148–51.

138. Raulin C, Greve B, Hammes S. Cold air in laser therapy: first experiences with a new cooling system. Lasers Surg Med 2000; 27: 404–10. Huang PS, Chang CJ. Cryogen spray cooling in conjunction with pulse dye laser treatment of port wine stains of the head and neck. Chang Gung Med J 2001; 24: 469–75.

139. Weiss RA, Sadick NS. Epidermal cooling crystal collar device for improved results and reduced side effects on leg telangiectasias using intense pulsed light. Dermatol Surg 2000; 26: 1015–18.

140. Tunnell JW, Nelson JS, Torres JH, Anvari B. Epidermal protection with cryogen spray cooling during high fluence pulsed dye laser irradiation: an ex vivo study. Lasers Surg Med 2000; 27: 373–83.

141. Chang CW, Reinisch L, Biesman BS. Analysis of epidermal protection using cold air versus chilled sapphire window with water or gel during 810 nm diode laser application. Lasers Surg Med 2003; 32: 129–36.

142. Muccini J, O'Donnell F, Fuller T, Reinisch L. Laser treatment of solar elastosis with epithelial preservation. Lasers Surg Med 1998; 23: 121–7.

143. Manstein D, Herron GS, Sink RK, Tanner H, Anderson RR. Fractional photothermolysis: a new concept for cutaneous remodeling using microscopic patterns of thermal injury. Lasers Surg Med 2004; 34: 426–38.

144. Zelickson B, Walgrave S, Al-Arashi M, et al. Evaluation of a fractional laser with optical compression pins. Lasers Surg Med 2011; 43: 137–42.

145. Rylander CG, Milner TE, Baranov SA, Nelson JS. Mechanical tissue optical clearing devices: enhancement of light penetration in ex vivo porcine skin and adipose tissue. Lasers Surg Med 2008; 40: 688–94.

146. Ross EV, Grossman MC, Duke D, Grevelink JM. Long-term results after CO_2 laser skin resurfacing: a comparison of scanned and pulsed systems. J Am Acad Dermatol 1997; 37: 709–18.

147. Svaasand LO, Aguilar G, Viator JA, et al. Increase of dermal blood volume fraction reduces the threshold for laser-induced purpura: implications for port wine stain laser treatment. Lasers Surg Med 2004; 34: 182–8.

148. Choi B, Tsu L, Chen E, et al. Determination of chemical agent optical clearing potential using in vitro human skin. Lasers Surg Med 2005; 36: 72–5.

149. Dolotov LE, Sinichkin YP, Tuchin VV, et al. Design and evaluation of a novel portable erythema-melanin-meter. Lasers Surg Med 2004; 34: 127–35.

150. Anderson RR. Polarized light examination and photography of the skin. Arch Dermatol 1991; 127: 1000–5.

151. Pitsillides CM, Joe EK, Wei X, Anderson RR, Lin CP. Selective cell targeting with light-absorbing microparticles and nanoparticles. Biophys J 2003; 84: 4023–32.

152. Reinisch L. Scatter-limited phototherapy: a model for laser treatment of skin. Lasers Surg Med 2002; 30: 381–8.

153. Berns MW. A possible two-photon effect in vitro using a focused laser beam. Biophys J 1976; 16: 973–7.

154. Haedersdal M, Katsnelson J, Sakamoto FH, et al. Enhanced uptake and photoactivation of topical methyl aminolevulinate after fractional CO_2 laser pretreatment. Lasers Surg Med 2011; 43: 804–13.

155. Gomez C, Costela A, Garcia-Moreno I, et al. Skin laser treatments enhancing transdermal delivery of ALA. J Pharm Sci 2011; 100: 223–31.

156. Kositratna G, Manstein D. Focused CO_2 laser radiation to create a gateway for transdermal light delivery. Lasers Surg Med 2010; 42: 28.

157. Boulnois JL. Photophysical processes in recent medical developments. Lasers Med Sci 1986; 1: 47–66.

2   Laser treatment of vascular lesions

E. Victor Ross and Andrew C. Krakowski

One of the first lesions to be treated using selective photo-thermolysis (SPT) was the port-wine stain (PWS), and vascular lesions were the first "test" case for SPT. Although Goldman accurately predicted that vascular lesions could be selectively heated, the pulsed dye laser (PDL) was the first laser to show that this selectivity was practical. The spectrum of oxy- and deoxy-hemoglobin (HgB) should be memorized by the laser surgeon (see Fig. 1.15 in chap. 1). Generally laser parameters should be applied that exploit the absorption peaks for oxy-HgB (roughly 70% of the total HgB, the remainder being mostly deoxy-HgB and met-HgB).

The first lasers to treat vascular lesions were CO_2 and argon lasers. The argon laser at 488 and 515 nm enjoyed a high absorption coefficient for HgB, but the pulse durations [continuous wave (CW)] were longer than the thermal relaxation time of the targeted blood vessels, and in the absence of surface/epidermal cooling, the high absorption by epidermal melanin resulted in a high risk of hypopigmentation and scarring (1). Scanners were adapted to limit the laser dwell time to 50 ms but even then collateral nonspecific thermal damage was observed. Although the importance of spatial and temporal selectivity had been known prior to the advent of the PDL, Anderson formulated a formal definition of SPT (2). The first real test of this theory was the use of the PDL in treatment of vascular lesions. The first PDLs were slow (0.5 Hz or less), equipped with only small diameter spot sizes (3–5 mm), lacked cooling, and used a 577 nm wavelength near one of the peaks of oxy-HgB absorption. Over the years from 1981 to 1990 the wavelength was changed to 585 nm; the rationale for the longer wavelength was deeper penetration of the laser beam (into the skin and the vessel) and enhanced dye life. Later, 7, 10, and 12 mm spots were introduced, and repetition rates approached 2 Hz. By the late 1990s, surface cooling devices were added and the laser wavelength was again increased to 595 nm to further enhance epidermal/vascular penetration. Epidermal cooling allowed treatment of darker skin and the use of higher laser energies. Larger spot size increased the number of photons that could penetrate deeper and increase the range of applications from discrete lesions to larger regions of the body where diffuse redness (i.e., neck and chest) was often observed.

In general, vascular laser technologies (where vessels are specifically targeted) can be divided into three spectral ranges. The first group comprises green-yellow (GY) light sources, such as PDL and frequency doubled neodymium:yttrium-aluminum-garnet (Nd:YAG) lasers (532 nm). The second group includes the 800 nm diode laser and alexandrite lasers. The third group, comprised of near infrared radiation (NIR) lasers with a smaller ratio of melanin to HgB absorption and deeper penetration

(940, 980, 1064 nm), complete the triad. In general, smaller lesions in lighter skin are treated with GY light sources and larger lesions in darker skin are treated with NIR lasers.

Intense pulsed light (IPL) sources cover all of the HgB peaks and cannot be "boxed" into one of the three aforementioned categories. However, if one were to analyze the thermal contribution from the range of wavelengths, small vessels in particular are coagulated by the GY light portion of the output spectrum.

So long as a lesion is a darker red than the surrounding tissue, a case can be made for HgB-selective technologies. Non-selective laser technologies can still be useful in vascular lesions [i.e., CO_2 laser in a pyogenic granuloma (PG)]; however, without a contrast agent, they require damage to the surface (a top-to-bottom injury) to adequately damage the underlying vessels. In designing optimal treatment algorithms, the microanatomy of the vascular lesion should always be considered.

LASER PARAMETERS OF IMPORTANCE IN THE TREATMENT OF VASCULAR LESIONS
Wavelength

More than any other parameter, wavelength determines the cutaneous tissue effect (see Fig. 1.15 in chap. 1). Ideally the ratio of absorption of the vascular target versus normal surrounding skin should exceed 10:1. The O_2 saturation of cutaneous blood ranges from 50% to 80% (3). The peaks of oxy-HgB absorption are 418, 542, and 577 nm with a smaller peak at 940 nm (2). However, all wavelengths from blue to NIR enjoy preferential heating of blood vessels over bloodless dermis (see Fig. 1.16 in chap. 1). Because epidermal pigment overlies the vessel, wavelength selections should be based on optimal ratios of vascular to pigment destruction. For example, the ruby laser would prove adequate (although one of the least selective choices) in treating a PWS in a vitiligo patient but would prove the poorest choice for vascular lesion destruction in any pigmented patient. Goldman did use the long pulsed ruby laser in a very fair-skinned patient with a PWS with only mild scarring.

A simple analysis of vascular to pigment absorption coefficient ratios, however, does not adequately characterize the laser–tissue interaction. For example, blue light, solely in terms of absorption coefficients, would be the best choice for vessels, even within the context of its high melanin absorption. However, because of scattering, blue light will almost invariably damage the epidermis at light doses sufficient to damage an underlying vessel (Fig. 2.1).

Pulse duration is another important parameter. Early PDLs generated very short pulses (as short as 1 µs) (2). The

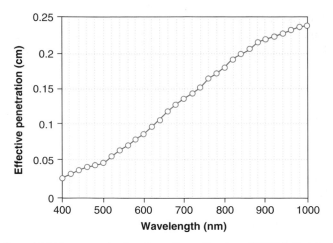

Figure 2.1 Light penetration into tissue. *Source*: Courtesy of ESC Medical, Inc.

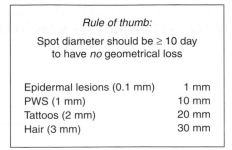

Figure 2.2 Rule of thumb for spotsize for various applications. Spot should be roughly 10× the target depth to minimize scattering losses. *Abbreviation*: PWS, port-wine stain.

Table 2.1 Approximate Thermal Relaxation Time for Vessels of Different Diameters

Diameter (μm)	Tr (ms)
10	0.048
20	0.19
50	1.2
100	4.8
200	19.0
300	42.6

Source: From Ref. 2.

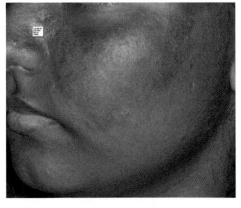

Figure 2.3 Arm one day after pulsed dye laser at 0.45 ms with three spot sizes (3, 5, 7 mm left to right) and four fluences (top to bottom: purple numerals 3, 5, 7, and 10 J/cm²). Note more intense surface effect with larger spot sizes (left to right) even with same fluences.

very short pulses confined heat not only to the vessel but also to the erythrocytes; accordingly, thermal confinement was excessive and localized vessel rupture and intravascular thrombosis were observed. With longer pulses (6–40 ms), intravascular thrombosis and spot-sized purpura were mitigated as gentle heating resulted in vessel wall stenosis and thrombosis of the larger vessels but not the microvessels that produce widespread purpura. As demonstrated with the IPL, pulse duration is very important in limiting the thermal effects to within the target (Table 2.1 gives the thermal relaxation times for various vessel sizes).

Spot Size

Larger spots increase the ratio of dermal-to-epidermal damage by increasing the number of photons that penetrate deeper into the dermis, so that as a general rule larger spots are better (Fig. 2.2) (4,5). However, despite the favorable *ratio* for larger spots, for the same fluence, a larger spot will produce more epidermal damage and pain (so long as all other parameters are held constant, i.e., surface cooling, pulse duration) so that in general, larger spots should be accompanied by smaller fluences than their small-spot counterparts. For example, in heating a PWS in an infant, the fluence with a 10 mm spot should be reduced about 10–15% versus a 7 mm spot to achieve the same degree for epidermal damage (Fig. 2.3). Larger spot size also speeds treatment time as well as minimizing the "polka dot" effect, which may occur with the use of nonoverlapped small spot sizes.

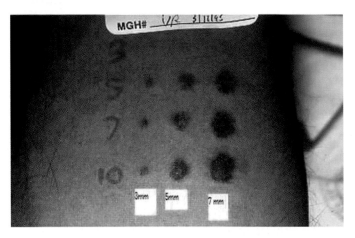

Figure 2.4 Note 5 mm depressed scar on nose 10 years after pulsed dye laser with no cooling; fluence was only 5.5 J/cm² at 0.45 ms.

Surface Cooling

Prior to the introduction of epidermal cooling devices, many vascular laser applications were associated with epidermal damage. Crusting after PDL treatment was not unusual, and scarring and/or hypopigmentation secondary to thermal damage of epidermal melanocytes occasionally occurred, particularly in darker-skinned patients (Fig. 2.4). Ice pre- and postoperatively was helpful but somewhat unreliable (6). In terms of cooling (see chap. 11), although the best cooling protection factor (CPF) among the leading technologies is achieved with cryogen spray, sapphire windows and refrigerated air cooling also are adequate in most cases. Disadvantages of the spray are the possibility of pigmentation changes (excessive cooling) and the need for purchasing cryogen canisters. Also, no bulk cooling is conferred with cryogen spray. Contact cooling typically includes either a sapphire window or copper plate (Fig. 2.5) where a temperature of about 5–15°C is maintained at the skin surface (normally about 30°C). Contact cooling risks include fogging and poor contact. Refrigerated air works well but requires a second hand to hold near the surface or an accessory that allows one-hand operation. Although inefficient and sometimes irritating near the nose and mouth, the long application times with refrigerated air provide for bulk cooling and reasonable epidermal protection.

PARTICULAR DEVICES

The PDL was the initial "test" for SPT. A review of the "older" literature (1981–1988) is instructive and still relevant for the modern practitioner. The early PDL evolved from very short pulses (300 ns and 1 μs) to 450 μs. Much of this was based on early experiences, where very short microsecond pulses showed steam bubble formation inside the erythrocytes, whereas longer pulses showed gentler heating of HgB and superior lightening

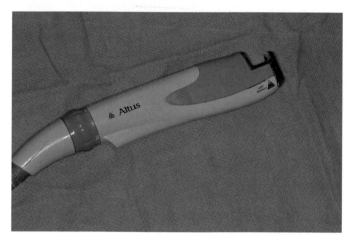

Figure 2.5 Note copper tip with popular neodymium:yttrium–aluminum–garnet laser.

of PWS (7). Garden et al, for example, compared 20- and 360-μs pulses and found superior lightening with the longer pulse. In this study they used 2× the purpuric threshold dose (about 2 and 4 J/cm², respectively, for the shorter and longer pulses). Typical purpuric thresholds with modern day 1.5-ms lasers in PWS are about 5–6 J/cm², partly because of epidermal cooling (8). Van Gemert et al. used a model to determine the best wavelength for PWS treatment. They showed that for vessels less than 14 μm in diameter, 577 nm is best, but for larger vessels, 585 nm might be better. The authors concluded that a number of wavelengths might be adequate for PWS. As PDL technology matured, 585 nm and later 595 nm were adopted as the optimal wavelengths; 585 nm has half the blood absorption of 577 nm—the decreased blood absorption allows for deeper penetration in the vessel and presumably deeper vessel clearing. In one study 585 nm showed about twice the depth of clearing (1.2 mm vs 700 μm) for PWS versus 577 nm. In theory 577 should be best for pink lesions where vessel thicknesses are less than 150 μm. Two manufacturers produce the PDL in the USA. Both permit a range or pulse durations (0.45–40 ms). The Candela laser deploys eight micropulses (Fig. 2.6) for durations exceeding 3 ms and the Cynosure laser counters with six micropulses. The use of micropulsing allows PDLs to create longer pulse durations (>3 ms). More micropulses have been shown to increase the purpura threshold as a gentler heating of the vessel is achieved (9). Although one study showed differences in beam profiles between the two lasers (10), the most recent versions from both manufacturers create almost flat-topped beam profiles. The optimal wavelength for PWS treatment has evolved over time. Generally longer wavelengths favor deeper treatment, but the associated lesser absorption coefficients for blood require higher fluences. Unfortunately commercially available PDLs today use only 595 nm. Some older versions allowed user selectively between 585 and 595 nm (11).

Potassium Titanyl Phosphate Laser

The term potassium titanyl phosphate (KTP) "laser" is not technically correct, as the laser is a frequency-doubled Nd:YAG laser; however, we use the term for the remainder of the chapter as its usage has become commonplace in esthetic dermatology. The KTP laser has been a workhorse in treatment of vascular

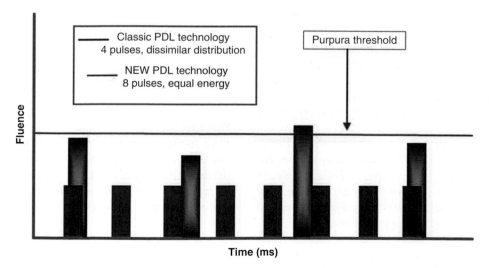

Figure 2.6 Schematic shows multiple pulsing and relationship to purpura threshold. *Abbreviation*: PDL, pulsed dye laser.

lesions. Both Iridex, Lutronic, ConBio, Cutera, and many others manufacture 532 nm sources. The larger Iridex device (Gemini) is an arc lamp drive device and the Cutera (Excel V) is driven by a flash lamp. Both the Gemini and the Excel V create high pulse energies over a range of pulse durations and spot sizes. The Cutera device enjoys a higher peak power. Both are equipped with sapphire contact cooling. Green light $HgBO_2$ absorption is roughly 5× that of 595 nm and shows only about 10% more melanin absorption. It follows that 532 nm enjoys a higher vascular to melanin damage ratio than 595 nm. For smaller vessels, user-selectable small spots (1–5 mm) can be applied. Larger 10–12 mm spots can be applied for larger areas (full faces and chest, arms, and others). With a 10 mm spot size and 2 Hz rep rate, coverage rates (cm^2/sec) are similar to some IPLs (Fig. 2.7).

Intense Pulsed Light

IPLs are increasingly useful in vascular applications. Since their development in 1992 and the US Food and Drug Administration clearance in 1995, refinement in power supplies, cooling, and filtering have increased their safety and efficacy (12–14). Modern IPLs rely on xenon flash lamps that, depending on the way they are pumped, emit an unfiltered spectrum. By appropriate filtering, one can customize the spectrum for

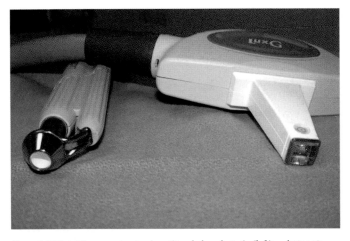

Figure 2.7 Note 10 mm spot potassium titanyl phosphate tip (left) and 12 × 12 mm intense pulsed light crystal (right).

specific disorders. For most vascular applications, shorter wavelength ranges are applied. There are two types of filtering: absorption and interference. Most devices use the latter where one slides a filter into the handpiece. The filters typically have a value that designates the shortest wavelength that is allowed through to the skin (Fig. 2.8). The cutoffs are not sharp. There are over 30 IPL devices available in the USA alone, and worldwide they account for a majority of vascular lesion treatments. Critics decry the IPL as the poor man's vascular tool; however, modern IPLs are sophisticated tools with tightly controlled power supplies, integrated surface cooling, variable pulse durations, and a variety of spot sizes. Some IPLs also allow for double and triple pulsing with variable pulse durations and pulse intervals to enhance efficacy and decrease the risk of nonspecific epidermal damage. Also, the multiple wavelength output spectrum of an IPL allows for heating of both superficial and deeper vessels (Fig. 2.9). Furthermore, by pumping the lamps less strongly, the spectra can be right shifted to favor deeper larger vessel heating and greater epidermal sparing (Fig. 2.10).

Alexandrite Laser

The long pulsed alexandrite laser has emerged as a valuable tool for vascular lesions. There is strong absorption for deoxy-HgB, and overall blood absorption is 2× that of the 1064 nm Nd:YAG laser. However, melanin absorption is also strong (about 3× that of the 1064 nm Nd:YAG laser) so that the laser is best used in lighter skin types and darker vessels. Darker-skinned patients (up to type IV) can be treated but test sites are advisable as are longer cooling times. Smaller darker red vessels can be treated but higher fluences might be required that risk not only epidermal damage but also bulk heating. We have studied the alexandrite laser for telangiectasia and found 6–8 mm spots the most useful (15). Depending on the device, a range of pulse durations can be used. Although 3 ms have been advocated in studies of PWS, we have found that 20 and 40 ms clear telangiectasia with a lower rate of purpura and epidermal damage. There are a number of alexandrite lasers (Candela, Sciton, Cynosure among them) with long pulsed capability. Cryogen spray, contact cooling, and refrigerated air are integrated into these devices, respectively.

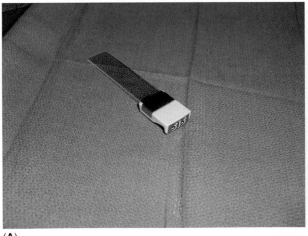

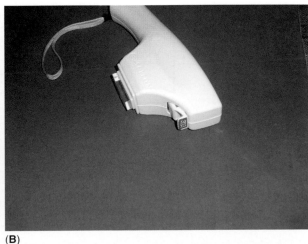

(A)   **(B)**

Figure 2.8 (**A**) Slide in filter 515 nm cutoff and (**B**) accompanying intense pulsed light handpiece with 15 × 45 mm sapphire crystal tip.

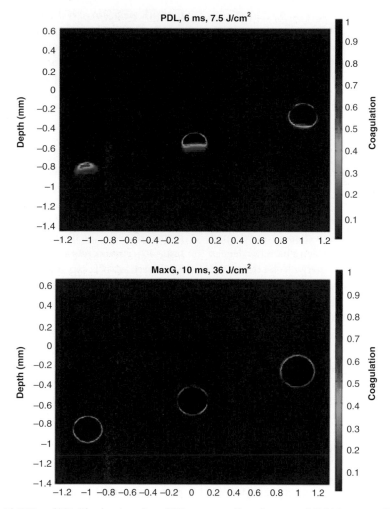

Figure 2.9 Depths of coagulation with PDL and IPL. The deeper option of IPL spectrum allows for greater full thickness vessel heating. *Abbreviations*: IPL, intense pulsed light; PDL, pulsed dye laser.

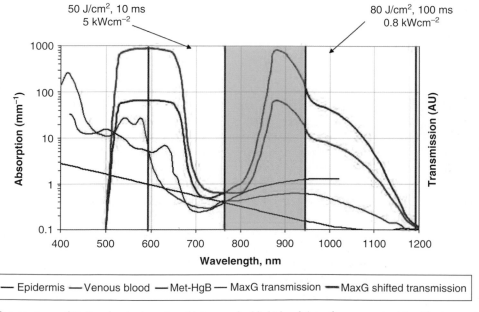

Figure 2.10 Note absorption spectrum of HgB and output spectra of intense pulsed light handpiece; the green output is with stronger lamp pumping and the orange output is the result of weaker lamp pumping. Deeper vessel heating should occur as spectrum shifts to right. *Abbreviation*: HgB, hemoglobin.

810 nm Diode Laser

This laser's effects are similar to those of the alexandrite laser. Like the alexandrite laser, 810 nm is best equipped for deeper vascular lesions in relatively fair-skinned patients (16). The laser can also be applied to reticular veins of the face.

1064 nm Nd:YAG Laser

The Nd:YAG laser is a good example of a "what you can't see can hurt you laser" (17). Although optimized for epidermal sparing, the relatively poor HgB absorption obliges the device to be used at higher fluences. Because there is some mild heating of tissue water, bulk heating can create significant pain. In general, the smallest spot size and smallest fluence sufficient for vessel closure should be used. The absorption coefficient for blood is about 1/10 that of GY light (see Table 1.2 in chap. 1) and dermal scattering is decreased versus shorter wavelengths. This deeper penetration allows a greater fraction of energy to be deposited in the deeper dermis. Also, compared with GY light, full thickness vessel heating is more likely with 1064 nm irradiation. Melanin absorption is much less than GY light. It follows that tanned and darker-skinned patients can be treated; however, bulk water heating is also possible with this wavelength such that large spots and high fluences can result in full thickness dermal injury and scarring. Also, visual endpoints in vascular lesions (i.e., PWS) are somewhat ambiguous (i.e., very slight transient bluing or very slight shrinkage of exophytic portions of a PWS) so that over treatment is not uncommon (Fig. 2.11). The higher oxy-HgB versus deoxy-HgB also permits deeper selective heating of arterioles (18). Pre– and post–pulse cooling enhances the safety associated with use of both alexandrite and Nd:YAG lasers, as thicker nodules require seconds to cool.

In addition to 1064 nm, 940 and 980 nm lasers have also been applied to vascular lesions—these wavelengths are near

the NIR peak for oxy-HgB. The advantage of these lasers is their portability; they are diode lasers. On the other hand, their peak powers are less than most solid-sate 1064 nm lasers and therefore are confined to small spots and discrete vessel heating and not treatment of larger confluent lesions.

FACIAL TELANGIECTASIA

For wavelengths from 520 to 800 nm, the primary absorbers are hemoglobin and melanin, so that improvement of telangiectasia is achieved by direct heating of HgB (either via a single wavelength or flash lamp). Devices targeting HgB/vessels are confined to pulsewidths (pw) ranging from 0.45 to 100 ms. Nanosecond lasers have been used at fluences from 1 to 4 J/cm^2 (5–10 ns) but purpura and possible postinflammatory hyperpigmentation make them suboptimal in clearance of telangiectasia (19). For discrete smaller (0.1–0.6 mm) telangiectases, PDL, KTP laser, or IPL can be applied. For larger vessels (>1 mm), the Nd:YAG laser or alexandrite laser is preferred, but care must be taken to apply the smallest fluence and smallest spot sufficient for closure. An alternative is the Cynergy™ laser (Cynosure, Chelmsford, Massachusetts, USA), which combines 595 and 1064 nm sequential pulses that can simultaneously address both smaller and larger telangiectases.

If a patient presents with telangiectases confined to very small areas, we typically use the long-pulsed KTP laser and use a small spot (1–3 mm) (Fig. 2.12). The ergonomic simplicity of this procedure and real-time assessment of vessel clearing are unsurpassed. Alternatively, we use nonpurpuric settings with the PDL or an IPL. The specific type of PDL determines the spot size, fluence range, and cooling type, and pw. Modern PDLs can generate effective fluences with 10 mm spots; moreover, the macropulses (pulse envelopes) are comprised of 6–8 micropulses, allowing for greater efficacy without a high risk of purpura (20). IPL can be applied as well; the optimal settings are machine specific.

IPLs are constantly improving with better cooling and variable pulse configurations. The advantages of IPL are the relatively large spot sizes, which can minimize the polka dot effect common to PDL and KTP lasers. IPLs are often based on platform designs, that is, a number of handpieces can be driven from the same base unit (similar to accessories on a vacuum cleaner); the handpieces share the power supply and other components. So long as we know the fluence, pulse profile, spot size, wavelength, pulse duration, and beam profile of a laser, tissue effects tend to be predictable. On the other hand, IPLs show spectral variability, and fluence measurement techniques

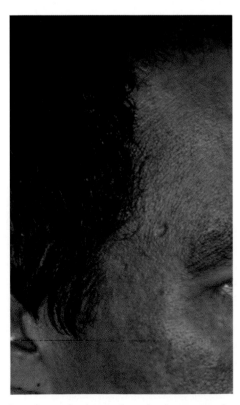

Figure 2.11 Scar after neodymium:yttrium–aluminum–garnet laser of nodule in port-wine stain.

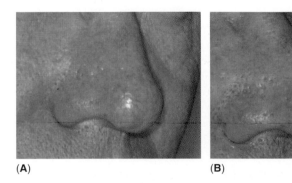

(A)   **(B)**

Figure 2.12 **(A)** A 0.3 mm vessel before treatment and **(B)** after treatment with potassium titanyl phosphate laser (9 J/cm^2, 15 ms, 5 mm spot, 4°C).

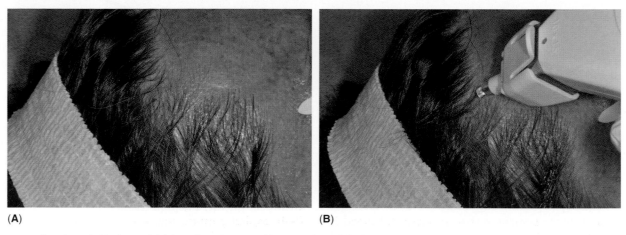

(A) **(B)**

Figure 2.13 Small angioma (**A**) before and (**B**) just after treatment with 4 mm adaptor that fits over 10 × 15 mm crystal. The adaptor allows for placement in hairline without damaging hair.

vary among manufacturers. Accordingly, comparison of settings between various manufacturers is difficult, as actual surface fluences will not always be equivalent among manufacturers even when the user interface indicates like-settings. In the case of IPL, changes in lamp pumping can affect the pulse profile and spectral emission, so that simple changes in the fluence typically will involve a change in another parameter (21–23). Also, various manufacturers' IPLs emit different output spectra and the "fluence" listed on the user interface is normally that of the whole output. Without knowledge of the exact spectrum and subsequent calculation of the laser equivalent tissue effect, predicting IPL responses in the skin is more difficult. Some physicians lament the IPL as a poor replacement for laser, even in the treatment of pigmented lesions and vascular lesions. However, modern IPLs can achieve very selective vascular and pigment heating; moreover, most IPLs incorporate cooling technologies (sapphire contact plate or cryogen spray), making them much safer than in previous years. For discrete lesions, IPLs can be optimized by using small spots. Cutera (Brisbane, California, USA) and Lumenis (Santa Clara, California, USA) manufactures a small spot IPL (Fig. 2.5), and Palomar manufactures a clip on adaptor that converts a 10 × 15 mm spot to a 4 mm round spot (Fig. 2.13). Another way to increase efficacy of millisecond technologies is to use a "mask" with an aperture that is roughly the size of the pigmented lesions or vessels. Accordingly, skin outside the hole in the plastic mask is preserved.

940 nm Diode-Pumped Laser

This laser (Medilas D SkinPulse; Dornier MedizinLaserGmbH, Germering, Germany) and Vari-lite (Cutera, California, USA) has been reported to be effective at clearing 1- to 3-mm-diameter periocular vessels in 86% of patients when used at 141 J/cm², 20-ms pulse through a 3-mm-diameter spot size (24). Also, a 980 nm miniaturized diode laser is available that weighs under four pounds (Fig. 2.14).

1064 nm Long Pulse Nd:YAG Laser

Using this wavelength requires fluences over 10 times that used with 532 and 595 nm lasers since the absorption of Hb and HbO₂ at 1064 nm is 10 times less. These higher fluences necessitate epidermal cooling. One laser uses cryogen spray cooling to achieve epidermal protection. A study using the CoolTouch

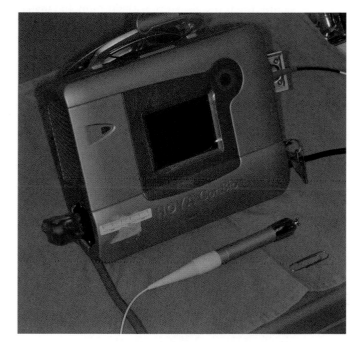

Figure 2.14 Small 980 nm laser for vessels. The whole unit weighs less than 5 pounds.

Varia laser (New Star Lasers, Rosemont, California, USA) found greater than 75% improvement in 97% of treated sites with a 125–150 J/cm² fluence through a 6-mm-diameter spot and 25-ms pulse duration for small diameter vessels and 75- to 100-ms pulse durations for facial reticular veins. All treated reticular veins including periorbital and temporal veins resolved 100%. One or two passes were required to achieve vessel spasm or coagulation (24).

Another long-pulse 1064 nm laser uses precooling through a copper contact probe and demonstrated moderate to significant vessel improvement in 80% of patients (25). This laser (Cool-Glide Excel/Xeo, Cutera, Burlingame, California, USA) is used at 120–170 J/cm² with a 3-mm-diameter spot size and 5- to 40-ms pulses until vessel blanching or coagulation occurs. These patients received two treatments 4 weeks apart to achieve therapeutic efficacy. Cutaneous blistering and scarring with 2- to 3-mm depressions and/or hypopigmentation were reported in this study. Bulk heating is (see figure 20 in chap. 1) likely in 1064 nm treatment of telangiectasia

Accordingly, treatment should be confined to very small spots (<2 mm) and to the smallest fluence sufficient to close the vessel. In this way the greatest fraction of incoming light is converted to vessel heating versus nonspecific dermal heating.

Intense Pulsed Light

This high-energy pulsed light source described previously is very effective in treating facial telangiectasia. Advantages are the almost complete lack of purpura and adverse sequelae. Fluences of 12–45 J/cm² are required for vessel ablation with the original machines using a double pulse of 2.4–6.0 ms each with a 10- to 30-ms delay between pulses (depending on skin type). A 550, 560, or 570 nm cutoff filter works best. Lesions usually clear in one treatment in 90% of patients. More modern IPLs, such as the Lumenis One and M22, use equal, double, or triple pulsing to enhance efficacy while minimizing excessive epidermal heating (26). Lesions are treated with one or two pulses until initial vessel spasm or slight purpura occurs. The only potential side effects are slight purpura, which lasts 2 to 4 days, or epidermal desquamation when treatment is performed on tanned or type III or IV skin. Epidermal desquamation in pigmented patients can be avoided by changing the filter to a longer wavelength or increasing the delay time between double or triple pulses (see chap. 8).

A dual-mode filtering IPL (Ellipse Flex, Danish Dermatologic Development, Hoersholm, Denmark) that restricts filtered light to between 555 and 950 nm (median wavelength of 705 nm) has been shown to provide more than 50% reduction in facial telangiectasia in 79% of patients after one to four treatments; 37.5% of patients had greater than 75% improvement (27). Another IPL light source [a.k.a. optimized pulse light (OPL)] uses dual filtering and enhanced cooling. The Max G handpiece (Palomar Medical Technologies, Burlington, Massachusetts, USA) uses a 10 × 15 mm spot to coagulate vessels (Fig. 2.15). Shorter pulses are optimal for light skin and smaller vessels and longer pulses area applied for deeper vessels in darker skin. A new addition is the Skintel, a builtin pigment meter with Bluetooth connectivity that transmits skin pigment levels back to the base unit and provides real-time test spot guidelines for safe clearance of vessels with epidermal sparing (Fig. 2.16) (28).

SPIDER TELANGIECTASIA

Spider telangiectasia represents telangiectasia with a central feeding arteriole. They typically appear in preschool and school-age children. The peak incidence appears to be between age of 7 and 10 years, and as many as 40% of girls and 32% of boys younger than 15 years have at least one lesion (29–31). The incidence in healthy adults is about 15%. The difference between these stated incidences implies that 50–75% of childhood lesions regress. However, this is not easily observable because most lesions seem to persist without change and become a source of cosmetic concern when present on the face. The PDL has proved to be a very effective treatment for these benign lesions (Fig. 2.17) (32). We also routinely use the IPL with a small tip adaptor or a small spot KTP laser.

GENERALIZED ESSENTIAL TELANGIECTASIA

Telangiectasia generally occurs on the legs but may also involve other cutaneous surfaces. Various treatments have been proposed, with variable efficacy (33). We also treated four patients with the PDL at fluences ranging from 6.0 to 7.5 J/cm². Two patients responded with total resolution, but two patients had almost no improvement in their appearance (34). We have also applied the large spot KTP laser with good results. Fluences of 6–8 J/cm² are applied with a 10 mm spot, cooling (contact) and pulse durations of 18–22 ms. IPL treatment has also been found to be effective (35).

ROSACEA

Rosacea is a cutaneous vascular disorder associated with follicular inflammation. A comprehensive review of the literature finds that of the 18 histologic studies on rosacea, 14 showed

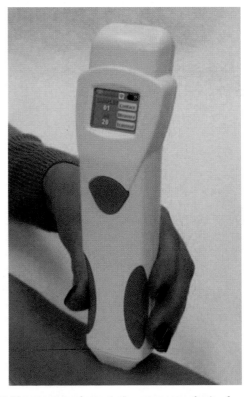

Figure 2.16 Pigment meter that optimizes parameter selection for vessel based on epidermal tolerance.

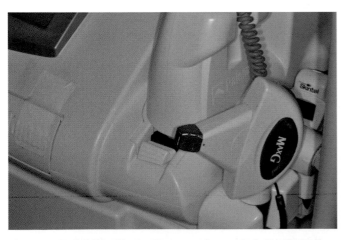

Figure 2.15 Typical IPL with 10 × 15 mm spot for vascular lesions. Unit allows for multiple other handpiece attachments for other applications.

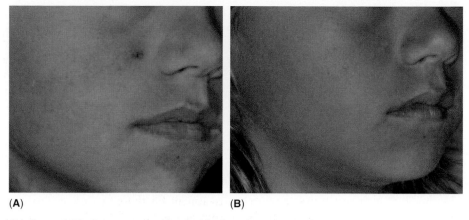

(A)   **(B)**

Figure 2.17 Angioma (**A**) before and (**B**) after treatment with pulsed dye laser (7 mm, 10 J/cm², 1.5 ms, 40 ms spray and 30 ms delay with cryogen spray).

an increase in Demodex mites (36). It is hypothesized that these mites may play a role in the inflammation of rosacea. Studies have demonstrated thermal destruction of these mites after IPL therapy, which may contribute to the therapeutic effects of IPL (37). Telangiectasia represents the later phase of vascularization and probably results from a reduction in mechanical integrity of the upper dermal connective tissue, allowing a passive dilatation of capillaries. Inflammation and associated angiogenesis may contribute to the telangiectasia. Interestingly, facial temperature is higher in rosacea and this has been associated with a difference in the nature and behavior of skin bacteria, particularly coagulase-negative staphylococci (38). Therefore, the elimination of excessive blood vessels may not only decrease the erythematous appearance of rosacea but also modify the bacterial flora further decreasing the cutaneous erythema. Erythema usually recurs within six months of laser treatment most likely due to a resurgence in Demodex population and/or associated inflammation. We advise our patients to plan on having at least two treatments a year to maximize control of their rosacea. Aminolevulinic acid-photodynamic therapy (ALA-PDT) has also been applied successfully to resistant rosacea regions (39).

Pulsed Dye Laser
Rosacea-associated telangiectasia and erythema respond well to treatment with the PDL (40–42). We have reported good-to-excellent results in 24 of 27 patients (89%). In addition to the cosmetic improvement resulting from elimination of the vascular component of this disorder, PDL treatment also appears to alter the pathophysiology of this condition because a decrease in papule and pustule activity occurs in up to 59% of patients. After PDL treatment, patients who responded to treatment with elimination of the vascular component required less or no topical or systemic antibiotic therapy to maintain disease resolution (43). The efficacy of the first-generation PDL was reproduced in a study of a 6-ms PDL at 595 nm with fluence between 7 and 9 J/cm² and cryogen spray cooling (44). Here, two of 12 patients had over 75% improvement with one treatment. Another two had 50–75% improvement; five had 25–50% improvement. These parameters did not produce significant purpura.

In assessing the overall success and potential risk of each laser used in the treatment of facial telangiectasia with rosacea, we believe that the PDL provides effective and relatively risk-free results. In addition, one study of 10 patients showed that only 50% had less papulopustular lesions after an average of 2.4 treatments with parameters of the PDL previously described above (45). However, even in this "negative" paper, two of the 10 treated patients had excellent results when evaluated five years after treatment.

Intense Pulsed Light
The IPL has been found to be effective in treating rosacea. As described previously, this light source has the advantage of relatively quick vessel elimination without significant purpura or crusting. Scanning Doppler evaluation demonstrated a 30% decrease in blood flow after five IPL treatments (46). In addition, a 21% decrease in erythema intensity as well as a 29% decrease in the actual size of the cheek with telangiectasia was noted in this study of four patients. A larger study of 60 patients were treated with the IPL with pulse durations of 4.3–6.5 ms and energy density of 25–35 J/cm² (47). A mean clearance of 77.8% was achieved and maintained for a follow-up period averaging 51.6 months. An additional study of 32 consecutive patients treated with an average of 3.6 IPL treatments similar to the above-mentioned parameters showed that 83% of patients had reduced redness, 75% experienced reduced flushing, and 64% noted fewer acne breakouts (48). We treat the entire facial area affected by the erythematous rosacea. Short pulses appear to be most effective. We typically use a 550 or 560 nm cutoff filter with a double pulse of 2.4 and 4.0 ms with a 10-ms delay and an energy density of 26 J/cm² with the Quantum SR, and 3.0 ms and 3.0 ms at 18 J/cm² with the Lumenis One, or 34 J/cm² and 10 ms with the Palomar MaxG device. Patients are retreated every 3 to 4 weeks until clear. We have found that most patients clear in two or three treatments (Fig. 2.18). A certain percentage of patients (20%) do not respond to the IPL and need to be treated with the PDL. Most of our patients need to return for re-treatment once or twice a year. We have also found the large spot KTP laser to be useful in rosacea.

POIKILODERMA OF CIVATTE
Poikiloderma was originally described by Civatte and represents a sun-induced dilation of blood vessels, sometimes accompanied by hyperpigmentation. The condition is best treated by IPL, large spot KTP laser, or extended pulse PDLs. Multiple sessions are necessary, and some cases are resistant to treatment. Interestingly, even in cases where both melanin and telangiectasia appear to be in excess, treatment of the ectatic

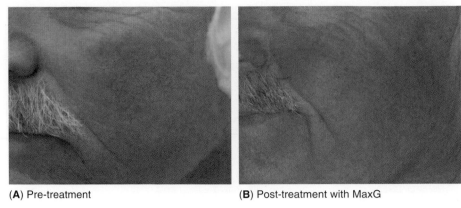

(**A**) Pre-treatment   (**B**) Post-treatment with MaxG

Figure 2.18 Telangiectasia (**A**) before and (**B**) after treatment with intense pulsed light (30 J/cm², 10 ms).

vessels alone will achieve marked clearance. The apparent paradox arises from the relative small percentage of neck discoloration that stems from melanin versus excess deoxy-HgB. Stamatas and Kollias found that a fraction of the apparent hyperpigmentation was deoxy-HgB being interpreted by the eye as melanin (they share a common reflectance pattern near the 560 nm deoxy-HgB peak) (49). Fractional lasers have recently been shown to reduce the redness and hyperpigmentation associated with poikiloderma. One investigator (50) applied the 1550 nm laser and reported a "significant" improvement using 8 mJ and 2000 MTZ/cm² after a single treatment. Tierney et al. (51) applied a fractional CO_2 laser and after one to three treatments found 65% reduction in red and brown dyschromias. One should use caution in treating the neck with ablative fractional lasers, as the recovery tends to be compromised in this very thin skin.

Pulsed Dye Laser

We recommend that if the PDL is used to treat poikiloderma of Civatte, it be used with a 10-mm-diameter spot size. In one scenario, fluence should be just strong enough to give a minimal purpuric response (about 5–6 J/cm², 1.5 ms and cooling). Patients must be told that three to five treatments will be necessary and that the treated area may appear to be polka-dotted until all treatments are given. An alternative nonpurpuric approach uses the same 10 mm spot and fluences ranging from 7 to 9 J/cm² with aggressive cooling and 10- to 20-ms pulse duration. This approach might require additional treatments but will be less likely to create the temporary honeycombed pattern that purpuric settings tend to cause. Also, most patients resist the objectionable appearance of purpura.

Intense Pulsed Light

Our results using an IPL have been favorable. With a pulsed light system, the target is both vascular and epidermal and dermal melanin. Various settings are applied that are device specific. Both single, double, and triple pulse configurations have been applied with good results. Multiple sessions are normally necessary to achieve an optimal clinical result. This experience has been detailed in a study in which 66 patients with typical changes of poikiloderma on the neck were treated with IPL at various settings every four weeks until desired improvement occurred. A 50–75% improvement in the extent of telangiectasia and hyperpigmentation comprising poikiloderma was observed in an average of 2.8 treatments. Incidence of hypopigmentation was 5% (52,53). A second expanded study of 135 patients randomly selected with typical changes of poikiloderma on the neck and/or upper chest were treated one to five times every four weeks with the IPL. Clearance of over 75% of telangiectasia and hyperpigmentation comprising poikiloderma was observed. Incidence of side effects was 5% including pigment changes. In many cases, improved skin texture was noted both by physician and patient.

Approximately 75% improvement occurs after one treatment. Side effects include transitory erythema from 24 to 72 hours. Purpura occurs only 10% of the time and only with some pulses in variable locations. This purpura is different from that seen with the PDL in that it is intravascular and resolution occurs within 3 to 5 days. A slight stinging pain during treatment is easily tolerated for up to 60 pulses per session. No anesthesia is required, and the entire neck and chest area can be treated during one treatment session (Fig. 2.19). Patients must be informed that "footprints" representing the shape of the contact crystal may be present after the first and even second treatment and is a normal response. One caution is the use of IPL in tanned and darker-skinned patients. Unlike PDL, where so long as cryogen cooling is applied, a sufficient fluence to close vessels is usually "epidermis-safe", the "sweet spot" for IPL, that being the fluence that closes vessels but spares the background epidermal melanin, is quite small. Test spots are advisable. Applying hydroquinone and waiting for the patient to "de-tan" over a month are other tools to increase the ratio of vascular-to-melanin heating.

CAPILLARY MALFORMATIONS (INCLUDING NEVUS SIMPLEX AND PORT-WINE STAINS)

Capillary malformations are among the most common vascular malformations of the skin, affecting 0.3–0.5% of newborns (54). They appear to have an equal sex distribution and, although familial cases have been described, most capillary malformations arise sporadically (55). These lesions are usually noted at birth appearing as pale pink macules and patches; they may be misdiagnosed as a bruise or erythema from birth trauma (56). They may be single or multiple lesions. They may present as small isolated patches or involve an entire limb or significant portion of the face or neck. Lesions on the face may extend to the lips, gingival, and/or oral mucosa.

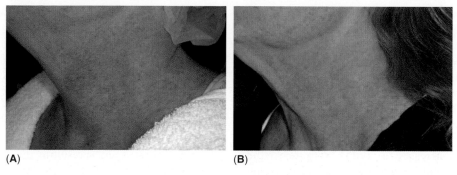

(A)   **(B)**

Figure 2.19 Poikiloderma (**A**) before and (**B**) after 2 treatments with intense pulsed light (30 J/cm², 10 ms).

The nevus simplex is a specific subset of capillary malformation that goes by a number of common names making its classification somewhat confusing. In general, nevus simplex may be referred to colloquially as a "salmon patch" (57). When located on the forehead/eyelid or nape of the neck, the terms "angel's kiss" or "stork bite" may be used, respectively. Such lesions have a characteristic predilection for the midline, mostly commonly affecting the nape of the neck and the central face (glabella, eyelids, nose, and upper lip); the occiput and lower back may also be affected (57).

The expected course of nevus simplex is to fade with maturity, with most lesions typically resolving within 1 or 2 years of age. Some lesions, particularly those located at the nape of the neck, have been known to persist without further darkening or thickening (58). Persistent glabellar and sacral lesions have also been referred to as "medial telangiectatic nevus" and "butterfly-shaped mark," respectively, and have further muddied the nomenclature waters (55).

PWSs ("nevus flammeus") are another subset of capillary malformations that are almost always congenital, although they may be acquired secondary to trauma and, thus, may develop in adolescence or adulthood (59). Unlike nevus simplex, PWSs persist throughout a patient's life. They may occur anywhere on the body. Typically, they grow proportionately with the child and may appear to lighten during the first three to six months of life. This is a physiologic change most likely due to the decrease in blood HgB concentration (typically 15–17 g/dL at birth to a nadir of 8–10 g/dL by age three months) and should not be interpreted as a sign of clinical resolution.

Videomicroscopy of PWS has demonstrated two patterns of vascular abnormality: type 1 consists of tortuous, superficial, dilated capillary loops (blobs or globular structures); type 2 consists of dilated ectatic vessels (rings) in the deeper horizontal vascular plexus or a mixed pattern. Vessel depth and number may correlate with anatomic location as one study demonstrated that PWSs in the V3, neck, and trunk locations were more likely to have a superficial type 1 pattern and typically responded well to laser treatment; on the other hand, lesions in V2 or distal extremity locations were more likely to have a deeper type 2 pattern and did not respond as well (60).

Although the exact molecular pathogenesis of capillary malformations remains unknown in the majority of cases, it is believed that localized defects in pathways controlling embryogenesis, vasculogenesis, and angiogenesis play key roles. Several specific mutations have recently been identified that have shed some light on possible etiologies. Mutations in *RASA1*, encoding p120-rasGTPase-activating protein (p120-rasGAP), along the Ras/MAPkinase pathway, have recently been identified in patients with atypical capillary malformations with or without concurrent arteriovenous malformations (AVMs) or arteriovenous fistulas; this protein appears to be crucial in controlling proliferation, migration, and cell death in a number of tissues, including vascular endothelium (61). Developmental endothelial locus-1 (Del-1), an extracellular matrix protein adhered to by human umbilical vein endothelial cells, is another protein being investigated for its potential to induce formation of a vascular plexus with increased number of capillaries (62).

ADVERSE MEDICAL EFFECTS

In addition to their abnormal cosmetic appearance, untreated PWSs tend to follow a predictable pattern of progression characterized by darkening in color (from pink-red to violaceous or deep purple), gradual thickening and nodularity (with possible bleb formation), and possible soft tissue hypertrophy and bone overgrowth (with subsequent deformation and functional impairment that may require surgical intervention) (63,64). One study found that two-thirds of patients develop hypertrophy and nodularity by age 46 years, with a mean age of 37 years for hypertrophy. Giant proliferative hemangiomas may also arise in PWSs and can develop without any prior history of trauma.

PWSs can also present with an inflammatory component consisting of scaling, excoriations, oozing, and crusting, resembling an eczematous dermatitis. Treatment with topical steroids to decrease the inflammation can help, and the PDL may be curative even after a single treatment (65,66).

The most serious extracutaneous findings of PWS may be glaucoma and the possible association with Sturge–Weber syndrome (SWS). A retrospective case–control study from a major ophthalmology referral center looked at 216 patients, mean age 3.25 years, with unilateral or bilateral PWSs in the ophthalmic (V1) and maxillary (V2) divisions of the trigeminal nerve. The authors identified the following risk factors for glaucoma: bilateral PWSs ($P = 0.0001$), upper and lower eyelid involvement ($P < 0.0001$), episcleral hemangioma ($P < 0.0001$), iris heterochromia ($P = 0.004$), or choroidal hemangioma ($P < 0.0001$) (67,68).

SWS is a sporadic congenital disorder characterized by the classic triad of facial PWS invariably involving V1 (although it may be more extensive) occurring in association with ipsilateral central nervous system vascular malformation (leptomeningeal angiomatosis) and vascular malformation of the choroid of the eye associated with glaucoma. The risk for SWS is determined by the distribution of the facial PWS, a fact that has been somewhat complicated by authors' definitions and anatomic variations in the distribution of V1 and V2 of the upper and lower eyelids (the so-called watershed areas). Overall, the risk of SWS with V1 PWS involving the upper eyelid approximates 10%; that risk increases to about 25% when either bilateral stains are present or when multiple dermatomes (V1, V2, V3) are involved (67,68). Because SWS can cause significant medical and ophthalmologic problems ranging from potential visual loss and hypothalamic–pituitary dysfunction (69) to seizures and mental retardation, the possibility of SWS should be considered in any infant with a PWS that includes the V1 distribution.

Other congenital syndromes include the Klippel–Trenaunay and Parkes–Weber syndromes (PWS with associated varicose vein and hypertrophy of skeletal tissue with or without AVMs, respectively) and Cobb syndrome (PWS with underlying AVM of the spinal cord). A PWS may be associated with an underlying venous malformation or occasionally an AVM, so the existence of these associated lesions should not cause confusion in diagnosis.

PSYCHOLOGIC IMPACT

In addition to producing physical deformity, a PWS carries a definite risk for lasting detrimental effects on a child's psychologic, social, interpersonal, and cognitive development. The exact age when psychosocial development is affected is speculative.

A common misperception regarding PWSs in adults is that if one has reached adulthood without psychologic damage from a cosmetic deformity, one does not require treatment. Adult PWS are known to impact social relationships. A questionnaire given to 186 patients who sought treatment for their PWS found that 29% thought the PWS was disadvantageous in forming interpersonal relationships with members of the opposite sex (70). A half rated their PWS as unattractive, although only 33% thought that other people perceived their PWS to be moderately to very unattractive. The true incidence of psychologic problems from PWS may be higher or lower because this study was obviously skewed to patients who were actively seeking treatment. Nevertheless, the survey does show that a significant number of adults with PWS would benefit psychologically from treatment.

Psychologic difficulties in interactions with others occur as often in adults as in children. The Soviet news agency, Tass, for example, famously airbrushed out former president Mikail Gorbachev's PWS from published photographs until *perestroika* as a means of hiding his "cosmetic handicap." Similarly, an experiment during the 1989 annual meeting of the American Academy of Dermatology dramatically demonstrates this point. A model had a PWS painted on her face and then feigned an illness that led to unconsciousness on a public bus. Not one passenger came to her aid. When the same model feigned the same illness on a bus without the facial PWS, all those present eagerly came to her aid. Pena Clementina Masclarelli (71), a senior occupational therapist who also has an extensive PWS, wrote a poignant chapter about her

interactions with others that should be required reading for all physicians.

Multiple studies have demonstrated an improvement in psychological health after successful treatment of PWS (72–76). We have noted a change in personal perceptions dramatically in our treated patients. On a personal level, a 12-year-old girl first sought treatment in our practice for a PWS on the right cheek. Initially, although of above-average intelligence, she was introverted and interacted sparingly with her classmates. After three treatment sessions, resulting in 75% clearance, she began dating, joined the school band, and excelled academically. These are the observations so gratifying to the physician and medical staff involved in laser treatment.

Despite the psychological and medical complications of PWS, insurance coverage in the United States for laser treatment of PWS varies from state to state. A study by McClean and Hanke (64) of insurance reimbursement in 18 states found that determination for approval of treatment was made on a case-by-case basis, with the majority requiring preauthorization. The percentage of requests approved for coverage varied from 50% to 100% without apparent reason. Some insurance carriers would only approve treatment if functional impairment existed and some only if the patient was less than 1 year of age. Only Minnesota has a law requiring all health insurance to cover the elimination or maximum feasible treatment of PWS.

Various support groups are available for children with congenital vascular abnormalities and their families. The Sturge–Weber Foundation (http://www.sturge-weber.org; Mt. Freedom, New Jersey, USA) publishes an excellent booklet for children that clearly explains the syndrome as well as multiple treatment options. The Klippel–Trenaunay Support Group (Edina, USA) publishes a useful quarterly newsletter and holds support group and educational meetings for the public. The National Congenital Port-Wine Stain Foundation (New York, USA) also provides information and support to patients and families of children with PWSs; www.birthmarks.com is an excellent website for patient information. Patients and parents should be encouraged to use these resources.

CHILDHOOD PORT-WINE STAINS

Because of the long-term physical and psychosocial comorbidities associated with PWSs, many specialists advocate for treatment of these lesions to begin as soon as possible after birth. Support for intervention at the earliest possible age is based on the fact that the lesions themselves are physically smaller in size and are comprised of vessels that are smaller in diameter and more superficial. Thus, early treatment may improve the responsiveness, decrease the number of treatments, and reduce the likelihood of permanent adverse sequelae (77–79).

Many therapeutic methods have been attempted to treat PWS. These include surgery (excision, grafts, flaps, dermabrasion) (80–82), radium implants, X-ray therapy (83), cryosurgery (84), electrocautery, sclerotherapy (85), tattooing (86), and cosmetic camouflage (Fig. 2.20). Vascular-targeted photodynamic therapy has also emerged as a potential option for patients with darker skin types (Fitzpatrick V) or for those patients with nodular lesions, with long-term studies in the Chinese population demonstrating 50% clearance in about 30% of patients receiving, on average, 2.6–8.2 treatment sessions (87). Many of these

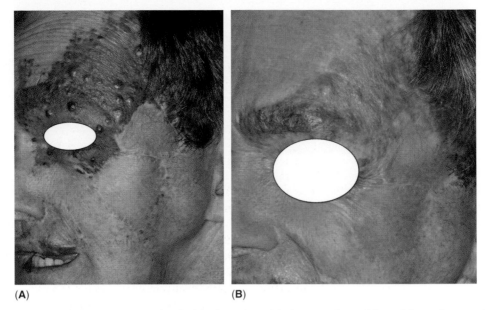

(A) (B)

Figure 2.20 (**A**) PWS before and (**B**) after 10 treatments with pulsed dye laser; alexandrite laser was also used for nodules on four occasions. Note skin graft that was placed to treat part of PWS while patient was youth. *Abbreviation*: PWS, port-wine stain.

methods have limited and/or unpredictable results as well as potentially serious complications.

PWSs, with their specifically targeted biologic structure, serve as ideal candidates for SPT with laser. Utilizing the careful selection of wavelength, fluence, and pulse duration coagulation can be induced while sparing surrounding tissue. While the CO_2 laser (88), Nd:YAG laser, copper vapor laser (89,90), and argon laser (89) have all previously been used to treat PWS in children, cosmetic results with these lasers have been poor in children, with the risk of scarring unacceptably high. Consequently, the PDL remains the gold standard of treatment for most PWS, although newer-generation IPLs and KTP lasers have evolved as reasonable options.

Prior to laser surgery, everyone in the treatment room should wear wavelength-appropriate safety goggles. Adults may use standard eye goggles for protection, but these may not fit properly on infants and young children. In such instances, white gauze may be used to cover the periorbital area (63). If the PWS is itself located around or near the eye, patients should also utilize opaque laser eye shields placed prior to treatment; this can be done immediately after the child is anesthetized if general anesthesia is used.

Anesthesia is an important concern when performing laser surgery in the pediatric population. Topical anesthetics that are commonly utilized include lidocaine 4% gel and eutectic mixture of local anesthetics (EMLA), which is 2.5% lidocaine and 2.5% prilocaine. EMLA has been known to cause local vasoconstriction that may impede visualization of the lesion itself and decrease effectiveness of treatment with laser (91). Additionally, its constituent, prilocaine, has a known risk of causing methemoglobinemia in children less than six months old as a result of immaturity of erythrocyte methemoglobin reductase, the enzyme that converts met-HgB to HgB. Children with glucose-6-phosphate dehydrogenase deficiency and other hemoglobinopathies may also be at particular risk. Consequently, alternatives to prilocaine anesthetics should be considered when possible (92). While older children may tolerate the laser procedure using topical anesthetics only, infants and young children may require general anesthesia.

General anesthesia affords the laser surgeon the ability to cover larger areas and to avoid the risk of unexpected movements during treatment of delicate anatomic areas requiring technical finesse. While the risk of general anesthesia on the developing infant's brain remains a controversial subject, most pediatric laser surgeons advocate for its use in younger children with larger lesions (93).

Cooling the skin is crucial to minimizing damage to surrounding tissues and for reducing the risk of postoperative complications such as swelling, scarring, and postinflammatory pigmentary changes (especially in darker-skinned patients). This may be accomplished using an attached cooling device that provides a targeted cryogenic spray to the superficial skin a fraction of a second before the laser energy is delivered (Fig. 2.21). Likewise, cool air machines can blow continuously cooled air across the treatment site. Cold compresses or bags of ice applied immediately to the treated area are another useful low-tech, low-cost tool that should not be underestimated.

Recent attention has been given to angiogenesis inhibitors as a novel means of preventing reformation and reperfusion of PWSs after photothermolysis. Angiogenesis inhibitors are a varied class of compounds that include cleaved proteins, monoclonal antibodies, and natural products used to prevent the development of malignancies. Rapamycin, an inhibitor of the mammalian target of rapamycin, has shown particular promise through its ability to inhibit proliferation of vascular endothelial cells. It has been well studied in transplant populations and appears to have a minimal side-effect profile (94–96). While long-term studies in humans with PWSs are lacking, vessel reperfusion has been effectively reduced in hamsters using laser with daily topical application of rapamycin versus laser alone (94). It is postulated that this is accomplished through suppression of vascular endothelial growth factor and hypoxia-sensitive gene transcriptional regulators, such as hypoxia-inducible factor 1-alpha (97). It remains to be seen whether other agents such as topical or oral beta-blockers (e.g., timolol or propranolol, respectively) have a role in decreasing PWS angiogenesis as has been demonstrated in hemangiomas of infancy (98,99).

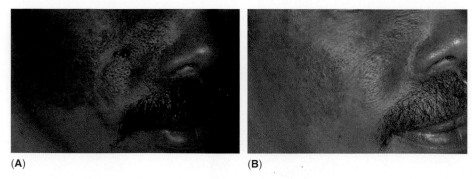

Figure 2.21 (**A**) Port-wine stain before and (**B**) after 12 treatments in type V skin with pulsed dye laser (10 mm, 7 J/cm², 1.5 ms, 50 ms spray, 30 ms delay with cryogen spray).

PULSED DYE LASER

The PDL remains the most studied device in PWS treatment. Over the years various pulse durations and wavelengths have been applied. Today, most PDLs emit 595 nm light over a range of pulse durations and pulse structures. The most commonly applied pulse duration is 1.5 ms; however, for lighter PWS, 0.45 ms has been advocated. Although the risk of general anesthesia (typically required in young children for larger lesions and lesions around the eye) increases risks to the patient, the typical course is to initiate treatment within three months of birth- the arguments for early intervention include the likeliness that the vessels are smaller and more superficial and the smaller overall size of the lesion (78,100,101). Those that argue for later intervention note that studies do not clearly show that earlier intervention is more effective than later treatments.

Treatment intervals are normally about 3 to 6 weeks apart. A recent study showed that more frequent treatments might be preferable (100,101). Treatment responses are variable according to anatomic areas and the gross and microscopic anatomy of the lesion. Facial lesions generally respond better than nonfacial lesions, and lesions on the mid-face respond more poorly that those lesions at lateral facial locations. There are multiple reasons for the multiple treatment requirements for PWS. One is the variable depth so the lesions and the likelihood that the most superficial vessels must be reduced first to allow for deeper light penetration and heating of deeper lesions. Also, angiogenesis between treatments might account for some resistance and is currently becoming a target of biologic strategies in PWS management. Some providers suggest that PWSs respond better once they are "broken up"; that is, the initial treatment creates islands or pixels in initially confluent lesions. Once the "break up" is achieved, light more readily propagates down the skin and can "hit" the PWS vessels from all sides (Fig. 2.22).

One study examined the use of multiple pulses (passes) in the same session (102), starting with a longer pulse and progressing to a shorter pulse. In this manner, a layered approach was suggested to accelerate PWS clearance and decrease the total number of treatment sessions. In the study, a first pass was made at 1.5 ms and 595 nm followed by treatment at 585 nm at 0.45 ms. In a recent study (103) the PDL was applied with two passes 30 minutes apart and with 0.45–3 ms and reducing the fluence by 0.5–2 J/cm² in the second pass (from, e.g., 12 J/cm² with 7 mm spot to 10 J/cm²). Tanghetti et al. found that multiple passes with a short interval (10 minutes) allowed for deeper injury in vessels. In all of these studies, epidermal damage was

avoided or mitigated by the dynamic cooling device (DCD) or contact cooling. Tanghetti et al. also found that by increasing the interpulse interval that the level of vascular damage was greater (104). Another study found that multiple passes might be superior to one pass in a single session (103). However, a more recent tightly controlled prospective study of PDL treatment of PWS found that two passes were not superior to one pass (105). Accessories to increase the efficacy of PWS clearance with PDL include vacuum assist (Serenty Pro, Candela, Wayland, Massachusetts, USA) (106–108). In one study the increase in blood fraction was significant and more purpura was observed after PDL; however, the vacuum chamber precludes the use of DCD and therefore would limit use in darker skin types.

PDLs contain a rhodamine dye excited by a xenon flash lamp that produces light at 585–600 nm; the most commonly used wavelength is 595 nm. A lack of controlled studies with a single parameter difference has made it difficult to optimize pediatric treatment settings (109). Pulses of 1.5 ms (long-pulsed) are most commonly applied; however, for lighter PWSs 0.45 ms (short-pulse PDL) has been advocated. Short-pulse widths (<3 ms) generally cause immediate purpura (a clinical endpoint), an effect that may take five to 10 days to resolve. Longer pulse widths tend to cause less bruising. Fluences range from 4 to 12 J/cm² and spot sizes range from 2 to 10 mm with 7 mm being a popular choice because of laser power limitations. In these ranges, light penetrates the dermis to approximately 1.2–1.5 mm in depth, with deeper penetration possible with higher wavelength and longer exposure durations.

While PDLs are a relatively safe and effective treatment, patient and parental anxiety will often require physician reassurance. Potential adverse events, including postinflammatory pigmentary changes (especially in darker-skinned patients), immediate postlaser purpura, recurrence, and infection should be addressed prior to treatment. Sun exposure can drastically affect pigmentary changes, and sun avoidance/protection is essential to optimizing outcomes. Blistering, crusting, and, rarely, hypertrophic or atrophic scarring may also occur. Surface cooling has markedly diminished this side effect. Swelling and erythema are frequently present immediately after treatment, especially around the eyes, but resolve within 24–48 hours. Hypopigmentation occurs infrequently and, in the absence of textural changes, usually resolves spontaneously over 3 to 6 months. Cutaneous depressions or atrophic scars have occurred in isolated laser impact sites and have been associated with excessive delivery of energy, absence of cooling, excessive

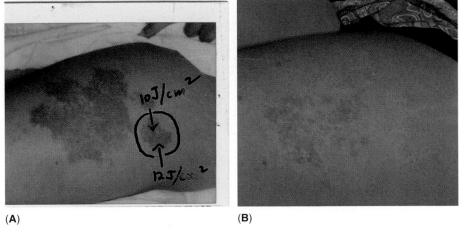

(A)   **(B)**

Figure 2.22 Port-wine stain (**A**) before and (**B**) after 25 treatments with potassium titanyl phosphate and pulsed dye laser.

spot overlap, or post-treatment trauma to the site. Almost all reported cases have resolved spontaneously within 1 year (77).

In terms of potential for laser treatments to disrupt local vascular flow and potentially cause glaucoma, initial evidence suggests that PDL treatments to periocular PWSs do not demonstrate clinically relevant effects on intraocular pressure (110). Similarly, the theoretical risk of hemoglobinemia that could result from photothermolysis does not appear to be clinically relevant. In this scenario, photothermolysis of blood vessels does result in the release of free HgB into the circulation with the resulting hemoglobinemia leading to renal impairment in a young patient. Fortunately, a study of 15 patients under age five years treated with the PDL-tested serum haptoglobin and urine hemosiderin postoperatively found that even though patients had a treatment region more than 3% of total body surface area and received 5-mm-diameter pulses more than 1500 in some cases, there was no evidence of urine HgB and serum haptoglobin levels were normal (111).

"Before" and "after" photos may be particularly useful tools for demonstrating efficacy and assuaging fears. If possible, a test area using a local anesthetic cream and about four to eight laser pulses (at the lower end of the energy range) may be performed prior to a full treatment session; this permits families to witness the entire treatment process and allows the laser surgeon to gauge the skin's response to laser treatment (109). Caregivers should always be informed of specific aftercare instructions, including follow-up clinic appointments and additional treatment sessions.

Generally, the smaller, more superficial vessels are targeted with GY light first. Deeper, larger caliber vessels may require longer pulse durations or longer wavelengths. Purpura (with GY light sources) is the clinical endpoint of successful laser treatment for most PWSs (77). However, studies have shown that purpura-free clearing of PWS is possible with PDL, KTP, and IPL devices. In all instances, graying of tissue is an indication of possible overtreatment.

It is not uncommon for an uneven response to PDL to be seen. Responses may vary according to the gross anatomic area, the local dermal blood fraction, and the microscopic anatomy of the lesion. Factors lending themselves to a more favorable response to treatment include younger age; lighter pink-red color (in contrast to deep purple); and certain anatomical sites, with lateral facial, periorbital, forehead, chest,

neck, and proximal aspect of arm lesions generally responding better than PWSs located on the center of the cheeks or on the more distal extremities (112).

Successful treatment also seems to correlate with timing, number, and frequency of laser treatment sessions. The first published reports of PDL for PWS noted complete clearing of pink-to-red macular PWS in 35 children younger than 14 years (mean age 7 years 2 months) with an average of 6.5 treatments (113). Subsequent clinical studies demonstrated notable efficacy and defined more reasonable expectations. Reyes and Geronemus (77) successfully treated 73 patients between age three months and 14 years. The overall average lightening after one treatment was 53%, and the percentage of lightening increased with subsequent treatments. More than 75% lightening was achieved with an average of 2.5 treatments in 33 patients.

Morelli and Weston advocate beginning treatment as early as 7–14 days of age so that three treatments can be done before the infant reaches six months of age. They noted a 50% resolution with this protocol by the third treatment. In their population of 132 patients, complete clearance was obtained in 25% of PWSs when treatment was begun before 18 months of age (average 7.8 treatment sessions) versus 7–10% having total clearance when treatment was begun between ages 11/2 and 18 years (average 7.0 treatment sessions). A follow-up evaluation of this patient population confirmed the authors' initial observations with 83 children: 32% of children who began treatment before 1 year of age had complete clearing of their PWS compared with 18% of children treated after 1 year of age. In this later study, 32% of patients with PWS less than 20 cm² in size completely cleared compared with an 8% complete clearance rate in patients with larger PWS (114–116).

Our studies on the treatment of 43 children between ages 2 weeks and 14 years with 49 lesions of capillary malformation confirm these results (117). Lesions treated in children under age 4 years had greater overall improvement with less treatment sessions compared with those in children over age 4½ years (Table 2.2). In general, improvement and clearance were gradual and required 5–10 treatments. However, very superficial lesions cleared more quickly, with four lesions reaching a level of 95% clearing in one or two treatments.

An additional study of 12 children 6–30 weeks of age confirmed that treatment of infants only a few weeks old can be

Table 2.2 Childhood Port-Wine Stains: Treatment Response by Age

No. of Patients	No. of Lesions	Average Range	Average Age (yr)	Average Treatments	Average Improvement (%)	Median Improvement (%)	95% Improvement No. of Lesions	Average Treatments
Age 0–4 yr								
21	25	2 wk to 4 yr	2.15	3.4	70	75	5 (20%)	3.8
Age 4.5–14 yr								
22	24	6–14 yr	10.3	4.0	68	75	3 (12.5%)	6.5
Total 0–14 yr								
43	49	2 wk to 14 yr	6.2	3.7	69	75	8 (16.3%)	4.8

Source: From Ref. 116.

undertaken safely and with an accelerated response: 45% demonstrated 75% or more lightening of their lesions after a mean of 3.8 treatments (118). Alster and Wilson (119) reported an 87% clearance rate in patients less than 2 years of age, 78% clearance in patients of ages three to eight, and 73% clearance rate in patients 16 years and older. All these studies demonstrate a better treatment outcome with younger patients.

One study of 23 facial PWS lesions in patients up to age 17 years showed no difference among different ages in the average number of treatments to obtain maximum lesion lightening (120). However, this study only evaluated four lesions in children less than 1 year of age and eight lesions in those 1 to 7 years of age.

This variation in response to treatment may be due to the variable depth of the lesions themselves and the likelihood that vessels located most superficially must be treated first to allow for deeper light penetration and, therefore, continued treatment of the deeper portion of the lesion. Additionally, vessel photocoagulation immediately following laser photothermolysis results in decreased blood supply to the skin, resulting in local hypoxia. Reactively, the normal wound healing response activates appropriate defense mechanisms such as angiogenesis. This normal reformation and reperfusion of blood vessels has been thought to interfere with subsequent laser photothermolysis and additional lightening of PWSs (121).

Another parameter is the interval between pulses (if one is applying more than one pulse). In the original proposal of SPT, calculations of thermal relaxation time (TRT) were based on theoretical considerations but measurements of actual temperature decay in vessels were not measured. Dierickx used 0.8x the purpura thresholds in PWS for various pulse delays to establish a real TRT, that is, the delay where the first and second pulses are almost decoupled thermally (122). They found longer TRTs than those theoretical values in the literature and that 1–10 ms was the ideal pulse duration for a single pulse based on their experimental data within the context of mathematical models of heat diffusion. Dual pulses (either comprised of one IPL or one wavelength of laser light, or sequential 595/1064 nm devices) have been applied to PWS—models predict that multiple pulses with 20–60 ms interpulse delays should allow for cumulative vessel heating during the pulse train with a smaller effect on the actively cooled and thinner epidermis. In some instances, nodular or hypertrophic PWSs

may require treatment with pulsed alexandrite laser or pulsed Nd:YAG laser (Fig. 2.20) (123).

Changing from a 585-nm dye to a 595-nm dye has resulted in enhanced clearing in some PWS. It appears that pink or red PWS do best with 585 nm, whereas blue or dark red PWS do better with 595-nm dyes. There is met-HgB production during heating of blood; this shifts the absorption spectrum during irradiation and just after irradiation. Met-HgB shows enhanced absorption for wavelengths greater than 600 nm versus oxy-HgB. The peaks for oxy-, deoxy-, and met-HgB are provided in (see Table 1.2 in chap. 1). Met-HgB has absorption peaks at 404, 508, and 635 nm. Following formation of met-HgB, decreases in oxy-HgB absorption peaks at 335, 415, 542, and 576 nm will occur (124). The changes suggest that 630 nm might be applied at the end of a laser pulse to enhance blood vessel heating. Another approach is sequential 595 or 532 nm then 1064 nm heating. Once again, the formation of met-HgB enhances light absorption, in this case in the NIR spectrum. The goal is epidermal sparing by decreasing the visible light fluence and adding a 1064 nm 10–50 ms later, thereby exploiting dynamic optical property changes in blood. Finally, other maneuvers, such as increasing the diameter of the blood vessels by using a proximal tourniquet, has also enhanced absorption with a 585-nm, 1.5-ms PDL.

The alexandrite laser has been advocated as a good choice for resistant PWS and some darker PWS. Fluences range from 25 to 80 J/cm^2 over pulse durations from 3 to 20 ms. Generally, smaller fluences (25–35 J/cm^2) are employed with larger 12–15 mm spots (likely a safer approach) and larger fluences (50–80 J/cm^2) with smaller 6–8 mm spots. The alexandrite laser should be used with surface cooling and care should be taken not to pulse stack or apply too many pulses in a small area. Bulk heating and overheating of the epidermis are likely if these precautions are not taken. Because of the deeper penetration of the laser versus PDL, deeper vessels can be treated, but also over treatment tends to result in scarring. Likewise, the 810 nm diode laser can be used with cooling with fluences ranging from 35 to 60 J/cm^2 with variably available spot sizes (usually ~1 cm^2).

The 1064 nm laser can be used for PWS but is best reserved for exophytic portions of the stain. Very small spot sizes should be applied (the same size as the nodule). Although test spots are not routinely performed in modern day treatment of PWS, a case can be made for such tests with 1064 nm given the unpredictability of responses and the potential for deep injury and subsequent scarring (125–127). Generally, smaller nodules are treated with a roughly 3 mm spot and fluence of about 60–120 J/cm^2 with cooling. The endpoint is a slight bluing of the lesion. Deep graying and complete shrinkage of the lesions often signal overtreatment and pandermal necrosis. In general, nodular lesions (larger than 3 mm in diameter) are best treated with the CO_2 laser, alexandrite laser, Nd:YAG laser, or the IPL. We have recently used a dual pulse with an IPL (Max G, Palomar Medical Technologies), with 30 J/cm^2, 10 ms then a 60 ms delay and second pulse of 60 J/cm^2 in 100 ms. Using this configuration, the deeper nodules are treated with relative epidermal sparing. The longer pulse IPL red shifts the output spectrum, which enhances deeper lesion heating.

With the millisecond CO_2 laser the lesion can be sculpted to reestablish a normal facial contour in addition to coagulate the ectatic blood vessels. The advantages of the CO_2 laser are its precise hemostasis and avoidance of nonspecific thermal damage. After normal contours are obtained, the PDL or IPL can be used to lighten the remaining erythema.

PDT has been applied to PWS, primarily outside the USA (87,128–130). Unlike ALA/PDT where ALA is converted to PpIX primarily in the epidermis and other very cellular structures (and where PDL/PDT for PWS has been shown to offer no advantage over PDL alone), PDT for PWS relies primarily on vascular-specific photosensitizers (131). The three necessary ingredients for any PDT procedure (see chap. 3) are O_2, photosensitizer (PS), and light, all co-located at the target. The dual selectivity of PDT relies on optimizing drug and light delivery. A critical component is the delay between drug and light administration (DLI). Qiu and others have shown that hematoporphyrin monomethyl ether [a refined derivative of hematoporphyrin derivative (HPD)] is an adequate PS with improved clearance and a more favorable vascular to skin damage ratio. The absorption peaks are 401, 500, 533, 569, and 613 nm. Most clinicians have used copper vapor and other lasers in quasi-CW mode. In the many studies over 20 years, they typically used a 9 cm spot and power density of 80–100 W/cm^2, and a 40- to 55-minute DLI after intravenous drug delivery. Most PWS cleared after two to three treatments 2 months apart. Photosensitivity generally lasted about 1 to 2 weeks. Complications have been reported after PDT for PWS including severe scarring. The light doses, DLI, wavelength, and power density must be carefully titrated for optimal outcomes. One study looked at intradermal ALA and PDT for PWS (132) and found some clearing of vessels in a chicken comb model; however, there was no selective PpIX formation in the vessels after intradermal administration.

Fractional lasers have been reported to lighten PWS through sequential cumulative destruction of vessels. The bulk of vessels in PWS lie within the range of most fractional lasers. Both nonablative and ablative lasers have been applied. Some practitioners advocate same-session treatment with a vascular-specific and fractional laser where one uses the GY light first followed by the fractional tool.

Adverse effects: Numerous retrospective studies have detailed adverse sequelae. Since the introduction of cooling, many of the adverse sequelae have been reduced. Before cooling crusting was not uncommon, occurring in as many as 50% of patients. The severity of purpura was also greater.

TREATMENT PROTOCOL

Prior to widespread use of epidermal cooling, test spots were advocated to optimize outcomes. Test spots were especially useful in treating darker skin, where 5.5 J/cm^2, for example, with a 0.45-ms PDL, would achieve an appropriate purpuric response and 6 J might result in graying, blistering, and dyschromia. When using a new device or in a tanned and/or darker patient, even in the presence of cooling, test spots can be useful. On the other hand, with modern day PDLs with cryogen spray, for example, one can apply fluence sufficient to cause purpura and still maintain a reasonable safety window (e.g., where 8 J/cm^2 is sufficient for purpura and 9.5 J/cm^2 might be required for unwanted crusting).

If the site does not discolor, too low a fluence may have been chosen. If graying occurs, too high an energy density may have been chosen. Generally, three or four fluences are tested and evaluated at approximately 3 to 4 weeks. The most effective one is then chosen for treatment. If none of the test sites shows improvement, a second series of test energies is chosen. With experience, the test period may be eliminated and the treatment energy chosen by evaluation of the laser's immediate effects.

Treatment of the entire lesion or a portion of the lesion may be accomplished by covering the treatment area with laser or IPL impacts that overlap 10%. Overlapping can minimize a mottled "egg crate" or "footprint" appearance. The use of overlapping pulses should be undertaken with caution, however, because biopsies of PWSs treated with single impact and consecutive double-impact therapy reveal an additive thermal effect resulting in nonspecific thermal damage to the superficial dermis and epidermis. This double-pulsing technique does promote greater resolution of nodular, thicker, and darker lesions but results in loss of specificity.

The reason for multiple treatments is the layered nature of ectatic vessels of a PWS. Modeling studies using the histologically correct layered vessel demonstrate that the more superficial vessels receive most of the delivered energy. The deeper vessels receive less energy and are therefore not coagulated because of mutual shadowing of the superficial vessels.

TREATMENT OF "RESISTANT" LESIONS

Multiple methods are available for treating PWS lesions that fail to respond to the PDL. The first option is to switch to the IPL, alexandrite, or KTP laser. In examining resistant PWS (133), Jasim and Handley noted many factors that might contribute to compromised clearance. They propose longer wavelengths with associated higher fluences, PDT, and optical clearing agents as possible optimizers for clearance.

RECURRENCE OF PORT-WINE STAINS

The use of the PDL in treating PWS has been widely practiced for almost 35 years. Recently, we and others have begun to evaluate our patients treated in the early years for signs of persistent or recurrent lesions. Although we have not seen a significant number of patients returning to our practice with progressing lesions, other physicians have reported recurrence after completion of treatment (134).

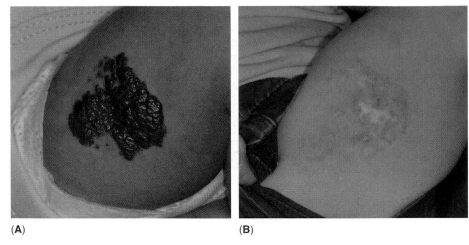

Figure 2.23 Congenital hemangioma (**A**) before and (**B**) after being treated in four sessions two months apart with alexandrite laser (8 mm, 3 ms, 45 J/cm², and 60 ms spray, 30 ms delay with cryogen spray). Note small scar after crusting in one area after laser.

clear" of IH at 1 year (169). Limitations of this study include a small spot size (5 mm), low fluences, the lack of use of a cooling handpiece, and a small number of treatments in the laser group. When considered in total, a 2011 Cochrane analysis found insufficient evidence to support PDL (and other laser) for uncomplicated IH (170).

Other lasers have been used to treat IH. This list includes the argon and Nd:YAG lasers, which may cause more significant scarring than PDL. A retrospective study comparing PDL (585 nm) and frequency-doubled Nd:YAG 532 nm (i.e., "KTP") lasers demonstrated less clinical efficacy (i.e., cessation of growth or regressive tendency) with KTP. Side effects, including purpura, crusting, and postinflammatory pigmentary changes, however, were less common with KTP than with PDL (171). Alexandrite lasers have also been applied to IH. We advise very conservative fluences with larger spots (25–30 J/cm² and 12 mm, or slightly higher fluence with smaller spots (8 mm)). In any case, aggressive cooling will limit the likelihood of ulceration and scarring (Fig. 2.23). Pain can be managed by topical anesthetics but the child will have to be restrained as well. One issue with alexandrite and Nd:YAG lasers is the potential for unwanted hair reduction, particularly in the area of the brow and scalp; therefore, their use in these areas should be confined to those cases where there is a clear benefit-to-risk ratio. Percutaneous treatment with a bare fiber Nd:YAG laser has been used to treat deep hemangiomas (172). Ablative fractional lasers are also being explored for their role in treating fibrofatty residua from involuted hemangiomas and scars secondary to previous surgical excision (173).

Venous Lakes

Venous lakes are 2–8 mm diameter red-blue nodules that typically occur on the lower lip. These "varicosities" of the lip respond to a number of lasers and/or IPLs. For very small lesions the KTP and PDL are helpful. For larger lesions, the depth exceeds the "reach" of the GY technologies so that longer wavelengths are favored. Our favorite newest approach is the 6 mm spot alexandrite laser with a 3-ms pulse and a fluence of 60–80 J/cm². Often one treatment session will reduce

the lesion by 80% in volume and occasionally the lesions will disappear after one treatment (Fig. 2.24). Surface cooling must be applied to prevent epidermal injury. The 810 nm diode laser can be used. We have also used the Nd:YAG laser with 3–5 mm spots and fluences ranging from 50 to 100 J/cm². With the 1064 nm laser, the endpoint should be very slight lesion shrinkage. Again, surface cooling must be applied. IPL can also be used with a range of pulse durations and fluences. Any device with contact cooling should be held against the skin surface with only gentle pressure lest the lesion be overcompressed and all of the chromophore is displaced. The PDL with compression has also been applied (using just enough compression to reduce the lesion thickness); however, in this scenario no cooling will be available.

Glomus Tumor

Small glomus tumors have been successfully treated with the PDL (174). We have found that the Nd:YAG laser achieves good resolution in deeper bluer lesions. Normally the Nd:YAG laser is applied with a 3 mm spot and cooling with fluences ranging from 120 to 200 J/cm² and about 50 ms. Larger lesions require smaller fluences and smaller lesions will require higher fluences. The endpoint is a slight immediate shrinkage of the lesion (175).

Blue Runner Bleb Nevus

We treat these lesions with the Nd:YAG laser with a 2–4 mm spot size, surface cooling, and fluences ranging from 80 to 130 J/cm².

Angiofibromas and Fibrous Papules

Angiofibromas are (176) associated with tuberous sclerosis. These lesions are best treated with a 1–2 mm spot CO_2 laser either in pulsed or CW mode. The lesions can be vaporized to a depth just beneath the skin surface. For CW mode we normally use powers from 2 to 5 W and for pulsed mode 200–400 mJ pulse energies. Very red individual lesions can be treated with the PDL or KTP laser. An article reported combining electrosurgery for individual lesion with fractional CO_2 laser and PDL (176).

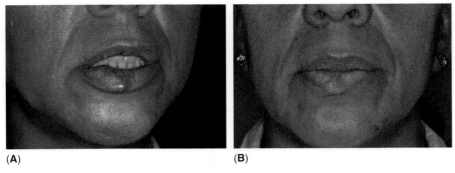

Figure 2.24 Venous lake (**A**) before and (**B**) after treatments with alexandrite laser (70 J/cm², 8 mm, 3 ms, 90 ms spray and 80 ms delay with cryogen spray).

Fibrous papules in adults can be treated with vascular-specific lasers or erbium:YAG/CO₂ lasers. More erythematous lesions respond well to KTP and PDL, whereas more flesh-colored lesions respond best to small spot applications of the erbium:YAG and CO₂ lasers.

Striae Rubra
These lesions respond well to purpuric settings with the PDL, particularly in lighter patients. We typically use 5–6 J/cm² with 1.5 ms, 595 nm, and a 10 mm spot. For narrower lesions, 5 and 7 mm spots can be applied.

Sebaceous Hyperplasia
These lesions may be treated with vascular lasers. In this case, one is exploiting the small telangiectasia that tends to course through the lesions, the blood vessel readily apparent upon dermoscopy. KTP and PDL have been used. We usually use the 3 mm spot PDL with purpuric settings (15 J/cm², 1.5 ms with DCD). Alternatively, we have used nonpurpuric settings with the PDL or the KTP laser with a 2 mm spot (15 J/cm², 15 ms; no cooling) with repeated stacked pulses at 1.5 Hz until the lesion undergoes a transition from yellow to a gray white color. The endpoint here is the production of a limited degree of nonspecific thermal damage to destroy the sebaceous gland. Photodynamic therapy is also useful in conjunction with the PDL. With PDT, the porphyrin (usually ALA or MALA) is absorbed by the sebaceous gland and is activated by the PDL and/or the blue, red, and/or IPL light sources (see chap. 3 on PDT).

Ecchymosis
Ecchymosis (177) has been treated with the PDL with nonpurpuric settings. Normally, a fluence of 5–6 J/cm² is applied at 595 nm with one to two passes (not stacked), 10 ms, and cooling. Care should be taken to not apply too high a fluence. The blood fraction in the dermis is quite high and these lesions are susceptible to blistering and even scarring. The most common application for this scenario is postfiller bruising. Early intervention (within 2 days of the bruise onset) will typically clear the purpura within 1 to 3 days. The IPL can also be used with similar minimally purpuric settings and has been shown to be as effective as the PDL.

Inflammatory Skin Diseases
A number of inflammatory skin diseases where the vasculature is the primary target have been treated with PDL. For example, lupus erythematosis, psoriasis, granuloma annulare, necrobiosis lipodica diabeticorum, granuloma faciale, lymphangioma circumscriptum, have all been treated with the PDL (178). We have found that purpuric settings work best for these conditions. Newer-generation IPLs with shorter pulse durations that allow for purpuric settings most likely could be used for all of these applications. Psoriasis has been treated in a number of studies. Typical settings are 5–9 J/cm² with the PDL at 0.45–1.5 ms. Hern et al. (179) studied the vascular response in plaques and found a reduction in vessel density and width. Most of these studies were conducted in the absence of surface cooling and pain was a limitation in some patients. On a practical level, PDL is best reserved for those patients with a few refractory red lesions.

Molluscum Contagiosum
In a study 19 patients were treated with PDL at setting ranging from 6 to 7 J/cm², 0.45 ms, 7 mm spot. Almost all patients responded to one treatment session (180).

Verrucous Hemangioma
Verrucous hemangioma normally occurs on the lower extremities. The lesions comprise a deeper hemangioma component and a more superficial angiokeratoma component. A recent report showed successful reduction (181) in the thickness and redness of the lesions after sequential CW CO₂ laser and 595–1064 nm laser.

Verruca Vulgaris
Verrucae represent benign tumors of epidermal cells induced by the human papillomavirus. They occur in about 10% of adults and children. To maintain a proliferative growth, neovascularization is stimulated. This is reflected histologically in prominent, dilated blood vessels in dermal papillae. Theoretically, vaporization and coagulation of the new capillaries should halt viral replication and promote verrucae resolution. The PDL has been used for about 18 years for warts. Multiple studies support its use (182–187). Biopsies suggest that both melanin at the dermal–epidermal junction and capillaries are the targets for 595 nm light. In our experience aggressive settings achieve the best results (12–15 J/cm² with 5 and 7 mm spots) without DCD (Fig. 2.25). Two to four pulses are given until the lesion turns gray. Flatter lesions in cosmetically conspicuous areas (face and backs of hands) should be treated at lower fluences and a smaller number of pulses, as scarring and long-term pigment changes are possible with PDL. We treat aggressively about the nails and on the palmar and planate surfaces as these areas tend to heal quickly and any long-term pigment changes are usually inconspicuous. Pain can be severe and can be mitigated by topical

32. Goldman MP, Sadick NS, Weiss RA. Treatment of spider veins with the 595 nm pulsed-dye laser. J Am Acad Dermatol 2000; 42: 849–50.

33. Goldman MP, Bennett RG. Treatment of telangiectasia: a review. J Am Acad Dermatol 1987; 17: 167–82.

34. Goldman M. Sclerotherapy: Treatment of Varicose and Telangiectatic Leg Veins, 2nd edn. Sr. Louis: CV Mosby, 1995.

35. Raulin C, Weiss RA, Schonermark MP. Treatment of essential telangiectasias with an intense pulsed light source (PhotoDerm VL). Dermatol Surg 1997; 23: 941–5; discussion 945–946.

36. Schmidt N, Gans E. Deodex and rosacea I: the prevalence and numbers of Demodex mites in rosacea. Cosmet Dermatol 2004; 17: 497–502.

37. Prieto VG, Sadick NS, Lloreta J, Nicholson J, Shea CR. Effects of intense pulsed light on sun-damaged human skin, routine, and ultrastructural analysis. Lasers Surg Med 2002; 30: 82–5.

38. Dahl MV, Ross AJ, Schlievert PM. Temperature regulates bacterial protein production: possible role in rosacea. J Am Acad Dermatol 2004; 50: 266–72.

39. Baglieri F, Scuderi G. Treatment of recalcitrant granulomatous rosacea with ALA-PDT: report of a case. Indian J Dermatol Venereol Leprol 2011; 77: 536.

40. Menezes N, Moreira A, Mota G, Baptista A. Quality of life and rosacea: pulsed dye laser impact. J Cosmet Laser Ther 2009; 11: 139–41.

41. Laube S, Lanigan SW. Laser treatment of rosacea. J Cosmet Dermatol 2002; 1: 188–95.

42. Tan SR, Tope WD. Pulsed dye laser treatment of rosacea improves erythema, symptomatology, and quality of life. J Am Acad Dermatol 2004; 51: 592–9.

43. Lowe NJ, Behr KL, Fitzpatrick R, Goldman M, Ruiz-Esparza J. Flash lamp pumped dye laser for rosacea-associated telangiectasia and erythema. J Dermatol Surg Oncol 1991; 17: 522–5.

44. Jasim ZF, Woo WK, Handley JM. Long-pulsed (6-ms) pulsed dye laser treatment of rosacea-associated telangiectasia using subpurpuric clinical threshold. Dermatol Surg 2004; 30: 37–40.

45. Berg M, Edstrom DW. Flashlamp pulsed dye laser (FPDL) did not cure papulopustular rosacea. Lasers Surg Med 2004; 34: 266–8.

46. Mark KA, Sparacio RM, Voigt A, Marenus K, Sarnoff DS. Objective and quantitative improvement of rosacea-associated erythema after intense pulsed light treatment. Dermatol Surg 2003; 29: 600–4.

47. Schroeter CA, Haaf-von Below S, Neumann HA. Effective treatment of rosacea using intense pulsed light systems. Dermatol Surg 2005; 31: 1285–9.

48. Taub AF. Treatment of rosacea with intense pulsed light. J Drugs Dermatol 2003; 2: 254–9.

49. Stamatas GN, Kollias N. Blood stasis contributions to the perception of skin pigmentation. J Biomed Opt 2004; 9: 315–22.

50. Behroozan DS, Goldberg LH, Glaich AS, Dai T, Friedman PM. Fractional photothermolysis for treatment of poikiloderma of Civatte. Dermatol Surg 2006; 32: 298–301.

51. Tierney EP, Hanke CW. Treatment of Poikiloderma of Civatte with ablative fractional laser resurfacing: prospective study and review of the literature. J Drugs Dermatol 2009; 8: 527–34.

52. Weiss RA, Goldman MP, Weiss MA. Treatment of poikiloderma of Civatte with an intense pulsed light source. Dermatol Surg 2000; 26: 823–7; discussion 828.

53. Goldman MP, Weiss RA. Treatment of poikiloderma of Civatte on the neck with an intense pulsed light source. Plast Reconstruct Surg 2001; 107: 1376–81.

54. Willenberg T, Baumgartner I. Vascular birthmarks. Vasa 2008; 37: 5–17.

55. Pasyk KA, Wlodarczyk SR, Jakobczak MM, Kurek M, Aughton DJ. Familial medial telangiectatic nevus: variant of nevus flammeus—port-wine stain. Plast Reconstr Surg 1993; 91: 1032–41.

56. Garzon MC, Enjolras O, Frieden IJ. Vascular tumors and vascular malformations: evidence for an association. J Am Acad Dermatol 2000; 42: 275–9.

57. Leung AK, Telmesani AM. Salmon patches in Caucasian children. Pediatr Dermatol 1989; 6: 185–7.

58. Juern AM, Glick ZR, Drolet BA, Frieden IJ. Nevus simplex: a reconsideration of nomenclature, sites of involvement, and disease associations. J Am Acad Dermatol 2010; 63: 805–14.

59. Adams DM, Lucky AW. Cervicofacial vascular anomalies. I. Hemangiomas and other benign vascular tumors. Semin Pediatr Surg 2006; 15: 124–32.

60. Eubanks LE, McBurney EI. Videomicroscopy of port-wine stains: correlation of location and depth of lesion. J Am Acad Dermatol 2001; 44: 948–51.

61. Eerola I, Boon LM, Mulliken JB, et al. Capillary malformation-arteriovenous malformation, a new clinical and genetic disorder caused by RASA1 mutations. Am J Hum Genet 2003; 73: 1240–9.

62. Hidai C, Zupancic T, Penta K, et al. Cloning and characterization of developmental endothelial locus-1: an embryonic endothelial cell protein that binds the alphavbeta3 integrin receptor. Genes Dev 1998; 12: 21–33.

63. Stier MF, Glick SA, Hirsch RJ. Laser treatment of pediatric vascular lesions: port wine stains and hemangiomas. J Am Acad Dermatol 2008; 58: 261–85.

64. McClean K, Hanke CW. The medical necessity for treatment of port-wine stains. Dermatol Surg 1997; 23: 663–7.

65. Syed S, Weibel L, Kennedy H, Harper JI. A pilot study showing pulsed-dye laser treatment improves localized areas of chronic atopic dermatitis. Clin Exp Dermatol 2008; 33: 243–8.

66. Sidwell RU, Syed S, Harper JI. Port-wine stains and eczema. Br J Dermatol 2001; 144: 1269–70.

67. Khaier A, Nischal KK, Espinosa M, Manoj B. Periocular port wine stain: the great Ormond street hospital experience. Ophthalmology 2011; 118: 2274–2278, e2271.

68. Tallman B, Tan OT, Morelli JG, et al. Location of port-wine stains and the likelihood of ophthalmic and/or central nervous system complications. Pediatrics 1991; 87: 323–7.

69. Comi AM, Bellamkonda S, Ferenc LM, Cohen BA, Germain-Lee EL. Central hypothyroidism and Sturge-Weber syndrome. Pediatr Neurol 2008; 39: 58–62.

70. Tan E, Vinciullo C. Pulsed dye laser treatment of port-wine stains: a review of patients treated in Western Australia. Med J Aust 1996; 164: 333–6.

71. Masclarelli P. Living with a port wine stain. In: Tan O, ed. Management and Treatment of Benign Cutaneous Lesions. Philadelphia: Lea and Febiger, 1992.

72. Schiffner R, Brunnberg S, Hohenleutner U, Stolz W, Landthaler M. Willingness to pay and time trade-off: useful utility indicators for the assessment of quality of life and patient satisfaction in patients with port wine stains. Br J Dermatol 2002; 146: 440–7.

73. O'Donnell J, Sell S, Rauso L, Goode J. Undisclosed port-wine stain—anesthetic implications and psychosocial considerations: a case report. Aana J 2001; 69: 206–10.

74. Troilius A, Wrangsjo B, Ljunggren B. Patients with port-wine stains and their psychosocial reactions after photothermolytic treatment. Dermatol Surg 2000; 26: 190–6.

75. Augustin M, Zschocke I, Wiek K, Peschen M, Vanscheidt W. Psychosocial stress of patients with port wine stains and expectations of dye laser treatment. Dermatology 1998; 197: 353–60.

76. Troilius A, Wrangsjo B, Ljunggren B. Potential psychological benefits from early treatment of port-wine stains in children. Br J Dermatol 1998; 139: 59–65.

77. Reyes BA, Geronemus R. Treatment of port-wine stains during childhood with the flashlamp-pumped pulsed dye laser. J Am Acad Dermatol 1990; 23: 1142–8.

78. Chapas AM, Eickhorst K, Geronemus RG. Efficacy of early treatment of facial port wine stains in newborns: a review of 49 cases. Lasers Surg Med 2007; 39: 563–8.

79. Chapas AM, Geronemus RG. Our approach to pediatric dermatologic laser surgery. Lasers Surg Med 2005; 37: 255–63.

80. Clodius L. Plastic surgery therapy of extensive port-wine stain of the face. Schweiz Med Wochenschr 1983; 113: 274–80.

81. Clodius L. Surgery for the extensive facial port-wine stain? Aesthetic Plast Surg 1985; 9: 61–8.

82. Clodius L. Surgery for the facial port-wine stain: technique and results. Ann Plast Surg 1986; 16: 457–71.

83. Natkunarajah J, Cliff S. Thorium X treatment: multiple basal cell carcinomas within a port-wine stain. Clin Exp Dermatol 2009; 34: e189–91.

84. Hidano A, Ogihara Y. Cryotherapy with solid carbon dioxide in the treatment of nevus flammeus. J Dermatol Surg Oncol 1977; 3: 213–16.

85. Wimmershoff MB, Schreyer AG, Glaessl A, et al. Mixed capillary/lymphatic malformation with coexisting port-wine stain: treatment utilizing 3D MRI and CT-guided sclerotherapy. Dermatol Surg 2000; 26: 584–7.

86. Conway H. The permanent camouflage of port-wine stain of the face by intradermal injection of insoluble pigments; tattooing. N Y State J Med 1948; 48: 2040–3.

87. Xiao Q, Li Q, Yuan KH, Cheng B. Photodynamic therapy of port-wine stains: Long-term efficacy and complication in Chinese patients. J Dermatol 2011; 38: 1146–52.

88. Buecker JW, Ratz JL, Richfield DF. Histology of port-wine stain treated with carbon dioxide laser. A preliminary report. J Am Acad Dermatol 1984; 10: 1014–19.

89. Jonell R, Larko O. Clinical effect of the copper vapour laser compared to previously used argon laser on cutaneous vascular lesions. Acta Derm Venereol 1994; 74: 210–11.

90. Kono T, Frederick Groff W, Chan HH, Sakurai H, Yamaki T. Long-pulsed neodymium:yttrium-aluminum-garnet laser treatment for hypertrophic port-wine stains on the lips. J Cosmet Laser Ther 2009; 11: 11–13.

91. McCafferty DF, Woolfson AD, Handley J, Allen G. Effect of percutaneous local anaesthetics on pain reduction during pulse dye laser treatment of portwine stains. Br J Anaesth 1997; 78: 286–9.

92. Peker E, Cagan E, Dogan M, et al. Methemoglobinemia due to local anesthesia with prilocaine for circumcision. J Paediatr Child Health 2010; 46: 362–3.

93. Davidson AJ. Anesthesia and neurotoxicity to the developing brain: the clinical relevance. Paediatr Anaesth 2011; 21: 716–21.

94. Jia W, Sun V, Tran N, et al. Long-term blood vessel removal with combined laser and topical rapamycin antiangiogenic therapy: implications for effective port wine stain treatment. Lasers Surg Med 2010; 42: 105–12.

95. Nelson JS, Jia W, Phung TL, Mihm MC Jr. Observations on enhanced port wine stain blanching induced by combined pulsed dye laser and rapamycin administration. Lasers Surg Med 2011; 43: 939–42.

96. Loewe R, Oble DA, Valero T, et al. Stem cell marker upregulation in normal cutaneous vessels following pulsed-dye laser exposure and its abrogation by concurrent rapamycin administration: implications for treatment of port-wine stain birthmarks. J Cutan Pathol 2010; 37: 76–82.

97. Hudson CC, Liu M, Chiang GG, et al. Regulation of hypoxia-inducible factor 1alpha expression and function by the mammalian target of rapamycin. Mol Cell Biol 2002; 22: 7004–14.

98. Bertrand J, Sammour R, McCuaig C, et al. Propranolol in the treatment of problematic infantile hemangioma: review of 35 consecutive patients from a vascular anomalies clinic. J Cutan Med Surg 2012; 16: 115–21.

99. Moehrle M, Leaute-Labreze C, Schmidt V, et al. Topical timolol for small hemangiomas of infancy. Pediatr Dermatol 2012. doi: 10.1111/j.1525-1470.2012.01723.x

100. Minkis K, Geronemus RG, Hale EK. Port wine stain progression: a potential consequence of delayed and inadequate treatment? Lasers Surg Med 2009; 41: 423–6.

101. Chapas AM, Geronemus RG. Physiologic changes in vascular birthmarks during early infancy: mechanisms and clinical implications. J Am Acad Dermatol 2009; 61: 1081–2.

102. Bencini PL. The multilayer technique: A new and fast approach for flashlamp-pumped pulsed (FLPP) dye laser treatment of port-wine stains (preliminary reports). Dermatol Surg 1999; 25: 786–9.

103. Rajaratnam R, Laughlin SA, Dudley D. Pulsed dye laser double-pass treatment of patients with resistant capillary malformations. Lasers Med Sci 2011; 26: 487–92.

104. Tanghetti EA, Sherr EA, Alvarado SL. Multipass treatment of photodamage using the pulse dye laser. Dermatol Surg 2003; 29: 686–90; discussion 690–681.

105. Peters MA, van Drooge AM, Wolkerstorfer A, et al. Double pass 595 nm pulsed dye laser at a 6 minute interval for the treatment of port-wine stains is not more effective than single pass. Lasers Surg Med 2012; 44: 199–204.

106. Franco W, Childers M, Nelson JS, Aguilar G. Laser surgery of port wine stains using local vacuum [corrected] pressure: changes in calculated energy deposition (Part II). Lasers Surg Med 2007; 39: 118–27.

107. Childers MA, Franco W, Nelson JS, Aguilar G. Laser surgery of port wine stains using local vacuum pressure: changes in skin morphology and optical properties (Part I). Lasers Surg Med 2007; 39: 108–17.

108. Kautz G, Kautz I, Segal J, Zehren S. Treatment of resistant port wine stains (PWS) with pulsed dye laser and non-contact vacuum: a pilot study. Lasers Med Sci 2010; 25: 525–9.

109. Mariwalla K, Dover JS. The use of lasers in the pediatric population. Skin Therapy Lett 2005; 10: 7–9.

110. Quan SY, Comi AM, Parsa CF, et al. Effect of a single application of pulsed dye laser treatment of port-wine birthmarks on intraocular pressure. Arch Dermatol 2010; 146: 1015–18.

111. Eppley BL, Sadove AM. Systemic effects of photothermolysis of large port-wine stains in infants and children. Plast Reconstr Surg 1994; 93: 1150–3.

112. Renfro L, Geronemus RG. Anatomical differences of port-wine stains in response to treatment with the pulsed dye laser. Arch Dermatol 1993; 129: 182–8.

113. Tan OT, Sherwood K, Gilchrest BA. Treatment children with port-wine stains using flashlamp pulsed tunable dye laser. N Eng J Med 1989; 320: 416.

114. Nguyen CM, Yohn JJ, Huff C, Weston WL, Morelli JG. Facial port wine stains in childhood: prediction of the rate of improvement as a function of the age of the patient, size and location of the port wine stain and the number of treatments with the pulsed dye (585 nm) laser. Br J Dermatol 1998; 138: 821–5.

115. Yohn JJ, Huff JC, Aeling JL, Walsh P, Morelli JG. Lesion size is a factor for determining the rate of port-wine stain clearing following pulsed dye laser treatment in adults. Cutis 1997; 59: 267–70.

116. Morelli JG, Weston WL, Huff JC, Yohn JJ. Initial lesion size as a predictive factor in determining the response of port-wine stains in children treated with the pulsed dye laser. Arch Pediatr Adolesc Med 1995; 149: 1142–4.

117. Goldman MP, Fitzpatrick RE, Ruiz-Esparza J. Treatment of port-wine stains (capillary malformation) with the flashlamp-pumped pulsed dye laser. J Pediatr 1993; 122: 71–7.

118. Ashinoff R, Geronemus RG. Flashlamp-pumped pulsed dye laser for port-wine stains in infancy: earlier versus later treatment. J Am Acad Dermatol 1991; 24: 467–72.

119. Alster TS, Wilson F. Treatment of port-wine stains with the flashlamp-pumped pulsed dye laser: extended clinical experience in children and adults. Ann Plast Surg 1994; 32: 478–84.

120. Orten SS, Waner M, Flock S, Roberson PK, Kincannon J. Port-wine stains. An assessment of 5 years of treatment. Arch Otolaryngol Head Neck Surg 1996; 122: 1174–9.

121. Katugampola GA, Lanigan SW. Five years' experience of treating port wine stains with the flashlamp-pumped pulsed dye laser. Br J Dermatol 1997; 137: 750–4.

122. Dierickx CC, Casparian JM, Venugopalan V, Farinelli WA, Anderson RR. Thermal relaxation of port-wine stain vessels probed in vivo: the need for 1-10-millisecond laser pulse treatment. J Invest Dermatol 1995; 105: 709–14.

123. Izikson L, Nelson JS, Anderson RR. Treatment of hypertrophic and resistant port wine stains with a 755 nm laser: a case series of 20 patients. Lasers Surg Med 2009; 41: 427–32.

124. Randeberg LL, Bonesronning JH, Dalaker M, Nelson JS, Svaasand LO. Methemoglobin formation during laser induced photothermolysis of vascular skin lesions. Lasers Surg Med 2004; 34: 414–19.

125. Civas E, Koc E, Aksoy B, Aksoy HM. Clinical experience in the treatment of different vascular lesions using a neodymium-doped yttrium aluminum garnet laser. Dermatol Surg 2009; 35: 1933–41.

126. Faurschou A, Olesen AB, Leonardi-Bee J, Haedersdal M. Lasers or light sources for treating port-wine stains. Cochrane Database Syst Rev 2011; 11: CD007152.

127. Geronemus RG. Long-pulsed neodymium:yttrium-aluminum-garnet laser treatment for port wine stains. J Am Acad Dermatol 2006; 54: 923.

128. Zhao Y, Zhou Z, Zhou G, et al. Efficacy and safety of hemoporfin in photodynamic therapy for port-wine stain: a multicenter and open-labeled phase IIa study. Photodermatol Photoimmunol Photomed 2011; 27: 17–23.

129. Lu YG, Wu JJ, Yang YD, Yang HZ, He Y. Photodynamic therapy of port-wine stains. J Dermatolog Treat 2010; 21: 240–4.

130. Huang N, Cheng G, Li X, et al. Influence of drug-light-interval on photodynamic therapy of port wine stains—simulation and validation of mathematic models. Photodiagnosis Photodyn Ther 2008; 5: 120–6.

131. Qiu H, Gu Y, Wang Y, Huang N. Twenty years of clinical experience with a new modality of vascular-targeted photodynamic therapy for port wine stains. Dermatol Surg 2011; 37: 1603–10.

132. Li W, Yamada I, Masumoto K, Ueda Y, Hashimoto K. Photodynamic therapy with intradermal administration of 5-aminolevulinic acid for port-wine stains. J Dermatolog Treat 2010; 21: 232–9.

133. Jasim ZF, Handley JM. Treatment of pulsed dye laser-resistant port wine stain birthmarks. J Am Acad Dermatol 2007; 57: 677–82.

134. Huikeshoven M, Koster PH, de Borgie CA, et al. Redarkening of port-wine stains 10 years after pulsed-dye-laser treatment. N Engl J Med 2007; 356: 1235–40.

135. Esterly NB. Cutaneous hemangiomas, vascular stains and malformations, and associated syndromes. Curr Probl Pediatr 1996; 26: 3–39.

136. Burton BK, Schulz CJ, Angle B, Burd LI. An increased incidence of haemangiomas in infants born following chorionic villus sampling (CVS). Prenat Diagn 1995; 15: 209–14.

137. Amir J, Metzker A, Krikler R, Reisner SH. Strawberry hemangioma in preterm infants. Pediatr Dermatol 1986; 3: 331–2.

138. North PE, Waner M, Mizeracki A, Mihm MC Jr. GLUT1: a newly discovered immunohistochemical marker for juvenile hemangiomas. Hum Pathol 2000; 31: 11–22.

139. Boscolo E, Bischoff J. Vasculogenesis in infantile hemangioma. Angiogenesis 2009; 12: 197–207.

140. Chang LC, Haggstrom AN, Drolet BA, et al. Growth characteristics of infantile hemangiomas: implications for management. Pediatrics 2008; 122: 360–7.

141. Bivings L. Spontaneous regression of angiomas in children; twenty-two years' observation covering 236 cases. J Pediatr 1954; 45: 643–7.

142. Garzon MC, Frieden IJ. Hemangiomas: when to worry. Pediatr Ann 2000; 29: 58–67.

143. Garzon M. Hemangiomas: update on classification, clinical presentation, and associated anomalies. Cutis 2000; 66: 325–8.

144. Chiller KG, Passaro D, Frieden IJ. Hemangiomas of infancy: clinical characteristics, morphologic subtypes, and their relationship to race, ethnicity, and sex. Arch Dermatol 2002; 138: 1567–76.

145. Haggstrom AN, Lammer EJ, Schneider RA, Marcucio R, Frieden IJ. Patterns of infantile hemangiomas: new clues to hemangioma pathogenesis and embryonic facial development. Pediatrics 2006; 117: 698–703.

146. Haggstrom AN, Drolet BA, Baselga E, et al. Prospective study of infantile hemangiomas: demographic, prenatal, and perinatal characteristics. J Pediatr 2007; 150: 291–4.

147. Tanner JL, Dechert MP, Frieden IJ. Growing up with a facial hemangioma: parent and child coping and adaptation. Pediatrics 1998; 101: 446–52.

148. Frieden IJ, Reese V, Cohen D. PHACE syndrome. The association of posterior fossa brain malformations, hemangiomas, arterial anomalies, coarctation of the aorta and cardiac defects, and eye abnormalities. Arch Dermatol 1996; 132: 307–11.

149. Ceisler EJ, Santos L, Blei F. Periocular hemangiomas: what every physician should know. Pediatr Dermatol 2004; 21: 1–9.

150. Goldberg NS, Hebert AA, Esterly NB. Sacral hemangiomas and multiple congenital abnormalities. Arch Dermatol 1986; 122: 684–7.

151. Geller JD, Topper SF, Hashimoto K. Diffuse neonatal hemangiomatosis: a new constellation of findings. J Am Acad Dermatol 1991; 24: 816–18.

152. Holden KR, Alexander F. Diffuse neonatal hemangiomatosis. Pediatrics 1970; 46: 411–21.

153. Enjolras O, Wassef M, Mazoyer E, et al. Infants with Kasabach-Merritt syndrome do not have "true" hemangiomas. J Pediatr 1997; 130: 631–40.

154. Frieden IJ, Haggstrom AN, Drolet BA, et al. Infantile hemangiomas: current knowledge, future directions. Proceedings of a research workshop on infantile hemangiomas; Bethesda, Maryland, USA, April 7-9, 2005. Pediatr Dermatol 2005. 22(5):383–406.

155. Kim HJ, Colombo M, Frieden IJ. Ulcerated hemangiomas: clinical characteristics and response to therapy. J Am Acad Dermatol 2001; 44: 962–72.

156. Morelli JG, Tan OT, Weston WL. Treatment of ulcerated hemangiomas with the pulsed tunable dye laser. Am J Dis Child 1991; 145: 1062–4.

157. David LR, Malek MM, Argenta LC. Efficacy of pulse dye laser therapy for the treatment of ulcerated haemangiomas: a review of 78 patients. Br J Plast Surg 2003; 56: 317–27.

158. Ezekowitz RA, Mulliken JB, Folkman J. Interferon alfa-2a therapy for life-threatening hemangiomas of infancy. N Engl J Med 1992; 326: 1456–63.

159. Barlow CF, Priebe CJ, Mulliken JB, et al. Spastic diplegia as a complication of interferon Alfa-2a treatment of hemangiomas of infancy. J Pediatr 1998; 132: 527–30.

160. Jiang C, Hu X, Ma G, et al. A prospective self-controlled phase II study of imiquimod 5% cream in the treatment of infantile hemangioma. Pediatr Dermatol 2011; 28: 259–66.

161. Bassukas ID, Abuzahra F, Hundeiker M. Regression phase as therapeutic goal of cryosurgical treatment of growing capillary infantile hemangiomas. Treatment decision, treatment strategy and results of an open clinical study. Hautarzt 2000; 51: 231–8.

162. Leaute-Labreze C, Dumas de la Roque E, Hubiche T, et al. Propranolol for severe hemangiomas of infancy. N Engl J Med 2008; 358: 2649–51.

163. Jinnin M, Medici D, Park L, et al. Suppressed NFAT-dependent VEGFR1 expression and constitutive VEGFR2 signaling in infantile hemangioma. Nat Med 2008; 14: 1236–46.

164. Pope E, Chakkittakandiyil A. Topical timolol gel for infantile hemangiomas: a pilot study. Arch Dermatol 2010; 146: 564–5.

165. Garden JM, Bakus AD, Paller AS. Treatment of cutaneous hemangiomas by the flashlamp-pumped pulsed dye laser: prospective analysis. J Pediatr 1992; 120: 555–60.

166. Barlow RJ, Walker NP, Markey AC. Treatment of proliferative haemangiomas with the 585 nm pulsed dye laser. Br J Dermatol 1996; 134: 700–4.

167. Hohenleutner U, Landthaler M. Laser treatment of childhood haemangioma: progress or not? Lancet 2002; 360: 502–3.

168. Batta K, Goodyear HM, Moss C, et al. Randomised controlled study of early pulsed dye laser treatment of uncomplicated childhood haemangiomas: results of a 1-year analysis. Lancet 2002; 360: 521–7.

169. Batta K, Goodyear HM, Moss C, et al. Randomised controlled study of early pulsed dye laser treatment of uncomplicated childhood haemangiomas: results of a 1-year analysis. Lancet 2002; 360: 521–7.

170. Leonardi-Bee J, Batta K, O'Brien C, Bath-Hextall FJ. Interventions for infantile haemangiomas (strawberry birthmarks) of the skin. Cochrane Database Syst Rev: CD006545.

171. Raulin C, Greve B. Retrospective clinical comparison of hemangioma treatment by flashlamp-pumped (585 nm) and frequency-doubled Nd:YAG (532 nm) lasers.[erratum appears in Lasers Surg Med 2001;29(3):293]. Lasers Surg Med 2001; 28: 40–3.

172. Berlien HP, Muller G, Waldschmidt J. Lasers in pediatric surgery. Prog Pediatr Surg 1990; 25: 5–22.

173. Alcantara Gonzalez J, Boixeda P, Truchuelo Diez MT, Lopez Gutierrez JC, Olasolo PJ. Ablative fractional yttrium-scandium-gallium-garnet laser for scarring residual haemangiomas and scars secondary to their surgical treatment. J Eur Acad Dermatol Venereol 2012; 26: 477–82.

174. Antony FC, Cliff S, Cowley N. Complete pain relief following treatment of a glomangiomyoma with the pulsed dye laser. Clin Exp Dermatol 2003; 28: 617–19.

175. Hughes R, Lacour JP, Chiaverini C, Rogopoulos A, Passeron T. Nd:YAG laser treatment for multiple cutaneous glomangiomas: report of 3 cases. Arch Dermatol 2011; 147: 255–6.

176. Weiss ET, Geronemus RG. New technique using combined pulsed dye laser and fractional resurfacing for treating facial angiofibromas in tuberous sclerosis. Lasers Surg Med 2010; 42: 357–60.

177. Karen JK, Hale EK, Geronemus RG. A simple solution to the common problem of ecchymosis. Arch Dermatol 2010; 146: 94–5.

178. Karsai S, Roos S, Hammes S, Raulin C. Pulsed dye laser: what's new in non-vascular lesions? J Eur Acad Dermatol Venereol 2007; 21: 877–90.

179. Hern S, Allen MH, Sousa AR, et al. Immunohistochemical evaluation of psoriatic plaques following selective photothermolysis of the superficial capillaries. Br J Dermatol 2001; 145: 45–53.

180. Binder B, Weger W, Komericki P, Kopera D. Treatment of molluscum contagiosum with a pulsed dye laser: Pilot study with 19 children. J Dtsch Dermatol Ges 2008; 6: 121–5.

181. Segura Palacios JM, Boixeda P, Rocha J, et al. Laser treatment for verrucous hemangioma. Lasers Med Sci 2012; 27: 681–4.

182. Sethuraman G, Richards KA, Hiremagalore RN, Wagner A. Effectiveness of pulsed dye laser in the treatment of recalcitrant warts in children. Dermatol Surg 2010; 36: 58–65.

183. Schellhaas U, Gerber W, Hammes S, Ockenfels HM. Pulsed dye laser treatment is effective in the treatment of recalcitrant viral warts. Dermatol Surg 2008; 34: 67–72.

184. Park HS, Kim JW, Jang SJ, Choi JC. Pulsed dye laser therapy for pediatric warts. Pediatr Dermatol 2007; 24: 177–81.

185. Borovoy MA, Borovoy M, Elson LM, Sage M. Flashlamp pulsed dye laser (585 nm). Treatment of resistant verrucae. J Am Podiatr Med Assoc 1996; 86: 547–50.

186. Webster GF, Satur N, Goldman MP, Halmi B, Greenbaum S. Treatment of recalcitrant warts using the pulsed dye laser. Cutis 1995; 56: 230–2.

187. Tan OT, Hurwitz RM, Stafford TJ. Pulsed dye laser treatment of recalcitrant verrucae: a preliminary report. Lasers Surg Med 1993; 13: 127–37.

188. Togsverd-Bo K, Gluud C, Winkel P, et al. Paring and intense pulsed light versus paring alone for recalcitrant hand and foot warts: a randomized clinical trial with blinded outcome evaluation. Lasers Surg Med 2010; 42: 179–84.

189. Han TY, Lee JH, Lee CK, et al. Long-pulsed Nd:YAG laser treatment of warts: report on a series of 369 cases. J Korean Med Sci 2009; 24: 889–93.

190. Kalil CL, Salenave PR, Cignachi S. Hand warts successfully treated with topical 5-aminolevulinic acid and intense pulsed light. Eur J Dermatol 2008; 18: 207–8.

191. Lai CH, Hanson SG, Mallory SB. Lymphangioma circumscriptum treated with pulsed dye laser. Pediatr Dermatol 2001; 18: 509–10.

192. Lee CT, Tham SN, Tan T. Initial experience with CO_2 laser in treating dermatological conditions. Ann Acad Med Singapore 1987; 16: 713–15.

193. Goldberg DJ, Sciales CW. Pyogenic granuloma in children. Treatment with the flashlamp-pumped pulsed dye laser. J Dermatol Surg Oncol 1991; 17: 960–2.

194. Tan O, Kurban A. Noncongenital benign cutaneous vascular lesions: pulsed dye laser treatment. In: Tan O, ed. Management and Treatment of Benign Cutaneous Vascular Lesions. Philadelphia: Lea and Febiger, 1992.

195. Gonzalez S, Vibhagool C, Falo LD Jr, et al. Treatment of pyogenic granulomas with the 585 nm pulsed dye laser. J Am Acad Dermatol 1996; 35: 428–31.

196. Hammes S, Kaiser K, Pohl L, et al. Pyogenic Granuloma: treatment with the 1,064-nm long-pulsed neodymium-doped yttrium aluminum garnet laser in 20 patients. Dermatol Surg 2012; 38: 918–23.

3   Laser treatment of benign pigmented lesions

Omar A. Ibrahimi and Suzanne L. Kilmer

INTRODUCTION

Significant advances in laser technology have increased the options available for the treatment of benign pigmented lesions. Lasers were first used in the treatment of pigmented lesions by Leon Goldman in the 1960s when he used the ruby laser (694 nm) to treat nevi and tattoos (1,2). The focus then shifted to the use of continuous-wave modalities such as CO_2 laser (10,600 nm) and argon laser (418 and 514 nm). These continuous-wave lasers were used to treat pigmented lesions via nonselective destruction. Due to the lack of selectivity, the results were often unpredictable, with frequent complications such as scarring and pigmentary changes.

A revolutionary advance in the laser treatment of pigmented lesions was made by R. Rox Anderson and John Parrish of the Wellman Center for Photomedicine at Massachusetts General Hospital with the elucidation of the theory of selective photothermolysis (3), which permitted precise and selective microsurgery of pigmented lesions. The Wellman group also developed fractional photothermolysis (4), which reintroduced the ability to nonselectively improve the appearance of certain types of undesirable pigment in a safe manner.

THE PRINCIPLE OF SELECTIVE PHOTOTHERMOLYSIS

Selective destruction of human epidermis with lasers using melanin as the target chromophore was first demonstrated in the early 1960s (1,2) using a normal-mode ruby laser (wavelength 694 nm and pulse width 500 µs). A subsequent study with the Q-switched (QS) ruby laser using a 50-ns pulse width showed the threshold radiant exposure to be 10–100 times lower, suggesting a more selective effect of the shorter pulse width (5). For the next 20 years, this work was largely overlooked, until the emergence of Anderson and Parrish's theory of selective photothermolysis (3,6–10). The theory of selective photothermolysis redirected attention to the concept of treating a specific target or chromophore (melanin and hemoglobin) with specific laser parameters (wavelength, pulse width, and energy level). Wavelength selectivity limits absorption to a specific target chromophore. Thermal damage is then confined to that target by limiting the pulse width to less than or equal to the thermal relaxation time of the target chromophore. Once the pulse width is determined, energy levels can be optimized to achieve a desired effect. Application of the theory of selective photothermolysis facilitates the selection of the most appropriate laser for various pigmented lesions, without the high rates of complications and recurrence noted with destructive, continuous-wave modalities. For example, melanocytes or melanin-containing keratinocytes are best

targeted with a QS laser with pulse widths in the nanosecond domain, whereas longer pulse widths used in lasers for hair removal better target clumped melanin such as hair shafts. In both cases, when appropriate settings are used the risk of dyspigmentation and scarring is rare.

CLINICAL TECHNIQUE
Lasers and Light Sources
Continuous-Wave Lasers

The continuous-wave lasers used include argon (488 and 514 nm), green light (532 nm), and CO_2 (10,600 nm) lasers. These continuous-wave lasers are useful only for epidermal lesions because the thermal injury that accompanies their use often leads to scarring when applied to dermal lesions. When each individual lesion is treated, a nonspecific thermal damage results in its destruction with subsequent denuding of the epidermis. The lesion's destruction may be followed by erythema as well as pigmentary and textural changes, but the skin generally heals with excellent cosmetic results.

QS Lasers

The QS laser systems used for the treatment of superficial pigmented lesions include the 532-nm frequency-doubled (FD) QS Nd:YAG, the 694-nm ruby, and the 755-nm alexandrite lasers. Strong absorption of light at these wavelengths by melanin and the nanosecond pulse duration make these lasers an excellent treatment modality for superficial and some dermal pigmented lesions in which the melanin is finely distributed. The QS ruby, alexandrite, and 1064-nm Nd:YAG lasers may be useful for treating deeper pigmented lesions such as nevi of Ota and tattoos (11). The 1064-nm QS Nd:YAG laser should be used when treating darker skin types, because it greatly reduces the risk of epidermal injury and pigmentary alteration. In addition to QS lasers, current research is focused on the development of picosecond lasers which may be beneficial in the treatment of pigmented lesions (12,13).

Long Pulsed Lasers

To better target hair follicles (which are larger melanin-containing targets), lasers with longer (millisecond range) pulse durations were developed. These systems include the long-pulsed ruby (694 nm), alexandrite (755 nm), diode (800 or 810 nm), and Nd:YAG (1064 nm) lasers. The millisecond pulse width more closely matches the thermal relaxation time of nested melanocytes, and the collateral thermal damage inflicts a lethal injury to melanocytes that are adjacent to the target area but that might not actually contain melanin at the time of treatment (9,10). Because scarring may result from thermal spread, care should be taken to minimize thermal damage to the surrounding collagen. Scarring is a particular concern in treating large, deeply pigmented lesions such as large congenital nevi, where the bulk of the dermis is taken up by nested melanocytes and an extensive collateral thermal damage can occur to the minimal normal dermis that remains (14,15).

Intense Pulsed Light

The noncoherent, broadband, intense pulsed light (IPL) source has also shown efficacy in the treatment of pigmented lesions. IPL is particularly effective in the treatment of epidermal pigmented lesions, such as lentigines. This modality can also be safely used on darker skin types when used in a double or triple pulsed mode that allows the epidermis to cool between light pulses as well as its low risk of postinflammatory hyperpigmentation.

Fractional Photothermolysis

Fractional photothermolysis is based on the use of laser microbeams to damage or remove an array of thousands of microscopic columns of skin. There are both ablative and non-ablative fractional resurfacing devices. Ablative fractional lasers include CO_2 (10600 nm wavelength) and erbium (Er:YAG, 2940-nm wavelength; Er:YSGG, 2790-nm wavelength), which vaporize an array of small channels through the skin, up to approximately 1.0–1.5 mm deep. Non-ablative fractional resurfacing devices are based on erbium (1540 and 1550 nm) and Nd:YAG lasers (1440 nm), and more recently the thulium laser (1927 nm). Because fractional photothermolysis removes or damages a portion of the treated area, it has the potential to improve certain types of pigmentary aberrations. Advances using this technology for pigmentary disorders are forthcoming.

LESION CLASSIFICATION

To effectively treat pigmented lesions, one must be proficient at diagnostic classification and also be familiar with the histopathological characteristics of the lesion. With this information, the lesion can effectively be categorized according to the depth of the target pigment distribution: epidermal, dermal, or a combination of both. The most suitable device can then be decided upon (Table 3.1).

Pigment Location

Epidermal pigmented lesions include lentigo, café-au-lait macule (CALM), ephelis, junctional nevus, nevus spilus, and seborrheic keratosis (SK). Dermal pigmented lesions include blue nevus and nevus of Ota or Ito. Some pigmented lesions, such as melasma, Becker's nevus, compound nevus, and congenital nevus have both an epidermal and a dermal component. For some pigmented lesions, the target is melanosomes in keratinocytes, whereas in most cases it is melanosomes in melanocytes or the whole melanocyte. In some cases, the spread of thermal damage from pigment-containing melanocytes may be advantageous in targeting adjacent melanocytes

that lack a significant melanin content [(i.e., dermal, compound, or congenital melanocytic nevi (CMN)].

The success of the QS lasers in the realm of pigmented lesions is based on the ability of these lasers to selectively target melanosomes situated within melanocytes and keratinocytes. The melanosome-specific damage is due to the absorption of high-energy, nanosecond laser pulses (6,7). Long-pulsed lasers in the millisecond domain were developed to target pigmented hair. These lasers can also be used to target epidermal and dermal pigment found in larger clumps such as those in nested melanocytes or confluent melanin in the epidermis (8–11,14).

Pigmented Lesion History

A principle that must be strictly adhered to by the laser surgeon is that a pigmented lesion with atypical features should never be treated with laser. Atypical features can be summarized by the acronym ABCDE:

> A = asymmetry
> B = border
> C = color
> D = diameter
> E = evolving

Lesions with atypical features should not be treated with laser and should be evaluated by a dermatologist. A patient with a personal or family history of melanoma or dysplastic nevi should be advised against laser treatment of nevi.

The treatment of CMN remains controversial (16,17), and should not be undertaken without an expertise in laser surgery. It remains unclear whether laser treatment of congenital nevi decreases the risk of malignant transformation, although some argue that decreasing the melanocytic burden reduces the overall risk of the lesion becoming malignant. However, large congenital nevi can also be cosmetically and psychologically challenging and improvement in the appearance of these lesions may greatly benefit the well being of patients with large sized congenital nevi.

LASER TREATMENT FOR EPIDERMAL LESIONS

Epidermal lesions are amenable to treatment with multiple modalities because of their superficial location; virtually all injuries confined to the epidermis heal without scarring. The 532-nm (FD Nd:YAG) and 694-nm (ruby) wavelengths are the most appropriate for epidermal lesions, followed by the 755-nm (alexandrite) and, least effective, the 1064-nm wavelength (long pulse Nd:YAG). Even though less penetrating, the shorter wavelengths are particularly useful because their greater melanin absorption best targets the superficial melanin in keratinocytes and melanocytes. In addition, lesions with less melanin such as lighter lentigines, freckles, or CALMs can still be effectively targeted. Longer pulsed pigment-specific lasers and ablative and non-ablative fractional photothermolysis lasers are also capable of treating epidermal pigmentation, although fractional photothermolysis would be used more appropriately in the context of a diffuse epidermal pigmentary aberration.

Table 3.1 Laser Selection for Different Types of Pigmented Lesions

Pathology	Lesion Type	Preferred Laser Choices
Epidermal	Lentigo	FD QS Nd:YAG (532 nm)
	Café-au-lait macule	QS ruby (694 nm)
	Ephelide	QS alexandrite (755 nm)
	Junctional nevus	LP alexandrite (755 nm)
	Nevus spilus	KTP (532 nm)
	Seborrheic keratosis	QS ruby (694 nm)
Epidermal–dermal	Melasma	QS ruby (694 nm)
		QS alexandrite (755 nm)
		FD QS Nd:YAG (532/1064 nm)
		Erbium (2940 nm)
		CO_2 (10,600 nm)
		IPL
	Becker's nevus	Combination of two lasers
		Hair removal laser appropriate for skin and hair type
		Pigment-specific laser such as QS ruby, alexandrite, or Nd:YAG
Dermal	Congenital nevus	Laser treatment should be undertaken with caution
	Acquired nevus	Laser treatment should be undertaken with caution
		QS ruby (694 nm)
		QS alexandrite (755 nm)
		FD QS Nd:YAG (532/1064 nm)
		LP alexandrite (755 nm)
		Diode (810 nm)
	Nevus of Ito/nevus of Ota	QS ruby (694 nm)
		QS alexandrite (755 nm)
		QS Nd:YAG (532/1064 nm)
	Blue nevus	Laser treatment should be undertaken with caution
		QS ruby (694 nm)
		QS alexandrite (755 nm)
		QS Nd:YAG (1064 nm)

Abbreviations: FD, frequency doubled; KTP, potassium titanyl phosphate; LP, long pulse; QS, Q-switched.

Lentigines

Lentigines are small, irregular but sharply marginated brown macules. Solar lentigo (lentigo senilis) is an acquired lentigo resulting from sun exposure. These lesions increase in number with advancing age and are usually related to the extent of past sun exposure, but are not premalignant. Histologically, these lesions have elongated rete ridges that extend into the underlying papillary dermis. The basal cell layer of the epidermis often shows hypermelanosis with an increased number of basal melanocytes.

Lentigines can also be a component of different cutaneous syndromes, including lentiginosis profusa, Peutz–Jeghers syndrome, Moynahan syndrome, and LEOPARD (multiple lentigines) syndrome. In these syndromes, the histology of the lentigo is identical to that of a normal lentigo simplex, or slightly different, with the finding that basal melanocytes are not always increased in number as with other lentigines. In addition, in Peutz–Jeghers syndrome, the melanosomes are deeply melanized. Giant macromelanosomes are found in the cells of the LEOPARD syndrome.

The three QS lasers and 532-nm potassium titanyl phosphate (KTP) laser have demonstrated efficacy in the clearance of lentigines (15,18–24), as well as the noncoherent, broadband, IPL source (25). For the QS lasers, one should utilize a 2- to 4-mm spot with a fluence that produces brisk whitening without epidermolysis. Owing to concomitant hemoglobin absorption when using the 532-nm wavelength, purpura may ensue. Although the purpura generally resolves, residual erythema may be noted for the first month postoperatively. The 532-nm KTP laser will immediately darken the lesion, which will then peel off approximately 7 days later if on the face and 10–14 days later if on the body. Purpura is not a factor as the longer pulse width does not cause bruising. The IPL should be set so that normal skin pigment is protected, but the treated lesions darken with treatment. A study on Asian patients with lentigines showed that both QS and microsecond, long-pulsed 755-nm alexandrite lasers were equally effective, although the longer pulse width was associated with less postinflammatory hyperpigmentation (26).

Case 1

Lentigo

A 28-year-old woman presented with a lentigo over her left cheek, which had failed to improve with topical hydroquinone and liquid nitrogen treatment (Fig. 3.1A). The treatment plan included IPL, daily application of sunblock, and nightly application of hydroquinone. The lesion was treated at the time of the initial visit with two passes of IPL; the first pass at 32 J/cm^2 and the second one at 36 J/cm^2. At the 5-week follow-up appointment, complete clearing of the lentigo was noted (Fig. 3.1B).

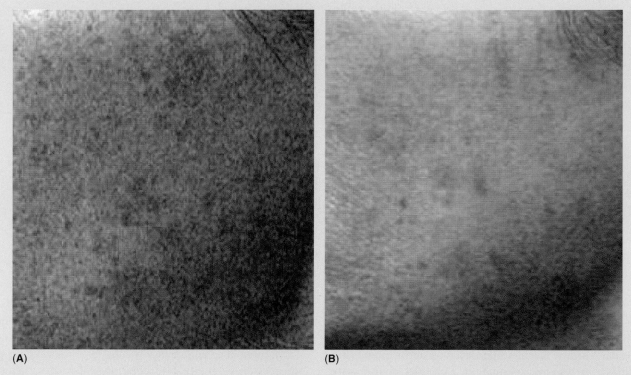

Figure 3.1 Lentigines. (**A**) Before and (**B**) 5 weeks after single intense pulsed light treatment.

Case 2

Lentigines

A 52-year-old man with numerous lentigines over bilateral dorsal forearms presented for discussion of treatment options (Fig. 3.2A). Treatment regimen included QS alexandrite (755 nm) treatment utilizing a 3-mm spot size at a fluence of 7 J/cm^2, in conjunction with strict sun protection. Dramatic clearing of lentigines over the right forearm was noted at 4 weeks post treatment (Fig. 3.2B).

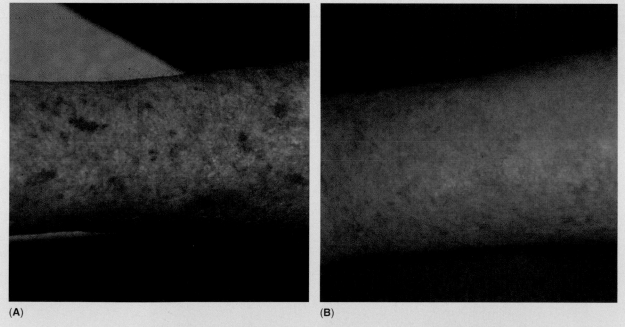

Figure 3.2 Lentigines. (**A**) Before and (**B**) 4 weeks after treatment with QS alexandrite (755 nm).

Case 3

Solar Lentigo

A 48-year-old woman presents with multiple solar lentigines (Fig. 3.3A). Figure 3.3B shows the clinical appearance after one treatment with a QS alexandrite laser at 9 J/cm^2.

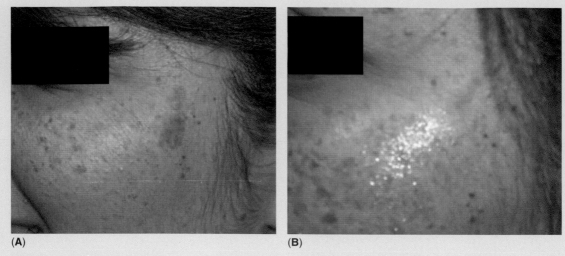

Figure 3.3 (**A**) Multiple solar lentigines. (**B**) Clinical appearance after treatment. *Source*: Photos courtesy of Mitchel P. Goldman, MD.

Ephelides

Ephelides (commonly known as freckles) are well demarcated, tan- to dark-brown macules that occur on sun-exposed skin and darken in response to sunlight. Ephelides appear early in childhood and increase in number during the summer. Their incidence decreases with age. Axillary freckling, the only type that appears on a non–sun-exposed skin, is seen in von Recklinghausen disease (neurofibromatosis).

Histologically, ephelides show normal epidermis without elongation or branching of the rete ridges, as in the case of lentigines. Hypermelanization is generally confined to the basal cell layer. The total number of basal melanocytes does not increase, but melanosomes and melanocytes grow in size and become more active than before (20–22).

Treatment of ephelides usually consists of sunscreen application and sun avoidance. Hydroquinone, alfahydroxy acids, and tretinoin can also diminish freckling if applied regularly. When requested for cosmetic purposes, similar to lentigines, the three QS lasers [QS ruby (694 nm), QS alexandrite (755 nm), and QS FD Nd:YAG (532 nm)] and KTP (532 nm) can be used to treat these lesions (22). Noncoherent, broadband IPL is also an effective modality in the treatment of ephelides (25). Re-exposure to ultraviolet light without adequate sun protection stimulates recurrence and occurrence of new ephelides.

Case 4

Ephelides

A 54-year-old woman with numerous ephelides presented for evaluation and discussion of treatment options (Fig. 3.4A). The ephelides were treated with the QS 532 nm Nd:YAG laser utilizing a 6-mm spot size and a fluence of 1.5 J/cm². Significant improvement was noted at the 6-week follow-up (Fig. 3.4B).

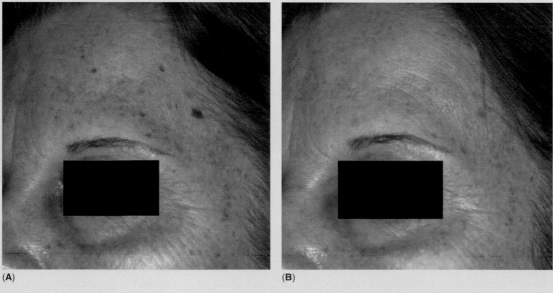

Figure 3.4 Ephelides (**A**) before and (**B**) 6 weeks after treatment with QS 532-nm Nd:YAG.

Seborrheic Keratoses

Seborrheic keratoses are common benign epidermal proliferations that evolve from light-yellow, smooth macules to verrucous pigmented papules or plaques. Although there are several histopathologic variants of SK, the acantholytic type is the most common, consisting of interweaving bands of keratinocytes associated with variable amounts of increased epidermal pigmentation. Dermatosis papulosa nigra is an entity that is clinically and histologically similar to SK and occurs in dark skin types. SK and DPN respond similarly to the lasers discussed for lentigines, but thicker lesions may require additional treatments (22–24). In addition, for thicker lesions, use of the long pulsed alexandrite laser is more effective and requires fewer treatments. However, it is important to note laser therapy has not been shown to be any more effective than treatment with non-laser destructive methods (cryotherapy and electrodessication) (27,28).

Case 5

Seborrheic Keratoses

A 51-year-old man with a history of numerous SKs scattered over his face presented for treatment (Fig. 3.5A). Treatment options were discussed, including liquid nitrogen, electrocautery, and laser treatment. Risks of possible pigmentary change secondary to treatment were emphasized to the patient. A test spot was performed using the QS alexandrite laser at 6.5 J/cm^2 with a 3-mm spot size. When the patient returned 3 weeks later, the treated area was noted to have complete clearance without residual pigmentary change. A larger area over the left forehead was therefore treated at the same settings. Patient returned 6 weeks following treatment and was noted to have significant improvement in his SKs (Fig. 3.5B).

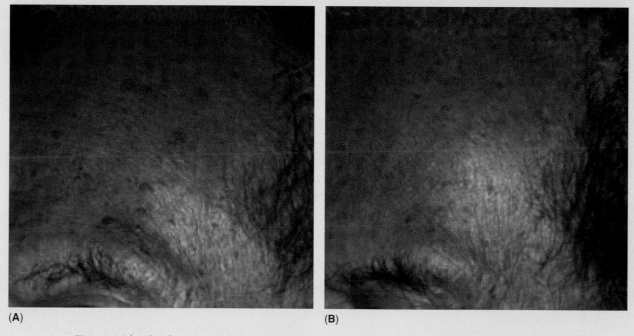

(A) **(B)**

Figure 3.5 Seborrheic keratoses (**A**) before and (**B**) 6 weeks after treatment with the QS alexandrite laser (755 nm).

Café-au-lait Macules

CALMs are light tan to brown hypermelanotic flat lesions that are sharply demarcated from the surrounding normal skin. Found in up to 13.8% of the population, CALMs may appear at birth or soon thereafter and increase in number over the first two decades of life. This lesion may be found in several syndromes, including von Recklinghausen disease, Albright syndrome, and Marfan syndrome.

Histologically, hypermelanosis is present in the basal layer of the epidermis in melanocytes and keratinocytes. Giant melanosomes, present in keratinocytes and basal melanocytes of CALMs in patients with neurofibromatosis, have not been reported in other CALM patients. These lesions are not associated with malignant potential and are commonly treated for cosmetic reasons. The QS ruby (5.0- to 6.5-mm spot size with 5–8 J/cm^2), QS alexandrite (3- to 5-mm spot size with 6–9 J/cm^2), and FD QS Nd:YAG lasers (3- to 4-mm spot size with 1–4 J/cm^2) have been used to treat CALMs (29,30). Longer pulsed alexandrite lasers have been used in hopes of decreasing the recurrence rate and also decreasing the number of treatment sessions required. It is possible that the longer pulse width allows for collateral thermal damage to non–pigment-containing melanocytes. CALMs may recur weeks to months after laser treatment, but are often responsive to re-treatment; in other cases, they can recur years later or can be very resistant to treatment. The variable behavior of CALMs implies a subset of lesions with unique biologic behavior. Repigmentation may occur from normal melanocytes in the normal surrounding skin or from melanocytes that were inactive at the time of treatment. Because the response of these lesions to laser treatment is unpredictable, it is advisable that a test spot be performed prior to treating the entire lesion.

Case 6

Café-au-Lait Macule

A 21-year-old woman with a history of large CALM on her left anterior neck presented for evaluation (Fig. 3.6A). Treatment plan included monthly sessions of treatment with the alexandrite laser (755 nm). At the first treatment session, the lesion was treated with an 8-mm spot and a 50 J/cm² fluence with multiple pulses. When she returned 6 weeks later, 50% clearance of the lesion was noted. The lesion was again treated with an 8-mm spot, 60 J/cm² fluence, and no cooling. When she returned 3 months later, the lesion was noted to be 90% cleared (Fig. 3.6B). The CALM was again treated with the alexandrite laser with an 8-mm spot, a fluence of 60 J/cm², and 50/20 cryogen cooling with three treatments approximately 6 weeks apart to treat the minimal amount of residual pigment.

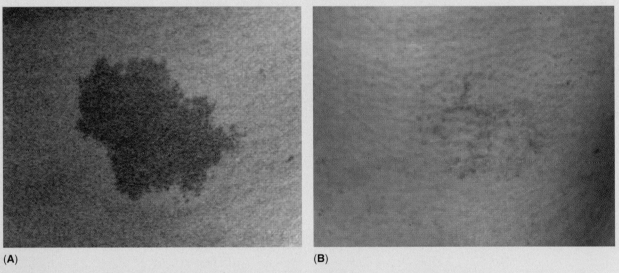

(A)   **(B)**

Figure 3.6 Café-au-lait. (**A**) Before and (**B**) after six treatment sessions with the 755-nm alexandrite laser.

Nevus Spilus

Nevus spilus is a lesion in which darkly pigmented macules or papules lie within a typical CALM. Estimated to occur in 2.3% of patients (male and female equally) visiting a dermatology practice, nevus spilus seems to be concentrated on the trunk and lower extremities. Although nevus spilus is generally not considered to be a precursor of malignant melanoma, several studies have reported cutaneous melanomas within these nevi.

Histologically, these lesions are composed of a lentiginous elongation and hyperpigmentation of rete ridges with an increase in melanocytes. Often a nesting of nevus cells occurs within the lesion. The clinically dark speckled areas are either junctional nevi or compound nevi. Although rare reports of nevus spilus undergoing malignant degeneration suggest exercising caution when treating them (31–34), many report a good response to QS-ruby, QS-alexandrite, and QS-FD

532-nm Nd:YAG lasers (35,36). Unfortunately, some patients respond poorly, and complete resolution may require four or more treatments. In addition, the longer pulsed diode and alexandrite lasers in the millisecond domain can be used on the discrete nevi within the nevus spilus. The underlying biology may explain the poor responders; not all the involved melanocytes are targeted because of insufficient melanin. The histology of these lesions reveals nothing that will further explain those with a poor response. Treatment is the same as for CALM.

LASER TREATMENT FOR EPIDERMAL–DERMAL LESIONS

Becker's Nevus

Becker's nevi usually appear in childhood or early adult life as a light- to medium-brown patch ranging in size from as small as 2 cm to encompassing an entire shoulder. Lesions are variably hyperkeratotic, with an increase in coarseness of hair occurring during puberty. Incidence has been calculated to be 0.5% of the population. Histologically, these lesions show rete ridge elongation and basal layer hyperpigmentation with variable amounts of acanthosis and hyperkeratosis. Although no nevus cells are found, melanocytes appear to be increased and the dermis tends to be thickened. In addition, hypertrophied sebaceous glands and bundles of smooth muscle fibers and enlarged pilar apparatus may be present. Therefore, this lesion is more correctly considered an organoid hamartoma (37,38).

Treatment of Becker's nevus requires therapeutic consideration of its two pathologic components: increased hair growth and increased pigmentation. The chromophore that must be targeted in its treatment is melanin. The fine clumping of melanin granules in the epidermis requires shorter pulse widths (nanosecond domain) than the larger hair follicles, which typically respond best to the millisecond pulse widths used in hair removal lasers.

Becker's nevi are notoriously difficult to clear, possibly because of their hamartomatous pathophysiology. The QS ruby, alexandrite, and FD Nd:YAG lasers can effectively target the increased pigmentation in Becker's nevi, but recurrence is common (39). The long pulsed alexandrite laser offers the best possibility for more permanent clearing of both pigmentation and increased hair growth. Settings are similar to those of CALM for the surrounding pigment and the hair removal lasers are used at their appropriate settings for hair color and shaft size (see chap. 5). Improvement in Becker's nevi with non-ablative fractional photothermolysis suggests another potential treatment modality, although the efficacy remains to be studied (40).

Melasma

Melasma is an acquired, usually symmetric, light- to dark-brown facial hypermelanosis that develops slowly. It may be idiopathic or more often associated with pregnancy or ingestion of oral contraceptives. This disorder, with a reported incidence of 50–70% in pregnant women, usually occurs in the second and third trimesters. It has an incidence of 8–29% in women taking oral contraceptives. The etiology and pathogenesis of melasma are unknown; however, a genetic predisposition is supported by a 21% familial occurrence in one series (41–43).

Two types of melasma exist on histologic examination. In the epidermal type, the major sites of melanin deposition are in the basilar and suprabasilar layers. The melanocytes have been found to contain highly melanized melanosomes. The dermal type is characterized by melanophages in the superficial and deep dermis in addition to the epidermal hyperpigmentation. A simple clinical differentiation between the two types can be made by using a Wood's lamp, which shows enhancement of pigmentation in the epidermal type and not in the dermal type.

Melasma is frustrating for both the patient and physician. Improvement in pigmentation is difficult and recurs easily, which reflects an inability to halt the underlying pathoetiologic mechanism. Laser is only an option as an adjunct to strict photoprotection and/or a topical regimen. Repigmentation can be minimized by strict sun avoidance and sun protection, as well as a regular use of hydroquinone. Strict sun avoidance and sun protection with UVA- and UVB-blocking sunscreens are of paramount significance. Treatment with QS lasers (ruby, alexandrite, and Nd:YAG), IPL, erbium, and CO_2 lasers has been reported to be of benefit in some patients, but subsequent repigmentation is a common occurrence, as is postinflammatory hyperpigmentation (44–52). Test sites help to predict which patient will respond to QS laser treatment. Those with a more superficial component are more likely to respond to the shorter wavelengths and those with a dermal component may respond better to longer wavelengths. Fractional photothermolysis has also been studied with great interest for the treatment of melasma (53–55); however, consistent and predictable improvement remains elusive for this refractory condition. A test site should be treated before undertaking treatment of the entire affected area, as some cases may be exacerbated by the treatment.

Nevocellular Nevi

Common Acquired Nevi

Common acquired nevi appear after the first 6–12 months of life and enlarge with body growth, reaching a peak average count in the third or fourth decade. Although the exact factors that influence the natural history of common nevi are not yet fully understood, a relationship exists between sun exposure and the number of nevi. The number of nevi increases with a greater concentration in sun-exposed areas. In addition, environmental factors, such as a propensity to burn rather than tan, a history of sunburn, a tendency to freckle, and a lifestyle involving increased sun exposure, are also related to the number of benign pigmented nevi in children. Unfortunately, an increased number of benign melanocytic nevi serves as an independent risk factor for malignant melanoma. Therefore, any treatment of common acquired nevi without histologic evaluation should be undertaken cautiously.

The efficacy of QS laser treatment of nevi is variable. Smaller and thinner nevi respond better; all three QS laser systems (QS ruby, alexandrite, and Nd:YAG lasers) are effective with minimal side effects. Unfortunately, many nevi recur or only partially respond. Long pulsed lasers (alexandrite and diode) have been shown to more effectively eradicate these nevi in fewer treatment sessions, using fluences of 40–60 J/cm², and 8- to 12-mm spot sizes; however, hypertrophic scarring can occur (56). Cooling may be turned off for better efficacy as long as the surrounding skin is protected. Settings should be determined with consideration of the nevus color, in the context of the patient's skin type. Ablative resurfacing with an Er:YAG laser has been reported in a small cohort to result in cosmetically satisfactory results (57).

Case 7

Nevi

A 24-year-old man with type IV skin presented with a history of dark compound melanocytic nevi on the face. (Fig. 3.7A). Initially he was interested in surgical treatment but did not want to have the lesions excised due to risk of scarring. Treatment plan included monthly sessions with the diode (810 nm) laser. Lesions were treated at 1-month intervals as follows: session 1, 40 J/cm² and 20-ms pulse width; session 2, 40 J/cm² and 20-ms pulse width (double pulsed); session 3, 60 J/cm² and 30-ms pulse width (double pulsed). Cooling was left on due to the patient's type IV skin type. Dramatic clearing was noted on follow-up at 11 weeks after the initial visit (Fig. 3.7B).

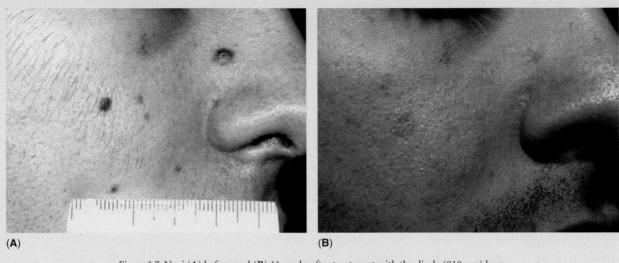

(A)   **(B)**

Figure 3.7 Nevi (**A**) before and (**B**) 11 weeks after treatment with the diode (810 nm) laser.

Congenital Melanocytic Nevi

Note: Laser treatment of CMN should be undertaken by those with expertise in both melanocytic lesions and laser surgery.

CMN occur with a prevalence of 1.0–2.5% of newborns. CMN are classified by size: small, medium, and large. Small CMN are those less than 1.5 cm; medium CMN are 1.5–19.9 cm and large or garment CMN are those greater than 20 cm in projected adult size. The risk of malignant progression to melanoma is a particular concern for large/garment congenital nevi, and classically has been estimated to be between 5 and 15%. However, data from a large meta-analysis suggest the risk for malignant transformation to be significantly lower at 2.5% for large/garment sized congenital nevi (58). In addition, nearly half of patients with a large/garment CMN have psychologic or social difficulties (59). Conflicting arguments have been made whether laser treatment of CMN elevates or decreases the risk of malignant transformation; however,

convincing evidence to either argument remains elusive. Thus treatment of these CMN can be done more so for cosmetic and psychosocial reasons.

QS lasers have been popular for treatment of congenital nevi because of their nanosecond pulse durations that closely match the thermal relaxation time of melanosomes. Reports of QS ruby and alexandrite lasers demonstrate responses ranging from poor to excellent. Multiple treatments are almost always required and there is likely to be persisting nevus cells in the deeper papillary dermis.

Long pulsed lasers have also been used to treat CMN due to their potential to better target nests of melanocytes. Like QS lasers, results have been variable to make definitive conclusions. Combination treatment with both QS and long pulsed lasers has also been reported with promising results (60). Ablative lasers such as the CO_2 and Er:YAG lasers have also been used alone or in combination with QS lasers.

Case 8

Congenital Nevus

This 7-year-old Asian girl presented with an unsightly nevus on her left upper lip. She was very self-conscious about its appearance. It measured 6 mm in diameter and was without any clinical atypicality (Fig. 3.8A). After a discussion with her mother regarding surgical excision and laser ablation, a decision was made to treat the lesion with a laser and watch it carefully for any atypical changes. The appearance after 4-monthly QS ruby laser treatments given at 4–5 J/cm² is shown in Figure 3.8B. Six months later (Fig. 3.8C), the lesion began to recur. After three separate QS alexandrite laser treatments at 6–7 J/cm² given over 2 years, the lesion had almost totally resolved (Fig. 3.8D). Further treatments with the 5-ms long pulsed alexandrite laser at 15–20 J/cm² were given to further improve the lesion and eliminate hairs within the lesion (Fig. 3.8E). The final appearance 6 years later—15 years after the first laser treatment—is shown in Figure 3.8F. The lesion was treated with a topical anesthetic cream (EMLA®, AstraZeneca, Luton, UK) prior to each treatment.

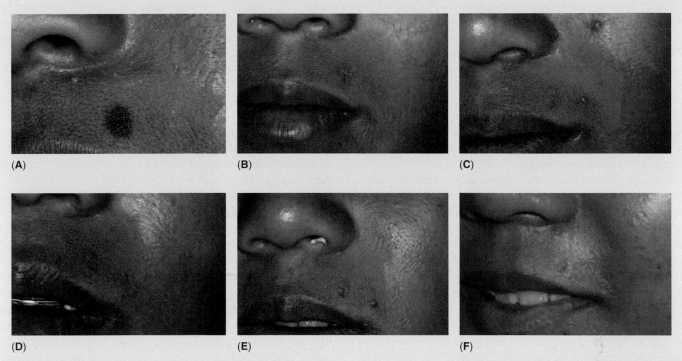

(A)   (B)   (C)

(D)   (E)   (F)

Figure 3.8 (**A**) Nevus on the left upper lip of a 7-year-old girl. (**B**) Appearance after 4-monthly Q-switched ruby laser treatments. (**C**) 6 months later the lesion began to recur. (**D**) After 3 separate Q-switched alexandrite laser treatments the lesion hass almost totally resolved. (**E**) Further treatment with the 5-ms long pulsed alexandrite laser further improved the lesion and eliminated hairs within the lesion. (**F**) The final appearance 10 years later. *Source*: Photos courtesy of Mitchel P. Goldman, MD.

Case 9

Congenital Hairy Nevus

This 12-year-old girl was concerned over the cosmetic appearance of a congenital hairy nevus on her left cheek (Fig. 3.9A). After a discussion with her parents regarding surgical excision versus laser treatment, a decision was made to treat the lesion with laser therapy and a close clinical follow-up. Figure 3.9B shows the clinical appearance after 11 separate laser treatments consisting of two Q-switched (QS) ruby laser treatments at 5 J/cm^2, one 510-nm 300-ms pigment lesion laser at 3 J/cm^2, one QS 532-nm Nd:YAG treatment at 4 J/cm^2, three QS alexandrite laser treatments at 7–8 J/cm^2, three treatments with the long-pulsed alexandrite laser at 5 ms and 20 J/cm^2, and one treatment with the Lumenis Vasculite IPL (Lumenis Aesthetic, Yokneam, Israel) with a 640-nm cut-off filter and a double pulse of 3 ms and 3 ms, 10-ms delay between pulses at an energy of 40 J/cm^2. The lesion has lightened and there is no more hair but the color has not resolved. Local anesthesia was performed with 1% lidocaine with epinephrine infiltrated into the lesion prior to each procedure to minimize pain.

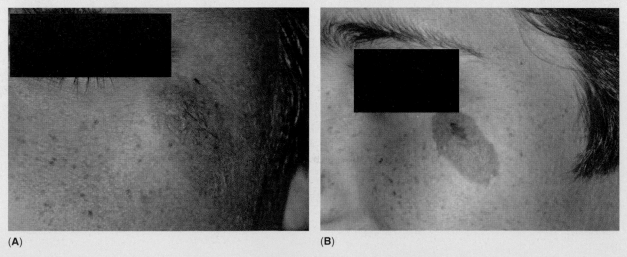

(A)   (B)

Figure 3.9 (**A**) A congenital hairy nevus on the left cheek of a 12-year-old girl. (**B**) Clinical appearance after 11 separate laser treatments. *Source*: Photos courtesy of Mitchel P. Goldman, MD.

Laser Treatment for Dermal Lesions

Nevus of Ota and Nevus of Ito

Nevus of Ota consists of bluish gray patches on the areas of the face innervated by the first and second divisions of the trigeminal nerve. It is frequently associated with ipsilateral ocular pigmentation and has been associated with glaucoma. This nevus is most often found in Asians and people of African ancestry and has a strong predilection for women. Incidence in the Japanese population is estimated at 1–2%. Hori nevus is a variant of nevus of Ota with a bilateral distribution. Nevus of Ito has a similar clinical and histologic appearance like nevus of Ota but is found in the areas innervated by the posterior supraclavicular and lateral brachial cutaneous nerves. The lesion is much rarer than nevus of Ota and the exact incidence is unknown. The clinical appearance resembles a powder blast, with poorly demarcated macules and patches blending readily with the normal surrounding skin. Lesions vary in color from brown to darker shades such as blue, gray, and purple.

Histologic examination of both lesions shows long, slender dermal melanocytes scattered largely in the upper half of the dermis. The normal dermal collagen architecture is well preserved. Although the epidermis is generally normal, focal basal hyperpigmentation may also be seen.

The lesions are usually benign, but rare cases of malignant melanoma arising in a nevus of Ota have been reported, and patients should be followed carefully. Development of new subcutaneous nodules within the lesion is particularly suggestive of malignant melanoma and the nodules should be biopsied. Ophthalmologic evaluation for possible glaucoma or ocular melanoma is necessary in patients with ocular involvement. The optimized ability of the QS ruby (694 nm), alexandrite (755 nm), and Nd:YAG (1064 nm) lasers to target the deeply situated melanocytes may be attributed to their longer wavelengths. Lesions containing more superficially located melanocytes may respond readily to treatment, whereas those that are deeper will likely be more resistant. The pulse width of the QS lasers is in the nanosecond range, thereby effectively targeting melanocytes and minimizing thermal injury to the surrounding collagen. Lesion clearance is generally noted with fluences ranging from 6 to 10 J/cm², after one to seven treatments (11). More resistant lesions generally continue to demonstrate improvement with successive treatments, though more slowly.

Conflicting reports of fluences necessary for treatment, as well as the necessary number of treatments and treatment intervals, probably result from the variability in lesions and the spot size used (61,62). Gradual clearing of lesions is noted after multiple treatments over several months. The optimal treatment interval between treatment sessions remains to be elucidated, however the current recommendation is to wait 3 months between treatment sessions to allow for pigment removal by melanophages and the resolution of all laser-induced hyperpigmentation, which can be facilitated by the use of zinc oxide sunblock and a hydroquinone preparation. Fractional photothermolysis was also reported in a case report, which resulted in the complete clearance of nevus of Ota with a single treatment (63).

Case 10

Nevus of Ota

An 18-year-old man with a history of nevus of Ota presented for discussion of treatment options (Fig. 3.10A). He was treated with QS Nd:YAG (1064 nm) laser using a 4-mm spot and 8.7 J/cm² fluence over the area with a total of four treatment sessions at 3-month intervals with significant improvement (Fig. 3.10B).

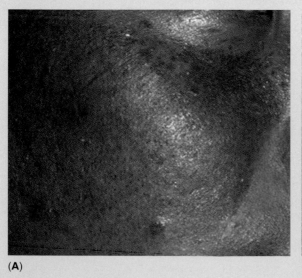 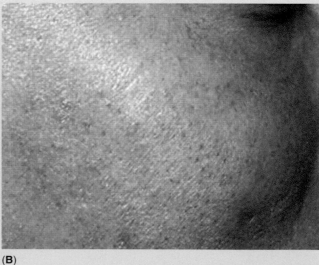

(A)   **(B)**

Figure 3.10 Nevus of Ota. (**A**) Before and (**B**) after 4 treatment sessions (at 3-month intervals) with Q-switched Nd:YAG (1064 nm) laser.

Case 11

Nevus of Ota

This 26-year-old woman is concerned about the pigmented lesion above and below the left eyelid (Fig. 3.11A). Because of the close proximity of the lesion to the eye, a stainless steel, internal eye shield was inserted into the eye prior to treatment. The patient required someone to drive her to and from the office in case of any blurry vision from the use of the topical anesthetic and lubrication required for inserting the eye shield. Local anesthesia was performed with 1% lidocaine with epinephrine infiltrated into the lesion prior to each procedure to minimize pain. Figure 3.11B shows the result after one treatment with the QS alexandrite laser at 9 J/cm^2; there is 75% resolution of the lesion. Figure 3.11C shows the result 6 months after a second treatment with the QS ruby laser at 5 J/cm^2: there is complete resolution of the lesion.

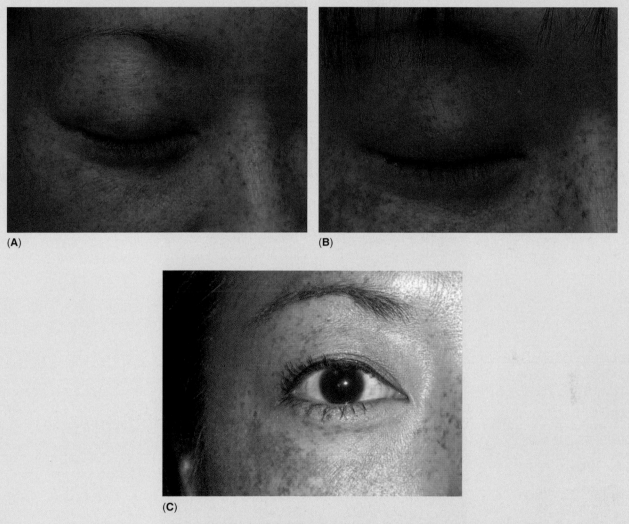

(A)

(B)

(C)

Figure 3.11 (**A**) Pigmented lesion above and below the left eyelid. (**B**) The result after one treatment with a Q-switched alexandrite laser at 9 J/cm^2; there is 75% resolution of the lesion. (**C**) 6 months after a second treatment with the Q-switched ruby laser at 5 J/cm^2. *Source:* Photos courtesy of Mitchel P. Goldman, MD.

Case 12

Nevus of Ito

This 3-year-old presented with a dark brown linear nevus on the lateral aspect of the neck extending to the left chin (Fig. 3.12A). Figure 3.12(B) shows the appearance 6 years after 3-monthly treatments with a QS ruby laser at 5 J/cm^2, or QS alexandrite laser at 8 J/cm^2, or QS 1064 nm Nd:YAG laser at 10 J/cm^2. All treatments were given after topical anesthesia with EMLA cream supplemented with local infiltration with 1% lidocaine with epinephrine. The appearance 10 years after the sixth and last treatment with a QS ruby laser at 5 J/cm^2: the lesion has lightened but is still persistent (Fig. 3.12C).

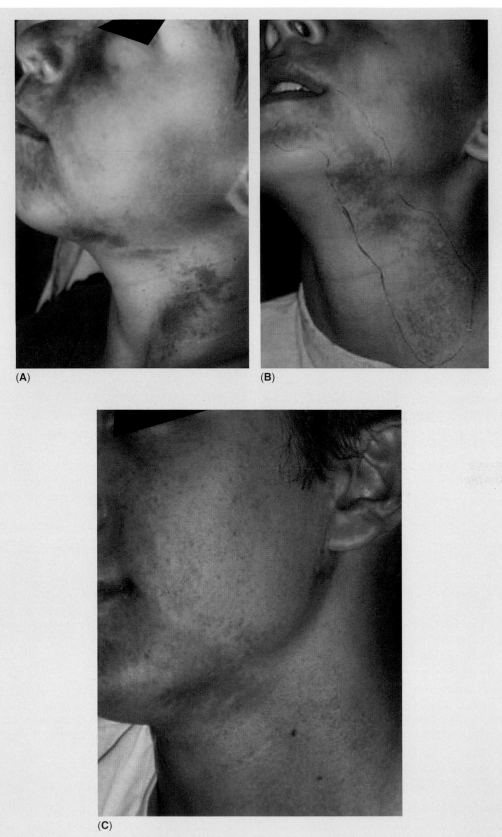

Figure 3.12 (**A**) A dark brown linear nevus on the lateral aspect of the neck of a 3 year old. (**B**) Appearance 6 years after 3-monthly treatments. (**C**) Appearance 10 years after the last treatment with a Q-switched ruby laser at 5 J/cm². *Source*: Photos courtesy of Mitchel P. Goldman, MD.

Blue Nevus

Blue nevi are usually solitary, discrete, well-circumscribed papules 1–8 mm in diameter that arise spontaneously, most often in children and young adults. The male–female ratio is approximately 2:1. The melanin-producing cells are deep within the dermis and their blue–black color results from the Tyndall light-scattering effect of the overlying tissues.

Histologic examination shows an extensive number of spindle-shaped, elongated melanocytes within the middle and lower dermis, occasionally extending into the fat. These cells may be grouped in fascicles between collagen bundles and tend to aggregate around adnexal structures, nerves, and blood vessels.

Because of their benign nature, blue nevi are usually removed for cosmetic reasons. Although extremely rare, malignant blue nevi have been reported. The primary method of removal of these lesions is local excision. Similar to treatment of nevi of Ota and Ito, the QS ruby, alexandrite, and Nd:YAG lasers should also be effective in removing these deep dermal melanocytes, as long as the lesion does not extend into the subcutaneous fat (64–69). Biopsy should be strongly considered for lesions which are new, multinodular, or plaquelike, or changing. Rare cases of malignant melanoma arising from cellular blue nevi have been reported. Cellular blue nevi should therefore be excised because of this rare but potential risk for malignant transformation.

The only mode of treatment mentioned in the literature is with the QS ruby laser (69), although all three QS lasers are efficacious, similar to their use with the nevus of Ota and Ito. Again, the longer-pulsed ruby and alexandrite lasers may prove effective.

Patient Selection

When determining whether a patient with a pigmented lesion is appropriate for laser treatment, the patient's dermatologic history must be evaluated. Consideration must be given to the patient's Fitzpatrick skin type and its innate tendency to hyperpigment in response to inflammation.

Patients should be educated regarding the laser procedure so that they have realistic expectations. Patients should be advised of potential side effects, including hyperpigmentation, hypopigmentation, temporary or permanent textural change, scarring, or recurrence. Showing patients photographs of similar lesions, immediately post treatment, after a few treatment sessions, and final clinical result, will increase their awareness of what to expect. It is also helpful to show examples of patients with average results, not complete clearing, so that patients are aware of the range of possible outcomes. It should be clearly stated that not all lesions can be removed completely and that successful lightening may require several treatment sessions at 6-week intervals. In addition, the unknown risk of melanoma formation must be addressed for all melanocytic lesions.

Laser Selection
Laser Technique

Most benign pigmented lesions respond fairly well to laser treatments. Those located more superficially can be treated with the shorter wavelengths of 510 and 532 nm, as well as 694 and even 755 nm. Deeper lesions require the longer wavelengths of 694, 755, and 1064 nm for better depth of penetration. Larger spot sizes also enhance the penetration depth. Unfortunately, pigmented lesions respond variably to lasers, and for any individual patient it is difficult to predict the treatment outcome.

Epidermal lesions treated with the QS lasers should have immediately visible superficial whitening, often associated with a slightly eroded surface, which heals over the course of approximately 7–10 days. The patient should be advised that the treated area may appear darker in color as it heals. If the lesion is treated with the QS Nd:YAG laser (532 nm), purpura may develop from the rupture of blood vessels due to the coincident absorption of hemoglobin and melanin at this wavelength. If an urticarial response to treatment is noted, the patient may require oral antihistamines and premedication with oral antihistamines should be considered prior to the next treatment session. The patient should be advised to wash the area daily with mild soap and water and cover with a layer of petrolatum or antibiotic ointment.

CLINICAL PEARLS

Atypical lesions should be carefully examined by a dermatologist and biopsied. When approaching pigmented lesions, a high level of suspicion should be maintained so that worrisome lesions are not overlooked, and appropriate treatment not delayed.

MANAGEMENT OF COMPLICATIONS

The risks of laser surgery include transient hyperpigmentation or hypopigmentation, scarring, permanent hyperpigmentation, incomplete clearance of treated lesion, and recurrence. Treatment of pigmented lesions is often done for cosmetic reasons. In selecting a therapeutic regimen, optimal esthetic result must be the goal in choosing the most appropriate treatment with minimal risk. Ideally, it must be both effective and free from the adverse sequelae of scarring and permanent pigmentary complications. This can be best achieved by selective targeting of pigment-containing cells. Should blistering of the treated area occur, local wound care should be administered. In an effort to minimize the risk of hyperpigmentation following laser treatment, the patient should be counseled on sun protection measures, including the use of broad spectrum physical sunblocks such as those containing micronized zinc dioxide.

If hyperpigmentation is noted within the healing irradiated sites, hydroquinone therapy should be used two times per day until it resolves. Avoidance of sun exposure and use of a UVA/UVB sunblock to minimize postinflammatory hyperpigmentation are recommended. If hypopigmentation does occur, it often resolves spontaneously with time. If not, the excimer laser or other narrow band UV source may be utilized. In the rare event of adverse sequelae such as scarring, it is best to implement early treatment with the pulsed dye laser.

FUTURE DIRECTIONS

The optimization of laser parameters, refinements in technique, and a better understanding of the underlying biology may further help clinicians to treat these lesions more effectively. The role of fractionated photothermolysis in improving certain types of pigmented lesions is forthcoming, and the potential use of picosecond lasers also holds promise for the treatment of pigmented lesions.

REFERENCES

1. Goldman L, Wilson R, Hornby P. Radiation from a QS ruby laser: effect of repeated impacts of power output of 10 megawatts on a tattoo of man. J Invest Dermatol 1965; 44: 69.
2. Goldman L, Rockwell J, Meyer R, et al. Laser treatment of tattoos: a preliminary survey of three years' clinical experience. JAMA 1967; 201: 841.
3. Anderson RR, Parrish JA. Selective photothermolysis: precise micro-surgery by selective absorption of pulsed irradiation. Science 1983; 220: 524.
4. Manstein D, Herron GS, Sink RK, Tanner H, Anderson RR. Fractional photothermolysis: a new concept for cutaneous remodeling using microscopic patterns of thermal injury. Lasers Surg Med 2004; 34: 426–38.
5. Goldman L. Optical radiation hazards to the skin. In: Sliney D, Wolbarsht M, eds. Safety with Lasers and other Optical Sources: A Comprehensive Handbook. New York: Plenum, 1983.
6. Anderson RR, Parrish JA. The optics human skin. J Invest Dermatol 1981; 77: 13.
7. Anderson RR, Margolis RJ, Watanabe S, et al. Selective photothermolysis of cutaneous pigmentation by QS Nd:YAG laser pulses at 1064, 532 and 355 nm. J Invest Dermatol 1989; 93: 28.
8. Margolis RJ, Dover JS, Polla LL, et al. Visible action spectrum for melanin-specific selective photothermolysis. Lasers Surg Med 1989; 9: 389.
9. Kurban AK, Scearbo ME, Morrison P, et al. Pulse duration effects on cutaneous pigment ablation. Lasers Surg Med 1990: 213A.
10. Parrish JA, Anderson RR, Harris T, et al. Selective thermal effects with pulsed irradiation from laser: from organ to organelle. J Invest Dermatol 1983; 80: 755.
11. Taylor CR, Flotte TJ, Gange RW, Anderson RR. Treatment of nevus of Ota by QS ruby laser. J Am Acad Dermatol 1994; 30: 743.
12. Ross V, Naseef G, Lin G, et al. Comparison of responses of tattoos to picosecond and nanosecond Q-switched neodymium: YAG lasers. Arch Dermatol 1998; 134: 167–71.
13. Herd RM, Alora MB, Smoller B, Arndt KA, Dover JS. A clinical and histologic prospective controlled comparative study of the picosecond titanium:sapphire (795 nm) laser versus the Q-switched alexandrite (752 nm) laser for removing tattoo pigment. J Am Acad Dermatol 1999; 40: 603–6.
14. Kilmer SL, Chotzen VA, McClaren M, et al. Diode (810 nm) laser treatment of pigmented lesions. Lasers Surg Med 2000; 23: 55.
15. Kilmer SL, Garden JM. Laser treatment of pigmented lesions and tattoos. Semin Cutan Med Surg 2000; 19: 232–44.
16. Alikhan A A, Ibrahimi OA, Eisen DB. Congenital melanocytic nevi: where are we now? Part I: clinical presentation, epidemiology, pathogenesis, histology, malignant transformation, and neurocutaneous melanosis. J Am Acad Dermatol 2012; 67: 495.e1–17.
17. Alikhan AA, Ibrahimi OA, Eisen DB. Congenital melanocytic nevi: where are we now? Part II: treatment options and approach to treatment. J Am Acad Dermatol 2012; 67: 515.e1–13.
18. Kurban AK, Morrison PR, Trainor S, et al. Pulse duration effects on cutaneous pigment. Lasers Surg Med 1992; 12: 282.
19. Watanabe S, Anderson RR, Brorson S. Comparative studies of femtosecond to microsecond laser pulses on selective pigmented cell injury in skin. Photochem Photobiol 1991; 53: 757–62.
20. Goldberg DJ. Laser treatment of pigmented lesions. Dermatol Clin 1997; 15: 397.
21. Kilmer SL, Wheeland RG, Goldberg DJ, Anderson RR. Treatment of epidermal pigmented lesions with the frequency-doubled Qswitched Nd:YAG laser: a controlled, single-impact, doseresponse, multicenter trial. Arch Dermatol 1994; 130: 1515.
22. Taylor CR, Anderson PR. Treatment of benign pigmented epidermal lesions by QS ruby laser. Int J Dermatol 1993; 32: 908.
23. Goldberg DJ. Benign pigmented lesions of the skin: treatment with the QS ruby laser. J Dermatol Surg Oncol 1993; 19: 376.
24. Tse Y, Levine VJ, McClain SA, Ashinoff R. The removal of cutaneous pigmented lesions with the QS ruby laser and the QS neodymium:yttrium-aluminum-garnet laser: a comparative study. J Dermatol Surg Oncol 1994; 20: 795.
25. Kawada A, Shiraishi H, Asai M, et al. Clinical improvement of solar lentigines and ephelides with an intense pulsed light source. Dermatol Surg 2002; 28: 504–8.
26. Ho SG, Yeung CK, Chan NP, Shek SY, Chan HH. A comparison of Q-switched and long-pulsed alexandrite laser for the treatment of freckles and lentigines in oriental patients. Lasers Surg Med 2011; 43: 108–13.
27. Kundu RV, Joshi SS, Suh KY, et al. Comparison of electrodesiccation and potassium-titanyl-phosphate laser for treatment of dermatosis papulosa nigra. Dermatol Surg 2009; 35: 1079–83.
28. Garcia MS, Azari R, Eisen DB. Treatment of dermatosis papulosa nigra in 10 patients: a comparison trial of electrodesiccation, pulsed dye laser, and curettage. Dermatol Surg 2010; 36: 1968–72.
29. Carpo GB, Grevelink JM, Grevelink SV. Laser treatment of pigmented lesions in children. Semin Cutan Med Surg 1999; 18: 233.
30. Shimbashi T, Kamide R, Hashimoto T. Long-term follow-up in treatment of solar lentigo and café-au-lait macules with Qswitched ruby laser. Aesthetic Plast Surg 1997; 21: 445–8.
31. Rhodes A, Mihm MC Jr. Origin of cutaneous melanoma in a congenital dysplastic nevus spilus. Arch Dermatol 1990; 126: 500.
32. Rutten A, Goos M. Nevus spilus with malignant melanoma in a patient with neurofibromatosis. Arch Dermatol 1990; 126: 539.
33. Cohen HJ, Minkin W, Frank S. Nevus spilus. Arch Dermatol 1970; 102: 433.
34. Stewart DM, Altman J, Megregan AH. Speckled lentiginous nevus. Arch Dermatol 1978; 114: 895.
35. Grevelink JM, Gonzalez S, Bonoan R, et al. Treatment of nevus spilus with the QS ruby laser. Dermatol Surg 1997; 23: 365.
36. Miyasaka M, Tanino R, Morita T, et al. Case 8.29: nevus spilus of the cheek; and case 8.30: nevus spilus of the left knee. In: Apfelberg DB, ed. Atlas of Cutaneous Laser Surgery. New York: Raven, 1992.
37. Chapel TA, Tavafoghi V, Mehregan AH. Becker's melanosis: an organoid hamartoma. Cutis 1981; 27: 405.
38. Haneke E. The dermal component in melanosis naeviformis Becker. J Cutan Pathol 1979; 6: 53.
39. Raulin C, Schonermark MP, Greve B, Werner S. QS ruby laser treatment of tattoos and benign pigmented skin lesions: a critical review. Ann Plast Surg 1998; 41: 555–65.
40. Glaich AS, Goldberg LH, Dai T, Kunishige JH, Friedman PM. Fractional resurfacing: a new therapeutic modality for Becker's nevus. Arch Dermatol 2007; 143: 1488–90.
41. Gilchrest BA, Fitzpatrick TB, Anderson RR, Parvish JA. Localization of melanin pigmentation on the skin with Wood's lamp. Br J Dermatol 1977; 96: 245.
42. Sanchez NP, Pathak MA, Sato S, et al. Melasma: a clinical, light microscopic, ultrastructural and immunofluorescent study. J Am Acad Dermatol 1981; 4: 698.
43. Resnick S. Melasma induced by oral contraceptive drugs. JAMA 1967; 199: 95.
44. Yoshimura K, Sato K, Aiba-Kojima E, et al. Repeated treatment protocols for melasma and acquired dermal melanocytosis. Dermatol Surg 2006; 32: 365–71.
45. Suh KS, Sung JY, Roh HJ, et al. Efficacy of the 1064-nm Q-switched Nd:YAG laser in melasma. J Dermatolog Treat 2011; 22: 233–8.
46. Cho SB, Kim JS, Kim MJ. Melasma treatment in Korean women using a 1064-nm Q-switched Nd:YAG laser with low pulse energy. Clin Exp Dermatol 2009; 34: e847–50.
47. Jeong SY, Shin JB, Yeo UC, Kim WS, Kim IH. Low-fluence Q-switched neodymium-doped yttrium aluminum garnet laser for melasma with pre- or post-treatment triple combination cream. Dermatol Surg 2010; 36: 909–18.
48. Angsuwarangsee S, Polnikorn N. Combined ultrapulse CO2 laser and Q-switched alexandrite laser compared with Q-switched alexandrite laser alone for refractory melasma: split-face design. Dermatol Surg 2003; 29: 59–64.
49. Nouri K, Bowes L, Chartier T, Romagosa R, Spencer J. Combination treatment of melasma with pulsed CO2 laser followed by Q-switched alexandrite laser: a pilot study. Dermatol Surg 1999; 25: 494–7.
50. Trelles MA, Velez M, Gold MH. The treatment of melasma with topical creams alone, CO2 fractional ablative resurfacing alone, or a combination of the two: a comparative study. J Drugs Dermatol 2010; 9: 315–22.
51. Manaloto RM, Alster T. Erbium:YAG laser resurfacing for refractory melasma. Dermatol Surg 1999; 25: 121–3.
52. Wanitphakdeedecha R, Manuskiatti W, Siriphukpong S, Chen TM. Treatment of melasma using variable square pulse Er:YAG laser resurfacing. Dermatol Surg 2009; 35: 475–81.

53. Lee HS, Won CH, Lee DH, et al. Treatment of melasma in Asian skin using a fractional 1,550-nm laser: an open clinical study. Dermatol Surg 2009; 35: 1499–504.

54. Rokhsar CK, Fitzpatrick RE. The treatment of melasma with fractional photothermolysis: a pilot study. Dermatol Surg 2005; 31: 1645–50.

55. Katz TM, Glaich AS, Goldberg LH, et al. Treatment of melasma using fractional photothermolysis: a report of eight cases with long-term follow-up. Dermatol Surg 2010; 36: 1273–80.

56. Reda AM, Taha IR, Riad HA. Clinical and histological effect of a single treatment of normal mode alexandrite (755 nm) laser on small melanocytic nevi. J Cutan Laser Ther 1999; 1: 209–15.

57. Baba M, Bal N. Efficacy and safety of the short-pulse erbium:YAG laser in the treatment of acquired melanocytic nevi. Dermatol Surg 2006; 32: 256–60.

58. Krengel S, Hauschild A, Schafer T. Melanoma risk in congenital melanocytic naevi: a systematic review. Br J Dermatol 2006; 155: 8.

59. Pers M. Naevus pigmentosus giganticus: Indikationer for operative behandling. Ungeskrift Laeger 1963; 125: 63.

60. Kono T, Erçöçen AR, Nozaki M. Treatment of congenital melanocytic nevi using the combined (normal-mode plus Q-switched) ruby laser in Asians: clinical response in relation to histological type. Ann Plast Surg 2005; 54: 494–501

61. Lowe NJ, Wieder JM, Sawcer D, Burrows P. Nevus of Ota: treatment with the high energy fluences of the QS ruby laser. J Am Acad Dermatol 1993; 29: 997.

62. Alster TS, Williams CM. Treatment of nevus of Ota by the Qswitched alexandrite laser. Dermatol Surg 1995; 21: 592.

63. Kouba DJ, Fincher EF, Moy RL. Nevus of Ota successfully treated by fractional photothermolysis using a fractionated 1440-nm Nd:YAG laser. Arch Dermatol 2008; 144: 156–8.

64. Patel BC, Egan CA, Lucius RW, et al. Cutaneous malignant melanoma and oculodermal melanocytosis (nevus of Ota): report of a case and review of the literature. J Am Acad Dermatol 1997; 38: 862.

65. Balmaceda CM, Fetell RM, O'Brian JL, Housepian EH. Nevus of Ota and leptomeningeal melanocytic lesions. Neurology 1993; 43: 381.

66. Chan HH, Leung RS, Ying SY, et al. A retrospective analysis of complications in the treatment of nevus of Ota with the Qswitched Alexandrite and QS Nd: YAG lasers. Dermatol Surg 2000; 26: 1000.

67. Rodriguez HA, Ackerman LV. Cellular blue nevus: clinicopathologic study of 45 cases. Cancer 1968; 21: 393.

68. Rubenstein N, Kopolovic J, Wexler MR, et al. Malignant blue nevus. J Dermatol Surg Oncol 1985; 11: 921.

69. Milgraum SS, Cohen ME, Auletta MJ. Treatment of blue nevi with the QS ruby laser. J Am Acad Dermatol 1995; 32: 307.

4 Tattoo removal

William T. Kirby

TATTOO HISTORY

In 1991, in the Alps mountain at the border of Austria and Italy, the frozen body of a tattooed man was found (1). The corpse was so well preserved that it was originally believed that the individual had only recently died. Subsequent carbon dating showed that this well-preserved human had died approximately 5300 years earlier. The now famous, Ötzi the Iceman, had 57 purposely placed skin markings (2–4), making this discovery one of the best-documented cases of tattoos in prehistoric man.

This was not an isolated incident however; prehistoric mummies with tattoos have also been found in Siberia, Peru, and Chile (5–7), and evidence of the ancient art of tattooing has been traced as far back as the Stone Age (12,000 BCE) (8). Primitive humans slashed their skin during bereavement ceremonies and rubbed ash (and conceivably the ashes of the deceased) into the cuts as a sign of grief and to possibly create a permanent reminder of their ancestors. Decorative tattooing has also been linked to the Bronze Age (8000 BCE) by the circumstantial evidence of crude needles and pigment bowls found in caves in France, Spain, and Portugal (9). People of this age decorated animal skins worn for warmth with ocher and plant pigments, and this may have eventually evolved into the decorative tattooing of their own skin as mummies dating from 4000 BCE have shown evidence of crude tattoos (10).

In 1796, Joseph Banks, a member of Captain James Cook's expedition, used the Samoan word "tatau," meaning to "to mark," to describe one of the earliest written records of purposeful tattoos. It is notably similar to the Tahitian word "tattau" and obviously the modern "tattoo" originates from these South Pacific island words. In 1891, Samuel O'Reilly modified an engraving device that was patented by Thomas Edison in 1876. With the edition of an electromagnetic oscillating unit that drove a solid steel needle and ink into the dermis, at a rate of 50–3000 injections per minute, the modern day tattoo "gun" was born.

In the 1980s, a surge in tattooing popularity occurred in the USA. Surveys in the early 2000s showed that 3–8% of the general population, 10–13% of adolescents, 19–35% of individuals in the 16- to 35-year-old age group, 11–28% of individuals in the 36- to 50-year-old age group, and 5–6% of Americans older than 50 years had tattoos (11–14). A 2006 study showed that 24% of Americans between 18 and 50 years of age were tattooed and that about 36% of Americans between 18 and 29 years of age had at least one tattoo (15), and a 2003 study estimated that 36% of those aged 25–29 have one or more tattoos (16). The average age of acquisition of a professional tattoo is 18 years (17) and that of a self-inflicted amateur tattoo is 14 years (18–20). However, one's quest for identity at the age of 14–18 years is often irrelevant or embarrassing by age 40 years, and 50% or more of individuals regret their tattoos (13,21).

Although most psychologic studies of individuals with tattoos have been restricted to psychiatric inpatients (22–24), prisoners in correctional institutions (21–23,25–27), military personnel (20,28–30), adolescents (31–34), and college students (35–38), and as such reflecting only specific populations, one common conclusion of these studies is that, of all the various motives for obtaining a tattoo, the quest for personal identity is central. The skin serves as a useful canvas on which to portray statements of individuality, sexuality, belonging, machismo, frustration, boredom, and anger. The most commonly stated reasons for obtaining a first tattoo are "to try something new or experimental" or "peer pressure" (39,40). Significantly, smokers are almost three times more likely than nonsmokers to have tattoos, and slightly more women than men on college campuses and entering military service have tattoos (10,12,13).

In a 1991 study of professional women with tattoos, 94% were pleased with the tattoo (41), although a potential bias exists in that those who were pleased may have been more likely to respond as 55% of respondents had friends with tattoos, a known influential factor. Despite this bias and stated satisfaction, 38% mentioned significant problems with having a tattoo and 28% were considering tattoo removal, and the desire for tattoo removal has probably been around nearly as long as tattoos themselves. In fact, Egyptian mummies from 4000 BCE show evidence of attempts at tattoo removal (42).

Motivation for tattoo removal may encompass not only internal regret and desire for more mature identity and self-expression but may be driven by external societal pressure (43). Although tattoos are far more accepted now than in the past, generally speaking, tattoos may not be well received by the public (44), and tattooed individuals may be perceived as antisocial, aggressive, or immature and unable to accept controls and authority (13). Moreover, tattoos may be a significant barrier to employment (45–47), social status, or religious acceptance (48,49).

TATTOO INK COMPOSITION

The US Food and Drug Administration identifies tattoo ink as a "color additive," and because ink manufacturers are not required to provide purchasers a list of ingredients, tattoo artists, patients, and physicians alike may not know the specific composition of a given tattoo (50,51).

That said, the composition of specific ink color and type is known and is shown in Box 4.1 (52).

Box 4.1 Tattoo Ink Composition

Tattoo Ink/Pigment Color	Ingredient
Black	Iron oxide
	Carbon
	Logwood
Brown	Ocher (ferric oxide)
Red	Cinnabar/mercuric sulfide
	Cadmium red
	Iron oxide/common rust
	Naphthol-AS pigment
Yellow	Cadmium yellow
	Ochers
	Curcuma yellow
	Chrome yellow (PbCrO$_4$, often mixed with PbS)
Green	Chromic oxide (Casalis green or Anadomis green)
	Lead chromate
	Phthalocyanine dyes
	Ferrocyanides and ferricyanides
Blue	Azure blue
	Cobalt blue
	Copper phthalocyanine
	Cobalt aluminate
Violet (purple)	Manganese ammonium pyrophosphate
	Various aluminum salts
	Dioxazine/carbazole
White	Lead carbonate
	Titanium dioxide
	Barium sulfate
	Zinc oxide
Henna	Henna dye and paraphenylene-diamine

Abbreviations: PbCrO$_4$, lead(II) chromate; PbS, lead sulfide. *Source*: From Ref. 52, by courtesy of Ravneet Ruby Kaur, William T. Kirby, and Howard Maibach and the publishers.

HISTOLOGY

Only recently have we begun to understand the natural history of an intradermally placed tattoo. A report of serial biopsy examinations of tattoos placed at 24 hours; at 1, 2, and 3 months; and at 40 years previously has given some insight into this process (53), as has an electron microscopic study of tattoos treated with the quality-switched (Q-switched) ruby lasers (54), argon lasers, and tunable dye lasers (55). Initially, ink particles are found within large phagosomes in the cytoplasm of both keratinocytes and phagocytic cells, including fibroblasts, macrophages, and mast cells (56–58). The epidermis, epidermal–dermal junction, and papillary dermis appear homogenized immediately after tattoo injection. At 1 month, the basement membrane is reforming and aggregates of ink particles are present within basal cells. In the dermis, ink-containing phagocytic cells concentrate along the epidermal–dermal border below a layer of granulation tissue closely surrounded by collagen. Pigment is not seen within mast cells, endothelial cells, pericytes, Schwann cells, in the lumina of blood and lymphatic vessels, or extracellularly. At 1 month, transepidermal elimination of ink particles through the epidermis is still in progress, with ink particles present in keratinocytes, macrophages, and fibroblasts. Reestablishment of an intact basement membrane prevents further transepidermal loss. In biopsies obtained at 2–3 months and at 40 years, ink particles are found only in dermal fibroblasts, predominantly in a perivascular location beneath a layer of fibrosis, which had replaced the granulation tissue (59).

Rabbit studies support that the fibroblast is responsible for the stable intracutaneous life span of the tattoo (45). Ink particle aggregates were usually surrounded by a single membrane, suggesting that they were partially free in the dermis; however, they were not found to be free in several studies (40,41,45), and in one study (42), they were present both extracellularly and within fibroblasts. The interpretation of free extracellular tattoo pigment may be a consequence of the difficulty in detecting the single membrane seen by some investigators (40,41,45), and in one study (42), tattoo particles are initially dispersed diffusely as fine granules in the upper dermis as well as in vertical foci at sites of injection but aggregate to a more focal concentrated appearance between 7 and 13 days (40,45). In another study (42), black ink granules have a mean diameter of 4.42 ± 0.72 mm (40) compared with a mean particle diameter of 4.024 ± 0.76 mm when embedded in agar. Taylor and colleagues (41) found black pigment granules in tattoos to be polymorphous, varying from 0.5 to 4.0 mm in diameter. Turquoise and red pigment particles are larger than black granules. In both amateur and professional tattoos, pigment ink depth and density are highly variable, although greater variability of size, shape, and location is noted with amateur tattoos. However, despite the diverse origins of tattoo pigment, the light and electron microscopic appearances of all pigments are remarkably similar, except for their color.

Tattoo pigment granules are composed of three kinds of loosely packed particles, ranging from 2 to 400 nm in diameter (41): most often 40 nm; much less often 2–4 nm (slightly more electron dense); and least frequently 400 nm (much more electron dense with a crystalline structure). A study of freshly implanted eyeliner tattoo ink revealed particle size in the extracellular matrix to be 0.1–1.0 nm, although the average particle size in the pigment vial before implantation was 0.25 nm (60). A prominent network of connective tissue surrounds each of the fibroblasts containing ink particles, effectively entrapping and immobilizing the cell. The life span of these fibroblasts is unknown and may persist for the individual's life.

Although these studies give considerable detail regarding the architectural morphology and physiology, they do not fully explain the natural history of dermal tattoo ink. It is common to observe that a tattoo becomes duller, bluer, more indistinct, and blurred with time, presumably a consequence of ink particles moving deeper into the dermis by the action of mobile phagocytic cells. Indeed, random biopsies of older tattoos demonstrate pigment in the deep dermis as opposed to a more superficial location of newer tattoos (61). Eventually tattoo ink appears in regional lymph nodes of tattooed patients (48,62).

SIDE EFFECTS OF TATTOO PLACEMENT

Tattoo pigment has been associated with occasional allergic granulomas (63–67) and sarcoid reactions (46,68–70). Infections (71) through cutaneous inoculation secondary to tattooing have included tuberculosis (72), HIV (73), leprosy (74,75), hepatitis (76–83), atypical mycobacteria (84), verucca (85–87), and zygomycosis (88). Coincidental lesions, including sarcoidosis, B-cell

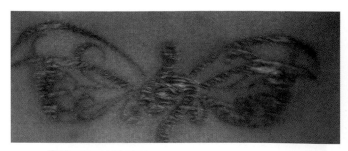

Figure 4.5 IPL. Hyperpigmentation, scarring, and ink retention following multiple IPL treatments of a tattoo. *Abbreviation*: IPL, intense pulsed light.

INTENSE PULSED LIGHT

Some novice practitioners have attempted to treat a tattoo with an intense pulsed light (IPL) device. The pulse duration of IPL, however, is much longer than the nanosecond times we see in the Q-switched devices (174) and thus selective photothermolysis does not occur. Instead of being destroyed, the tattoo ink particles heat up and nonspecific tissue injury occurred resulting in hypopigmentation, hyperpigmentation, ink retention, and scarring (Fig. 4.5). This source of significant medical liability is not an acceptable means by which to remove a tattoo, and the treatment of tattoo ink with an IPL device should be avoided.

CONTINUOUS WAVE LASERS

The first medical lasers to be developed were continuous wave (CW) lasers that, as the name suggests, produced a continuous beam of radiation that was subsequently absorbed by a target. Although this constant laser light could effectively destroy tattoo ink, its use was limited by the fact that the laser energy not only altered the target but also "spilled over" into adjacent tissue structures, causing unwanted collateral damage including hypertrophic scarring. Two CW devices that were used for tattoo removal were the argon and carbon dioxide (CO_2) lasers.

ARGON LASER

The argon laser uses the noble gas argon as the active medium, and reports of its use for tattoo removal in 28 patients first appeared in 1979 (175). Although hypertrophic scarring occurred in 21% and half of the patients had residual tattoo pigment, the complete removal of tattoo pigment in eight patients (29%) with acceptable, reportedly scarless, cosmetic results led the authors to recommend this laser enthusiastically for tattoo removal at the time. In their subsequent study, 20 of 60 patients had complete removal of tattoo pigment without scarring, with amateur tattoos responding slightly better than professional tattoos (42% vs. 29%) (176). However, hypertrophic scarring occurred in 35% of patients and residual tattoo pigment remained in 67% of patients. Biopsy studies showed obliteration of the dermis to a depth of 1 mm, and the authors stressed the preservation of adnexal structures to aid wound healing and avoid scarring (120,121,177).

The initial use of the argon laser for treatment of tattoos was based on selective absorption of energy with vaporization from its 488 and 514 nm wavelengths by complementary tattoo pigment colors (121,122,178). However, the clinical usefulness of this factor is severely limited by melanin and hemoglobin absorption of laser energy, resulting in unwanted thermal damage to tissue (42,123). It was also originally thought that selective heating of tattoo pigments and their immediate surroundings would elicit an inflammatory response and help remove or obscure the pigment. Although nonspecific heat absorption resulted in diffuse tissue necrosis, this was thought to be necessary for successful pigment removal (42).

A histologic study was performed to determine whether it was possible to oxidize or fragment tattoo pigment, confining thermal necrosis to a zone immediately adjacent to tattoo particles and thus avoiding widespread thermal necrosis of the dermis (42). The argon laser was used with powers ranging from 1.0 to 3.5 W and shuttered pulses of 0.2 seconds and 50 ms in addition to a continuous beam, using a 1-mm spot size. At 48 hours, subepidermal blisters overlying necrotic papillary dermal collagen appeared with all treatment parameters. At 3 months, fibrosis was present in the papillary and upper reticular dermis. Pigment-laden macrophages were present at the junction of fibrotic and nonfibrotic dermis, with pigment present at a deeper level within the dermis. Thus, although these authors were able to demonstrate somewhat selective absorption of laser energy by tattoo pigment (the threshold being 6.25 J/cm^2 for black and red tattoos, compared with 20 J/cm^2 for injury to normal skin), the 50- to 200-ms pulses allowed extensive diffusion of heat from all absorbing chromophores, resulting in nonselective thermal destruction. The inflammatory response was found to be a minor factor; clinical improvement depended on widespread necrosis that removed pigment and resulted in fibrosis thus altering light transmission through the dermis to obscure underlying residual pigment. Fitzpatrick et al. (179) confirmed these results and the lack of a specific laser-induced change in tattoo pigment particles as a result of argon laser therapy. Although Apfelberg and colleagues (180) reported the argon laser to be comparable with the CO_2 laser for tattoo removal, the relatively low-power emission of the argon laser results in inefficient removal of tattoo pigment, requiring multiple treatment sessions and a high incidence of hypertrophic scarring.

CARBON DIOXIDE LASER

The CO_2 laser emits a continuous beam at 10,600 nm, a wavelength completely absorbed by water, limiting penetration to a depth of 0.1–0.2 mm. Initial reports of the successful removal of tattoos with the CO_2 laser appeared in 1978 (123,181,182) with other reports following soon thereafter (183–186). Instantaneous transfer of heat from laser absorption by tissue (cellular) water results in immediate vaporization. The physics of this interaction was initially misinterpreted to imply that this always results in confinement of thermal damage to the 30- to 50-mm layer of laser impact. In reality, thermal diffusion can be quite extensive when a continuous beam is used. Even with pulses of 50–200 ms, great caution must be used to avoid unwanted thermal necrosis. The original objective in CO_2 treatment of tattoos was to vaporize tissue containing tattoo pigment, using visual control to remove all tattoo pigments in one treatment session. Attempts were made to confine the depth of tissue vaporization to the precise level of tattoo pigment, which often varies from one portion of the tattoo to another, resulting in a variable wound depth.

Histologic evaluation of the created wounds revealed loss of dermis and subcutaneous tissue up to a depth of 5 mm (128). Because of the slow healing time (4.5 ± 1.5 weeks) (123) and resultant thick, unsightly scars, most did not attempt complete pigment removal in one session and instead treated more conservatively, relying on macrophage engulfment and transepidermal removal of tattoo pigment during the healing phase (128).

Originally used as a continuous beam, repetitive pulses of 50–200 ms or superpulsed CO_2 lasers became more acceptable, with reports of good results in 29 of 30 tattoos after an average of 2.4 treatments. Although only a 7% incidence of hypertrophic scarring was noted, vaporization confined to the tattoo may result in a scar in its original shape; therefore feathering into normal tissue is recommended. Power settings of 8–25 W were common for repetitive treatments, with higher powers more rapidly vaporizing the tissue.

Because of the common occurrence of residual tattoo pigment after more superficial CO_2 laser vaporization, together with the increasing risk of hypertrophic scarring with subsequent treatments, methods to improve the results of a single treatment were explored. Although the concomitant use of 2% gentian violet to prolong the exudative phase following superficial CO_2 laser vaporization did not increase efficacy, 50% urea paste did improve results (187), as was reported with the argon laser (188).

In summary, the CO_2 laser removes tattoo pigment in much the same way as the argon laser, although with higher fluencies and more efficient tissue vaporization with the CO_2 laser is more efficient. Tattoo pigment is removed by direct tissue vaporization, as well as by thermal necrosis of adjacent tissue and through loss of pigment in the exudative healing phase. Dermal tissue is reconstituted by fibrosis and scar tissue, and although acceptable results can occasionally be obtained, because there is a level of unpredictability and some scarring usually occurs, the CO_2 is no longer a viable option for treating unwanted tattoos.

QUALITY-SWITCHED LASER TREATMENT OF TATTOOS

Anderson and Parrish's principle of selective photothermolysis revolutionized the treatment of tattoos (189). The word "photothermolysis" is derived from the Greek word "photo" meaning light, "thermo" meaning heat, and "lysis" meaning destruction. Thus, selective photothermolysis therefore refers to the precise targeting of a structure using a specific wavelength of light with the intention of absorbing light into that target area alone. They proposed that if a wavelength was well absorbed by the target and the pulse width was equal to or shorter than the target's thermal relaxation time, the heat generated would be confined to the target and allow the surrounding area to remain relatively untouched. The thermal relaxation time is the time it takes a given target chromophore (in this case, tattoo ink) to lose 50% of its absorbed heat energy.

In one of the earliest studies, Diette et al. (55) examined the effects of a tunable dye laser at three wavelengths (505, 577, and 680 nm) using a 1-ms pulse to remove black, blue, red, and white tattoo pigments. They found that the threshold dose to induce the same histologic changes was much less than that required for the argon laser and that each wavelength reacted only with complementary colors of tattoo pigment. However, despite the short 1-ms pulse, widespread tissue necrosis was observed, and tattoo lightening occurred only as a result of significant dermal necrosis and resultant fibrosis. The authors postulated that an even shorter pulse in the nanosecond domain would interact best with the micrometer-sized pigment granule's approximate thermal relaxation time.

To destroy tattoo ink selectively, the best wavelength is chosen to achieve selective absorption for that ink color while minimizing the nonspecific thermal effects from the primary endogenous chromophores, hemoglobin, and melanin. After laser treatment, a small portion of the ink may be partially extruded through the scale crust that forms following epidermal injury. A greater proportion of the ink particles may be fragmented, released into the extracellular space, and eliminated into the lymphatics or rephagocytosed as laser-altered residual tattoo particles, perhaps with altered optical properties. With the advent of Q-switched lasers operating in the nanosecond (billionth of a second, 10^{-9}) range, the promise of scarless tattoo removal became a reality.

Q-SWITCHED RUBY LASER

The ruby laser uses a synthetic ruby crystal as the active medium and emits a wavelength of light at 694 nm, which has a deep red color. In 1965, the earliest reports of tattoo–pigment interaction with short-pulsed lasers were documented by Goldman et al. (190,191) who compared the reaction of a dark-blue tattoo to a Q-switched ruby laser with nanosecond pulses with a microsecond-pulsed ruby laser. They found nonspecific thermal necrosis with microsecond impacts, whereas nanosecond impacts produced only transient edema accompanied by a peculiar whitening of the impact area, lasting about 30 minutes. No thermal necrosis was present but tattoo fragments remained in the dermis. The mechanism of this reaction was unknown but was not thought to be thermal because of normal measurements taken with a thermistor. Because of the reported retention of tattoo pigment, this modality was originally interpreted as a failure. Goldman, however, followed the patient's progress and noted continued fading of the treated area. Goldman was unable to continue this work because his engineer was fatally electrocuted, and subsequently he abandoned the project. Only 3 years later, however, other investigators confirmed and expanded these results (192,193) using a Q-switched ruby laser to remove blue and black tattoo pigments successfully without tissue damage. Biopsies performed after 3 months showed absence of tattoo pigment and no evidence of thermal damage. These effects were dose dependent, with fluences of 5.6 J/cm² or less, showing absence of thermal damage but incomplete pigment removal. Higher fluences led to subepidermal blisters similar to a second-degree burn and dermal fibrosis at 3 months, although pigment removal was more complete. Subsequent studies (123,194) concluded that this treatment modality was impractical because of the small target areas and the risk of coagulation necrosis of tissue surrounding the tattoo pigment.

Reid and coworkers (195) continued to study the Q-switched ruby laser and in 1983 published an additional report on removal of black pigment in professional and amateur tattoos.

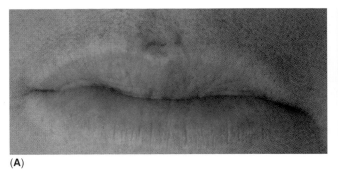
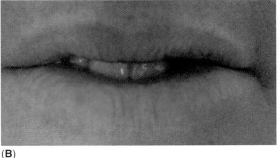

(A)   (B)

Figure 4.12 Traumatic tattoo before and traumatic tattoo after. (**A**) Traumatic tattoo at the Cupid's bow secondary to a fall on asphalt; (**B**) significant ink resolution 8 weeks after a single treatment with a neodymium-doped:yttrium-aluminum-garnet laser.

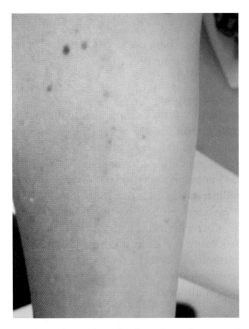

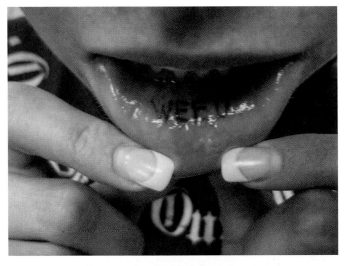

Figure 4.14 Lip. Orolabial mucosal tattoo.

Figure 4.13 Track marks. Unintentional track mark tattoos in a former intravenous heroin user.

Q-switched lasers or punch biopsies. Many cancer survivors feel that these tattoos are a sign of strength and survival and may choose to forgo tattoo removal treatment.

Fluorescent Tattoos
Rarely a patient will present with a tattoo composed of pigment that is invisible in normal light but becomes observable with exposure to black light or a Wood's lamp. Patients refer to these tattoos as "fluorescent" tattoos, but they are also known as "glow-in-the-dark" or "ultraviolet (UV)" tattoos. Because the photoluminescent ingredient in many of these tattoos is unknown and since this ink is often not responsive to Q-switched laser treatment, the safest removal option for these tattoos, if possible, is often surgical excision.

Henna Tattoos
Coming from a south Asian tradition that has now become common at many tropical vacation destinations, henna tattoos are a form of a temporary tattoo that uses a dye made from the leaves of the henna plant, *Lawsonia inermis*. After being painted on and left to dry, a paste made from the powdered leaves of the plant binds with keratin in skin. No treatment is

warranted as a henna tattoo will gradually fade away over the course of a few days to weeks as the skin naturally sloughs off.

FUTURE DEVELOPMENTS IN TATTOO REMOVAL
Although Q-switched lasers provide a dramatic improvement over previous tattoo removal modalities and are now considered the "gold standard" treatment option, it is possible that we will see even more efficient removal techniques in the future.

Some dermatologists are beginning to combine Q-switched laser technology with fractional resurfacing in hopes of increasing ink clearance (261). Additionally, the exploration of picosecond (10^{-12}) lasers has begun (262). Theoretically, this would allow for more effective treatment utilizing lower fluences, thereby decreasing thermal energy transfer to surrounding tissues and minimizing the risk of adverse events, including tissue texture changes, scarring, and discoloration. The possibility of the use of femtosecond (10^{-15}) technology to treat tattoos exists in theory as well, but the viability of its practical application on a wide scale is yet to be determined.

Changes to current treatment protocols using existing technology could theoretically provide faster ink resolution. A small study on 12 patients in Greece was performed using a single Q-switched laser with four treatment passes separated by 20 minutes (263). The authors of this "R20" method noted that this treatment protocol was more effective than conventional laser treatment with the same incidence of side effects. It should be acknowledged, however, that the device used in this study was an alexandrite laser, which, as noted above, is less powerful than Nd:YAG devices. Thus, the question remains to be answered if the finding of this study could be reproduced with other Q-switched lasers such as an Nd:YAG or ruby with the same low level of adverse events. These findings have yet to be corroborated, but the author of this chapter has begun a proof of concept study with a larger patient population.

Eventually it may be possible to quantify tattoo pigment absorption characteristics more specifically and then choose an appropriate wavelength of laser light that will facilitate clearing of multicolored tattoos and tattoos resistant to treatment. This could also conceivably result in a faster treatment regime. Additionally, future lasers may fire even more rapidly and the use of picosecond lasers could further enhance our ability to remove tattoos rapidly without damaging surrounding tissue (195,197,264–266).

As Cohen and Goldman first hypothesized in 1994, macrophage-stimulating factors can be used for adjuvant therapy with laser tattoo removal (267) and nonsurgical tattoo removal in animal models has been demonstrated using topical imiquimod cream (268–271). Thus, topical immune response modifier molecules may serve as an accepted adjuvant therapy in future treatment regimes.

Lastly, tattoo removal may one day become more efficient not by the device used but by the tattoo pigment itself. Multiple companies have proposed tattoo inks packaged in microscopic, transparent, biocompatible capsules that theoretically require fewer treatments with a Q-switched laser to remove and still others claim that their ink remains in the dermis after exposure to laser but that the color becomes transparent after a single-treatment session. Studies supporting these claims are not yet available and the question of whether these inks will be embraced by the tattoo artist community remains to be answered.

ACKNOWLEDGMENTS

Dr. Kirby would like to thank the following individuals for their assistance with this chapter: Cynthia Chen, DO; Ian Andrew Kirby; Emily Holmes, RN; Tejas Desai, DO, FAOCD; and Alpesh Desai, DO, FAOCD

REFERENCES

1. Hammond N. Iceman was wearing earliest snowshoes. The Times 2005. [Available from: http://www.thetimes.co.uk/tto/life/courtsocial/article1814891.ece].
2. Höpfel F, Platzer W, Spindler K, eds. Der Mann im Eis Vol. 1. Innsbruck. Austria: Veröffentlichungen der Universität Innsbruck, 1992.
3. Seidler H, Berhard W, Teschler-Nicola M, et al. Some anthropological aspects of the prehistoric Tyrolean Ice Man. Science 1992; 258: 455–7.
4. Spindler K. The Man in the Ice. The Preserved Body of the Neolithic Man Reveals the Secrets of the Stone Age. London: Weidenfeld and Nicolson, 1994.
5. Rudenko SI. Frozen tombs of Siberia. London: J M Dent & Sons, 1970.
6. Allison MJ. Early mummies from coastal Peru and Chile. In: Spindler K, Wilfing H, Rastbichler-Zissernig E, zur Nedden D, Nothdurfter H, eds. The Man in the Ice, vol. 3: Human Mummies. Vienna, Austria: Springer Verlag, 1996: 125–9.
7. Dorfer L, Moser M, Bahr F, et al. A medical report from the Stone Age? Lancet 1999; 354: 1023–5.
8. Hambly WD. The History of Tattooing and Its Significance. London: H.F. & G. Witherby, 1925.
9. Scutt R, Gotch C. Art, Sex and Symbol: The Mystery of Tattooing. Cranbury, NJ: Barnes, 1974.
10. Ebensten H. Pierced Hearts and True Love. London: Verschoyle, 1953.
11. Stephens MB. Behavioral risks associated with tattooing. Fam Med 2003; 35: 53–4.
12. Carroll ST, Riffenburgh RH, Roberts TA, Myhre EB. Tattoos and body piercings as indicators of adolescent risk-taking behaviors. Pediatrics 2002; 109: 1021–7.
13. Forbes GB. College students with tattoos and piercings: motives, family experiences, personality factors, and perception by others. Psychol Rep 2001; 89: 774–86.
14. Rooks JK, Roberts DJ, Scheltema K. Tattoos: their relationship to trauma, psychopathology, and other myths. Minn Med 2000; 83: 247.
15. Laumann AE, Derick AJ. Tattoos and body piercings in the United States. J Am Acad Dermatol 2006; 55: 413–21; Epub 2006 Jun 16.
16. Sever JM. 2003. "A Third of Americans With Tattoos Say They Make Them Feel More Sexy." The Harris Poll: #58, Harris Interactive Web site. 2003. [Available from: http://www.harrisinteractive.com/harris_poll/index.asp ?PID=407] [Accessed July 17, 2011]
17. Hellgren L. Tattooing: the Prevalence of Tattooed Persons in a Total Population. Stockholm: Almquist & Wiksell, 1967.
18. Hamburger E. Tattooing as a psychic defence mechanism. Int J Soc Psychiatry 1966; 12: 60.
19. Lepine A. Tattooing in approved schools and remand homes. Health Trends 1969; 1: 11.
20. Scutt RWB. The chemical removal of tattoos. Br J Plast Surg 1972; 25: 189.
21. Goldstein N. Psychological implications of tattoos. J Dermatol Surg Oncol 1979; 5: 883.
22. Pers M, von Herbst T. Tatovering af umyndige. Ugeskr Laeg 1965; 31: 973.
23. Pers M, von Herbst T. The demand for removal of tattoos: a plea for regulations against tattooing of minors. Acta Chir Scand 1966; 131: 201.
24. Gittleson N, Wallen G, Dawson-Butterworth K. The tattooed psychiatric patient. Br J Psychiatry 1969; 115: 1249.
25. Taylor A. A search among Borstal girls for the psychological and social significance of their tattoos. Br J Criminol 1968; 8: 170.
26. Hamburger E, Lacovara D. A study of tattoos in inmates at a federal correctional institution: its physical and psychological implications. Milit Med 1963; 128: 1205.
27. Roe A, Howell R, Payne I. Comparison of prison inmates with and without juvenile records. Psychol Rep 1974; 34: 1315.
28. Lander J, Kohn A. A note on tattooing among selectees. Am J Psychiatry 1943; 100: 326.
29. Youniss R. The relationship of tattoos to personal adjustment with a second, larger tattoo of another bird. Initially, the among enlisted submarine school volunteers. US Naval Med tattoo was divided into three sections (Figure 4.38). Section Res Lab 1959; 18: 1; Report no 319.
30. Armstrong ML, Murphy KP, Sallee A, Watson MG. Tattooed Army soldiers: examining the incidence, behavior, and risk. Mil Med 2000; 165: 135–41.
31. Armstrong ML, Murphy KP. Tattooing: another adolescent health risk behavior warranting health education. Appl Nurs Res 1997; 10: 181–9.
32. Roberts TA, Ryan SA. Tattooing and high-risk behavior in adolescents. Pediatrics 2002; 110: 1058–63.
33. Armstrong ML, McConnell C. Tattooing in adolescents: more common than you think—the phenomenon and risks. J Sch Nurs 1994; 10: 26–33.
34. Brown KM, Perlmutter P, McDermott RJ. Youth and tattoos: what school health personnel should know. J Sch Health 2000; 70: 355–60.
35. Armstrong ML, Murphy KP, Sallee A, Watson MG. Tattooed Army soldiers: examining the incidence, behavior, and risk. Mil Med 2000; 165: 135–41.
36. Greif J, Hewitt W, Armstrong ML. Tattooing and body piercing. Body art practices among college students. Clin Nurs Res 1999; 8: 368–85.
37. Mayers LB, Judelson DA, Moriarty BW, Rundell KW. Prevalence of body art (body piercing and tattooing) in university undergraduates and incidence of medical complications. Mayo Clin Proc 2002; 77: 29–34.

38. Roberti JW, Storch EA, Bravata EA. Sensation seeking, exposure to psychosocial stressors, and body modifications in a college population. Pers Individ Dif 2004; 37: 1167–77.

39. Smith SR, Matheson BK, Riffenburgh RH. Trends in tattooing. Dermatol Surg 1996; 22: 485–6.

40. Grumet GW. Psychodynamic implications of tattoos. Am J Orthopsychiatry 1983; 53: 482.

41. Armstrong ML. Career-oriented women with tattoos. J Nurs Schol 1991; 23: 215.

42. Cohen M. Tattooing: some medical and psychological aspects. Br J Dermatol 1927; 39: 290.

43. Varma S, Lanigan SW. Motivation for tattoo removal. Arch Dermatol 1996; 132: 1516.

44. Swami V, Furnham A. Unattractive, promiscuous and heavy drinkers: Perceptions of women with tattoos. Body Image 2007; 4: 343–52; Epub 2007 Sep 20.

45. Armstrong ML. Career-oriented women with tattoos. Image J Nurs Sch Winter 1991; 23: 215–20.

46. Varma S, Lanigan SW. The psychological, social, and financial burden of tattoos [Abstract]. Br J Dermatol 1996; 135: 37–8.

47. Bekhor PS, Bekhor L, Gangrabur M. Employer attitudes toward persons with visible tattoos. Australas J Dermatol 1995; 36: 75–7.

48. Armstrong ML, Roberts AE, Koch JR, et al. Motivation for tattoo removal. Arch Dermatol 1996; 132: 412–16.

49. Lapidoth M, Aharonowitz G. Tattoo removal among Ethiopian Jews in Israel: tradition faces technology. J Am Acad Dermatol 2004; 51: 906–9.

50. Tope WD. State and territorial regulation of tattooing in the United States. J Am Acad Dermatol 1995; 32: 791–9.

51. Armstrong ML. Tattooing, body piercing, and permanent cosmetics: a historical and current view of state regulations, with continuing concerns. J Environ Health 2005; 67: 38–43; 54,53.

52. Kaur R, Kirby W, Maibach H. Cutaneous allergic reactions to tattoo ink. J Cosmet Dermatol 2009; 8: 304–9.

53. Lea PJ, Pawlowski A. Human tattoo: electron microscopic assessment of epidermis, epidermal–dermal junction, and dermis. Int J Dermatol 1987; 26: 453.

54. Taylor CR, Anderson R, Gange W, Michaud NA, Flotte TJ. Light and electron microscopic analysis of tattoos treated by Q-switched ruby laser. J Invest Dermatol 1991; 97: 131.

55. Diette KM, Bronstein BR, Parrish JA. Histologic comparison of argon and tunable dye lasers in the treatment of tattoos. J Invest Dermatol 1985; 85: 368.

56. Patipa M, Jakobiec FA, Krebs W. Light and electron microscopic findings with permanent eyeliner. Ophthalmology 1986; 93: 1361.

57. Christensen HE, Schmidt H. The ultrastructure of tattoo marks. Pathol Microbiol Scand 1972; 80A: 573.

58. Mann R, Klingmuller G. Electron-microscopic investigation of tattoos in rabbit skin. Arch Dermatol Res 1981; 271: 367.

59. Goldstein AP. Histologic reactions in tattoos. J Dermatol Surg Oncol 1979; 5: 896.

60. Tse T, Folberg R, Moore K. Clinicopathologic correlate of a fresh eyelid pigment implantation. Arch Ophthalmol 1985; 103: 1515.

61. Goldstein N, Sewell M. Tattoos in different cultures. J Dermatol Surg Oncol 1979; 5: 857.

62. Everett MA. Tattoos: abnormalities of pigmentation. In: Clinical dermatology, vol 2, units 11–21. Hagerstown, MD: Harper & Row, 1980.

63. Yang DS, Kim SC, Lee S, Chung Y. Foreign body epithelioid granuloma after cosmetic eyebrow tattooing. Cutis 1989; 43: 224.

64. Ravits HG. Allergic tattoo granuloma. Arch Dermatol 1962; 86: 287.

65. Tope WD, Arbiser JL, Duncan LM. Black tattoo reaction: the peacock's tale. J Am Acad Dermatol 1996; 35: 477–9.

66. Duke D, Urioste SS, Dover JS, Anderson RR. A reaction to a red lip cosmetic tattoo. J Am Acad Dermatol 1998; 39: 488–90.

67. Schwarze HP, Giordano-Labadie F, Loche F, Gorquet MB, Bazex J. Delayed-hypersensitivity granulomatous reaction induced by blepharopigmentation with aluminum-silicate. J Am Acad Dermatol 2000; 42: 888–91.

68. Dickinson JA. Sarcoidal reaction in tattoos. Arch Dermatol 1969; 100: 315.

69. Farzan S. Sarcoidal reaction in tattoos. NY State J Med 1977; 77: 1477.

70. Jones MS, Maloney ME, Helm KF. Systemic sarcoidosis presenting in the black dye of a tattoo. Cutis 1997; 59: 113–15.

71. Nishioka Sde A, Gyorkos TW, Joseph L, Collet JP, Maclean JD. Tattooing and risk for transfusion-transmitted diseases: the role of the type, number and design of the tattoos, and the conditions in which they were performed. Epidemiol Infect 2002; 128: 63–71.

72. Horney DA, Gaither JM, Lauer R, Norins AL, Mathur PN. Cutaneous inoculation tuberculosis secondary to 'jailhouse tattooing'. Arch Dermatol 1985; 121: 648–50.

73. Doll DC. Tattooing in prison and HIV infection. Lancet 1988; 1: 66–7.

74. Singh G, Tutakne MA, Tiwari VD, Dutta RK. Inoculation leprosy developing after tattooing—a case report. Indian J Lepr 1985; 57: 887–8.

75. Sehgal VN, Jain S, Bhattacharya SN, Chouhan S. Borderline tuberculoid (BT) leprosy confined to a tattoo. Int J Lepr Other Mycobact Dis 1991; 59: 323–5.

76. Haley RW, Fischer RP. Commercial tattooing as a potentially important source of hepatitis C infection. Clinical epidemiology of 626 consecutive patients unaware of their hepatitis C serologic status. Medicine (Baltimore) 2001; 80: 134–51.

77. Alter MJ, Kruszon-Moran D, Nainan OV, et al. The prevalence of hepatitis C virus infection in the United States, 1988 through 1994. N Engl J Med 1999; 341: 556–62.

78. Hayes MO, Harkness GA. Body piercing as a risk factor for viral hepatitis: an integrative research review. Am J Infect Control 2001; 29: 271–4.

79. Thompson SC, Goudey RE, Breschkin AM, Carnie J, Catton M. Exposure to hepatitis B and of tattooists in Victoria in 1984. J Viral Hepat 1997; 4: 135–8.

80. Mowat NAG, Brunt PW, Albert-Recht F, Walker W. Outbreak of serum hepatitis associated with tattooing. Lancet 1973; 1: 33–4.

81. Goh KT. Hepatitis B surveillance in Singapore. Ann Acad Med Singapore 1980; 9: 136–41.

82. Abildgaard N, Peterslund NA. Hepatitis C virus transmitted by tattooing needle. Lancet 1991; 338: 460.

83. Thompson SC, Hernberger F, Wale E, Crofts N. Hepatitis C transmission through tattooing: a case report. Aust N Z J Public Health 1996; 20: 317–18.

84. Wolf R, Wolf D. A tattooed butterfly as a vector of atypical Mycobacteria. J Am Acad Dermatol 2003; 48: S73–4.

85. Miller DM, Brodell RT. Verruca restricted to the areas of black dye within a tattoo. Arch Dermatol 1994; 130: 1453–4.

86. Ragland HP, Hubbell C, Stewart KR, Nesbitt LT Jr. Verruca vulgaris inoculated during tattoo placement. Int J Dermatol 1994; 33: 796–7.

87. Baxter SY, Deck DH. Tattoo-acquired verruca plana. Am Fam Physician 1993; 47: 732.

88. Parker C, Kaminski G, Hill D. Zygomycosis in a tattoo, caused by Saksenaea vasiformis. Australas J Dermatol 1986; 27: 107–11.

89. Armiger WG, Caldwell EH. Primary lesion of a non-Hodgkin's lymphoma occurring in a skin tattoo: case report. Plast Reconstr Surg 1978; 62: 125–7.

90. Khan IU, Moiemen NS, Firth J, Frame JD. Malignant melanoma disguised by a tattoo. Br J Plastic Surg 1999; 52: 598.

91. Kirsch N. Malignant melanoma developing in a tattoo. Int J Dermatol 1972; 11: 16–20.

92. Kircik L, Armus S, van den Broek H. Malignant melanoma in a tattoo. Int J Dermatol 1993; 32: 297–8.

93. Paradisi A, Capizzi R, De Simone C, et al. Malignant melanoma in a tattoo: case report and review of the literature. Melanoma Res 2006; 16: 375–6.

94. Stinco G, De Francesco V, Frattasio A, Quinkenstein E, Patrone P. Malignant melanoma in a tattoo. Dermatology 2003; 206: 345–6.

95. Soroush V, Gurevitch AW, Peng SK. Malignant melanoma in a tattoo: case report and review of the literature. Cutis 1997; 59: 111–12.

96. Bartal AH, Cohen Y, Robinson E. Malignant melanoma arising at tattoo sites used for radiotherapy field marking. Br J Radiol 1980; 53: 913–14.

97. Wolfort FC, Hoopes JE, Filtzer HS, Cochran TC. Superficial melanoma in a tattoo. Br J Plast Surg 1974; 27: 303–4.

98. Kirsch N. Malignant melanoma developing in a tattoo. Arch Dermatol 1969; 99: 596–8.

99. Wiener DA, Scher RK. Basal cell carcinoma arising in a tattoo. Cutis 1987; 39: 125–6.

100. Earley MJ. Basal cell carcinoma arising in tattoos: A clinical report of two cases. Br J Plast Surg 1983; 36: 258–9.

101. Doumat F, Kaise W, Barbaud A, Schmutz JL. Basal cell carcinoma in a tattoo. Dermatology 2004; 208: 181–2.

102. Omidian M, Esad-Mostofi N. Basal cell carcinoma arising from traditional tattoo. Arch Iran Med 2009; 12: 198.

103. Birnie AJ, Kulkarni K, Varma S. Basal cell carcinoma arising in a tattoo. Clin Exp Dermatol 2006; 31: 820–1.

104. Bashir AH. Basal cell carcinoma in tattoos: report of two cases. Br J Plastic Surg 1976; 29: 288–90.

105. Kleinerman R, Greenspan A, Hale EK. Mohs micrographic surgery for an unusual case of keratoacanthoma arising from a longstanding tattoo. J Drugs Dermatol 2007; 6: 931–2.

106. Chorny JA, Stephens FV, Cohen JL. Eruptive keratoacanthomas in a new tattoo. Arch Dermatol 2007; 143: 1457–8.

107. Kluger N, Minier-Thoumin C, Plantier F. Keratoacanthoma occurring within the red dye of a tattoo. J Cutan Pathol 2008; 35: 504–7.

108. Fraga GR, Prossick TA. Tattoo-associated keratoacanthomas: a series of 8 patients with 11 keratoacanthomas. J Cutan Pathol 2010; 37: 85–90.

109. Goldenberg G, Patel S, Patel MJ, Williford P, Sanqueza O. Eruptive squamous cell carcinomas, keratoacanthoma type, arising in a multicolor tattoo. J Cutan Pathol 2008; 35: 62–4.

110. Ortiz A, Yamauchi PS. Rapidly growing squamous cell carcinomas from permanent makeup tattoo. J Am Acad Dermatol 2009; 60: 1073–4.

111. McQuarry DG. Squamous cell carcinoma arising in a tattoo. Minn Med 1966; 49: 799.

112. Nicolle E, Bessis D, Guihou JJ. Seborrheic keratosis erupting in a tattoo. Ann Dermatol Venereol 1998; 125: 261–3.

113. Pack GT, Tabah EJ. Dermatofibrosarcoma protuberans: a report of 39 cases. Arch Surg 1951; 62: 391–411.

114. Kluger N, Cotton H, Magana C, Pinguier L. Dermatofibroma occurring within a tattoo: report of two cases. J Cutan Pathol 2008; 35: 696–8.

115. Reddy KK, Hanke CW, Tierney EP. Malignancy arising within cutaneous tattoos: case of dermatofibrosarcoma protuberans and review of the literature. J Drugs Dermatol 2011; 10: 837–42.

116. West CC, Morritt AN, Pedelty L, Lam DG. Cutaneous leiomyosarcoma arising in a tattoo—'a tumour with no humour'. J Plast Reconstr Aesthet Surg 2009; 62: e79–80.

117. Jacob CI. Tattoo-associated dermatoses: a case report and review of the literature. Dermatol Surg 2002; 28: 961–5.

118. Silberberg I, Leider M. Studies of a red tattoo. Arch Dermatol 1970; 101: 299.

119. Abel EA, Silberberg I, Queen D. Studies of chronic inflammation in a red tattoo by electron microscopy and histochemistry. Acta Dermatol Venereol (Stockh) 1972; 52: 453.

120. Rostenberg A, Brown RA, Caro MR. Discussion of tattoo reactions with report of a case showing a reaction to a green color. Arch Dermatol Syph 1950; 62: 540.

121. Anderson RR. Tattooing should be regulated. N Engl J Med 1992; 326: 207.

122. Ballin DB. Cutaneous hypersensitivity to mercury from tattooing: report of case. Arch Dermatol Syph 1933; 27: 292.

123. Bonnell JA, Russell B. Skin reactions at sites of green and red tattoo marks. Proc R Soc Med 1956; 49: 823.

124. Harper & Row; 1980. Bjornberg A. Reactions to light in yellow tattoos from cadmium sulfide. Arch Dermatol 1963; 88: 267.

125. Tindall JP, Smith JG Jr. Unusual reactions in yellow tattoos: microscopic studies on histologic sections. South Med J 1962; 55: 792.

126. Loewenthal LJA. Reactions in green tattoos: the significance of valence state of chromium. Arch Dermatol 1960; 82: 237.

127. Bjornberg A. Allergic reactions to chrome in green tattoo markings. Acta Derm Venereal 1959; 39: 23.

128. Tazelaar DJ. Hypersensitivity to chromium in a light-blue tattoo. Dermatologica 1970; 141: 282.

129. Rorsman H, Brehmer-Andersson E, Dahlquist I, et al. Tattoo granuloma and uveitis. Lancet 1969; 11: 27.

130. Swinny B. Generalized chronic dermatitis due to tattoo. Ann Allergy 1946; 4: 295.

131. Novy FG. A generalized mercurial (cinnabar) reaction following tattooing. Arch Dermatol 1944; 49: 172.

132. Goldstein N. Complications for tattoos. J Dermatol Surg Oncol 1979; 5: 869.

133. England RW, Vogel P, Hagan L. Immediate cutaneous hypersensitivity after treatment of tattoo with Nd:YAG laser: a case report and review of the literature. Ann Allergy Asthma Immunol 2002; 89: 215–17.

134. Bjornberg A. Reactions to light in yellow tattoos from cadmium sulfide. Arch Dermatol 1963; 88: 267.

135. Boo-Chai K. The decorative tattoo: its removal by dermabrasion. Plast Reconstr Surg 1963; 32: 559.

136. Clabaugh W. Removal of tattoos by superficial dermabrasion. Arch Dermatol 1968; 98: 515.

137. Clabaugh W. Tattoo removal by superficial dermabrasion. Plast Reconstr Surg 1975; 55: 401.

138. Bunke HJ, Conway H. Surgery of decorative and traumatic tattoos. Plast Reconstr Surg 1957; 20: 67.

139. Colver GB, Jones RL, Cherry GW, Dawber RP, Ryan TJ. Precise dermal damage with an infrared coagulator. Br J Dermatol 1986; 114: 603.

140. Colver GB, Cherry GW, Dawber RP, Ryan TJ. The treatment of cutaneous vascular lesions with the infrared coagulator: a preliminary report. Br J Plast Surg 1986; 39: 131.

141. Colver GB, Hunter JAA. Venous lakes: treatment by infrared coagulation. Br J Plast Surg 1987; 40: 451.

142. Dorn B, Christophers E, Kietzmann H. Treatment of port-wine stains and haemangiomas by infrared contact coagulation. 17th World Congress of Dermatology Abstracts 1987; 2: 307.

143. Groot DW, Arlett JP, Johnston PA. Comparison of the infrared coagulator and the carbon dioxide laser in the removal of decorative tattoos. J Am Acad Dermatol 1986; 15: 518.

144. Colver GB, Cherry GW, Dawber RP, Ryan TJ. Tattoo removal using infrared coagulation. Br J Dermatol 1985; 112: 481.

145. Venning VA, Colver GB, Millard PR, Ryan TJ. Tattoo removal using infrared coagulation: a dose comparison. Br J Dermatol 1987; 117: 99.

146. Colver GB. The infrared coagulator in dermatology. Dermatol Clin 1989; 7: 155.

147. Leopold PJ. Cryosurgery for facial skin lesions. Proc R Soc Med 1975; 68: 606.

148. Zacarian SA. Cryosurgery for cutaneous carcinoma. Dermatol Dig 1970; 9: 49.

149. Colver GB, Dawber RPR. Tattoo removal using a liquid nitrogen cryospray. Clin Exp Dermatol 1984; 9: 364.

150. Dvir E, Hirshowitz B. Tattoo removal by cryosurgery. Plast Reconstr Surg 1980; 66: 373.

151. Colver GB, Dawber RPR. The removal of digital tattoos. Int J Dermatol 1985; 24: 567.

152. Goldstein N. Tattoo removal. Dermatol Clin 1987; 5: 349.

153. Gupta SC. An investigation into a method for the removal of dermal tattoos: a report on animal and clinical studies. Plast Reconstr Surg 1965; 36: 354.

154. Ruiz-Esparza J, Fitzpatrick RE, Goldman MP. Tattoo removal: selecting the right alternative. Am J Cosmet Surg 1992; 9: 171.

155. Variot G. Nouveau procede de destruction des tatouages. Compte Rendu Societe Biologie (Paris) 1888; 8: 836.

156. Goldstein N, Penoff J, Price N, et al. Techniques of removal of tattoos. J Dermatol Surg Oncol 1979; 5: 901.

157. Van der Velden EM, Van der Walle HB, Groot AD. Tattoo removal: tannic acid method of Variot. Int J Dermatol 1993; 32: 376–80.

158. Penoff JH. The office treatment of tattoos: a simple and effective method. Plast Reconstr Surg 1987; 79: 186.

159. Rudlinger R. Successful removal by ruby laser of darkened ink after ruby laser treatment of mismatched tattoos for acne scars. J Cut Laser Ther 2000; 2: 37–9.

160. Fogh H, Wulf HC, Poulsen T, Larsen P. Tattoo removal by overtattooing with tannic acid. J Dermatol Surg Oncol 1989; 15: 1089–90.

161. Lindsay DG. Tattoos. Dermatol Clin 1989; 7: 147.

162. Piggot TA, Norris RW. The treatment of tattoos with trichloroacetic acid: experience with 670 patients. Br J Plast Surg 1988; 41: 112.

163. Hudson DA, Lechtape-Gruter RU. A simple method of tattoo removal. S Afr Med J 1990; 78: 748.

164. Crittenden FM. Salabrasion: removal of tattoos by superficial abrasion with table salt. Cutis 1971; 7: 295.

165. Koerber WA, Price NM. Salabrasion of tattoos. Arch Dermatol 1978; 114: 884.

166. Morgan BDG. Tattoos. Br Med J 1974; 3: 34.

167. Strong AMM, Jackson JT. The removal of amateur tattoos by salabrasion. Br J Dermatol 1979; 101: 693.

168. Wentzell JM, Robinson JK, Wentzell JM, Schwartz DE, Carlson SE. Physical properties of aerosols produced by dermabrasion. Arch Dermatol 1989; 125: 1637.

169. Bailey BN. Treatment of tattoos. Plast Reconstr Surg 1976; 40: 361.

170. Ceilley RI. Curettage after dermabrasion: techniques of removal of tattoos. J Dermatol Surg Oncol 1979; 5: 905.

171. Robinson J. Tattoo removal. J Dermatol Surg Oncol 1985; 11: 14.

172. Apfelberg DB, Manchester GH. Decorative and traumatic tattoo biophysics and removal. Clin Plast Surg 1987; 14: 243.

173. Wheeler ES, Miller TA. Tattoo removal by split thickness tangential excision. West J Med 1976; 124: 272.

174. Wenzel S, Landthaler M, Raumler W. Recurring mistakes in tattoo removal: A case series. Dermatology 2009; 218: 164–7.

175. Apfelberg DB, Maser MR, Lash H. Argon laser treatment of decorative tattoos. Br J Plast Surg 1979; 32: 141.

176. Apfelberg DB, Rivers J, Maser MR, Lash H. Update on laser usage in treatment of decorative tattoos. Lasers Surg Med 1982; 2: 169.

177. Apfelberg DB, Laub DR, Maser MR, Lash H. Pathophysiology and treatment of decorative tattoos with reference to argon laser treatment. Clin Plast Surg 1967; 7: 369.

178. Reid R. Muller S. Tattoo removal with laser. Med J Aust 1978; 1: 389.

179. Fitzpatrick RE, Goldman MP, Ruiz-Esparza J. The use of the alexandrite laser (755 nm, 100 msec) for tattoo pigment removal in an animal model. J Am Acad Dermatol 1993; 28: 745.

180. Apfelberg DB, Maser MR, Lash H, White DN, Flores JT. Comparison of argon and carbon dioxide laser treatment of decorative tattoos. a preliminary report. Ann Plast Surg 1985; 14: 6.

181. McBurney EI. Carbon dioxide laser treatment of dermatologic lesions. South Med J 1978; 71: 795.

182. Brady SC, Blokmanis A, Jewett L. Tattoo removal with the carbon dioxide laser. Ann Plast Surg 1978; 2: 482.

183. Beacon JP, Ellis H. Surgical removal of tattoos by carbon dioxide laser. J R Soc Med 1980; 73: 298.

184. Bailin PL, Ratz JL, Levine HL. Removal of tattoos by CO_2 laser. J Dermatol Surg Oncol 1980; 6: 997.

185. Reid R, Muller S. Tattoo removal by CO_2 laser dermabrasion. Plast Reconstr Surg 1980; 65: 717.

186. Dixon J. Laser treatment of decorative tattoos. In: Arndt KA, Noe JM, Rosen S, eds. Cutaneous Laser Therapy: Principles and Methods. New York: John Wiley & Sons, 1983.

187. Ruiz-Esparza J, Goldman MP, Fitzpatrick RE. Tattoo removal with minimal scarring: the chemo-laser technique. J Dermatol Surg Oncol 1989; 14: 1372.

188. Dismukes DE. The 'chemo-laser technique' for the treatment of decorative tattoos: a more complete dye-removal procedure. Lasers Surg Med 1986; 6: 59.

189. Anderson RR, Parrish JA. Selective photothermolysis: precise microsurgery by selective absorption of pulsed irradiation. Science 1983; 220: 524.

190. Goldman L, Blaney DJ, Kindel DJ Jr, Richfield D, Franke EK. Pathology of the effect of the laser beam on the skin. Nature 1965; 197: 912.

191. Goldman L, Wilson RG, Hornby P, Meyer RG. Radiation from a Q-Switched ruby laser. Effect of repeated impacts of power output of 10 Megawatts on a Tattoo of Man. J Invest Dermatol 1965; 44: 69.

192. Yules RB, Laub DR, Honey R, Vassiliadis A, Crowley L. The effect of Q-switched ruby laser radiation on dermal tattoo pigment in man. Arch Surg 1967; 95: 179.

193. Laub DR, Yules RB, Arras M, et al. Preliminary histopathological observation of Q-switched ruby laser radiation on dermal tattoo pigment in man. J Surg Res 1968; 5: 220.

194. Goldman L. Laser surgical research. Ann NY Acad Sci 1970; 168: 649.

195. Reid WH, McLeod PJ, Ritchie A, Ferguson-Pell M. Q-switched ruby laser treatment of black tattoos. Br J Plast Surg 1983; 36: 455.

196. Polla LL, Margolis RJ, Dover JS, et al. Melanosomes are a primary target of Q-switched ruby laser irradiation in guinea pig skin. J Invest Dermatol 1987; 89: 281.

197. Dover JS, Margolis RJ, Polla LL, et al. Pigmented guinea pig skin irradiated with Q-switched ruby laser pulses: morphologic and histologic findings. Arch Dermatol 1989; 125: 43.

198. Scheibner A, Kenny G, White W, Wheeland RG. A superior method of tattoo removal using the Q-switched ruby laser. J Dermatol Surg Oncol 1990; 16: 1091.

199. Taylor CR, Anderson R, Gange RW, Michaud NA, Flotte TJ. Light and electron microscopic analysis of tattoos treated by Q-switched ruby laser. J Invest Dermatol 1991; 97: 131.

200. Ho DD, London R, Zimmerman GB, Young DA. Laser-tattoo removal—a study of the mechanism and the optimal treatment strategy via computer simulations. Lasers Surg Med 2002; 30: 389–97.

201. Geronemus RG, Ashinoff R. Use of the Q-switched ruby laser to treat tattoos and benign pigmented lesions of the skin. Lasers Surg Med 1991; 3: 64.

202. Ashinoff R, Geronemus RG. Rapid response of traumatic and medical tattoos to treatment with the Q-switched ruby laser. Plast Reconstr Surg 1993; 91: 841.

203. Lowe NJ, Luftman D, Sawcer D. Q-switched ruby laser: further observations on treatment of professional tattoos. J Dermatol Surg Oncol 1994; 20: 307.

204. Levins PC, Grevelink JM, Anderson RR. Q-switched ruby laser treatment of tattoos. Lasers Surg Med 1991; 3: 63.

205. Bernstein LJ, Palaia DA, Bank D, Geronemus RG. Tattoo formation from absorbable synthetic suture and successful removal with Q-switched ruby laser. Dermatol Surg 1996; 22: 1040–2.

206. Ashinoff R, Tanenbaum D. Treatment of an amalgam tattoo with the Q-switched ruby laser. Cutis 1994; 54: 269–70.

207. Achauer BM, Nelson JS, Vander Kam VM, Applebaum R. Treatment of traumatic tattoos by Q-switched ruby laser. Plast Reconstr Surg 1994; 93: 318–23.

208. Kilmer SL, Anderson RR. Clinical use of the Q-switched ruby and the Q-switched Nd:YAG (1064 nm and 532 nm) lasers for treatment of tattoos. J Dermatol Surg Oncol 1993; 19: 330.

209. DeCoste SD, Anderson RR. Comparison of Q-switched ruby and Q-switched Nd:YAG laser treatment of tattoos. Lasers Surg Med 1991; 3: 64.

210. Kilmer SL, Lee M, Farinelli W, Grevelink JM. Q-switched Nd:YAG laser (1064 nm) effectively treats Q-switched ruby laser resistant tattoos. Lasers Surg Med Suppl 1992; 4: 72.

211. Pay AD, Kenealy JM. Laser transmission through membranes using the Q-switched Nd:YAG laser. Lasers Surg Med 1999; 24: 48–54.

212. Kilmer SL, Lee MS, Grevelink JM, Flotte TJ, Anderson RR. The Q-switched Nd:YAG laser (1064 nm) effectively treats tattoos: a controlled, dose–response study. Arch Dermatol 1993; 129: 971.

213. Ferguson JE, August PJ. Evaluation of the Nd/YAG laser for treatment of amateur and professional tattoos. Br J Dermatol 1996; 135: 586.

214. Naverson DN, Igelman JD. Q-switched laser management of an explosion tattoo. J Am Acad Dermatol 2004; 50: 479–80.

215. Suzuki H. Treatment of traumatic tattoos with the Q-switched neodynium:YAG laser. Arch Dermatol 1996; 132: 1226–9.

216. Wong SS, Goh KS. Successful treatment of traumatic tattoos with the Q-switched neodymium:YAG laser: a report of two cases. J Dermatol Treat 1998; 9: 193–5.

217. Jones A, Roddey P, Orengo I, Rosen T. The Q-switched Nd:YAG laser effectively treats tattoos in darkly pigmented skin. Dermatol Surg 1996; 22: 999.

218. Grevelink JM, Duke D, Van Leeuwen RL, et al. Laser treatment of tattoos in darkly pigmented patients: efficacy and side effects. J Am Acad Dermatol 1996; 34: 653.

219. Geronemus RG. Surgical pearl: Q-switched Nd:YAG laser removal of eyeliner tattoo. J Am Acad Dermatol 1996; 35: 101–2.

220. Kilmer SL, Lee MS, Anderson RR. Treatment of multi-colored tattoos with the frequency-doubled Q-switched Nd:YAG laser (532 nm): a dose-response study with comparison to the Q-switched ruby laser. Lasers Surg Med 1993; 5: 262.

221. Kilmer SL, Farinelli WF, Tearney G, Anderson RR. Use of a larger spot size for the treatment of tattoos increases clinical efficacy and decreases potential side effects. Lasers Surg Med 1994; 6: 51.

222. Fitzpatrick RE, Goldman MP. Tattoo removal using the alexandrite lasers. Arch Dermatol 1994; 130: 1508.

223. Alster TS. Q-switched alexandrite laser treatment (755 nm) of professional and amateur tattoos. J Am Acad Dermatol 1995; 33: 69.

224. Stafford TJ, Lizek R, Tan OT. Role of the alexandrite laser for removal of tattoos. Lasers Surg Med 1995; 17: 32.

225. Garcia C, Clark RE. Tattoo removal using the alexandrite laser. NC Med J 1995; 56: 336.

226. Dozier SE, Diven DG, Jones D, et al. The Q-switched alexandrite laser's effects on tattoos in guinea pigs and harvested human skin. Dermatol Surg 1995; 21: 237–40.

227. Moreno-Arias GA, Camps-Fresneda A. The use of Q-switched alexandrite laser (755 nm, 100 ns) for eyeliner tattoo removal. J Cut Laser Ther 1999; 1: 113–15.

228. Moreno-Arias GA, Camps-Fresneda A. Cosmetic tattoo refractive to Q-switched alexandrite laser. J Cut Laser Ther 1999; 1: 117–19.

229. Moreno-Arias GA, Camps-Fresneda A. Use of the Q-switched alexandrite laser (755 nm, 100 ns) for eyebrow tattoo removal. Lasers Surg Med 1999; 25: 123–5.

230. Moreno-Arias GA, Casals-Andreu M, Camps-Fresneda A. Use of Q-switched alexandrite laser (755 nm, 100 ns) for removal of traumatic tattoo of different origins. Lasers Surg Med 1999; 25: 445–50.

231. Levine VJ, Geronemus RG. Tattoo removal with the Q-switched ruby laser and the Q-switched Nd:YAG laser: a comparative study. Cutis 1995; 55: 291–6.

232. McMeekin TO, Goodwin DP. A comparison of the alexandrite laser (755 nm) with the Q-switched ruby laser (694 nm) in the treatment of tattoos. Lasers Surg Med Suppl 1993; S5: 43.

233. Kaufman R, Boehncke WH, Konig K, Hibst R. Comparative study of Q-switched Nd:YAG and alexandrite laser treatment of tattoos. Lasers Surg Med 1993; S5: 54.

234. Zelickson BD, Mehregan D, Zarrin AA, et al. Clinical, histologic, and ultrastructural evaluation of tattoos treated with three laser systems. Lasers Surg Med 1994; 15: 364–72.

235. Leuenberger ML, Mulas MW, Hata TR, et al. Comparison of the Q-switched alexandrite, Nd:YAG, and ruby lasers in treating blue-black tattoos. Dermatol Surg 1999; 25: 10–14.

236. Goyal S, Arndt KA, Stern RS, O'Hare D, Dover JS. Laser treatment of tattoos: a prospective, paired, comparison study of the Q-switched Nd:YAG (1064 nm), frequency-doubled Q-switched Nd:YAG (532 nm), and Q-switched ruby lasers. J Am Acad Dermatol 1997; 36: 122–5.

237. Boehncke WH, Hibst R, Kaufman R. Within-individual comparison of Q-switched Nd:YAG and alexandrite lasers in the treatment of monochromatic black amateur tattoos. J Dermatol Treat 1994; 5: 29–32.

238. Kirby W, Desai A, Desai T. The Kirby–Desai scale: A proposed scale to assess tattoo-removal treatments. J Clin Aesthet Dermatol 2009; 2: 32–7.

239. Kirby W, Koriakos A, Desai A, Desai T. Undesired pigmentary alterations associated with quality-switched laser tattoo removal treatment: a retrospective study and review of the literature. Skin Aging 2010; 18: 38–40.

240. Fusade T, Toubel G, Grognard C, Mazer JM. Treatment of gunpowder traumatic tattoo by Q-switched Nd:YAG laser: an unusual adverse effect. Dermatol Surg 2000; 26: 1057–9.

241. Alora MB, Arndt KA, Taylor CR. Scarring following Q-switched laser treatment of "double tattoos". Arch Dermatol 2000; 136: 269–70.

242. Kirby W, Kartono F, Desai A, Desai T. Treatment of Bulla in three patients after treatment with a Q-switched laser. J Clin Aesthet Dermatol 2010; 3: 39–41.

243. Sowden JM, Byrne JP, Smith AG, et al. Red tattoo reactions: X-ray microanalysis and patch-test studies. Br J Dermatol 1991; 124: 576–80.

244. Ashinoff R, Levine VJ, Soter NA. Allergic reactions to tattoo pigment after laser treatment. Dermatol Surg 1995; 21: 291.

245. Vasold R, Naarmann N, Ulrich H, et al. Tattoo pigments are cleaved by laser light—the chemical analysis in vitro provide evidence for hazardous compounds. Photochem Photobiol 2004; 80: 185–90.

246. Bäumler W, Eibler ET, Hohenleutner U, et al. Q-switch laser and tattoo pigments: first results of the chemical and photophysical analysis of 41 compounds. Lasers Surg Med 2000; 26: 13–21.

247. Kirby W, Kaur R, Kartono F, Desai A, Desai T. Research letter: Paradoxical Darkening and Removal of Pink Ink Tattoo. J Cosmet Dermatol 2010; 9: 149–51.

248. Swanson VS. Tattoo ink darkening of a yellow tattoo after Q-switched laser treatment. Clin Exp Dermatol 2002; 27: 461–3.

249. Cotton FA, Wilkinson G. The transition elements. In: Cotton FA, Wilkinson G, eds. Advanced Inorganic Chemistry. New York: Interscience, 1972.

250. Anderson RR, Geronemus R, Kilmer SL, Farinelli W, Fitzpatrick RE. Cosmetic tattoo ink darkening. A complication of Q-switched and pulsed-laser treatment. Arch Dermatol 1993; 129: 1010–14.

251. Ross V, Naseef G, Lin G, et al. Comparison of responses of tattoos to picosecond and nanosecond Q-switched neodymium:YAG lasers. Arch Dermatol 1998; 134: 167.

252. Shelley WB, Shelley ED, Burmeister V. Tattoos from insulin needles. Ann Intern Med 1986; 105: 549–50.

253. Balsam MS, Sagarin E, eds. Cosmetics: Science and Technology, 2nd edn. New York: Wiley-Interscience, 1974.

254. Angres GA. Angres permalid-liner method: a new surgical procedure. Am J Ophthalmol 1984; 16: 145.

255. Farber MG, Lamberg RC, Smith ME. A histologic study of eyelid pigment eight weeks after implantation (eyelid tattoo). Arch Ophthalmol 1986; 104: 1434.

256. Angres GG. Blepharo and dermapigmentation techniques for facial cosmesis. Ear Nose Throat J 1987; 66: 344.

257. Putterman AM, Migliori ME. Elective excision of permanent eyeliner. Arch Ophthalmol 1988; 106: 1034.

258. Dedio RM, Henry WJ, Scipione CR. Surgical removal of blepharopigmentation. Am J Cosmet Surg 1990; 7: 93.

259. Kirby W, Chen C, Desai A, Desai T. Successful treatment of cosmetic mucosal tattoos via Q-switched laser. Dermatol Surg 2011; 37: 1767–9.

260. Shah G, Alster TS. Treatment of amalgam tattoo with a Q-switched alexandrite (755 nm) laser. Dermatol Surg 2002; 28: 1180–1.

261. Weiss ET, Geronemus RG. Combining fractional Resurfacing and q-switched Ruby laser for tattoo removal. Dermatol Surg 2011; 37: 97.

262. Herd RM, Alora MB, Smoller B, Arndt KA, Dover JS. A clinical and histologic prospective controlled comparative study of the picosecond titanium:sapphire (795 nm) laser versus the Q-switched alexandrite (752 nm) laser for removing tattoo pigment. J Am Acad Dermatol 1999; 40: 603–6.

263. Aschwanden A, Lorenser D, Unold HJ, et al. 2.1 Picosecond passively mode-locked external-cavity semiconductor laser. Opt Lett 2005; 30: 272–4.

264. Audebert P, Renaudin P, Bastiani-Ceccotti S, et al. Picosecond time-resolved X-ray absorption spectroscopy of ultrafast aluminum plasmas. Phys Rev Lett 2005; 94: 025004; Epub 2005.

265. Izikson L, Farinelli W, Sakamoto F, et al. Safety and effectiveness of black tattoo clearance in a pig model after a single treatment with a novel 758 nm 500 picosecond laser: a pilot study. Lasers Surg Med 2010; 42: 640–6.

266. Kossida T, Rigopoulos D, et al. Optimal tattoo removal in a single session based on the method of repeated exposures. J Am Acad Dermatol 2012; 66: 271–7.

267. Cohen PR, Goldman MP. The adjuvant use of macrophage colony stimulating factor in tattoo removal using laser. Med Hypotheses 1995; 45: 83–5.

268. Ramirez M, Magee N, Diven D, et al. Triweekly topical 5% imiquimod cream fades experimental tattoos in guinea pigs. Cosmet Dermatol 2005; 18: 155–61.

269. Solis RR, Diven DG, Colome-Grimmer MI, Snyder N IV, Wagner RF Jr. Experimental nonsurgical tattoo removal in a guinea pig model with topical imiquimod and tretinoin. Dermatol Surg 2002; 28: 83–7.

270. Berman B, Poochareon VN, Villa AM. Novel dermatologic uses of the immune response modifier imiquimod 5% cream. Skin Therapy Lett 2002; 7: 1–6.

271. Magee NS, Zamora JG, Colome-Grimmer MI, Wagner RF Jr. Triweekly topical 5% imiquimod cream fades experimental tattoos in guinea pigs. Cosmet Dermatol 2005; 18: 155–61.

5 Hair removal

Omar A. Ibrahimi and Suzanne L. Kilmer

INTRODUCTION

The ability of lasers to nonspecifically damage hair follicles was noted nearly 50 years ago in the first reports on the use of lasers on human skin (1,2). However, it was not until the theory of selective photothermolysis was proposed by Rox Anderson and John Parrish at the Wellman Center for Photomedicine at Harvard Medical School that the concept of selectively targeting a particular chromophore based on its absorption spectra and size was realized (3). Several years later, this group also reported one of the first successful uses of a normal-mode ruby laser for long-term and permanent hair removal (4,5).

Today, removing unwanted body hair is a worldwide trend, and photoepilation by laser or other light-based technology is one of the most highly requested procedures in cosmetic dermatology (6). Alternative methods for removing unwanted hair include bleaching, plucking, shaving, waxing, and chemical depilatories. Threading is a common practice in some cultures. Unfortunately, these methods do not provide a permanent solution to unwanted hair, and can be inconvenient and tedious (7,8). Electrolysis is a method for hair removal in which a fine needle is inserted deep into the hair follicle and uses electrical current, thereby destroying the hair follicle and allowing for permanent hair removal of all types of hair (9,10). However, this technique is extremely operator dependent and efficacy in achieving permanent hair removal is variable among patients (9,10). It is also impractical in terms of treating large areas. Eflornithine is a topical inhibitor of ornithine decarboxylase that slows the rate of hair growth and is effective for decreasing unwanted facial hair (8), and is currently indicated for the removal of unwanted facial hair in women. Eflornithine can be combined with lasers and intense pulsed light (IPL) for hair removal (11,12). In this chapter, we provide a detailed overview on laser hair removal (LHR), including discussion of hair follicle biology, the science behind LHR, key factors in optimizing treatment, and future directions.

THE HAIR FOLLICLE

The hair follicle is a complex, hormonally active structure with a programed growth pattern (Fig. 5.1). It is anatomically divided into the infundibulum (hair follicle orifice to insertion of the sebaceous gland), isthmus (insertion of the sebaceous gland to the insertion of the arrector pili muscle), and inferior (insertion of the arrector pili to the base of the hair follicle) segments. The dermal papilla, a neurovascular structure that supplies the cells of the proliferating matrix at the base of the follicle, helps form the hair shaft.

Each hair follicle consists of a permanent (upper) and nonpermanent (lower) part, with the follicular bulge forming the lowermost aspect of the permanent part. In periods of active growth (anagen) the rapidly developing bulbar matrix cells differentiate into the hair shaft and the hair lengthens. A transition period follows in which the bulbar part of the hair follicle undergoes degradation through apoptosis (catagen). A resting period (telogen) phase ensues, and regrowth is started once again in early anagen. Stem cells within the hair follicle regenerate the follicle within or near the hair bulb matrix. Slow-cycling stem cells have also been found in the follicular bulge arising off the outer root sheath at the site of arrector pili muscle attachment. The duration of each growth phase is body site dependent.

There are three main types of hair: lanugo, vellus, and terminal hairs. Lanugo hairs are fine hairs that cover a fetus and are shed in the neonatal period. Vellus hairs are usually nonpigmented, and have a diameter of roughly 30–50 μm. Terminal hair shafts range from 150 to 300 μm in cross-sectional diameter. The type of hair produced by an individual follicle is capable of change (e.g., vellus to terminal hair at puberty or terminal to vellus hair in androgenic alopecia).

Hair color is determined by the amount of pigment in the hair shaft. Melanocytes produce two types of melanin—eumelanin, a brown-black pigment, and pheomelanin, a red pigment. Melanocytes are located in the upper portion of the hair bulb and outer root sheath of the infundibulum.

Excessive and unwanted body hair ranges in severity, depending on cultural mores, and can usually be classified as either hypertrichosis or hirsutism (13). Hirsutism is defined as the abnormal growth of terminal hair in women in male-pattern (androgen-dependent) sites, such as the face and chest. Hypertrichosis refers to excess hair growth at any body site that is not androgen dependent (13). Additionally, the use of grafts and flaps in dermatologic and reconstructive surgery can often introduce hair to an area that causes a displeasing appearance or functional impairment.

MECHANISM OF LHR

The theory of selective photothermolysis enables one to selectively target pigmented hair follicles by using the melanin of the hair shaft as a chromophore (3). Melanin is capable of functioning as a chromophore for wavelengths in the red and near-infrared (NIR) portion of the electromagnetic spectrum (14).

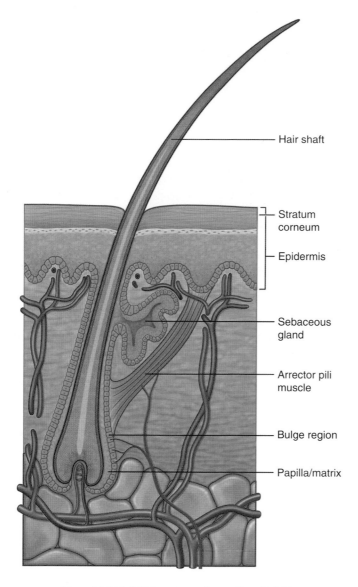

Hair shaft

Stratum corneum

Epidermis

Sebaceous gland

Arrector pili muscle

Bulge region

Papilla/matrix

Figure 5.1 Hair follicle anatomy. *Source*: From Ref. 66.

However, to achieve permanent hair removal the biological "target" is likely the follicular stem cells located in the bulge region and/or dermal papilla. Based on the slight spatial separation of the chromophore and desired target, an extended theory of selective photothermolysis was proposed, which requires diffusion of heat from the chromophore to the desired target for destruction (15). This requires a laser pulse duration that is longer in duration than if the actual chromophore and desired target were identical. Temporary LHR can result when the follicular stem cells are not completely destroyed, primarily through induction of a catagen-like state in pigmented hair follicles. Temporary LHR is much easier to achieve than permanent removal, using lower fluences. Long-term hair removal depends on hair color, skin color, and tolerated fluence. Roughly 15–30% long-term hair loss may be observed with each treatment when optimal treatment parameters are used (16). The remaining hairs are also thinner and lighter in color (Fig. 5.2). A list of laser and light devices that are commercially available at the time of this publication for hair removal are summarized in Table 5.1.

KEY FACTORS IN OPTIMIZING TREATMENT

The ability to selectively target hair follicles with lasers and light sources has revolutionized the ability to eliminate unwanted hair temporarily and permanently in many individuals. As laser technology advances, the ability to treat individuals of all skin types and all hair colors broadens. Proper patient selection, preoperative preparation, informed consent, understanding of the principles of laser safety, and laser and light source selection are key to the success of laser treatment. An understanding of hair anatomy, growth, and physiology, together with a thorough understanding of laser–tissue interaction, in particular within the context of choosing optimal laser parameters for effective LHR, should be acquired before using lasers for hair removal.

Patient Selection

Despite the seemingly cosmetic nature of LHR, a complete medical history, physical examination and informed consent, including setting realistic patient expectations and potential risks, should be preformed prior to any laser treatment (Table 5.2). Any patient with evidence for endocrine or menstrual dysfunction should be appropriately worked up. Similarly, patients with an explosive onset of hypertrichosis should be evaluated for paraneoplastic etiologies. Treatment of a pregnant woman for nonurgent conditions is discouraged, although there is no evidence suggesting a potential risk to pregnant women undergoing LHR. The past medical history should be reviewed to identify patients with photosensitive conditions, such as the autoimmune connective tissue disorders, or disorders prone to the Koebner phenomenon. A history of recurrent cutaneous infections at or in the vicinity of treatment area might warrant the use of prophylactic medications. Any past history of keloid or hypertrophic scar formation should be elicited as well. Previous methods for hair removal, including any past laser treatments, should be reviewed. Any methods of epilation, such as waxing or tweezing, that entirely remove the target chromophore, render LHR less effective for at least 2 weeks. Although there is little evidence for the time frame a patient must wait after complete epilation of the hair shaft and laser treatment, we recommend a minimum of 6 weeks. Shaving and depilatory creams can be used up to the day of laser treatment as they do not remove the entire hair shaft.

A thorough medication history should be obtained. Any history of gold intake is a contraindication for laser therapy. The use of any photosensitizing medications or over-the-counter supplements should also delay treatment until these medications can be safely discontinued. There is controversy as to whether patients on isotretinoin should be treated with laser, although conventionally most practitioners recommend a 6-month to 1-year washout period prior to ablative resurfacing laser treatment (17–19). Whether this recommendation is appropriate for other laser procedures is speculative at best. Topical retinoids used in the treatment area should be discontinued 1–2 days prior to treatment.

The physical examination should evaluate the patient's Fitzpatrick skin phototype. This will help determine which lasers and light sources are safe to use for that patient (Table 5.1), because epidermal melanin in darkly pigmented patients can compete with the melanin within hair follicles as

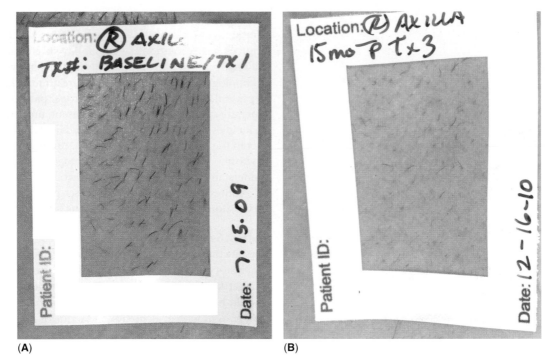

Figure 5.2 Visual decrease in hair thickness and color in a study subject. (**A**) baseline and (**B**) 15-month follow-up visit. This subject had a 60% decrease in hair thickness and a 40% decrease in hair color (44).

the target chromophore. Importantly, every patient should always be evaluated for the presence of a tan, and if present, laser treatment should be delayed or the treatment parameters appropriately adjusted until the tan has faded. Finally, the patient's hair color should be noted as the chromophore for LHR is melanin. Black and brown hairs contain sufficient amounts of melanin to serve as a chromophore for LHR. In contrast the lack of melanin, paucity of melanin or presence of eumelanin in the hair follicle, which clinically correlates to white, gray, or red/blonde hair is predictive of a poor response to LHR. For patients with little to no melanin in their hair follicles, attempts have been made to use an exogenous chromophore that can be topically delivered to the hair follicles, thereby making the removal of white, gray, red, and blonde hair hypothetically possible. This concept was first demonstrated with a topical carbon solution dissolved in mineral oil (20). However, we have noticed very little efficacy of topical chromophores in our vast experience.

Informed Consent

An explanation of the potential risks of LHR should be reviewed as part of the informed consent process. The risks include but are not limited to temporary and permanent hypo/hyperpigmentation, blister formation, scar formation, ulceration, hive-like response, bruising, infection, acne flare, and folliculitis. For those patients with Fitzpatrick skin type IV or greater or of Mediterranean, Middle Eastern, Asian, or South Asian descent, the low risk of paradoxical hypertrichosis (conversion of vellus hairs to terminal hairs), especially when treating the lateral face and jaw, should be reviewed (21–24). Patients should be counseled that permanent and complete hair removal is not likely, but that with multiple treatments, significant long-term reduction can be achieved. Hirsute women with hormonal abnormalities may require continued

maintenance therapy and should be advised of this possibility. Procedural pain is expected with LHR but can be minimized with topical anesthetics and the use of cold air cooling. Erythema and edema are also expected with treatment and may last up to 1 week. Patients should be aware of the need for strict sun avoidance for a minimum of 6 weeks before and after each treatment.

Preoperative Preparation and Laser Safety

The need for topical anesthesia is variable among patients and particular anatomic sites. Various topical anesthetics, including lidocaine, lidocaine/prilocaine, and other amide/ester anesthetic combinations, can be used to diminish the procedural discomfort, and should be applied 30 minutes to 1 hour before treatment under occlusion. Care should be taken when using lidocaine or prilocaine to apply these medications to a limited area to diminish the risk of lidocaine toxicity or methemoglobulinemia, respectively.

Patients should be placed in a room with a treatment chair that makes the desired treatment area easily accessible. The room should be adequately cooled to keep the laser device from overheating and be free of any hanging mirrors or uncovered windows. A fire extinguisher should be readily available, especially if oxygen is being used. Having a vacuum device on hand during treatment can minimize the plume and unpleasant odor created by each laser pulse. Because the retina contains melanin which can be damaged by all LHR devices, proper eye protection is absolutely critical for both the patient and the laser surgeon. Each device requires the use of protective goggles that are unique to the device's particular wavelengths. Goggles cannot be interchangeably used with laser or IPL devices of other wavelengths. Furthermore, because of the risk of retinal damage, it is the authors' strong opinion that one should never treat a patient for LHR within the bony orbit.

Table 5.1 Commercially Available Lasers and Light Sources for Hair Removal[a]

Laser/Light Source	Wavelength (nm)	System Name	Pulse Duration (ms)	Fluence (J/cm²)	Spot Size (mm)	Other Features
Long-pulsed ruby	694	RubyStar and Ruby Star+	4	Up to 24	8, 10, 12, 18	Contact cooling
Long-pulsed alexandrite	755	Apogee (Cynosure)	0.5–300	25–50	5–15	Cold air or integrated cooling, can add 1064-nm Nd:YAG module to form Apogee Elite
		Arion (Quantel Derma)	5–140	Up to 40	6–16	Cold air unit
		ClearScan YAG (Sciton)	Up to 200	Up to 140	3, 6, and 30 × 30	Contact cooling
		Coolglide (Cutera)	0.1–300	5–300	10	Contact cooling
		Elite (Cynosure)	0.5–300	25–50	5–15	Cold air cooling, available with 1064-nm Nd:YAG, EliteMPX model can simultaneously treat with 755-nm Alexandrite and 1064-nm Nd:YAG
		EpiCare LP/LPX (Light Age)	3–300	22–40	7–16	Dynamic cooling
		GentleLASE, (Candela)	3	Up to 100	6–18	Dynamic cooling, comes with 1064-nm Nd:YAG
		GentleMax (Candela)	0.25–300	Up to 600	1.5–18	Dynamic cooling
		Ultrawave 755/II/III (AMC Aesthetics and Advance Aesthetic Concepts)	Up to 100	Up to 125	Up to 16	Available with 532-, 1064-, and 1320-nm Nd:YAG
Diode	805	Advantage (Lutronic, Freemont, California, USA)	5–400	Up to 100	10 × 10, 10 × 30	Contact cooling
	800–810	F1 Diode (Opusmed)	15–40	Up to 40	5, 7	Chiller tip
	808, 980	Leda (Quantel Derma)	6–60	Up to 60	50 × 12, 10 × 12	Contact cooling
	810, 940	MeDioStar XT (Aesclepion)	5–500	Up to 90	6, 12	Integrated scanner with cold air cooling device
	800	LightSheer Duet (Lumenis)	5–400	10–100, 4.5–12	9 × 9, 22 × 35	Chilltip for smaller handpiece, vacuum skin flattening for larger handpiece
	810	Soprano XL (Alma Lasers)	10–1350	Up to 120	12 × 10	Contact cooling
Long-pulsed Nd:YAG	1064	Acclaim (Cynosure)	0.4–300	35–600	1.5–15	Cold air or integrated cooling, can add 755-nm alexandrite module to form Apogee Elite (Cynosure)
		ClearScan YAG (Sciton)	0.3–200	Up to 400	3, 6, and 30 × 30	Contact cooling
		CoolGlide CV/XEO/Excel/Vantage (Cutera)	0.1–300	Up to 300	3–10	Contact cooling
		Cynergy (Cynosure)	0.3–300	Up to 600	1.5–15	Cold air
		Dualis XP, XP Plus and XS Max (Fotona)	5–200	Up to 600	2–10	N/A
		GentleYAG (Candela, Wayland, MA)	0.25–300	Up to 600	1.5–18	Dynamic cooling
		Gemini (Iridex)	1–100	Up to 990	2, 10	Available with 532-nm KTP
		LightPod Neo (Aerolase)	0.65–1.5	Up to 312	2	Builtin cooling system
		Lyra (Iridex)	20–100	5–900	1–5, 10	Contact cooling
		MultiFlex (Ellipse, Atlanta, GA)	N/A	Up to 600	1.5–5	Equipped with IPL device
		Mydon (Quantel)	0.5–90	10–450	1.5–10	Integrated air cooling
		NaturaLase 1064/LP (Focus Medical)	0.5–100	Up to 400	3–15	Integrated air cooling
		Profile (Sciton)	0.1–10000	Up to 75	N/A	Contact cooling, 2940-nm Er:YAG and 410- to 1400-nm flashlamp in same device
		SmartEpil (Deka)	Up to 20	11	2.5, 4, 5, 6	
		SP Plus (Fotona)	Up to 300	Up to 600	1–42	
		Synchro_FT (Deka)	2–30	Up to 50	2.5–13	Available with IPL handpiece

(Continued)

Table 5.1 Commercially Available Lasers and Light Sources for Hair Removal[a] (*Continued*)

Laser/Light Source	Wavelength (nm)	System Name	Pulse Duration (ms)	Fluence (J/cm²)	Spot Size (mm)	Other Features
Intense pulsed light sources	520–1200	Ultrawave II/III (AMC Aesthetics, and Advance Aesthetic Concepts)	Up to 300	5–500	Up to 12	Pulsed cryogen cooling
		Varia (CoolTouch)	0.6	Up to 500	2–10	Dynamic cryogen cooling
	420–1400	Axiom (Viora)	25–75 and 2.2–12.5	Up to 39	50 × 25, 35 × 15, 20 × 10	Builtin cooling system
	560–590	BBL (Sciton)	Up to 200	Up to 30	15 × 45	Builtin cooling system
	400–1200	Cynergy (Cynosure)	0.3–300	Up to 600	N/A	Builtin cooling system
	600–950	Duet/SkinStation/SpaTouch II (Radiancy)	3–10	35	22 × 55	
	400–1400	Ellipse I2PL/MultiFlex (Ellipse)	2.5–88.5	4–26	10 × 48	MultiFlex model with long-pulsed Nd:YAG
	650–950	EsteLux (Palomar Medical Technologies)	10–100	Up to 28	N/A	
	530–1200	Harmony XL (Alma Lasers)	30–50	Up to 40	30 × 30	Available with 755-nm alexandrite and 1064- and 1320-nm Nd:YAG
	390–1200	iPulse (Dermavista)	5–120	Up to 20	89 sq	Air cooling
	525–1200	Med Flash II (General Project)	Up to 100	Up to 45	N/A	
	500–1200	MediLux/StarLux Y, Ys, R, Rs (Palomar)	5–500	Up to 70	28 × 12, 46 × 16	1064 Nd:YAG handpiece for StarLux 500
	400–1200	MiniSilk_FT (Deka)	3–8	Up to 160	48 × 13, 23 × 13	Contact cooling
	640–1400	Mistral (Radiancy)	Up to 80	4–15	25 × 50, 13 × 50, 13 × 35, 12 × 12	
	640–1200	NannoLight MP50 (Sybaritic)	1–30	2.8–50	40 × 8	Nd:YAG handpiece, optional cooling
	750–1100	NaturaLight (Solamed)	Up to 500	Up to 50	10 × 40	
	550–950	Solera Opus (Cutera)	auto	3–24	10 × 30	Nd:YAG handpiece
	770–1100	PhotoSilk/PhotoLight/MiniSilk (Cyanosure)	Up to 30	10–340	21 × 10, 46 × 10, 46 × 18	
	500–1200	ProWave (Cutera)	auto	5–35	10 × 30	
	695–1200	Quadra Q4 (DermaMed)	48	10–20	33 × 15	Builtin cooling system
	560–950	Quantum HR (Lumenis)	15–100	25–45	34 × 8	
	530–1200	SmoothCool (Eclipse)	1–60	10–45	8 × 34	
		Trios (Viora)	25	Up to 22	15 × 50	Automatic temperature control system
Fluorescent pulsed light	615–920	OmniLight/NovaLight (Medical Bio Care)	2–500	Up to 90	7 × 15, 10 × 20, 30 × 30	Sapphire tip cooling
Optical energy combined with RF electrical energy	580–980	eMax/eLight (Syneron)	Up to 100	Up to 50 optical; up to 50 J/cm² RF	12 × 15	Contact cooling
Diode combined with RF electrical energy	800	eLaser (Syneron)	Up to 100	Up to 50 optical; up to 50 J/cm² RF	12 × 15	Contact cooling
	810	MeDioStar Effect (Aesclepion, Jena, Germany)	Up to 500	Up to 90	10, 12, 14	Acoustic wave technology, integrated scanner with cold air cooling device, 940 nm simultaneously

[a]This table is intended only as a reference aid. The authors have made every attempt to provide an exhaustive list of available devices for laser hair removal but do not guarantee comprehensiveness.

Abbreviations: Er:YAG, erbium-doped:yttrium-aluminum-garnet; IPL, intense pulsed light; Nd:YAG, neodymium-doped:yttrium-aluminum-garnet; N/A, not available; RF, radiofrequency.

Table 5.2 Pertinent History for Laser/Light Device Hair Removal

- Presence of conditions that may cause hypertrichosis:
  ○ Hormonal
  ○ Familial
  ○ Drug (i.e., corticosteroids, hormones, immunosuppressives, self or spousal use of minoxidil)
  ○ Tumor
- History of local or recurrent skin infection
- History of herpes simplex, especially perioral
- History of herpes genitalis, important when treating the pubic or bikini area
- History of keloids/hypertrophic scarring
- History of koebnerizing skin disorders, such as vitiligo and psoriasis
- Previous treatment modalities—method, frequency, and date of last treatment, as well as response
- Recent suntan or exposure to tanning or light cabinet
- Onset of hair regrowth (recent)
- Tattoos or nevi present
- Patient's expectations
- Patient's hobbies or habits that might interfere with treatment
- Present medications:
  ○ Photosensitizing medications
  ○ Isotretinoin intake within the past year
  ○ Gold therapy

Device Variables

Wavelength

The chromophore for LHR is melanin. Within the hair follicle, melanin is principally located within the hair shaft, although the outer root sheath and matrix area also contain melanin. Melanin is capable of functioning as a chromophore for wavelengths in the red and NIR portion of the electromagnetic spectrum (14) and can be targeted by ruby, alexandrite, diode, and neodymium-doped:yttrium-aluminum-garnet (Nd:YAG) lasers, as well as IPL devices.

The long-pulsed ruby laser (694 nm) was the first device used to selectively target hair follicles (5), and result in long-term (follow-up at 2 years) hair loss (6-mm spot size, 270-µs pulse duration, and fluences 30–60 J/cm^2) (4). The long-pulsed ruby laser can be safely used in Fitzpatrick skin phototypes I–III. A large multicenter trial of nearly 200 patients showed that the majority of patients had >75% hair loss on 6-month follow-up after an average of four treatments (25). Table 5.1 lists the long-pulsed ruby lasers that are commercially available.

The long-pulsed alexandrite (755 nm) laser has been shown to be effective for hair removal in multiple studies (26). The long-pulsed alexandrite laser can be safely used in Fitzpatrick skin phototypes I–IV, although some experts limit the use of the long-pulsed alexandrite laser to Fitzpatrick skin phototypes I–III. A few studies have demonstrated the safety of the long-pulsed alexandrite laser in a large cohort of patients with Fitzpatrick skin phototypes IV–VI (27,28). A randomized, investigator-blinded clinical trial (29) of subjects with Fitzpatrick skin phototypes III and IV treated with a long-pulsed alexandrite laser (12- and 18-mm spot size, 1.5-ms pulse duration, and fluences of 20 or 40 J/cm^2) for four sessions at 8-week intervals showed 76–84% hair reduction 18 months after the last treatment and provides the best evidence for long-term hair removal efficacy with the alexandrite laser. A randomized controlled trial of 144 Asian subjects with Fitzpatrick skin types III–V with a long-pulsed alexandrite laser (12.5-mm spot size, pulse duration of 40 ms, and fluences of 16–24 J/cm^2) found that subjects with three treatments had a 55% hair reduction compared with subjects treated two times with a 44% hair reduction and subjects treated one time had a 32% hair reduction at 9-month follow-up (30). A combination treatment of alexandrite and Nd:YAG lasers provides no added benefit over the alexandrite laser alone (31). The commercially available long-pulsed alexandrite devices are summarized in Table 5.1.

The long-pulsed diode (800–810 nm) laser has also been extensively used for LHR (26,32). The diode laser can be safely used in patients with Fitzpatrick skin phototypes I–V. Two long-term nonrandomized controlled studies showing roughly 40% hair reduction at a mean follow-up of 20 months after one or two treatments (9-mm spot size, pulse duration of 5–30 ms, fluences of 15–40 J/cm^2) (33), and 84% hair reduction at 1-year follow-up after four treatments (9-mm spot size, pulse duration of 5–30 ms, fluences of 12–40 J/cm^2) (34) demonstrate the efficacy of the diode laser for long-term hair removal.

The long-pulsed Nd:YAG laser has been thought to offer the best combination of safety and efficacy for Fitzpatrick skin phototype VI patients. In our vast experience, we have found the Nd:YAG to offer good efficacy but with higher relative fluences relative to the above wavelengths. A nonrandomized trial reported a 70–90% reduction of facial, axillary, and leg hair growth one year after three monthly treatments with an Nd:YAG laser (5-mm spot size, pulse duration of 50 ms, fluences of 40–50 J/cm^2) (35). A small study of axillary LHR comparing long-pulsed alexandrite, diode, and Nd:YAG lasers showed that both the alexandrite and diode lasers were significantly more efficacious than the Nd:YAG laser for LHR (36).

IPL is composed of polychromatic, noncoherent light ranging from 400 to 1200 nm. Various filters can be used to target particular chromophores, including melanin. Long-term (>1 year) hair removal has not been convincingly demonstrated to date. Various reports have demonstrated some short-term efficacy (37,38). One study of patients treated with a single IPL session reported 75% hair removal 1 year after treatment (39). Two studies providing a head-to-head comparison of IPL versus either the long-pulsed alexandrite laser (40) or Nd:YAG laser (41) both found the IPL to be inferior to laser devices for hair removal. In contrast, a study of hirsute women, some with a diagnosis of polycystic ovarian syndrome, who underwent a split face treatment with six IPL or long pulsed diode laser (LDPL), shows statistically equivalent reductions in hair counts at 1 (77% vs. 68%, respectively), 3 (53% vs. 60%, respectively), and 6 months (40% vs. 34%, respectively) after the final treatment (42).

Fluence

Fluence is defined as the amount of energy delivered per unit area and is expressed as J/cm^2. Higher fluences have been correlated with greater permanent hair removal (5,43), however are also more likely to cause untoward side effects. Recommended treatment fluences are often provided with each individual laser device for nonexperienced operators. However, a more appropriate method of determining the optimal treatment fluence for a given patient is to evaluate for the desired clinical endpoint of perifollicular erythema and edema (Fig. 5.3). The highest

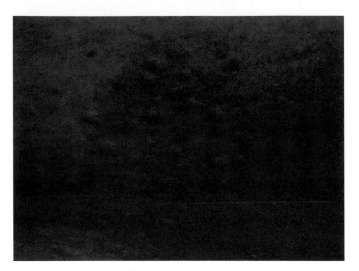

Figure 5.3 Transient perifollicular eythema and edema is a desired endpoint to occur immediately after hair removal treatment.

possible tolerated fluence which yields this endpoint, without any adverse effects, is often the best fluence for treatment.

Pulse Duration

Pulse duration is defined as the duration in seconds of laser exposure. The theory of selective photothermolysis (3) enables the laser surgeon to select an optimal pulse duration based on the thermal relaxation time (TRT). Terminal hairs are roughly 300 μm in diameter, and thus the calculated TRT of a terminal hair follicle is roughly 100 ms. However, unlike many other laser applications, the hair follicle is distinct in that there is a spatial separation of the chromophore (melanin) within the hair shaft and the biological "target" stem cells in the bulge and bulb areas of the follicle. The expanded theory of selective photothermolysis (15) takes this spatial separation into account and proposes a thermal damage time, which is thought to be longer than the TRT. Shorter pulse widths are also capable of removing hair, and it is unclear which is more effective in producing permanent hair removal. Longer pulse widths are likely more selective for melanin within the hair follicle and can minimize epidermal damage as the pulse widths are greater than the TRT of the melanosomes and melanocytes within the epidermis.

Spot Size

The spot size is the diameter in millimeters of the laser beam. As photons within a laser beam penetrate the dermis, they are scattered by collagen fibers, and those that are scattered outside the area of the laser beam are essentially wasted. Photons are more likely to be scattered outside of the beam area for smaller spot sizes, whereas in a larger spot size, the photons are likely to remain within the beam area following scatter. A double-blind, randomized controlled trial of a long-pulsed alexandrite device for LHR of the axillary region comparing 18- and 12-mm spot sizes at otherwise identical treatment parameters showed a 10% greater reduction in hair counts with the larger spot size (43). Recently, a prospective study (44) using an LDPL with a large 22 × 35 mm handpiece at low fluences and no skin cooling was shown to have similar long-term hair removal efficacy to published studies of LPDLs with smaller spot sizes using higher fluences and skin cooling. Thus, larger spot sizes are preferable to smaller spot sizes.

Skin Cooling

The presence of epidermal melanin, particularly in darker skin types, presents a competing chromophore to hair follicle melanin, which can be damaged during LHR. Cooling of the skin surface can be used to minimize epidermal damage, while permitting treatment with higher fluences (45). All of the skin cooling methods function by acting as a heat sink and removing heat from the skin surface. The least effective type of cooling is the use of an aqueous cold gel, which passively extracts heat from the skin and then is not capable of further skin cooling. Alternatively, cooling with forced chilled air can provide cooling to the skin before, during, and after a laser pulse. However, today, most of the commercially LHR devices have a builtin skin cooling system, which either consists of contact cooling or dynamic cooling with a cryogen spray. Contact cooling, usually with a sapphire tip, provides skin cooling just before and during a laser pulse. It is most useful for treatments with longer pulse durations (>10 ms) (46). Dynamic cooling with cryogen liquid spray (47) precools the skin with a millisecond spray of cryogen just before the laser pulse. A second spray can be delivered just after the laser pulse for postcooling, but parallel cooling during the laser pulse is not possible as the cryogen spray interferes with the laser beam. Dynamic cooling is best suited for use with pulse durations shorter than 5 ms.

Postprocedure Care

It is expected for the patient to have perifollicular erythema and edema in the treatment area following LHR. This generally persists for 2 days but can last for up to 1 week. Ice and application of a topical corticosteroid can be used to shorten the duration of these desired clinical findings. Patients will often find that a single treatment of LHR with shorter pulse durations results in nearly total epilation of the hair follicles in the treatment area. It is important to counsel the patient that a majority of these hairs will likely regrow, and this is not considered a treatment failure. Generally, only about 15% of hairs are permanently removed with each laser treatment. On the other hand, LHR treatments with longer pulse durations may leave behind many hairs which appear to "grow" following treatment. It is important to reassure the patient that these "growing" hairs are dislodged from the hair follicle and require 1–2 weeks to be completely shed. Nearly any method of epilation can be used to hasten their removal.

The importance of strict sun precaution following LHR treatments cannot be overemphasized. This can be achieved by the use of topical sunscreens, ultraviolet light impermeable garments, and sun avoidance.

Long-Term Efficacy

Dierickx et al. followed up 7 of 13 subjects from the seminal study demonstrating the first example LHR (5), 2 years after a single treatment with the normal mode ruby laser. Of the seven subjects, four had evidence of persistent permanent hair reduction at 2-year follow-up, whereas three subjects experienced complete regrowth. Lou et al. reported that 18 out of

50 original study subjects showed roughly a 25–33% and 36–46% hair reduction at a mean follow-up of 20 months after one or two treatments (9-mm spot size, pulse duration of 5–20 ms, fluences of 15–40 J/cm², single or triple pulsed), respectively, with an LPDL device (33). Eremia et al. in a head-to-head trial comparing an LPDL to a long-pulsed alexandrite laser found a 49–94% hair reduction at 1-year follow-up after four treatments (9-mm spot size, pulse duration of 20 ms, fluences of 12–40 J/cm²) (34) with the LPDL in 15 subjects. Similar results were achieved with the alexandrite laser used in this study. Fifteen of 20 subjects with Fitzpatrick skin phototypes III and IV treated with a long-pulsed alexandrite laser (12- and 18-mm spot size, 3-ms pulse duration, fluences of 20 or 40 J/cm²) or a long-pulsed Nd:YAG laser (12-mm spot size, 3-ms pulse duration, fluence of 40 J/cm²) for four sessions at 8-week intervals showed 76–84% and 74%, respectively, hair reduction 18 months after the last treatment (29). Braun reported a head-to-head trial of a high fluence LPDL (9-mm spot size, pulse duration of 30 ms, fluences of 20–50 J/cm²) versus a low fluence LPDL (12 × 10 mm spot size, pulse duration of 20 ms, fluences of 5–10 J/cm²) in 22 subjects and showed similar, 94% and 90%, respectively, hair reduction at 18-month follow-up following five treatments spaced 6–8 weeks apart (48). Finally, we recently reported statistically significant hair clearance, 54% and 42%, at 6- and 15-month followup visits following three monthly treatments using an LPDL using a large handpiece in the largest prospective trial to date (44). Remaining hairs were found to also grow back less thick and lighter.

CASE STUDIES

Case 1

A 37-year-old woman was diagnosed with polycystic ovary syndrome (PCOS). Her symptoms of PCOS are as follows: infrequent menstrual periods; increased growth of hair on the face, fingers and toes; oily skin and acne; obesity; and type 2 diabetes. Current therapy consists of maintaining a healthy weight and treatment of her diabetes with insulin. Although the male hormones are elevated, she refuses to take any androgen-blocking drugs. She consulted for treatment of her facial hirsutism, characterized by increased growth of black terminal hairs in the submandibular area, which she shaves daily (Fig. 5.4A). She was looking for a more efficient treatment modality of hair removal. As this patient was diagnosed with an underlying endocrine abnormality, she was alerted to the potential limitations of LHR treatment. Initially, she was treated with an 800-nm diode laser [LightSheer, Lumenis (San Jose, California, USA)] at 30–35 J/cm², 30 ms, and a 12 × 12 mm spot. Once the regrowing hairs became lighter and finer, treatment was continued with a 3 ms, 755-nm alexandrite laser [GentleLase, Candela (Wayland, Massachusetts, USA)] 8-mm, at 40 J/cm² for an 8-mm spot with dynamic cooling device (DCD) cooling (30 ms on, 30 ms off time).

The patient underwent eight treatment sessions in total, at 2- to 3-month intervals. A very satisfying result with 90% reduction of the hair regrowth was obtained (Fig. 5.4B). Because of the continued hormonal stimulation, she continues to be treated once a year for the few regrowing hairs.

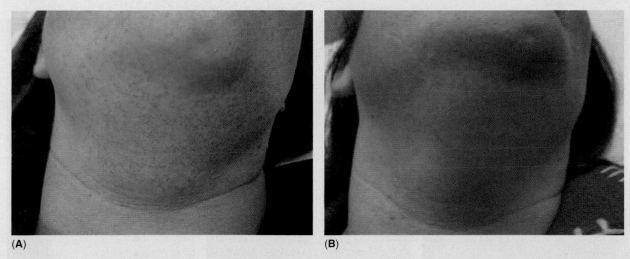

(A)   (B)

Figure 5.4 (**A**) Patient with hirsutism due to polycystic ovary syndrome. (**B**) Significant reduction of hair growth at 9 months after the eighth laser hair removal treatment.

Case 2

A 44-year-old female patient consulted for LHR of her axillae (Fig. 5.5A). Previous treatment modality consisted of shaving or the use of depilatory creams. She received four treatments with an 800-nm LightSheer diode laser (30 ms, 30 J/cm², 12 × 12 mm) and one final treatment of the remaining fine, regrowing hairs with a 3-ms, 755-nm GentleLase, alexandrite laser (40 J/cm², 8-mm spot, 30/30 DCD cooling). Except for a few occasional regrowing hairs, a very satisfactory result was obtained 5 years after the last treatment (Fig. 5.5B).

As an alternative to pulsed delivery, a CW CO_2 laser may be used with a scanning system that sweeps the beam across tissue rapidly enough that the tissue-dwell time is less than the thermal relaxation time of the tissue, simulating the tissue effects of a pulsed delivery system (4,97).

The laser beam may be delivered using a focused system, in which the beam is focused with lenses to a point having maximal fluence or irradiance. The distance from that focal point is a major determinant of tissue reaction, resulting in decreasing energies with increased handpiece-to-tissue distances. Alternatively, the beam may be delivered in a collimated manner, in which the beam is parallel and nondivergent, having the same fluence or irradiance independent of handpiece-to-tissue distances.

Although several new pulsed lasers were introduced in the mid-1990s, two laser systems have been used to pioneer this field and have generated virtually all the published data available: the UltraPulse laser (Coherent) and the SilkTouch scanner (Sharplan). The UltraPulse laser can deliver up to 500 mJ in a single pulse with a duration of less than 1 ms. This energy is delivered with a 3-mm collimated beam, generally used with 3–5 W resulting in a repetition rate of 6–10 Hz. Rapid, precise placement of these high-energy pulses ensuring single-pulse tissue interaction is achieved with a computer pattern generator (CPG) (91–94), using a 2.25-mm beam, 300 mJ per pulse, and a power of 60 W resulting in a placement of 81 pulses in one of six patterns at a rate of 220 Hz and with pulse densities varying from no overlap to 60% overlap (Fig. 6.3). While the original names of these lasers have been presented above for historical interest, there has been a consolidation in the ablative pulsed CO_2 lasers such that the Sharplan devices and Coherent devices have been acquired by Lumenis and marketed as a single device known as the UltraPulse system.

The Sharplan system uses a standard CW CO_2 beam focused to a 200-μm spot that is manipulated through rotating mirrors to scan tissue rapidly, resulting in a tissue dwell time of less than 1 ms. Scanning patterns of 4, 6, or 9 mm may be chosen.

In clinical use, two passes with the Sharplan SilkTouch systems appear to be approximately equal to three passes with the UltraPulse laser in terms of the amount of tissue removed and the depth of residual thermal necrosis (95).

Experimental data and theoretic calculations reveal the necessary pulse fluence to vaporize epidermal tissue to be approximately 5 J/cm² (72) To utilize a large spot size and deliver a pulse less than 1 ms in achieving this threshold fluence, a very high irradiance is necessary. When a spot size of 2.5 mm is used, 250 mJ must be delivered in less than 1 ms (73). This is generally delivered with a Gaussian beam, so a peripheral ring of about

10% may exist in which this threshold may not be reached. This suprathreshold energy will immediately vaporize intracellular water, leaving behind cellular proteinaceous debris. The depth of vaporization is proportional to the pulse energy. However, when the laser is interacting with the dermis, a new situation exists. Water is now primarily extracellular, in the dermal matrix, which is dominated by the structural proteins collagen and elastin. Type I collagen will melt at temperatures greater than 60°C but requires fluences much greater than 5 J/cm² for vaporization. Nonvaporization heating of the dermis will have little adverse effect as long as the pulse width is less than 1 ms and pulses are delivered to the same tissue spot at rates less than 5 Hz. If the delivery rate is greater than this, heat will accumulate between pulses, and thermal damage by diffusion may occur. This can result in poor wound healing or scarring.

Histologic studies have revealed a relationship between depth of ablation and pulse energy as well as the number of passes (72,79,80–85,96). A comparison between the CO_2 laser used with various pulse energies and numbers of passes and TCA peeling, dermabrasion, and Baker's phenol peel on a porcine model showed that typical pulse energies at one to three passes produced a wound depth intermediate between a 35% TCA peel and dermabrasion, but much more superficial than a phenol peel (79). Most histologic studies have shown the first CO_2 laser pass to result in epidermal ablation and subsequent passes to result in variable depths of dermal ablation and necrosis. The amount of residual thermal necrosis has also been shown to correlate with both pulse energy and number of passes, with each pass delivering the same amount of energy with less vaporization and more extensive heat absorption because of the layer of desiccated tissue at the treatment surface (Table 6.1 and Fig. 6.4) (79–83,85).

Table 6.1 Residual Thermal Necrosis with CO_2 Laser Treatment[a]

Laser Passes	Area of Necrosis (μm)
One	15.5 ± 7.0
Two	53.0 ± 21.2
Three	40.0 ± 21.7
Four	50.2 ± 26.4

Data from E. Bernstein, UltraPulse CO_2 Multicenter Clinical Trial.
[a]Pulse width less than 1 ms, fluence 7.1 J/cm².

	Face				Eyelids			
	Pulse energy	Pattern	Size	Density	Pulse energy	Pattern	Size	Density
First pass	300 mJ	3	9	6	200 mJ	5	9	5
Second pass	300 mJ	3	9	5	200 mJ	5	8	4
Third pass	300 mJ	3	8	4	None			

Figure 6.3 Computer pattern generator settings should not use densities greater than 6 if cumulative thermal damage from excessive pulse overlap is to be avoided.

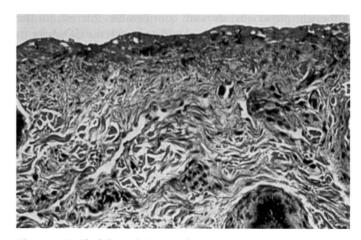

Figure 6.4 Residual thermal damage after two or three passes of UltraPulse CO_2 laser averages approximately 70 μm.

Published reports have correlated clinical signs with anatomic depths of ablation (98). A pink color of tissue was found to correlate with superficial papillary dermis, chamois-cloth appearance for deeper papillary dermis, and waterlogged cotton-thread appearance for reticular dermis. We have found this to be true, but only in deep ablation, such as with treatment of plantar warts or basal cell carcinoma of the back. When thinner layers of ablation are used, as in resurfacing, these subtle clinical signs are not seen. Unfortunately, a second report that has received a tremendous amount of attention stated that color was an indication of depth of ablation: pink indicating epidermis, gray indicating papillary dermis, and chamois yellow indicating reticular dermis (99). These color changes are actually a misinterpretation of anatomic changes and not a reliable indicator of tissue depth. If little residual thermal necrosis (less than 30 μm) exists, thermal reaction will not be sufficient to coagulate fine papillary vessels, and the tissue will be pink because of the visible capillary blood flow. This is typical of the appearance of the tissue after a single laser pass removing the epidermis. After a second or third laser pass, the laser is reacting with the dermis and leaves 70–100 μm of thermal necrosis, adequate for hemostasis and resulting in whitish gray tissue. Further laser passes tend to leave more thermal injury, resulting in progressive yellow-brown discoloration, which is a sign of thermal injury, not an indication of penetration into the reticular dermis.

These color changes probably do correlate to some degree with depth of injury, but many inexperienced physicians have interpreted this report too literally and spend much wasted time attempting to recognize subtle color changes, when attention to the laser–tissue interaction with better comprehension would be much more informative.

One study used posttreatment biopsies to compare three pulsed CO_2 lasers with a CW CO_2 laser. After one, two, and three passes, the depth of residual thermal damage measured 30, 80, and 150 μm, respectively, with the SilkTouch laser; 30, 100, and 150 μm with the SurgiPulse laser; and 20, 50, and 70 μm with the UltraPulse laser (80). The CW CO_2 laser left a 400-μm layer of thermal necrosis.

Although early studies appeared to show a relatively constant amount of tissue to be ablated per pass (approximately 75 μm) (79), it became clear in clinical use that a decreasing amount of tissue was ablated per pass. To investigate this hypothesis, as well as the effects of single-pulse vaporization versus multipulse vaporization, or "pulse stacking", and its possible relationship to scarring, a study on excised tissue was done (100). Skin excised for "face-lift" surgery was treated with one through ten passes, wiping with saline between passes and using single-pulse, double-pulse, and triple-pulse impacts at 10 Hz on the same impact site. Biopsies were done to study the depth of ablation as well as residual thermal necrosis. Be it a single, or double, or a triple pulse used at either 250 mJ or 500 mJ per pulse, a similar curve was generated showing that an ablation plateau was reached after three or four passes at 225–250 μm in the dermis (Fig. 6.5).

Residual thermal necrosis showed a linear relationship to both pulse energy and number of passes, with single-pulse vaporization gradually increasing to a maximum of 100 μm at pass no. 7. However, pulse stacking had a marked impact on residual thermal necrosis, because double pulses added significantly more thermal injury per pass and triple pulses even more per pass, about 30 μm (Fig. 6.6). This additional thermal injury may

significantly affect wound healing and result in a much deeper wound than what is intended. Pulse stacking may occur intentionally by concentrating repeated laser impacts on the same tissue site or unintentionally by moving the handpiece at too slow a pace or by using a CPG density that results in too much pulse overlap (densities 7, 8, and 9) corresponding to 40%, 50%, and 60% overlap. This may be a significant factor in causing scarring, hypopigmentation, or poor wound healing (Fig. 6.7).

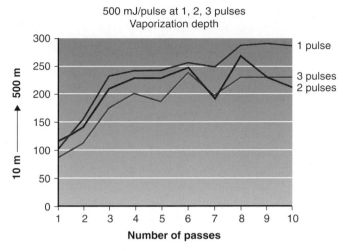

Figure 6.5 With pulsed CO_2 laser ablation, using one, two, or three pulses per impact site at 10 Hz, ablation plateau is reached in three to four passes, limiting the ablation depth to approximately 250 μm.

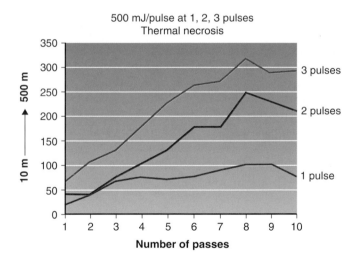

Figure 6.6 When multiple pulses impact the same site at 10 Hz (double or triple sets), a cumulative thermal effect occurs resulting in an increasing loss of control of residual thermal necrosis. Single-tissue impacts, however, result in excellent control of residual thermal damage, even after 10 laser passes.

Density	Overlap	Average fluence (J/cm²)					
1	–10%	2.4	3.3	4.1	4.9	6.5	8.2
2	0%	3.0	4.0	4.9	5.9	7.9	9.9
3	10%	3.7	4.9	6.1	7.3	9.8	12.2
4	20%	4.6	6.2	7.7	9.3	12.3	15.4
5	30%	6.0	8.1	10.1	12.1	16.1	20.2
6	35%	7.0	9.4	11.7	14.0	18.7	23.4
7	40%	8.2	11.0	13.7	16.5	21.9	27.4
8	50%	11.9	15.8	19.8	23.7	31.6	39.5
9	60%	18.5	24.7	30.9	37.0	49.4	61.7
Pulse energy		150 mJ	200 mJ	250 mJ	300 mJ	400 mJ	500 mJ

Figure 6.7 Most effective fluences for treatment are 5–18 J/cm², corresponding to green and yellow zones of this chart. CPG settings of 9 can result in a fluence as high as 60 J/cm².

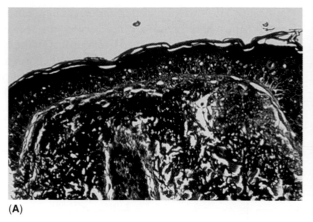

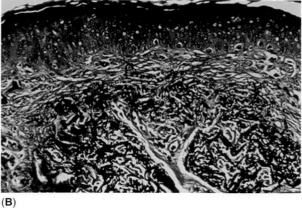

(A)   **(B)**

Figure 6.8 (**A**) Before treatment. (**B**) Using elastic tissue stains, a 600% increase in Grenz zone is noted 90 days after resurfacing, indicating new collagen formation. In addition, layer of solar elastosis is reduced.

Another finding from this study is that in using single-pulse vaporization with a fluence of 3–7 J/cm² and a pulse width of less than 1 ms, CO_2 laser resurfacing is a self-limiting procedure, plateauing at a depth of 250–300 μm in the dermis, too superficial a wound to result in scarring because of depth alone. Therefore adherence to proper treatment techniques is critical in avoiding excessive thermal injury.

Previous histologic studies of dermabraded skin revealed a new, orderly epidermis overlying an upper papillary dermal band of new collagen or "scar." Similar results (increased collagen I formation in the papillary dermis) have been reported after 10 months of treatment with topical tretinoin for photoaged skin. Biopsy specimens obtained at baseline and 3 and 12 weeks after dermabrasion were analyzed and correlated with clinical assessment. Clinical reduction in wrinkling correlated significantly with an increase in fibroblast procollagen-1 mRNA and an increase in procollagen-1 protein, suggesting that clinical improvement might be a result of increased collagen synthesis. Similar increases in Grenz zone collagen were reported after laser resurfacing (81,82,86). This new collagen production and remodeling may be a significant factor in achieving rejuvenation of facial photodamage, as well as in improvement in atrophic acne scars (Fig. 6.8). Continued improvement in facial wrinkling has been noted to occur for as long as 6 months postoperatively and in acne scars for 12 months or more. Long-term biopsies (up to 4 years postoperatively) have shown reversal of epidermal dysplasia, maintenance, and continued thickening of the Grenz zone, and marked improvement in the layer of solar elastosis underlying the Grenz zone, with reduction in overall depth and development of a more fibrillar character (Figs 6.9 and 6.10).

A further consideration is that consecutive passes with the laser result in the laser encountering desiccated, thermally denatured collagen with little water to act as a target for the laser. This results in a progressively decreased depth of vaporization per pulse. When less of the pulse energy goes into vaporization, progressively more energy is deposited into the tissue, potentially causing thermal necrosis by diffusion. In this situation, the pulse width and repetition rate become critical.

In addition to the vaporization and coagulation effects of these lasers removing up to 250–300 μm of tissue in the

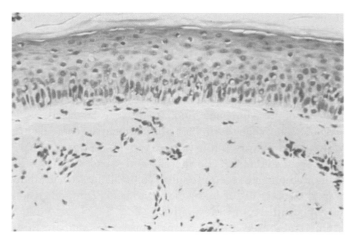

Figure 6.9 Ultraviolet light damage to skin results in epidermal atrophy and flattening of rete ridges with the development of precancerous and cancerous epidermal cells. Amorphous elastotic material (solar elastosis) replaces normal collagen and elastin. Capillaries become reduced in number with thin fragile walls.

dermis, with decreasing tissue ablation with each sequential pass, a second mechanism of laser–tissue interaction appears to be important in achieving the desired clinical results. A discernible shrinkage of the skin is visible as the laser reacts with the dermis, tightening the loose folds of skin. This is thought to be a result of heat-induced collagen shrinkage (101).

When the CO_2 laser interacts with tissue, three distinct zones of tissue alteration correlate to the degree of tissue heating. The zone of direct impact results in vaporization of intracellular water and tissue ablation. Underlying this is a zone of irreversible thermal damage and denaturation resulting in tissue necrosis. Below this layer is a zone of reversible, nonlethal thermal damage (Fig. 6.11), in which collagen shrinkage is thought to occur, accounting for the visible tissue tightening observable as the CO_2 laser interacts with the dermis.

Skin Rejuvenation
Clinical observations have confirmed the value of collagen shrinkage in the rejuvenation of photodamaged skin. This is a significant component of the clinical improvement seen in laser resurfacing. Its exact mechanism and relative importance have been debated. We have hypothesized that the shortened

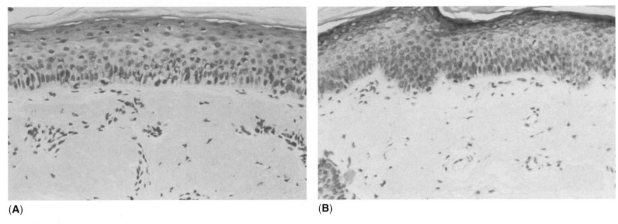

(A)   (B)

Figure 6.10 (**A**) Pretreatment biopsy. (**B**) Long-term biopsies (2 years or more postoperatively) have demonstrated normalization of epidermis, continued gradual thickening of Grenz zone, and reduction of solar elastosis. In addition, solar elastosis was found to become progressively less homogeneous and amorphous with a much greater fibrillar content (see also Figure 6.9).

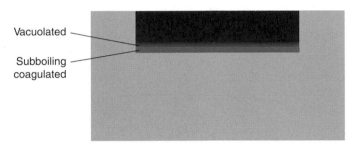

Figure 6.11 Zones of thermal damage in tissue instantaneously heated above 70°C but below 100°C. Normal tissue has a temperature of 37°C. Between this 70°C layer and normal 37°C tissue is a gradient of temperature in which collagen shrinkage occurs, ideally at 63°C.

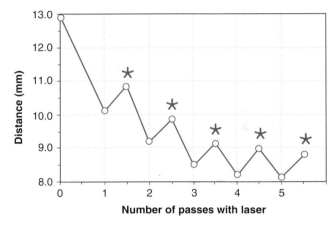

Figure 6.12 Collagen shrinkage as seen per pass with UltraPulse CO_2 laser. *Asterisks* represent rehydration between passes. *Source*: From Ref. 86.

collagen fibers result in a shrunken matrix on which collagen remodeling occurs, resulting in the preservation of this tightened skin. That the tightened skin does persist to variable degrees is confirmed by study of photographs over time, as well as by the occurrence of laser-induced ectropion, a condition of excessive tissue tightening.

Tissue contraction is grossly visible on impact of the pulsed CO_2 laser with skin during resurfacing being most profound on the first and second dermal passes after removal of the epidermis. Although some component of this tissue contraction is undoubtedly secondary to tissue volume loss as a consequence of vaporization of tissue water, a large portion is thought to be from collagen contraction. Gardner et al. (86) found a positive linear correlation between the number of passes and the degree of skin shrinkage. A linear regression model showed a 6% size reduction per pass with the SilkTouch laser and a 5% reduction per pass with the Ultra-Pulse laser. Rehydrating the tissue between passes resulted in only slight correction of the shrinkage (Fig. 6.12). Analysis of a single specimen treated with the SilkTouch laser for five consecutive passes with rehydration between passes revealed about 15% reduction on the first pass and a plateau at about 31% reduction after three to five passes. Temperature elevation in the tissue was approximately 20°C and unchanged with each pass. Ross et al. (102) observed a positive correlation between contraction of the treated area and both fluence and the number of laser passes in their studies on pig skin.

CO_2 LASER SKIN RESURFACING

The most important factor in performing CO_2 laser resurfacing is single-pulse laser–tissue interaction (Fig. 6.13). If vaporization is accomplished in a single pulse, the heat of the laser–tissue interaction is released in the vapor created, and thermal diffusion deep into the treated tissue will not occur. If the tissue cannot be vaporized (i.e., the threshold for vaporization is not reached), it is critical that the pulse duration be less than the thermal diffusion time. In this situation, the laser–tissue interaction site will cool off before there is time for thermal diffusion to occur. If laser pulses are stacked one on top of another, additive thermal effects will occur because of heat retention. For the CO_2 laser, the pulse repetition rate must be less than an estimated 5 Hz to allow tissue cooling between pulses and to avoid cumulative thermal effects (103). The technique used with the Lumenis UltraPulse is described here.

UltraPulse Technique

When performing resurfacing procedures by hand with a 3-mm collimated beam, it is critical to move the handpiece at a rate that allows single-pulse laser–tissue interaction, with minimal overlapping (generally a rate of 4–10 Hz). When using the CPG, the patterns should not be overlapped, and the

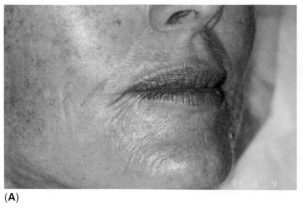

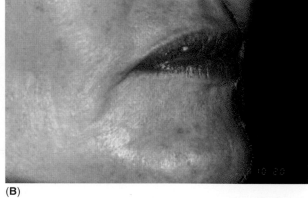

(A)   **(B)**

Figure 6.13 (**A**) Relatively superficial lines may be completely removed by ablating to depth of wrinkle line. (**B**) Improvement depends on ablation of solar elastosis and wound healing. Collagen shrinkage and new collagen formation are not necessary for this improvement to occur.

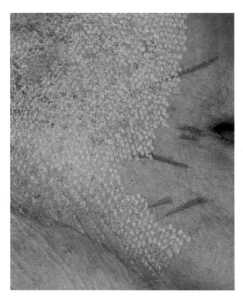

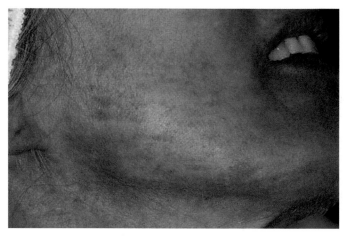

Figure 6.15 Single pass of computer pattern generator may result in linear streaks of hyperpigmentation, resulting from differential thermal effects leaving a mixture of non–sun-damaged cells and sun-damaged cells. To prevent this, a second pass is performed at 90° to first pass.

Figure 6.14 Initial CO_2 laser pass effectively removes epidermis by vaporizing a 40- to 50-µm layer and causing a subepidermal vesicle to form. Surface is covered with white, desiccated, proteinaceous debris from epidermis immediately after first pass. This needs to be wiped away with saline-soaked gauze.

individual laser impacts within the pattern should have minimal overlap (generally densities of 3–6).

The surface is covered with a single pass of laser impacts, resulting in white, desiccated debris composed of proteinaceous epidermal tissue remaining after intracellular tissue water vaporization (Fig. 6.14). This tissue debris should be wiped away with saline-moistened gauze to remove the remaining epidermis. The first pass generally removes the epidermis and leaves only minimal residual thermal damage (10–30 µm) depending on epidermal thickness, with more thermal damage in thin epidermis, such as eyelid or neck skin. This procedure is repeated over the entire surface to be treated for the second pass. The only difference is that during this pass, the CPG is oriented at 90° to the direction used for the first pass. The reason for this is to avoid the appearance of linear pigment streaks that may be associated with the pattern of the CPG (Fig. 6.15).

Generally, the third pass is applied more selectively to areas of more significant photodamage and wrinkling. If photodamage

remains visible over the entire treatment area, the entire area is treated again. In general, however, the third pass is confined to the glabellar area, upper lip, nasolabial folds, and lateral cheeks. A fourth pass with the Lumenis CPG is only rarely needed except in cases of advanced, severe photodamage and is therefore not recommended (Fig. 6.3).

Generally, after the third pass with the Lumenis CPG, treatment with the 3-mm beam is used in selective areas to flatten high tissue points by vaporization and to tighten loose skin or ablate wrinkles by pulling the base of wrinkle lines up and achieving as smooth a surface as possible to act as a base for new collagen formation.

In performing resurfacing, clinicians should keep in mind the following:

1. Always "feather" the peripheral areas by decreasing the density of pulse application as well as the pulse energy (decrease to 200–250 mJ), or angle the beam at 45° to spread the fluence over a larger surface area.
2. Feather into the hairline a distance of 5–15 mm and well under the jawline (3–5 cm) (Fig. 6.16).

3. Use feathering parameters to treat the eyelid surfaces; use no more than two passes in the immediate periorbital area except isolated spot application to persisting folds of tissue.

4. Carefully observe the laser–tissue interaction of the eyelids to avoid excessive tightening of tissue and possible scleral show or ectropion, especially in patients with a prior blepharoplasty.

5. Use the 3-mm beam to make a single pass along the vermilion borders of the upper and lower lips, because this is the most common area of persistence of wrinkle lines. This also helps to emphasize the vermilion border.

6. Do not routinely cross the vermilion border. Treat up to the border, because this will make the lips appear fuller and emphasize the vermilion border as a result of the collagen tightening of the lip.

7. Treat lines that cross the vermilion border individually by tracing over the line with the laser once all the other areas have been treated, rather than treating the entire vermilion surface.

8. After completion of treatment with the CPG, carefully search the treatment surface for signs of residual seborrheic keratoses, actinic keratoses, or SCC in situ and for thickened scars, and vaporize these to a flat surface using the 3-mm beam with pulse-stacking treatment technique or with the Er:YAG laser.

9. Always carefully observe the immediate tissue response regarding contraction or yellow-brown discoloration. If this discoloration persists after wiping with saline, this is a sign of thermal necrosis (Fig. 6.17).

10. Use the 3-mm spot in placing impact sites at 3- to 5-mm intervals to achieve tightening of the skin without significant thermal risk (concentric lines of these treatment spots moving away from a site to be tightened is effective). This is particularly useful on the eyelids and midcheeks.

The endpoint of treatment is when one of the following conditions is seen:

1. The wrinkle or scar is removed.
2. A yellow-brown discoloration indicating thermal damage is seen.
3. No further skin tightening is observed.

No reason exists to continue treating an area when any of these signs is observed. Leave that area untreated from that point on and concentrate on other tissue sites.

Collagen Shrinkage and Skin Tightening

It was not initially anticipated that collagen shrinkage would be a component of the laser–tissue interaction. However, unexpected improvement in redundant folds of the eyelids, loose skin of the cheeks, nasolabial folds, and the other deep wrinkle lines, coupled with the visible skin tightening observable with the laser–tissue interaction, has led to the use of heat-induced collagen shrinkage for clinical benefit (Box 6.1).

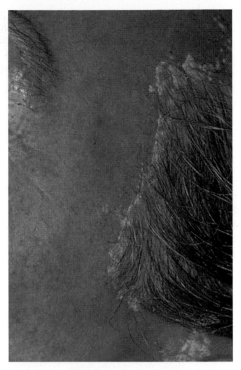

Figure 6.16 "Feathering" into hairline 5–15 mm to avoid leaving a line of contrast anterior to hairline. Hair will regrow normally in this feathered zone, but it is not possible to treat the inside scalp without coagulating shaft of hairs.

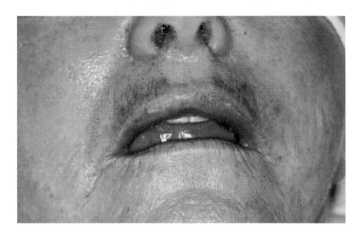

Figure 6.17 Persistent yellow-brown discoloration of dermis after wiping with saline is a sign of thermal injury that may be extending deeper into dermis.

This skin-tightening effect allows achievement of comparable clinical results at a more superficial level of tissue removal than is necessary with other resurfacing modalities, such as dermabrasion and chemical peels. The amount of tightening observed depends on the number of passes delivered, unknown specific tissue factors (possibly the numbers and health of intact collagen fibers), tissue thickness, and anatomic location. Thin tissue such as eyelid and neck skin tightens very readily and often profoundly, even to the point of causing ectropion in eyelid skin. Temporal skin is generally thinner compared with other facial skin and also tightens more significantly. Tightening of cheek skin may be important in reducing nasolabial fold prominence and "jowls" under the jawline. Tightening may be used very selectively to achieve desired clinical

Box 6.1 Collagen Shrinkage with CO_2 Laser

Collagen Molecule

- Three polypeptide chains in helical conformation result from repetitive positioning of glycine at every third amino acid locus
- Intermolecular cross-links provide tensile strength and are inhibited by heat
- Heat dissociates interpeptide bond; molecules remain intact
- Hydrothermal shrinkage occurs through molecular structure transition from a triple helix to a random coil
- Immediate contraction of fibers occurs to about one-third their original length
- Collagen is progressively more cross-linked with time, so new collagen is less stable and contracts at lower temperature

Collagen–Heat Reaction

- Polypeptide strands of heated tissue have capacity to resume the original intrachain characteristics
- Collagen readily self-assembles into fibrils, which cross-link in a spontaneous, progressive manner
- A myriad of molecular conformations are possible
- Denaturation process is both time and temperature dependent; in general, a 2°C rise in temperature reduces shrinkage time by 50%
- Very narrow temperature range exists for shrinkage without destroying fibrils
- Instantaneous shrinkage temperature of human collagen was found to be 62.9°C, with a range of 57–65°C
- As temperature rises, more and more cross-link bonds are broken until denaturation and loss of structure occur
- Percent shrinkage is directly proportional to heat applied while not exceeding threshold for denaturation

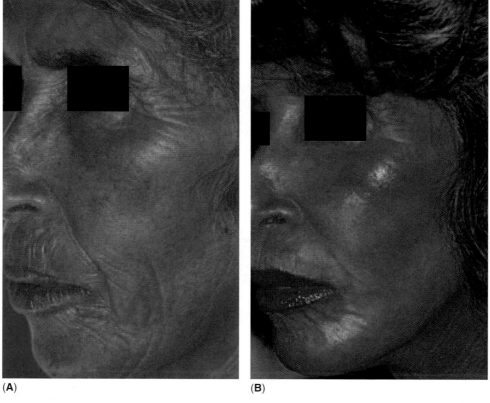

(A)   **(B)**

Figure 6.18 Skin tightening and collagen shrinkage result in clinical improvement in nasolabial folds and cheeks. (**A**) Before treatment; (**B**) 1 year after full-face CO_2 laser resurfacing.

effects (Fig. 6.18). Precise tightening of folds of loose eyelid tissue (Fig. 6.19) or atrophic scars (Fig. 6.20) can dramatically improve clinical results without significant risk if careful clinical observation is used.

By targeting high points of glabellar and forehead lines, better smoothing of these areas may be achieved. This type of tissue change has been shown to persist 4 years or more and is thought to be a permanent structural change in the skin once the new collagen formation has occurred.

New Collagen Formation and Collagen Remodeling

To avoid excessive thermal injury, it is recommended that the laser resurfacing procedure be discontinued when signs of

thermal injury are seen, that is, yellow-brown discoloration of the skin. Often, when treatment is discontinued because of visible thermal effects, visible wrinkle lines are still present, particularly on the glabella, forehead, and upper lip (Fig. 6.21A,B). These lines may gradually improve during the healing process and may gradually subside over 6–12 weeks (Fig. 6.21C,D). This occurs as a consequence of new collagen formation and collagen remodeling.

A multicenter study demonstrated that UltraPulse laser resurfacing results in up to a 600% increase in the Grenz zone layer. A new layer of healthy, fine collagen fibrils is laid down parallel to the epidermis and measures 100–400 μm in depth, replacing the layer of solar elastosis vaporized by the laser.

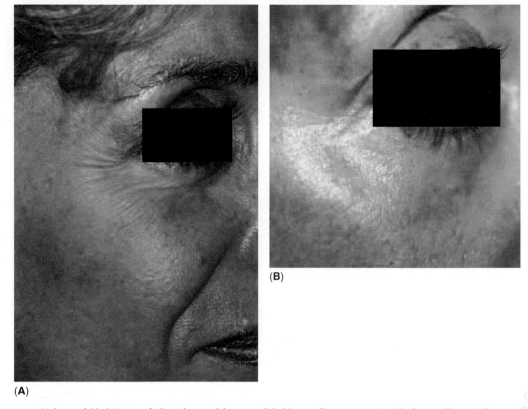

Figure 6.19 Improvement in loose, folded tissue of photodamaged lower-eyelid skin usually occurs primarily from collagen tightening. (**A**) Before therapy; (**B**) 4 months after CO_2 laser resurfacing.

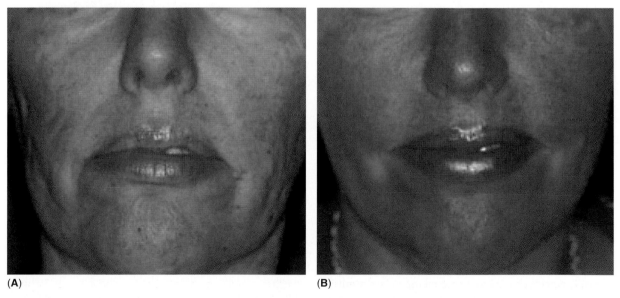

Figure 6.20 Atrophic acne scars may respond dramatically to a single treatment with CO_2 laser by using collagen tightening selectively and artfully to elevate scars. (**A**) Before treatment; (**B**) 4 months after CO_2 laser resurfacing.

Multipulse Coagulation

The most efficient fluences for vaporizing the epidermis have been shown to be in the range of 5–19 J/cm^2. Single-pulse vaporization generally uses fluences of about 7 J/cm^2. However, when one pulse is stacked on top of another without sufficient tissue cooling time, additive thermal effects occur. When using the CPG with the UltraPulse laser, a density of 9 results in as high an energy density as 60 J/cm^2 to be delivered to the tissue. It has been clinically observed that after making three or four passes with the UltraPulse laser using CPG densities of 4–6, nothing visible appears to occur to the tissue. Neither the depth of vaporization nor the thermal injury appears to be increasing. Biopsy studies confirm this impression as long as single-pulse vaporization is being used (100).

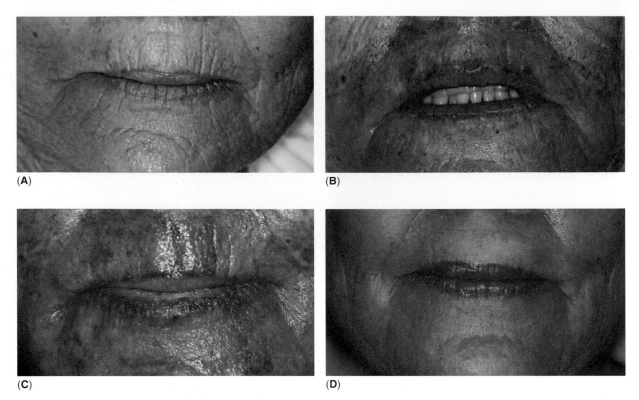

(A)   (B)

(C)   (D)

Figure 6.21 Clinical improvement often occurs in a delayed manner secondary to new collagen formation and collagen remodeling. (**A**) Deep upper-lip lines before treatment. (**B**) Immediately after treatment, these lines remain very visible. (**C**) 3 days after treatment, swelling intensifies visibility of some lines. (**D**) 6 months later, lines are gone.

However, these same tissue studies have shown that with stacking pulses on top of one another, the zone of thermal necrosis gradually increases and may increase to greater than 300 μm, although the depth of vaporization remains basically unchanged. The procedure of vaporization appears to level off because the tissue target (i.e., water) changes as the procedure progresses. In the first pass, the laser is interacting with intracellular water. Once the epidermis has been stripped away, however, the laser is acting primarily with extracellular water in the dermis. In addition, the water content of the epidermis is closer to 80%, whereas in the dermis it is closer to 60%. The dermis is made up primarily of protein fibrils of collagen and elastic tissue. These fibers have a much higher threshold of vaporization than water. Therefore, the amount of tissue vaporized with each pass becomes less and less.

Complicating the situation even further is the layer of thermal necrosis, which measures generally between 50 and 100 μm, is desiccated, and has very little water. Therefore, it is difficult to vaporize deeper than 200–300 μm using single-pulse vaporization with a collimated beam. However, stacking pulses result in cumulative thermal effects and may allow deeper vaporization because of the higher fluence that results from rapid pulse succession.

This is a hazardous procedure because the residual thermal damage is greater with pulse stacking and may progress to the point of interfering with wound healing, which may cause scarring. This occurs without obvious clinical signs of potential problems, but subtle signs may be distinguished by experienced observation. When stacking pulses on top of each other, a yellow-brown discoloration of the tissue is observed clinically. This is initially subtle and clears with saline wiping.

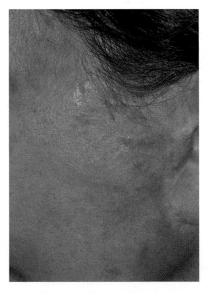

Figure 6.22 Failure to adhere carefully to single-pulse vaporization may result in inadvertently stacking pulses and extending thermal necrosis deeply into dermis. This may result in delayed wound healing and scarring.

As further passes are performed, the yellow color gradually deepens to brown and will not get wiped away. When this yellow-brown discoloration is seen, the physician can be certain that this area will be the last to heal and that this tissue will slough. Although this pulse-stacking technique can be used to resurface deeper because of the resultant tissue slough, it is a potentially dangerous technique that can result in poor wound healing and scarring (Fig. 6.22).

If a decision is made to use this technique clinically, it is imperative to learn the signs of depth of injury by observation of tissue healing with variable levels of treatment on repeated occasions. As mentioned earlier, the three end points of treatment are elimination of the wrinkle or scar, a yellow-brown discoloration indicating thermal damage, and no further collagen shrinkage or tightening. When any one of these is reached, the laser procedure should be terminated in that area of the face. It is much safer to re-treat residual lines after an adequate healing time of 6 months or longer.

FACIAL WRINKLING

To evaluate the severity of wrinkling and photodamage present and therefore achieve some degree of predictability of response to resurfacing, a clinical classification and numeric scoring system have been adapted from other photodamage assessment systems. Although other wrinkling and photodamage assessment scales exist, the need for a system related purely to visible wrinkling and visible textural changes secondary to solar elastosis was thought to be more relevant to the topic of wrinkle eradication (101).

Use of this scoring system allows broad classification into mild, moderate, and severe categories as well as a subjective numeric severity score (Table 6.2). Assessing patients both before and after treatment in a study with an average follow-up of about 90 days revealed that the average patient's preoperative score decreased approximately 50% as a consequence of resurfacing (104). This means that mild wrinkles generally resolve completely, moderate wrinkles become mild, and severe wrinkles become moderate.

Other studies (3,4,97) using different assessment systems have come to basically the same conclusion: wrinkles generally improve 50–70%, with superficial lines eliminated, deeper lines softened, skin texture normalized, precancerous lesions eliminated, and lentigines and seborrheic keratoses eliminated. These are realistic expectations for the patient although, occasionally, even severe wrinkles may completely resolve. The treated area may continue to improve for several months after laser resurfacing as collagen remodeling takes place.

Our studies of patients with an average follow-up of 2 years postoperatively (range 1–4 years) have revealed an excellent preservation of these results. Generally, as anticipated, the lines first to recur are those caused by muscle motion ("crow's feet," glabellar, and forehead). Excellent preservation of results was seen, however, because 3-month versus 25-month scores revealed an average improvement in preoperative photodamage scores periorally of 49% versus 38%, respectively, while periorbital scores were 46% versus 31% improved (Fig. 6.23). Interestingly, patient satisfaction for these two areas was 55% for the perioral area and 80% for the periorbital area. Overall, 94 of 104 patients (90%) considered laser resurfacing to be a beneficial procedure that they would recommend to others (105). This may be true because the laser removes the textural and pigmentary abnormalities (the "weathered" look) although the muscles may still be able to fold the skin into wrinkles.

Other investigators have found similar results. Burns (personal communication) had independent observers grade 95 consecutive full-face resurfacing procedures at 90 days and 1 year postoperatively using a scale of 1–8 and found an average decrease in photodamage scores (Table 6.3). No difference was seen in outcome whether patients were treated with the previously used Coherent or Sharplan systems.

Ross et al. (106) reported the long-term results of 28 patients treated with either the SilkTouch or the UltraPulse laser and found that their pretreatment photodamage scores continued to improve from 60 days to the reassessment point at 1 year. Scores improved 43% in the SilkTouch group and 34% in the UltraPulse group, but no statistical difference was seen between the two groups. The immediate thermal damage was found to be about 30% greater in the SilkTouch group, with a wider zone of fibroplasia (220 vs. 150 µm in the UltraPulse group) at 1 year postoperatively. No statistical difference was seen in adverse effects for the two groups, although focal hypopigmentation

Table 6.2 Facial Wrinkling: Clinical Classifications

Class	Wrinkling	Score	Degree of Elastosis
I	Fine wrinkles	1–3	Mild: fine textural changes with subtly accentuated skin lines
II	Fine-to-moderate depth wrinkles	4–6	Moderate: distinct popular elastosis (individual papules with yellow translucency under direct lighting) and dyschromia; moderate number of lines
III	Fine-to-deep wrinkles; numerous	7–9	Severe: multipapular and confluent elastosis (thickened, yellow, and pallid) lines; with or without redundant skin folds approaching or consistent with cutis rhomboidalis

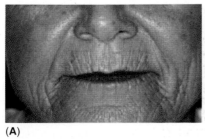 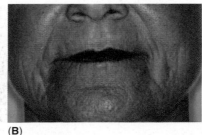 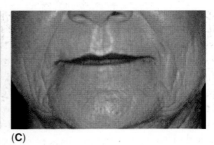

(A)   **(B)**   **(C)**

Figure 6.23 Excellent long-term results after CO_2 laser resurfacing of facial wrinkles. (**A**) Before surgery: class III, level 8. (**B**) 14 months postoperatively: class II, level 4. (**C**) 39 months postoperatively: class II, level 4. Note progression of photoaging of medial cheeks, which were not treated.

Table 6.3 The Average Decrease in Photodamage at 90 days and 1 year after Full-Face Resurfacing

Area	90 Days (%)	1 Year (%)
Perioral	69	64
Cheeks	89	72
Forehead	80	48
Periorbital	79	52

was noted in two patients treated with the SilkTouch laser and one patient treated with both. Weinstein (107) reports that follow-up of her patients for as long as 5 years after resurfacing has shown that improvement visible at 6 months was still present at 5 years and that the overall results are indeed long lasting.

In addition, 24 subjects were treated with the SilkTouch laser on one side of the face and 35% TCA on the opposite, for correction of periorbital wrinkling. Using a scoring system of 1–5, pretreatment scores were found to diminish 56% with laser treatment versus 20% with chemical peeling at 6 months. The outcome difference was statistically significant. Posttreatment erythema, however, lasted 4.5 months versus 2.5 months for the respective groups.

Long-term follow-up of 12 patients having photodamage treated with dermabrasion and followed for 6 months to 8 years showed that not only did cosmetic improvement persist over these time periods, but the need for continued treatment of premalignant and malignant lesions was virtually eliminated. All patients were noted to have maintained a smooth, supple skin with pigmentation slightly lighter than the adjacent nondermabraded skin. The problem of course is that although this laser resurfacing can improve the appearance of wrinkling by over 50%, the patient continues to age. We typically are seeing our patients back after 10 years asking for a second laser resurfacing procedure.

OTHER INDICATIONS OF THE CO_2 LASER
Acne
Laser resurfacing can achieve significant improvement in acne scarring. The procedure can be made very precise by sculpting the edges of the scars and vaporizing more tissue away only in the areas of scar tissue while doing only superficial resurfacing in the rest of the cosmetic unit being treated. The tissue-tightening effects can achieve dramatic improvement in soft atrophic scars with sloping walls (Fig. 6.20). Some "ice pick" and bound-down scars should first be removed with punch excision, punch elevation, or punch grafting, with laser resurfacing performed 6–12 weeks later if maximum improvement is desired (Fig. 6.24) (108). Those not treated first with excision will improve, but the degree of improvement achieved will depend on the scar's depth and the operator's skill. In general, a 30–50% improvement is the treatment goal. However, a study using the Coherent UltraPulse CO_2 laser to treat moderate-to-severe atrophic acne scars in 50 patients revealed an average clinical improvement of 81% at 6 months after treatment, with progressive improvement occurring during that period (18).

We always treat acne scars with the Er:YAG laser after resurfacing with the CO_2 laser. The use of the Er:YAG allows for continued sculpting of the acne scar without an increase in nonspecific thermal damage.

Patients should be advised that acne scars are always difficult to treat by any method, and the patient rarely reaches the level of satisfaction desired in a single surgical procedure. The same is true for laser resurfacing, but additional laser procedures add significant degrees of improvement.

Scars
Crateriform varicella scars and isolated acne scars can be improved with spot laser resurfacing. The area around and over the scar is vaporized with one laser pass. Additional passes with the Er:YAG laser are concentrated along the edge of the scar crater until it has been completely effaced.

Postsurgical (Fig. 6.25) and traumatic scars and skin grafts (Fig. 6.26) can be dramatically improved if resurfaced (66,67,109). It is best to wait until the scar has completely healed (3–6 months) (Fig. 6.27). This is an artistic endeavor and involves the vaporization of elevated tissue high points, as well as skin tightening to elevate loose atrophic tissue. This is often a process of trial and error, attempting various maneuvers in small selective areas with observation of tissue effects before deciding to use an approach in a larger surface area.

Actinic Cheilitis
Actinic cheilitis has proved to be a condition for which CO_2 laser therapy is considered the treatment of choice (69,110–119). It can be successfully treated by performing a laser vermilionectomy using any of the resurfacing lasers (108). This procedure usually requires only one pass with the laser over the vermilion surface and then spot treatment of persistently visible actinic damage. This has significantly reduced postoperative healing to approximately 10 days, in contrast to the 4 weeks required when the conventional CO_2 laser was used in the past (69,110–119).

Also, the risk of scarring is greatly reduced because the extent of thermal damage is much less.

Actinic keratoses unresponsive to conventional treatment with liquid nitrogen and topical 5-fluorouracil can be treated by removing the epidermis with one pass and then concentrating treatment on visible dermal extensions using one of the resurfacing lasers. This is especially useful on the dorsal hands and scalp but may be a primary or sole indication for laser resurfacing.

Pigmentation
Pigmentation irregularities such as postinflammatory hyperpigmentation or melasma can sometimes be improved with laser resurfacing. It is very important to use tretinoin (Retin-A) and hydroquinone for an extended period before and after the procedure (120,121). Other lasers more specific for melanin or medium-depth chemical peels are often preferable because they do not require anesthesia and recovery time is much shorter (122–126). Melasma responds variably, in a similar manner to its response to other modalities (127). Usually these pigment abnormalities are a secondary component of treatment and not the primary treatment objective. If they are the primary reason for treatment, care must be taken to ensure that other, more pigment-specific therapies are not desirable for whatever reason.

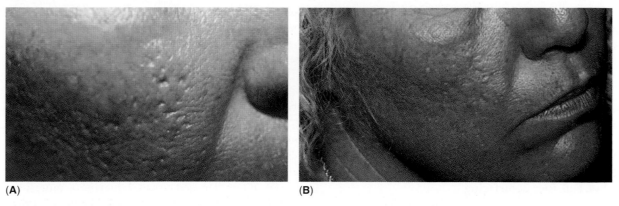

(A)　　　　　　　　　　　　　　　　　　**(B)**

Figure 6.24 "Ice pick" or bound-down scars will improve greatly if scar excisions are performed before CO_2 laser resurfacing. (**A**) Before excision; (**B**) 1 year after laser resurfacing.

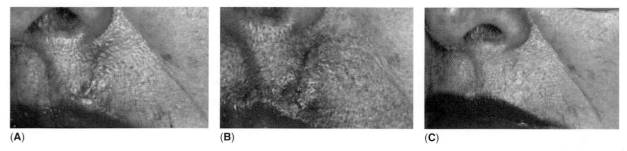

(A)　　　　　　　　　**(B)**　　　　　　　　　**(C)**

Figure 6.25 (**A**) Linear scar 6 weeks after repair of Mohs surgical defect. (**B**) Immediately after resurfacing with an UltraPulse CO_2 laser at 500 mJ, 3-mm-diameter spot size, with three passes given to vaporize the scar. (**C**) 9 months after resurfacing, virtual disappearance of the scar.

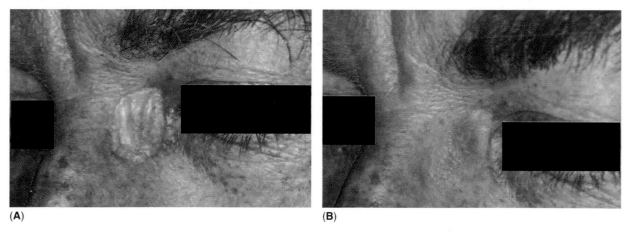

(A)　　　　　　　　　　　　　　　　　　**(B)**

Figure 6.26 (**A**) 6 weeks after full-thickness skin graft repair of Mohs surgical defect. (**B**) 4 months after laser resurfacing of skin graft with laser parameters identical to those in Figure 6.27.

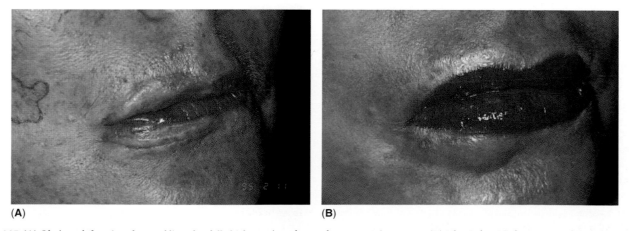

(A)　　　　　　　　　　　　　　　　　　**(B)**

Figure 6.27 (**A**) Obvious deformity of scarred lips after full-thickness tissue loss and reconstructive surgery. (**B**) UltraPulse CO_2 laser was used to sculpt scar tissue and normalize lip contours.

Rhinophyma and Benign Growths

Rhinophyma (128,129) and various small benign growths such as syringoma (130), trichoepithelioma (131), dermatosis papulosa nigra, xanthelasma (132), adenoma sebaceum (133), sebaceous hyperplasia, and epidermal nevi (134,135) have traditionally been treated with the conventional CO_2 laser and respond in an even more excellent manner to the resurfacing CO_2 lasers.

CO_2 LASER RESURFACING: SURGICAL CONSIDERATIONS

Regional vs. Full-Face Resurfacing

The two areas of photodamage and wrinkling that have been shown to respond dramatically well to laser resurfacing are the perioral and periorbital regions (101). These areas are not improved by face-lifting procedures, and although blepharoplasty may improve the skin laxity, it does not smooth out the wrinkle lines and textural changes of the periorbital region. Chemical peels and dermabrasion have given disappointing results in both these regions after treatment by the average practitioner. Treatment success in these regions has given laser resurfacing its popularity. Either of these areas may be successfully treated as an isolated region, but if both areas are to be treated, it is far better to treat the entire face.

In general, full-face resurfacing will give a better clinical result in all patients, because treatment of the full cheeks results in better tightening of the nasolabial lines, lateral "crow's feet," and midcheek creases. The same is true of treating the entire forehead and its effects on glabellar lines, lateral temporal lines, and upper aspects of crow's feet. In addition, the even pigmentation and smoothing of the skin result in a much more pleasant cosmetic appearance than blending new, smooth skin to photodamaged skin and creating a patchwork pattern. From a practical standpoint, it is also much easier for the patient to deal with postoperative erythema that is uniform over the full face rather than patchy erythema with multiple borders to blend. We rarely treat only a single anatomic unit, almost never treat an isolated wrinkle or scar, and never treat two isolated anatomic units simultaneously without treating the intervening skin. In our office, 90–95% of patients receive full-face treatment.

Timing of Treatment

Whether to treat early or later is an issue that frequently arises. The potential advantages of treating early, rather fine, subtle wrinkle lines are that the procedure can be done more superficially and with less risk of prolonged erythema, pigment changes, or scarring. Also, greater potential exists for removing all the photodamaged tissue, achieving a more long-lasting result, and providing a preventive benefit regarding future wrinkling. However, these early changes are usually relatively subtle clinically and, even when fully removed, result in only modest cosmetic benefits. The primary benefit may be in halting the progression of photodamage. The pros and cons of performing a relatively aggressive procedure for a relatively minor cosmetic problem need to be discussed in detail and a decision made with realistic expectations (Table 6.4).

Degree of Photodamage and Pigmentation

When dealing with more advanced photodamage, full-face resurfacing is almost always necessary. Complete removal of deep lines in a single procedure may not be possible, as previously discussed. The anticipated improvement is 50–70% (Fig 6.28) (3,4,97,101,104,136). If further improvement is desired, a second treatment may be done after 6–12 months to allow new collagen formation and collagen remodeling. Patients with more advanced photodamage are usually very pleased with their clinical improvement although it may not be complete eradication of wrinkle lines. Complete elimination of wrinkle lines is usually not the patient's goal, and overaggressive treatments may result in prolonged healing or hypopigmentation from deep levels of tissue ablation and deep resurfacing. The physician must effectively communicate to the patient that some degree of decreased pigmentation is a consequence of treatment.

Table 6.4 Early vs. Later CO_2 Laser Treatment of Wrinkles[a]

Pros	Cons
Treatment of early wrinkling	
More superficial resurfacing necessary	Use of relatively aggressive treatment for relatively minor cosmetic problem
Less risks of scarring, prolonged erythema, and pigment loss	Must weigh risk–benefit ratio
Complete elimination of wrinkles typically achieved	Patients often very demanding and critical of less-than-perfect results
Long-lasting results achieved with good maintenance program	Deeper resurfacing procedure and more aggressive therapy necessary
Dramatic improvement often achieved	Greater risks of scarring, prolonged erythema, and pigment loss
	Improvement might be subtle
Treatment of late wrinkling	
Medical benefit (e.g., removal of actinic keratoses, squamous cell carcinoma in situ) common	More than one procedure necessary for complete elimination of wrinkles
Significant psychologic benefit	Persistence of benefits variable, depending on the depth of preexisting damage as well as maintenance program
Patient satisfied with improvement, with no expectation of complete eradication of wrinkles	

[a]Both are successful. Both patient and physician must have realistic expectations. In general, earlier treatment is preferable to later treatment because of decreased risks and enhanced ability to achieve excellent results.

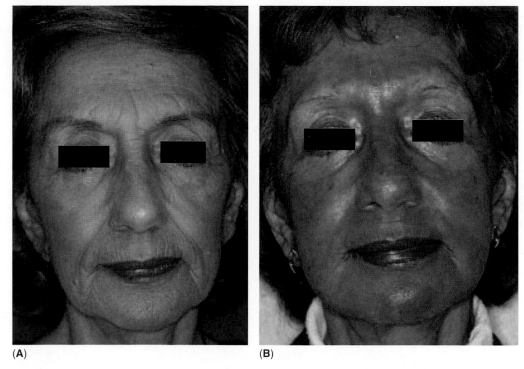

(A)   (B)

Figure 6.28 Anticipated improvement results for full-face resurfacing are 50–70%. Complete elimination of some wrinkle lines definitely will occur, but other lines may only soften. (**A**) Before surgery; (**B**) 3 months postoperatively.

Sun-damaged skin, with a history of decades of sun exposure, has a different pigmentation than non–sun-damaged skin that is related to the depth of resurfacing. Removal of the epidermis alone may result in healing with a population of melanocytes derived from the most superficial aspect of the follicular epithelium. These melanocytes have a significant history of prior sun damage and may produce persistent dyspigmentation. Deeper resurfacing results in progressive elimination of this sun-exposed subset of follicular epithelial melanocytes, yielding a more uniform pigmentation. An effective means of communicating this to patients is to have them compare the pigment of a non–sun-exposed area, such as the skin of the medial upper arms, to that of their face. This is likely to be the color of their newly healed skin, with non–sun-exposed epithelium and papillary dermis having developed during the healing process. If a strong color contrast is seen, a decision must be made regarding (*i*) selection of epidermal resurfacing only, which can be accomplished with a 20% TCA peel or Er:YAG laser resurfacing and (*ii*) consideration of forming the transition zone from treated to nontreated skin.

The natural shadowing under the jawline makes this area a good transition area. For some patients, the contrast will be too great if they do not wear makeup. It may be preferable, however, to have this contrast occur at the jawline rather than at midneck (chosen by some physicians because the upper neck heals better than the lower neck and can be treated more aggressively), the clavicular level, or the V of the neck or upper chest. Resurfacing of the neck to the clavicles or down to the middle anterior chest is difficult and should only be performed by those who are experienced and have a mastery of laser–tissue interaction (Fig. 6.29) (40). The erbium laser may also be used successfully in this regard with proper technique.

Some physicians use 20–25% TCA applied in a light coat, with only spotty frosting occurring. The latter two choices may be appropriate for a woman who always wears a collared shirt and rarely or never has her entire upper chest and shoulder area visually exposed. When these areas are more visible from the clothing worn, especially in those frequently involved in athletics, women may prefer more superficial resurfacing and a transition zone at the jawline.

To preserve normal pigmentation, although it may be reduced in contrast to sun-damaged skin, it is necessary to avoid deep, midreticular dermal tissue removal. This type of pigment loss is considered a complication and is usually associated with prolonged erythema (Fig. 6.30). It should be avoidable through adherence to our recommended techniques.

Lines of Expression
Lines of expression—forehead lines, glabellar lines, and, particularly, "crow's feet" lateral canthal lines—are caused by muscle contraction and will always recur, even if completely erased after the procedure. As long as the muscles involved continue to fold the skin, a crease is formed. Several surgical procedures may be used to denervate or demuscle some of these areas. However, a very useful adjunctive procedure is the injection of botulinum toxin type A (Botox/Dysport/Xeomin) to block nerve transmission to these muscle groups (137–140). These injections should be performed 1–2 weeks preoperatively to block these muscle groups and prevent motion in these areas for 3–4 months during the time of new collagen formation and remodeling. Enhanced results are seen and should give a more lasting clinical improvement (Fig. 6.31). We recommend continuing with Botox injections every 3–4 months for 1 year to achieve longer-lasting results.

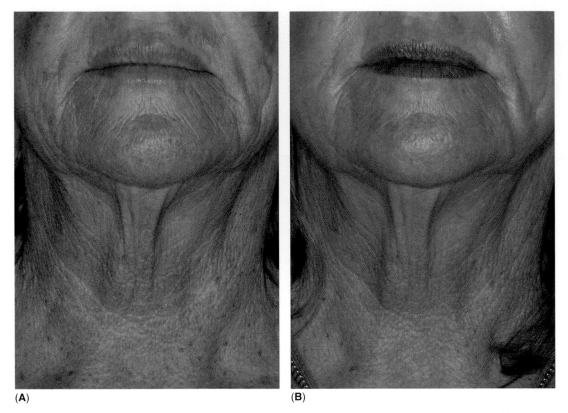

(A)   (B)

Figure 6.29 (**A**) Before and (**B**) 3 weeks after a single-pass CO_2 laser with topical EMLA for hydration. It cannot be overstated that ablative CO_2 resurfacing of the neck should be performed only by those with a mastery of laser–tissue interaction.

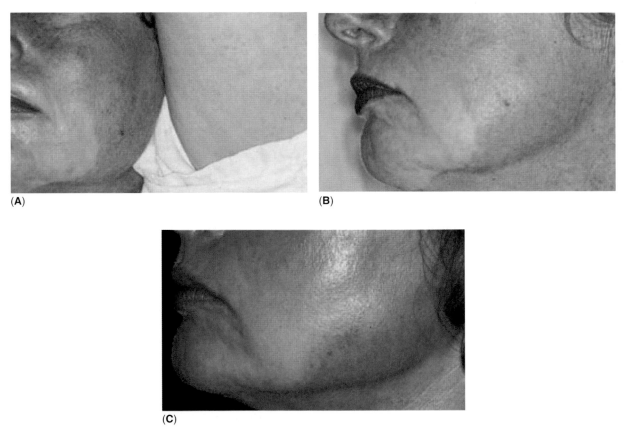

(A)   (B)

(C)

Figure 6.30 (**A**) True hypopigmentation occurs with loss of melanocytes and results in pigment loss that is usually more significant than that of non–sun-exposed skin. (**B**) This type of pigment loss contrasts sharply with photodamaged skin. (**C**) Treatment of this condition is oriented toward removal of contrasting photodamaged skin.

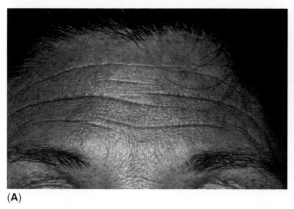
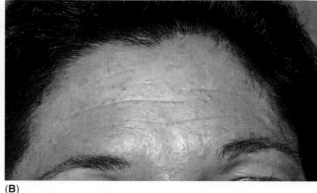

(A)   **(B)**

Figure 6.31 (**A**) Deep lines of forehead, glabella, and lateral canthi caused by muscle movement frequently recur after laser resurfacing. (**B**) Pretreatment with Botox results in more significant, longer-lasting improvement.

Contraindications
Box 6.2 lists possible contraindications to resurfacing.

PREOPERATIVE CARE
Currently, there is no consensus on what the most appropriate preoperative skin care regimen is to prepare the skin for cutaneous laser resurfacing (42,120,121). In fact, many studies have questioned the need for a preoperative skin care regimen at all.

Topical tretinoin has been shown by a number of studies to stimulate epithelial proliferation and regeneration and to decrease epidermal melanin content (140,141). Additionally, topical tretinoin acid has been shown in a number of studies to speed reepithelialization and improve clinical outcome when used to prime the skin before dermabrasion and chemical peels.

Extrapolation from the literature reporting the benefits of tretinoin acid when used prior to dermabrasion and chemical peels led to its widespread use by cosmetic surgeons prior to laser skin resurfacing. In a 1998 survey of physician members of the American Society of Laser Medicine and Surgery, 80% of the 116 responders reported that they pretreated cutaneous laser resurfacing patients with topical tretinoin (2).

However, the widespread use of tretinoin preoperatively was not based on well-controlled clinical studies. Investigations have questioned the benefit of pretreatment with topical tretinoin before cutaneous laser resurfacing. In a randomized, side-by-side comparative study, Orringer et al. pretreated patients who underwent CO_2 laser skin resurfacing of the forearms with topical tretinoin (0.05%) for 3 weeks. Posttreatment biopsy specimens were obtained at baseline and at various times (1 day to 6 months). They found no evidence of enhanced collagen formation, accelerated reepithelialization, or quicker resolution of postoperative erythema with tretinoin pretreatment before CO_2 laser resurfacing (142).

Moreover, adverse side effects secondary to tretinoin pretreatment have been reported. Some authors believe that topical application of tretinoin before cutaneous laser resurfacing may contribute to prolonged erythema postoperatively (143). Skin irritation and exacerbation of facial telangiectasias are also potential hazards of tretinoin therapy according to other authors (144,145). Given the lack of well-controlled clinical trials showing a benefit, and the risk, albeit small, of adverse side effects, it seems judicious to reexamine the current widespread use of tretinoin as a pretreatment medication for the laser resurfacing patient.

Box 6.2 Relative Contraindications to Skin Resurfacing

Possible Abnormal Wound Healing
- Prior isotretinoin (Accutane) treatment within 1–2 years
- Keloids/hypertrophic scars
- Scleroderma/collagen vascular diseases
- Immunosuppressive drugs

Decreased Adnexal Structures of Skin
- Prior radiation therapy
- Prior deep phenol peel
- Burn scars

Infectious Diseases
- HIV/AIDS
- Hepatitis C
- Active herpes simplex
- History of recurrent infections/anergy

Koebnerizing (Isomorphic) Diseases
- Labile psoriasis
- Severe eczema
- Vitiligo

Medical Conditions
- Significant diabetes
- Problematic hypertension
- Significant cardiovascular/pulmonary disease

Up to one-third of patients experience postinflammatory hyperpigmentation after laser resurfacing (16). The risk of hyperpigmentation after laser resurfacing parallels the degree of a patient's natural skin pigmentation and it is most prevalent in patients with Fitzpatrick skin phototypes greater than III (5). To reduce the incidence of postinflammatory hyperpigmentation, many laser surgeons routinely pretreat patients with skin phototypes III–VI with a combination of topical skin lightening agents, including tretinoin, hydroquinone, kojic acid, azelaic acid, and alfa-hydroxy acids, for 4–8 weeks prior to cutaneous laser resurfacing (121).

The widespread use of these skin lightening agents before cutaneous laser resurfacing was highlighted by a 1998 survey of physician members of the American Society of Laser Medicine and Surgery; 80% of the 116 responders reported that they routinely pretreated their patients with topical tretinoin, 69% pretreated with hydroquinone, and 10% pretreated with glycolic acid cream.

Hydroquinone inhibits tyrosinase, a key enzyme in the melanin synthesis pathway, and is directly toxic to melanocytes. Tretinoin promotes melanosome transfer and keratinocyte turnover and decreases epidermal melanin content. Azelaic acid, kojic acid, and glucosamine also inhibit tyrosinase and pigment synthesis. Reported benefits of alfa-hydroxy acids (i.e., glycolic acid) include increased epidermal thickness, decreased stratum corneum thickness, and reversal of basal cell layer atypia.

Despite their widespread use, currently there is a great debate over whether pretreatment with these skin bleaching agents helps prevent hyperpigmentation after cutaneous laser resurfacing (Table 6.5). Data from several studies suggest that these agents are ineffective in the prophylaxis of hyperpigmentation after cutaneous laser resurfacing. West et al. randomized 100 consecutive CO_2 laser skin resurfacing patients (skin phototypes I–III) to receive pretreatment with 10% glycolic acid cream b.i.d. or a combination of tretinoin 0.025% cream b.i.d. and hydroquinone 4% q.h.s. or no pretreatment at all. The overall incidence of postinflammatory hyperpigmentation was 11.1%, 32.3%, and 50% in patients with skin phototypes I, II, and III, respectively. Most importantly, they observed no significant difference in the incidence of postinflammatory hyperpigmentation between those patients who received pretreatment and those who did not (54).

Postinflammatory hyperpigmentation is largely caused by the migration of melanocytes from deep within the adnexal epithelium or from cutaneous wound edges after resurfacing. Because of their limited penetration depths, topical bleaching agents may not exert any effect on these deeply situated melanocytes. Instead, they most likely affect superficially located melanocytes that are generally removed by the initial passes of the resurfacing laser. Topical bleaching agents such as tretinoin and hydroquinone may be most effective, not as prophylactic agents during the preoperative period, but rather as therapeutic agents during the postoperative period once melanocyte and keratinocyte migration has taken place (3–4 weeks postoperatively) and hyperpigmentation has manifested itself clinically (54,55).

To reduce the risk of hyperpigmentation, patients are encouraged to avoid having a suntan at the time of the laser resurfacing procedure. Daily application of a full-spectrum sunscreen containing broad-spectrum physical blockers such as micronized zinc is an important, noncontroversial, aspect of the pre- and postoperative care of the cutaneous resurfacing patient.

Table 6.5 Agents to Treat Hyperpigmentation

Agent	Mechanism of Action
Hydroquinone	Cytotoxic to melanocytes
Azelaic acid	Inhibits tyrosinase and pigment synthesis
Kojic acid	Inhibits tyrosinase and pigment synthesis
Glucosamine	Inhibits tyrosinase and pigment synthesis
Tretinoin	Promotes melanosome transfer and keratinocyte turnover
Alfa-hydroxy acids	Promotes keratinocyte turnover

ANTIBIOTIC PROPHYLAXIS

The use of antibiotic prophylaxis for cutaneous laser resurfacing remains a controversial issue. A number of studies have found antibiotics to be effective in the prevention of infection after cutaneous laser resurfacing.

Bernstein et al. observed no infections in a series of 50 patients who underwent full-face resurfacing and were treated with 250 mg of dicloxacillin q.i.d., starting the day before resurfacing and continuing for 1 week (146). Nanni et al. reported no bacterial infections in 500 consecutive cases of full-face cutaneous laser resurfacing, using 1 g intravenous (IV) cefazolin intraoperatively followed by 500 mg of azithromycin on postoperative day 1 and 250 mg for at least 4 days (147). Waldorf et al. found three instances of clinical infection in a series of 47 patients undergoing facial laser resurfacing that were prescribed 250 mg of dicloxacillin q.d. or 333 mg of erythromycin b.i.d. for 1 week throughout the reepithelialization period. The patients who developed infection were not taking antibiotics nor receiving aggressive wound care (148). Ross et al. reported that two of four patients without antibiotic prophylaxis undergoing full-face laser resurfacing developed *Staphylococcus aureus* infection, whereas none of four patients with gram-positive antibiotic prophylaxis developed infection. Notably, they also reported a gram-negative infection in a patient who had received gram-positive antibiotic prophylaxis (46).

Gaspar et al. performed a randomized prospective study of 31 patients undergoing full-face CO_2 laser resurfacing and found four culture-positive clinical infections in the group of patients not receiving antibiotic prophylaxis ($n = 14$) and no cases of infection in the group of patients ($n = 17$) treated with cephalexin 500 mg PO b.i.d. started the day before surgery and continued for 5–10 days. The most common pathogen found in this study was *S. aureus*. An occlusive dressing was used postoperatively in their patients (149). Sriprachya-Anunt et al. retrospectively found a 4.3% rate of culture-positive infection in a series of 395 patients undergoing facial skin laser resurfacing. However, the rate of infection increased sevenfold (from 1.35% to 9.82%) with a change from oral antibiotic prophylaxis (azithromycin 250 mg q.d. or a similar antibiotic for 7 days) to intranasal mupirocin and gentamicin otic solution, and the use of occlusive dressings rather than an open wound care technique postoperatively. The most common organism found was *Pseudomonas aeruginosa*, followed by *S. aureus* and *S. epidermidis*. Several combinations of gram-positive and gram-negative organisms were found in their study. Prophylactic ciprofloxacin (500–750 mg) b.i.d. for 5–7 days, starting the morning of surgery, was recommended by these authors, especially when an occlusive dressing technique was used (43). Manuskiatti et al. reported on the infection rates of a large series of 356 patients who underwent facial skin resurfacing with the CO_2 laser. They observed an 8.2% bacterial infection rate when antibiotic prophylaxis was not given and a closed wound care technique was utilized. The infection rate decreased to 4.3% in the group of patients who received antibiotic prophylaxis with ciprofloxacin. Of note, infections in the group of patients who received prophylaxis occurred almost exclusively after discontinuation of ciprofloxacin (45).

The "pseudo-tissue culture" environment maintained by occlusive dressings is an ideal growth medium not only for host cells that will carry out reepithelialization but also for pathogenetic bacteria that can cause infection. As the studies described earlier suggest that antibiotic prophylaxis can help reduce the rate of infection after ablative laser skin resurfacing, especially when a closed wound care technique is utilized postoperatively. Furthermore, many authors believe that both gram-positive and gram-negative antibiotic coverage should be instituted when occlusive dressings are utilized for wound care after cutaneous laser skin resurfacing (43,150).

There are some authors, however, who have not found antibiotic prophylaxis effective in reducing rates of infection after cutaneous laser resurfacing. In a retrospective study of 133 consecutive patients undergoing CO_2 laser resurfacing, Walia et al. found a significantly higher rate of infection in patients receiving intraoperative (cephalexin 1 g IV) or postoperative (azithromycin 1.5 g PO for 5 days) antibiotics. The most common pathogens found were *Pseudomonas* and *Enterobacter* species. The authors concluded that prophylactic antibiotics are not necessary, especially if good postoperative care is followed (151,152).

The literature shows that staphylococcal infection may be prevented by the prophylactic use of systemic antibiotics such as dicloxacillin, azithromycin, or ciprofloxacin (16,45,121). The use of intranasal mupirocin (Bactroban®) (153), however, has not proved to be advantageous and may even worsen the situation. All staphylococcal infections occurred in the group of patients using intranasal Bactroban in a study of patients randomly assigned to use or not to use Bactroban for 3 days preoperatively and 7 days postoperatively (100).

The prevention of bacterial infections should not be taken lightly, because toxic shock syndrome has been reported after a benign cutaneous infection with *S. aureus* after laser resurfacing in three patients to date. Also, scarring secondary to disruption of wound healing has resulted from *S. aureus* and *Pseudomonas* infection.

Another postoperative infection that may result from the moist wound environment is cutaneous candidiasis. This has been found to correlate with a prior history of vaginal yeast infection (43). Prophylaxis with a single dose of fluconazole (400 mg) on the day of surgery is recommended. To date, we have not seen a yeast infection occur in a patient who received this prophylactic treatment preoperatively. The presentation of this infection postoperatively may include typical signs and symptoms of cutaneous candidiasis but also may be atypical and present only as slow wound healing, itching, and erythema. It should always be suspected in a patient with unexplained poor wound healing. A potassium hydroxide preparation from a scraping of a suspicious area or a culture usually confirms the diagnosis.

In contrast to the controversial nature of antibacterial prophylaxis, most authors today advocate antiviral prophylaxis for herpes simplex virus for all patients undergoing full-face or perioral skin laser resurfacing (42,44,47). Resurfacing laser-induced epidermal trauma and thermal injury can reactivate latent labial herpes simplex virus. The de-epithelialized surface left behind after cutaneous laser resurfacing is highly susceptible to rapid dissemination of the herpes simplex virus. The incidence of herpetic outbreak in the postoperative period has been reported in the range of 2–7% (2,16). All patients should be administered prophylaxis for herpes simplex virus, because patients with no known prior history of herpes

simplex infection have been noted to develop an acute episode in the immediate postoperative period (101). Dissemination over the treatment area with resultant scarring has been observed to occur in these patients (Fig. 6.32).

Patients should be treated with an antiviral agent such as valacyclovir (Valtrex®) or famcyclovir (Famvir®) starting a day or two preoperatively if they have a prior history of herpes simplex infection or starting on the day of the procedure if no prior history. This treatment should be continued at least through the reepithelialization phase of wound healing (an additional 10 days). An acute treatment dose rather than a suppressive dose should be used. Valtrex (500 mg twice daily) and Famvir (250 mg twice daily) provide higher and longer-lasting blood drug levels than does acyclovir (Zovirax®, 400 mg four times daily).

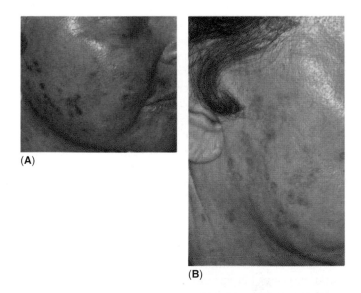

(A)

(B)

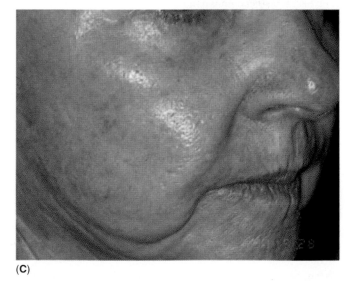

(C)

Figure 6.32 (**A**) Dissemination of herpes simplex occurred on day 4 postoperatively in a patient with no prior history of herpes simplex infection, despite pretreatment with acyclovir (Zovirax). Valacyclovir (Valtrex) has been found to be superior as a preventive medication because much higher drug blood levels are achieved. (**B**) 10 months postoperatively, scarring from infection is apparent. (**C**) 8 months later, marked improvement has been achieved with pulsed dye laser treatment of scars.

IMMEDIATE PREOPERATIVE MEASURES

The skin should be prepped with Techni-Care, a broad-spectrum, nontoxic microbicide that is antiviral, antifungal, and effective against both gram-positive and gram-negative bacteria; 30-s contact use has been shown to result in 99.99% bacterial reduction. Flammable agents such as chlorhexidine gluconate (Hibiclens®) and isopropyl alcohol should not be used in the immediate preoperative stage unless thoroughly washed off with water preoperatively. Hibiclens and alcohol also have ocular toxicities, especially in a sedated patient (Table 6.6).

Metal eye shields should be inserted to protect the eyes (154). Tetracaine (Tetracaine HCl Ophthalmic 0.5%) or a similar ophthalmic anesthetic solution is first placed in the eyes. Metallic eye shields with an external etching coated with sterile ophthalmic petrolatum should be used. Cox laser eye shields (Delasco, Council Bluffs, Iowa, USA), which are available in three sizes, are inserted with a rubber vacuum plunger and have proved to be the most effective of those available because of the ease of insertion and the ability to close the lids over them without distorting the overlying skin. When the eye shields are removed at the end of the procedure, the eyes should be flushed with sterile saline to wash out the remaining petrolatum. This minimizes blurry vision postoperatively. If the periorbital area is not to be treated, the eyes may be protected with moistened gauze pads rather than eye shields.

The periphery of the patient's face should be draped with wet cloths before the procedure so that errant laser impacts do not contact a flammable surface or skin unintended for treatment. The teeth may be protected by placement of wet gauze under the lips and over the teeth, but we have not found this to be necessary, except in patients with extensive porcelain crowns.

ANESTHESIA

For CO_2 laser resurfacing of the face, as for any surgical procedure, the goals of anesthesia are to provide optimal conditions for the surgeon while ensuring the patient's safety and comfort (41). Facial resurfacing is a highly stimulating and painful procedure requiring significant analgesia and alteration of consciousness level for optimal results. Muscle relaxation and loss of all reflexes are unnecessary and may be undesirable.

The sensory innervation of the face is complex and in some areas overlapping, making it difficult to attain adequate anesthesia using only nerve blocks. Even with perfect technique, the numerous nerve blocks required for facial anesthesia often leave areas of the face without adequate anesthesia (155). Supplementation of the nerve blocks that are easily performed (infraorbital, mental, supraorbital, and supratrochlear) with local infiltration is painful and only partially effective.

Some physicians treat with only the use of topical anesthetic creams, such as lidocaine-prilocaine (EMLA cream), lidocaine 4% (LMX), or potent concentrations of lidocaine or lidocaine/tetracaine. Another alternative is tumescent anesthesia: using a much diluted infiltration of 0.1–0.2% lidocaine (Xylocaine) in saline to distend the tissue subcutaneously, as is done with liposuction. This undoubtedly may produce adequate anesthesia but also may cause tissue distortion and alterations of the skin's mechanical properties. This interferes with the identification of tissue laxity and its elimination through collagen shrinkage and skin tightening. Skin tightening depends not only on the pliability and ease of movement of the collagen but also on that of immediately adjacent tissue.

Some compromise in results would be anticipated with the use of these local anesthetic techniques, either from inability to treat adequately because of incomplete anesthesia or alterations in the laser–tissue interaction. Local anesthesia techniques are generally supplemented with sedatives such as diazepam (Valium®), midazolam (Versed®), or lorazepam (Ativan®) and analgesics such as meperidine (Demerol®) or hydromorphine (Dilaudid®), generally given orally or intramuscularly. Possible side effects from these drugs must be considered as well in the choice of anesthesia.

General anesthesia with endotracheal (ET) intubation for full-face laser resurfacing is an acceptable technique and has certain advantages. It ensures airway control, is safe and quickly administered, and allows the administration of adequate narcotic analgesia without concern for respiratory depression. However, not all facilities are equipped to provide general anesthesia and it is not without significant risks. Also, patients or physicians may be reluctant to use general anesthesia for this procedure. A method of deep IV sedation combined with the use of the laryngeal mask

Table 6.6 Antimicrobials and Microbicides as Prophylaxis Before Skin Resurfacing

	Chlorhexidine Gluconate (Hibiclens)	Povidone Iodine (Betadine)	Linear Alcohol	Techni-Care
Substantivity (hours)	>6	3	None	>6
Ocular irritation	Yes	Yes	Yes	Minimal
Scrub time (minutes)	8	3.5	11	0.5
Dermatitis potential	30%	30%	High	<1%
Formulation dependent	Yes	Yes	Variable	Yes
Amount needed (mL)	10	10	–	2.5
Tissue contraindications	Yes	Yes	Yes	None
Toxicity/chemical burns	Eyes, ears	Skin, genitalia	Eyes	Nontoxic[a]
Denatured by organic material	Minimal	Yes	No data	Minimal
Transdermal penetration/absorption	No	Yes	No	Yes
pH measurement	5.86	4.0	6.8	7.2

Data from a variety of sources.

[a]Safe for mucous membranes.

airway (LMA) allows the procedure to be accomplished without ET intubation or an anesthesia machine.

Propofol is the primary agent used and provides rapidly induced, easily maintained, and quickly terminated loss of consciousness. IV midazolam is used to provide initial sedation and amnesia, while analgesia is provided by fentanyl (Sublimaze®) supplemented intermittently with ketamine (Ketalar®). To counteract potentially troublesome side effects of ketamine, all patients receive glycopyrrolate (Robinul®) as a drying agent and midazolam and propofol before receiving ketamine. By using this regimen and limiting the total ketamine dose to about 1 mg/kg, patients have had no problems with "bad dreams" or adverse psychic experiences (155).

The requisite equipment for this technique consists of an electrocardiogram (ECG), blood pressure monitor, pulse oximeter, supplemental oxygen source, LMA, and an intravenous infusion pump, as well as an anesthesiologist to administer the anesthesia. Capnohepatography, while optional, is desirable to monitor adequacy of ventilation. Prudence dictates that any facility administering narcotics or sedatives has appropriately trained medical personnel, a fully stocked resuscitation cart, intubation equipment (laryngoscope, blades, ET tubes), a method for delivering positive-pressure ventilation (Ambubag or Jackson–Rees circuit), and a charged and functional defibrillator. A recovery area staffed with qualified nursing personnel should have the capacity to monitor ECG, blood pressure, and pulse oximetry.

Concern over the safety of laser energy in proximity to oxygen and the patient's face is understandable. All modern inhaled anesthetics are nonflammable, and although oxygen and nitrous oxide support combustion, neither is by itself flammable. It is imperative that flammable liquids not be used in the facial preparation. The patient must be instructed not to use hairspray or other topical skin and hair products before surgery to avoid the introduction of unknown chemicals into the surgical field.

The oxygen delivery system consists of the LMA and the tubing from a green oxygen mask connecting the oxygen cylinder and the LMA, which includes a small pilot tube used to inflate the pharyngeal cuff. The LMA is very resistant to damage from the laser. An informal study performed in our facility revealed it to be resistant to penetration or inflammation despite 60 consecutive laser impacts while oxygen was flowing to enrich the immediate open-air vicinity. The pilot tube is also very resistant to laser damage, requiring 22 impacts before it was cut through, but never ignited. The green oxygen tubing, on the other hand, is easily damaged, and a few pulses will melt it. However, the oxygen flowing through the tube will not ignite, although any flammable object present in the field (e.g., dry gauze and dry hair) will ignite. ET tubes and LMA tubes can be fully protected by wrapping them with saline-soaked gauze or towels. With proper procedures and caution that no combustible liquids or other products are used near surgical areas, laser resurfacing in the presence of oxygen and an anesthetic delivery system such as an ET tube or LMA is safe.

ANESTHESIA FOR Er:YAG LASER RESURFACING

While a topical-only anesthesia approach has been found impractical for CO_2 laser skin resurfacing, topical anesthetics such as LMX-5 (Ferndale Laboratories, Ferndale, Michigan, USA) have been able to provide an effective level of anesthesia for superficial resurfacing with the Er:YAG laser. For deeper resurfacing with the short-pulsed Er:YAG laser, regional nerve blocks (supraorbital, supratrochlear, infraorbital, and mental nerve blocks can be easily performed) and/or local infiltration with 1–2% lidocaine with 1:100,000 epinephrine can be used. However, for ablation into the dermis or full-face resurfacing with the Er:YAG laser, a more potent topical cream or IV sedation performed by an anesthesiologist as described earlier under careful monitoring is generally required.

WOUND HEALING

Observations in animal models and clinical studies suggest a general sequence of events that occur in wound healing, largely controlled by fibroblasts (156–162). This has been divided into three phases: inflammatory, proliferation, and maturation.

Inflammatory Phase

The inflammatory phase lasts 3–10 days (159,162). After dermal trauma, blood vessels constrict, and leakage of plasma proteins (fibrinogen, fibronectin, and plasminogen) and platelets occurs. Plasma and blood clot when exposed to tissue factors (163) and form a gel-like fibrin–fibronectin matrix. Inflammatory cells, new capillaries, and fibroblasts derived from the wound edges migrate into this matrix. Activated macrophages are probably the most important cells in this phase of healing, particularly for wound debridement (164–167).

The fibrin–fibronectin matrix is degraded by inflammatory cells. Fibroblasts synthesize fibronectin, interstitial collagens, and GAGs to form a new fibrovascular connective tissue or granulation tissue, within 2–4 days of injury (157,168,169).

Proliferation Phase

The prominent collagen formed during the inflammatory phase is type III collagen, which has a gel-like consistency (170). Its synthesis is maximal between 5 and 7 days. The proliferation phase occurs over the next 10–14 days and is dominated by the proliferation of fibroblasts and synthesis of collagen as well as regeneration of the epidermis and neoangiogenesis. Reepithelialization is heralded by mitoses at wound edges and at appendages within 24 hours (160). Epidermal proliferation is maximal at 24–72 hours (161). Direct contact with fibronectin and type I collagen guides and stimulates epithelial cell migration in culture (162). Soluble substances such as growth factors derived from platelets, macrophages, dermal parenchymal cells, and keratinocytes stimulate reepithelialization in animal models (169). Continued collagen synthesis proceeds, stimulated by macrophage-derived and platelet-derived factors (171), followed by capillary resorption and disappearance of fibroblasts (172).

Lymphokines, complement, native collagens of types I to V, fibronectin, and platelet-derived growth factor may be potent mitogens and chemotactants for fibroblasts (156,173). In addition, macrophages may be activated by blood and may play a key role in inducing a fibroproliferative response when there is significant blood within the healing wound (156,165,174).

In the biosynthesis of collagen, procollagen is formed intracellularly by fibroblasts and secreted into the extracellular space (172). It is then biochemically transformed into tropocollagen by proteases (175–177). The tropocollagen molecules aggregate into immature soluble collagen fibrils, which are then cross-linked by the action of lysyl oxidase to form mature, stronger collagen fibers (178).

Maturation Phase

The total amount of collagen in a wound reaches a maximum at 2–3 weeks, but collagen remodeling continues over months to years (179). This characterizes the third phase of wound healing, the maturation phase. The earliest collagen fibers are thin and unorganized, becoming thicker, cross-linked, and parallel to skin tension lines with time. As new collagen is formed, abnormal or damaged collagen is broken down by collagenases and proteases produced by fibroblasts, macrophages, and inflammatory cells. Proteoglycans, responsible for water storage in the healing wound, decrease, and water is reabsorbed as the wound heals (180,181).

Remodeling of the collagen matrix ends up in gradual shrinkage, thinning, and paling of the scar. Once the collagen bed is established as a stable matrix, collagen production, and resorption continue in a steady, balanced state in a normally healed scar. Tensile strength increases from 5% of original strength at 2 weeks to 80% in a mature scar (182). Contraction of a scar, which begins 1 week after wounding, is not caused by excessive deposition of collagen, but rather by the effects of transformation of fibroblasts to myofibroblasts (183,184). These cells produce contractile proteins with characteristics of smooth muscle cells. Granulation tissue has been shown to contain as much actomyosin as an equivalent weight of smooth muscle (185). Furthermore, it has been demonstrated that contraction of myofibroblasts can be inhibited by smooth muscle relaxants (159,183). It has been proposed that migrating fibroblasts interact with their surrounding matrix components to reorganize connective tissue fibers to induce shrinkage (186). These factors can result in as much as a 45% reduction in wound surface area (159).

POSTOPERATIVE CARE

If the patient develops noticeable intraoperative swelling, usually detected in the periorbital area, dexamethasone (Decadron®, 10–12 mg by IV push) may be administered. Although some physicians routinely use a Decadron Dospak, oral prednisone (20 mg every day for 7 days), or triamcinolone (Kenalog®, 40 mg IM) postoperatively, the effects on suppression of fibroblast activity and infection surveillance must be considered. Single-dose IV Decadron is rapidly cleared and thus should not interfere with wound healing. Because postoperative swelling generally clears rapidly (2–5 days), the choice of the shorter-acting corticosteroids is preferable.

Minimal thermal damage that results in poor coagulation of dermal blood vessels and poor hemostasis characterizes treatment with the short-pulsed Er:YAG laser. Application of wet gauze compression is useful to deal with the bleeding that is typically seen after resurfacing with the short-pulsed Er:YAG laser (12). Patients are told to expect a mild burning sensation for the first 1–3 days and significant swelling for the first 2–5 days postoperatively. The edema that develops in the first 48 hours postoperatively can be controlled with icepacks, head elevation at night, and in severe cases, with oral corticosteroids.

During the first 3–5 days, significant serous exudate is present as well, related to the swelling and absence of an epithelial barrier. Use of topical antibiotics and other topical drugs should be particularly avoided during this phase, because the incidence of contact irritant and allergic dermatitis is enhanced by the absence of epithelium (187). We have found the incidence to increase from about 3% to 4% when topical agents are used in non–laser-treated skin to 20% or higher when they are used after laser skin resurfacing. Bacitracin is a frequent sensitizer, with a fivefold increase in dermatitis reported from 1990 to 1994 (188). In addition, a compound such as petrolatum, which usually does not cause contact sensitivity, has a greater potential to sensitize in this situation (100,189).

WOUND CARE

The benefits of wound occlusion have been well documented (52,190,191). Wound occlusion creates a moist environment that protects the wound from exogenous bacteria, inhibits crust formation, enhances reepithelialization, and reduces patient discomfort. Occlusion can be achieved by either open or closed wound care techniques.

Open wound care techniques facilitate surveillance of the laser wound for clinical signs of infections or other complications. Additionally, they are relatively inexpensive and do not elicit the feeling of claustrophobia that some patients can experience with occlusive dressings. However, to achieve the healing benefits of occlusion, open wound care techniques demand around-the-clock wound care by the patient and thus are largely dependent on patient compliance.

Open-wound care generally consists of frequent soaking with cool distilled water containing a small amount of white vinegar. One teaspoon per cup is generally the starting concentration (0.25% acetic acid). The mildly acidic pH has an antibacterial effect, which is especially important in suppressing *Pseudomonas* species. The skin should be soaked for 20 minutes every 1–2 hours. The objective is to soak away the serous exudate and any necrotic tissue on the skin surface. Just patting the skin with a moist gauze pad is not adequate. Between soakings, the skin should be liberally and continuously coated with petrolatum (Vaseline®), Aquaphor® (Beiersdorf, Charlotte, North Carolina, USA), or Theraplex®. This coating may be gently removed with gauze or facial tissue before the next soaking. Ice packs or frozen peas may be applied during this period for symptomatic pain relief.

The application of petrolatum to the wound surface results in a semiocclusive, moist environment. Studies have shown that wounds treated with petrolatum compared with those treated with a topical antibiotic have no increased incidence of infection and heal at the same rate (182). In contrast, in a study of accidental burns treated with either petrolatum mesh gauze or nitrofurazone, 75% of the petrolatum group had bacteria reported as "too numerous to count" compared with only 10% of the nitrofurazone group (192).

The composition of a bland emollient apparently may have an effect on wound healing. A U.S.P. petrolatum ointment decreased wound healing by 17%, a white petrolatum cream increased wound healing by 24%, and a lotion with propylene glycol without petrolatum increased wound healing by 15% (193).

Wound-healing studies have shown that vehicles with the proper combination of fatty acids result in faster healing than do petrolatum or Aquaphor (194). Fatty acids that reflect the composition of fatty acids in human membranes are required for the proliferation of epithelial cells (195,196).

This mixture of fatty acids also significantly enhances the ability of pyruvate and vitamin E to inhibit reactive oxygen production and improve membrane function and cellular viability. These three components, vitamin E, pyruvate, and essential fatty acids, have been shown to be synergistic in reducing oxidative stress to keratinocytes and enhancing wound healing (194).

Patients treated with an open wound care regimen are seen on the first and third day postoperatively, and any excess crust is gently removed with saline. The frequency of soaks and ointment application is tapered off as reepithelialization progresses. Once reepithelialization is complete, a mild facial cleanser (i.e., Neutrogena fresh foaming cleanser or Cetaphil facial cleanser) and a daily moisturizer-sunscreen are introduced.

The benefit of occlusive dressings in accelerating wound healing was first demonstrated in 1962 (197) and confirmed in numerous studies (190,198–208). Reepithelialization was shown to occur 30–45% more quickly, with decreased pain and inflammation and more cosmetically acceptable scar formation. In addition, new collagen formation has been shown to begin 3 days earlier than in open wounds (209), with an increased rate of collagen synthesis (210). The increased rate of reepithelialization produced by occlusive dressings is generally attributed to the moist wound environment and the absence of a crust that may impede cellular movement. In addition, occlusive dressings provide an environment that maximizes exposure to various endogenous growth factors. Continued exposure to epidermal growth factor has been shown to quicken epidermal resurfacing (211).

Studies of varying the time of application or removal of an occlusive dressing have shown that for optimal healing, dressings need to be applied within 2 hours after wounding and should be left in place for at least 24 hours (212). Waiting 24 hours before application almost precludes the occlusive dressing's effect on wound healing, but it still may have benefit in pain reduction. Early removal of the dressing greatly reduces the occlusive effects, but not if 24 or 48 hours has passed.

Moreover, several studies have demonstrated that closed wound care techniques utilizing occlusive dressings for the first 48–72 hours after laser skin resurfacing reduce crusting, erythema, and edema (Fig. 6.33). Moreover, occlusive dressings have been reported to significantly decrease postoperative pain and patient discomfort and simplify wound care for patients compared with open wound care techniques (42,48–52).

The most popular commercially available closed-occlusive dressings for laser skin resurfacing wounds belong to one of the following categories: composite foams, polymer films, polymer meshes, hydrogels, hydrocolloids, and alginates. These closed-occlusive dressing categories are summarized in Table 6.7.

Some studies have shown that bacterial colonization under occlusion does not impair wound healing (213–216), and that wound fluid and exudate collecting under an occlusive dressing have bactericidal activity (217,218). Oliveria-Gandia et al. demonstrated that occlusive dressings can act as barriers to invading wound organisms and that dressing composition can influence the growth of various pathogens (219). Moreover, several studies found that wounds covered with occlusive dressings had reduced infection rates when compared with nonocclusive dressings (193,206,208,218,220–224).

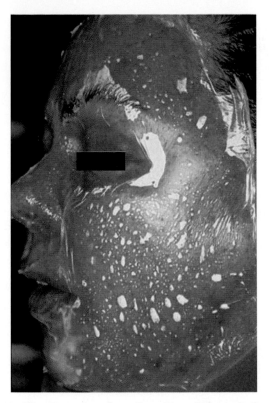

Figure 6.33 Silon II, a polyurethane film with multiple small slits, allows soaking directly through film and enhances wound healing during first 72 hours.

Christian et al. reported four cases of culture-positive infections among 354 patients who underwent full-face CO_2 laser resurfacing (1.13% rate of infection) and were treated with occlusive dressings and empiric oral cephalexin. Three of the four infections developed 3–5 weeks after the laser resurfacing (225). Newman et al. evaluated the efficacy and safety of four different types of closed dressings following full-face laser resurfacing in 40 patients and observed no cases of infection (50).

However, a study comparing semiocclusive dressings exposed to open air showed not only an increased number of microorganisms, but also a shift toward gram-negative organisms (213). Other investigators have shown a similar pattern on normal skin occluded with a plastic film (216,223). Moreover, an increased incidence of infection after laser skin resurfacing has been reported in some studies when antibiotics have not been used (43,100).

An increased susceptibility to gram-negative infections in resurfacing patients would reflect our clinical experience as well. If semiocclusive dressings are to be used postoperatively, most physicians now would advise that (*i*) antibiotic coverage should include gram-negative organisms; (*ii*) dressings should be changed frequently, if not daily; and (*iii*) occlusive dressings should be used for no more than 72 hours.

After reepithelialization, the next phase of wound healing lasts another 7–10 days. During this phase, no further weeping occurs and swelling has usually resolved. Maturation of the epithelium still requires a moist environment. Of note, continued use of occlusive ointments such as petrolatum beyond complete re-epithelialization has been associated with the occurrence of folliculitis in some patients (121). Lighter

Table 6.7 Biosynthetic Dressings

Classification	Composition	Examples	Transmits oxygen
Polyurethane films	Polyurethane *or* co-polyester with adhesive backing	Op-Site Bioclusive, Opraflex, Uniflex, Blisterfilm, Visulin, Ensure, Clingfilm, Viofilm, Acuderm, Omniderm, Dermafilm, Silon II, Tegaderm	Fluid retention may be problem Difficult to handle Omniderm or Silon II better suited for exudative wounds
Hydrocolloids	Hydrophilic colloidal particles bound to polyurethane foam	DuoDerm, Actiderm, Tegasorb, Cutinova Hydro, Ultec, Comfeel Ulcus, Restore, Hydrapad, Granulfex E, Intrasite, Intact, Flexzan	
Hydrogels	60–99% water cross-linked polymer, such as polyethylene or polyvinyl	Vigilon, Second Skin, Biofilm, Geliperm, Cutinova Gel, Elasto-Gel, Intrasite Gel, Span Gel, ClearSite	Gel formed by dressing often purulent in appearance and acrid in odor If a wound is very exudative, gel will leak beyond dressing
Calcium alginate	Composite of fibers from calcium alginate	Sorbsan	Capable of significant fluid absorption
Foams	Hydrophilic or hydrophobic polyurethane or gel film	Kaltostat	Require frequent dressing change Significant hemostatic properties
Others			
Biobrane	Silicone rubber with nylon and porcine collagen bilaminate	Cutinova Plus Ulcer Care, Lyofoam, Sythaderm Allevin, Epigard	Very high absorbency Similar to hydrogels
N-Terface	Monofilament plastic		Can become incorporated in wound if wound dries May delay reepithelialization
Cellophane wrap (contains 65% glycerin)	Cellulose with glycerin	Saran Wrap	Excessive fluid accumulation occurs Wick effect transfers fluids to outer membrane Oxygen transmission increases 1000-fold when material is wet

preparations such as Theraplex emollient, Cetaphil moisturizer (Galderma Laboratories, Inc., Fort Worth, Texas, USA), Norwegian Formula emulsion (Neutrogena), and Curel (Bausch and Lomb, Inc., Rochester, New York, USA) are preferred during this phase. Biologic agents, such as vitamin C, essential fatty acids, hyaluronic acid, aloe vera, and topical photoprotective antioxidants such as green tea extract, idebenone, or ferulic acid, may be beneficial in this phase. After the second week, a lighter, high-moisture cream containing these biologic agents can be used and continued. Preoperative topical agents are restarted at 2–3 weeks postoperatively.

To minimize postoperative erythema, we use 0.1% fluocinolone ointment (Synalar®, Medicis, Scottsdale, Arizona, USA) applied to the face at night from postoperative day 5–21. We have not noted any decrease in wound healing or allergic reactions as this topical steroid ointment does not contain any preservatives or stabilizers. In addition, the addition of a topical steroid decreases postoperative pruritus and edema. Aquanil HC lotion (Person & Covey, Glendale, California, USA) is recommended for daytime use during the same period. This mild topical steroid is in a light, moisturizing, nonsensitizing base.

Close surveillance of patients during the postoperative period is important to provide emotional support and to detect abnormalities in the healing process at the earliest manifestation. Ideally, patients are seen 1 day, 3 days, 1 week, 3 weeks, 6 weeks, 3 months, 6 months, and 1 year postoperatively.

COMPLICATIONS OF CO_2 LASER RESURFACING

As with all resurfacing procedures, the incidence of complications is related to both the depth of resurfacing and the patient's preexisting skin pigment type. Complications include infection, pigmentary changes, acne and milia, scarring, and ectropion. Swelling, erythema, petechiae, and itching are normal postoperative sequelae that may be more prominent in some patients (120).

Postoperative Swelling

Postoperative swelling is generally mild to moderate, peaking on day 2–3 and most often resolving by day 5–7. At times, however, dramatic swelling may occur that is frightening and uncomfortable for the patient. Although we do not routinely use steroids in the postoperative course, in this situation of excessive swelling, IM Celestone® (6–9 mg) or oral prednisone (40–60 mg daily for 3–5 days) may be valuable. Patients are also advised to soak their face frequently and use ice packs or frozen peas as frequently as needed.

Erythema

Erythema occurs to some degree in all patients and reflects the increased blood flow and angiogenesis associated with dermal healing. The degree and persistence of erythema relate to the depth of resurfacing performed and the amount of nonspecific thermal injury produced, as well as to unidentified individual variables and possibly to preoperative and postoperative regimens. The regimens outlined previously appear to enhance wound healing and decrease erythema. In addition, the inflammatory reaction related to slough of thermal necrotic tissue may be a factor in prolonging erythema. Removal of this layer with the Er:YAG laser has been shown to be effective both in reducing erythema and infection and in enhancing the healing process and speeding its conclusion.

Itching

Itching is a common postoperative complaint, particularly during the second postoperative week. It can indicate infection, particularly candidiasis, but is then often accompanied by other signs, such as poor wound healing, beefy erythema in patches, and exudate. Contact dermatitis must be considered as well when pruritus occurs, particularly if any topical medications are being used. If these conditions are excluded, generally the itching will respond well to an antihistamine such as diphenhydramine (Benadryl, 10 or 25 mg) or loratadine (Claritin®, 10 mg) or a topical steroid such as Synalar, as described earlier.

Infection

The combined incidence of bacterial, viral, and candidal infection has been found to be 4.7% in a multicenter study (226) and 4.3% in a retrospective study (43), 12% in Burns' study (personal communication), 7.6% in Goldman and Fitzpatrick's study, and 8.4% in the study of Waldorf et al. (97). Multiple organisms are typically found, and the microorganisms identified (*Staphylococcus* and *Pseudomonas* species) are similar to those found in burn injuries (227–229).

The moist wound care and the layer of thermal necrosis provide an environment conducive to bacterial and candidal growth. The absence of the protective epidermal barrier further invites infection and allows dissemination of the infection across the surface of the treatment area. Bio-occlusive dressings further complicate the situation by trapping bacteria and increasing the incidence of infection (43).

Infection should be suspected in the following situations:

1. Patient complains of persistent or new onset of pain.
2. Burning or intense itching is reported after day 2 or 3.
3. Patient has patchy, intense erythema, yellow exudate or crust, papules, pustules, or erosions.
4. "Reversal of healing" is seen; that is, previously reepithelialized areas become eroded.

Eighty percent of infections become symptomatic within 7 days and pain is the most common complaint, reported by 50% of patients. However, as previously mentioned, the use of antibiotics may alter this pattern, and antibiotics used for 10–14 days may eliminate postoperative bacterial infections. A sensation of burning and itching is the second most common symptom, reported by a third of patients.

When an infection is suspected, direct smears and cultures for bacteria, yeast, and herpes virus should be taken, because the physical findings of infection may be atypical, with the absence of the epithelium and presence of a necrotic layer and edema. Correct diagnosis requires proper identification of the infectious agent.

All patients should be given appropriate antiviral medication at surgery, because the laser resurfacing procedure may be a potent factor in herpetic reactivation (44). Should this occur despite antiherpetic prophylaxis, it is best to switch from valacyclovir to famciclovir, or vice versa, and to increase the dosage.

When candidal infections are encountered, a 400-mg dose of fluconazole should be given and occlusive topical regimens discontinued.

Bacterial infections should be treated according to culture and sensitivity results. Serious consideration should be given to prophylactic use of ciprofloxacin (500 mg twice daily) starting the evening before surgery and continuing for 10–14 days postoperatively.

Acne and Milia

Many physicians report an unusually high incidence of milia formation after laser resurfacing as well as increased or exacerbation of acne. Although the use of petrolatum-based ointments may be an exacerbating factor in many patients, particularly those with a prior history of acne, the incidence of this complication appears to parallel the degree of thermal injury to the tissue. Thermal injury may lead to a shock effect on sebaceous glands, causing their disruption and dedifferentiation of adnexal structures and producing an aberrant re-formation of the canal (230). Dermabrasion, by contrast, generally results in improvement in acne; some physicians believe this is an invariable consequence of dermabrasion, although degree of improvement may vary.

Treatment of acne and milia is that traditionally used for acne: minimize occlusive ointments, reinstitute tretinoin and AHAs, and administer systemic tetracycline or minocycline. Gentle acne surgery performed at 2- to 4-week intervals may be beneficial as well. Isotretinoin (Accutane®) may be started if the acne fails to respond to more conservative measures.

Hyperpigmentation

Hyperpigmentation is generally related to the degree of natural pigmentation and occurs in 20–30% of those with Fitzpatrick type III skin and nearly 100% of patients with type IV skin if treatment is performed without preoperative preparation (104). Almost all episodes will resolve within 2–4 months if aggressively treated. Strict sun avoidance is a fundamental aspect of treatment and is enhanced by daily use of full-spectrum sunscreens containing titanium dioxide or Parsol 1789. Hydroquinone is cytotoxic to melanocytes and is the mainstay of treatment. Tretinoin promotes melanosome transfer and keratinocyte turnover and is almost always beneficial as well. Azelaic acid, kojic acid, and glucosamine inhibit tyrosinase and pigment synthesis and may be added to the regimen when patients are responding slowly. Topical vitamins C and E function as free-radical scavengers and help prevent further stimulation of melanocytes by UV radiation. Pretreatment with these agents will minimize the occurrence of hyperpigmentation, as well as its degree of severity and its favorable response to therapy.

Hypopigmentation

Hypopigmentation is a delayed phenomenon, generally not apparent for 6–12 months. True hypopigmentation must be differentiated from pseudohypopigmentation, a situation in which the resurfaced area has normal pigmentation reflective of non–sun-exposed skin, but contrasts distinctively with the more darkly pigmented sun-damaged skin. True hypopigmentation reflects a diminished melanocyte content of the skin and correlates with both the depth of resurfacing and the degree of thermal injury. These patients generally have long-lasting erythema, often have had problems with milia and acne as well, and may have areas of scarring. These patients typically have been treated with free-hand techniques allowing pulse stacking or with CPG patterns having greater than 50% overlap. These patients often have received more than three laser passes as well.

Treatment of hypopigmentation has been difficult, including the use of PUVA, excimer laser, or UVB flashlamps. When segmental hypopigmentation or pseudohypopigmentation is present, resurfacing the remainder of the face will blend the area and decrease its visibility (Fig. 6.30). An incidence of about 20% has been reported for hypopigmentation, but this must be examined carefully and pseudohypopigmentation separated as a different phenomenon, because it may not be preventable. In a review of 104 patients 1–4 years postoperatively, we found hypopigmentation in 19.2% (20 of 104). Pseudohypopigmentation was present in 65% of these patients and true hypopigmentation in 35%. Hypopigmentation was classified as mild in 85% of these patients. When examined more closely, these 20 patients with hypopigmentation were also the patients having the worst photodamage preoperatively, those with the most significant clinical improvement, and those who were most pleased with their results. Pseudohypopigmentation should be viewed as a consequence of resurfacing in significantly photodamaged skin rather than a complication. However, patients should be forewarned of this aspect of the procedure.

Petechiae

Although of almost no long-term significance, the appearance of small petechiae is often a source of much concern to the patient. They appear just as reepithelialization is complete, conflicting with the patient's desire to return to public view. Small subepithelial hemorrhages from the immature basement membrane and undeveloped rete appear to be the cause. These factors render the skin more fragile and easily damaged with minor trauma from rubbing or scratching. Petechiae may continue for several weeks after the procedure but clear quickly without treatment.

Scarring

Erythematous and hypertrophic scars often result from excessive depth of tissue injury. This is usually caused by excess tissue heating and residual thermal damage well beyond the depth of tissue vaporized by the laser. Incorrect "off" times, high scanner densities (greater than 40%), and failure to keep the handpiece moving during resurfacing are some of the treatment methods that lead to inadvertent overlap or "stacking" of pulses, with the resultant accumulation of heat and residual thermal damage.

Scarring is also seen more frequently in patients who develop a postoperative infection, particularly in those who have had multiple prior surgical procedures, altering the anatomy of the region. In addition, patients treated more aggressively, resulting in a thicker layer of thermal necrosis, may be more prone to infection. Careful preoperative history taking to rule out predisposing factors and immediate treatment of postoperative infections are mandatory.

Scarring is much more frequently seen in treatment of nonfacial areas, such as the neck. Decreased adnexal structures, thinner dermis, and increased tissue tension and traction secondary to motion are predisposing factors. In a trial of 10 patients receiving a single-laser pass of 300 mJ with a CPG density of 6, we encountered scarring of the lower one-third of the neck in three patients and patchy hypopigmentation in four patients (Fig. 6.34).

The earliest evidence for the development of a scar is usually erythema and pruritus. At this point, the affected area should be cultured to rule out infection, and topical high-potency corticosteroids should be applied two or three times daily. If the affected area begins to thicken, intralesional injection of triamcinolone (10 mg/mL) with 5-fluorouracil (50 mg/mL) in a 1:9 dilution (1-mg triamcinolone with 45-mg 5-fluorouracil) should begin every 2–3 days. Topical silicone dressings should also be applied. If further progression occurs, we advise using the 585-nm flashlamp pumped pulse dye laser (PDL) or other vascular lasers or intense pulsed light (IPL) every 4 weeks. With these techniques, permanent scarring has been avoided (Fig. 6.35).

Ectropion

Contraction of previously scarred tissue of the lower eyelid leads to excessive tightening and exposure of the conjunctiva. This avoidable complication usually occurs in patients who

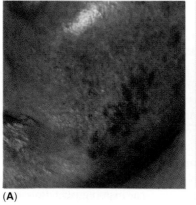 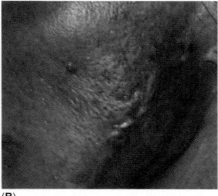 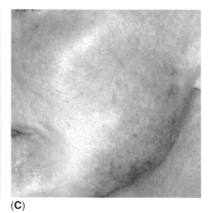

(A)   **(B)**   **(C)**

Figure 6.34 (**A**) *Pseudomonas* infection developed on day 8 after single-pass laser resurfacing, resulting in nonhealing erosions on lower cheek. (**B**) Although this area initially healed very well, at 4 months an obvious hypertrophic scar was developing, corresponding to site of infection. (**C**) Intensive treatment with intralesional 5-fluorouracil (45 mg/mL) and triamcinolone (Kenalog, 1 mg/mL) followed by pulsed dye laser (6 J/cm²) resulted in scar resolution after approximately 1 year.

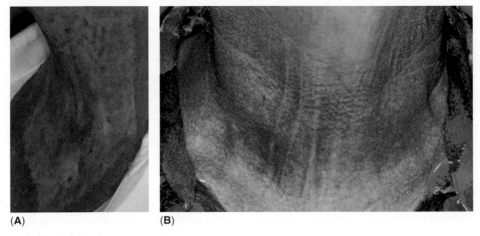

Figure 6.35 (**A**) Treatment of the neck in the same manner as the face may result in severe scarring. (**B**) Treatment goals must be much more conservative, but even a single pass with the same laser parameters used for the face may result in scarring of the lower neck.

have undergone resurfacing after a lower-lid blepharoplasty without stabilizing the lateral canthal tendon. It may also occur if laser resurfacing is performed too aggressively in this region without attention to the laser–tissue interaction.

To minimize the occurrence of ectropion, we recommend that the patient's skin elastic recoil be tested, the so-called snap test, with close observation for loose tissue folds and the effect on the lid margin when tightened. If the lid margin moves easily, close observation during the procedure is essential to avoid excessive tightening of the lid. In addition, laser density should not exceed 20–30% in this region to limit nonspecific thermal damage of dermal tissue, and only one or two passes should be performed with careful attention to the tightening effect. The cheeks should be treated before the periorbital area so that the additive tightening effects of this area are known before periorbital resurfacing. Scleral show was found in 3% of patients less than 4 months postoperatively and in 2% more than 4 months postoperatively in a report of 1000 procedures (231). Ectropion occurred in 0.3% of patients in this series.

Synechiae
Synechiae are adhesions that occur when two adjacent areas of de-epithelialized skin are in contact with each other in a fold and a bridge of epithelium develops over the top of the fold. This occurs primarily on the lower eyelid and has the appearance of an unusual crease or a faint white line 1–2 weeks postoperatively. Treatment consists of cutting the epidermal bridge with a fine-tipped scissors, lancet, or scalpel. The patient then must carefully roll a moist cotton-tipped applicator over the area frequently to avoid recurrence. Synechiae almost always resolve without problems (231).

Er:YAG LASER
Er:YAG Laser–Tissue Interaction
The short-pulsed Er:YAG laser is a flashlamp-pumped YAG crystal laser system doped with atoms of the element erbium. Laser energy is generated within a cavity containing the flashlamp-excited YAG crystal rod, mirrors at each end, and a cooling system. On exiting the cavity, the laser light is focused into a beam delivery system that typically incorporates an articulated arm, which allows the use of handpieces capable of producing highly collimated beams. Er:YAG lasers used in cutaneous

resurfacing typically have a bell-shaped Gaussian laser beam profile (232).

The Er:YAG laser produces light in the near-infrared (NIR) portion of the electromagnetic spectrum at 2.94 mm. The broad water-absorption band extends from just under 2 mm to beyond 10 mm, ensuring superficial absorption of NIR light. The Q-switched Er:YAG laser ablates approximately 15–20 μm of skin and leaves such a thin layer of thermal damage (5 μm) that it is not hemostatic. The Er:YAG laser has been investigated using a Q-switched pulse of 90 μs, but pulse-to-pulse instability and a low-intensity tail of a Gaussian beam have made this beam profile undesirable. Instead, the laser is used in its normal-spiking mode, emitting a macropulse of approximately 250 μs, made up by a train of 1-ms micropulses with pulse-to-pulse stability of ±2% (233). The Er:YAG laser was first studied in this mode to determine whether it could be an effective resurfacing device.

When the coefficient of absorption for water is compared directly, that for the CO_2 laser (10.6 mm) is approximately 790 μm^{-1}, whereas the erbium laser peak at 2.94 mm is approximately 13,000 μm^{-1}, more than 16 times greater than that of the CO_2 laser (Fig. 6.36). This results in its energy being absorbed much more readily in a thinner layer of tissue than with the CO_2 laser. In fact, calculations of the absorption coefficient, assuming tissue to be 70% water, show this energy to be absorbed in about 1 μm of tissue (11,24,233–239). This results in efficient tissue ablation with very little scattering of the beam and minimal residual thermal damage. However, actual clinical and experimental data reveal deeper tissue penetration than this calculated optical penetration (239).

The ablation threshold for the Er:YAG laser is about 1.5 J/cm^2 (233,235,240), and the ablation efficiency about 2–3 $\mu m/pulse/J/cm^2$ up to about 10 J/cm^2 (24,233,235,237). However, ablation rates per pulse of 16 (235), 30 (238), and 400 μm (at 80 J/cm^2) (233) have been reported, which seem inconsistent with the reported optical penetration depth of the Er:YAG laser of about 1 μm.

This deeper ablation process occurs because ablation at 2.94 μm is an explosive process caused by rapid heating, vaporization, and consequent high-pressure expansion of irradiated tissue (233,239). Explosive particle ejection occurs when a gradient exists between the atmospheric pressure of the

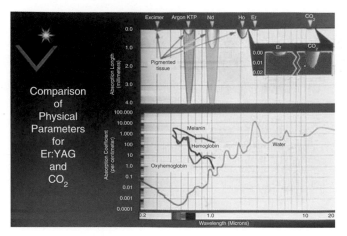

Figure 6.36 Er:YAG laser wavelength of 2.94 μm is absorbed 16 times more readily than that of CO_2 laser.

environment and pressure within tissue. When tissue water is evaporated and prevented from escaping from tissue fast enough, tissue pressures may exceed atmospheric pressures when temperatures exceed 100°C. Because the tissue surface is cooled by expansion of the vapor, temperature and pressure may then be higher in a subsurface layer. The steam pressure of water increases rapidly with increasing temperature. Indeed, these high-temperature, high-pressure gases forming at the absorption site are thought to result in explosive tissue removal (233,239). High-speed photography has shown ablated material to leave the surface at supersonic velocities (103 m/s) (241).

The ablation of tissue during the pulse of the Er:YAG laser is a dynamic process during which material heated at the beginning of the pulse is removed during the pulse, clearing a path for radiation to be deposited deeper in tissue during the same pulse (233). High-speed photography has shown that tissue removal begins within 200 μs after the beginning of the pulse (242). The explosive ejection of this ablated material removes it from the beam pathway. Furthermore, water vaporized by the pulse has a much lower coefficient of absorption than does liquid water and therefore does not interfere with the beam, because it is essentially transparent (233,239). The explosive ejection of ablated material from the tissue surface causes the characteristic "popping" sound heard during Er:YAG laser skin resurfacing.

Interestingly, lower fluences (less than 10 J/cm²) of a thermal energy analyzer CO_2 laser using 2-μs pulses result in the same ablation efficiency, supporting this instantaneous vaporization model (233). This in-depth absorption explains the tearing of tissue seen in vascular tissue, the large ablation depths per pulse, and the zones of residual thermal damage that increase greatly at high fluences (233,239).

The CO_2 laser is operated near its tissue ablation threshold (5 J/cm²) in most resurfacing applications. This means that a large fraction of its energy is invested to heat, rather than ablate the target tissue. Therefore, the CO_2 laser produces relatively large residual thermal damage zones of up to 150 μm and causes significant desiccation of the target tissue after only a few passes. With each subsequent pass of the CO_2 laser, the amount of vaporized tissue diminishes while the extent of thermal necrosis increases and a "plateau" of ablation is typically reached after the fourth pass.

In contrast to the CO_2 laser, the Er:YAG laser has 16 times greater affinity for water and a significantly lower tissue ablation threshold (1.6 J/cm²), which allows the Er:YAG to be operated at 8–10 times above its ablation threshold in most resurfacing applications (6). Therefore, most of the energy delivered with the Er:YAG laser is utilized to ablate rather than heat the tissue, and residual thermal damage zones not exceeding 30–50 μm have been confirmed both in vitro and in vivo with the Er:YAG laser (23,24,235,238–240).

Given the narrow zone of residual thermal damage produced by the Er:YAG laser, tissue desiccation does not significantly increase with each subsequent pass and the ablation plateau characteristic of CO_2 laser resurfacing is not reached. In contrast to the coagulative, desiccating effect of the CO_2 laser on dermal blood vessels and dermal tissue, the Er:YAG laser causes vasodilation of dermal blood vessels and transudation of fluid that maintains a high water content in the target tissue and allows the Er:YAG laser to continue with efficient ablation (10). The absence of tissue coagulation, however, results in bleeding as the vessels of the superficial dermal plexus are severed. This may limit the depth of ablation that is achievable (23,24,240).

Clinical use of high-fluence, small-diameter beams is undesirable, because it may result in an irregular surface because of the deep instantaneous ablation.

This energy is delivered with a pulse duration that is far below the 1-ms thermal relaxation time calculated for that layer of human skin heated by the pulsed CO_2 laser, with the pulse generally in the range of 250–350 μs. However, because of the short penetration depth of the 2.94-mm wavelength, the laser-heated layer of tissue is only 1-μm thick and this layer has a thermal relaxation time of approximately 1 μs (89,239,242). Single pulses of less than 1-μs duration are needed to minimize thermal diffusion during the laser pulse. In the normal-spiking mode, the Er:YAG laser emits approximately twenty 1-μs micropulses in a macropulse burst of approximately 200 μs. Because of efficient tissue vaporization and interpulse cooling time, minimal thermal damage occurs. Each micropulse can ablate tissue and act independently (232,243), but in general the thermal damage from normal-spiking-mode irradiation is more extensive than that of Q-switched irradiation.

Most erbium lasers now available can deliver 1–3 J per pulse, at repetition rates of 1–10 Hz, so very high irradiances may be achieved, particularly with a focused beam. Although physicians and manufacturers typically report results as pulse energy and spot size, it would be much more meaningful and allow easier comparison if treatment parameters were discussed in fluence (J/cm²) (Table 6.8).

Thermally induced dermal collagen contraction is thought to underlie the superior clinical results achieved with the CO_2 laser. In contrast to the CO_2 laser (15–40% reported intraoperative collagen contraction), first-generation low-power short-pulsed Er:YAG lasers did not produce significant tissue contraction. The development of a second generation of more powerful Er:YAG lasers allowed investigators to demonstrate small but measurable degrees of tissue contraction after Er:YAG laser skin resurfacing. In 1998, Hughes et al. demonstrated an immediate 4% linear tightening of the skin immediately after two or three passes with a short-pulsed (250 μs) Er:YAG laser (5-mm spot diameter, fluences of up to 4.6 J/cm²), which increased to a maximum of 14% 16 weeks postoperatively (244).

Table 6.8 Er:YAG Laser Fluences (J/cm²)

Spot Size (mm)	Pulse Energy (J)					
	0.5	1.0	1.2	1.7	2.0	3.0
0.2	1592.4	3184.7	3821.7	5414.0	6369.4	9554.1
0.5	254.8	509.6	611.5	866.2	1019.1	1528.7
1	63.7	127.4	152.9	216.6	254.8	382.2
2	15.9	31.8	38.2	54.1	63.7	95.5
3	7.1	14.2	17.0	24.1	28.3	42.5
4	4.0	8.0	9.6	13.5	15.9	23.9
5	2.5	5.1	6.1	8.7	10.2	15.3
6	1.8	3.5	4.2	6.0	7.1	10.6

Because of the high coefficient for absorption of water, very little tissue water is necessary for tissue reaction, allowing deep or very superficial vaporization, but both being done with minimal thermal injury. Its high affinity for tissue water and its ability to yield a narrow zone of residual thermal damage make the Er:YAG laser an exceptionally efficient and precise ablative laser with a side effect profile that is considerably more favorable than that of the CO_2 laser (11).

Er:YAG Laser—Indications
The indications for Er:YAG laser resurfacing are discussed next.

Rhytides
Mild-to-moderate photo-induced rhytides and mildly atrophic facial scars can be effectively treated with the short-pulsed Er:YAG (245). Severe rhytides (Fitzpatrick–Goldman class III or greater) and severely photodamaged skin respond better to treatment with one of the modulated Er:YAG lasers with coagulative capabilities that facilitate deeper dermal ablation and induce a greater degree of collagen contraction and collagen remodeling. Static facial rhytides in the periorbital, perioral, cheek, and forehead areas respond particularly well to Er:YAG laser resurfacing (246). To preserve clinical correction of dynamic rhytides (e.g., periorbital, glabella, and forehead), botulinum toxin A can be safely used (as previously described) in conjunction with Er:YAG laser resurfacing (247).

Acne Scars
Modest improvement of mild-to-moderate acne scarring can be achieved with the short-pulsed Er:YAG laser resurfacing. Deep acne scars have a better chance of improvement when resurfaced with a modulated Er:YAG laser. However, even with the modulated Er:YAG lasers, the reported improvement has been moderate at best (28). Adjunctive treatment with other modalities (e.g., subcision, punch excision, fillers, and grafts) is usually required to achieve significant correction of this difficult-to-treat condition (248–250).

Posttraumatic and Surgical Scars
When performed during the phase of collagen remodeling (i.e., within 90 days of the original trauma), Er:YAG laser resurfacing can significantly improve the cosmetic appearance of posttraumatic and surgical scars. Linear facial scars tend to respond the best. Kwon et al. reported 50% improvement of 9 of 12 hypertrophic scars, 17 of 20 depressed scars, and 4 burn scars treated with a short-pulsed Er:YAG laser (2-mm handpiece, 500–1200 mJ/pulse, 3.5–9 W) (29). Additionally, immediate

postoperative resurfacing of Mohs surgery defects with the Er:YAG laser has been shown to significantly improve the outcome of second intention healing in anatomical areas that typically do not heal well by second intention (i.e., convex nasal surfaces) (251).

Benign Epidermal and Dermal Lesions
The Er:YAG laser has been used to safely and effectively treat a number of benign cutaneous lesions including syringomas (42), trichoepitheliomas, sebaceous hyperplasia, seborrheic keratoses (252), actinic keratosis (253), epidermal nevi (254), Becker's nevi (255), xanthelasma palpebrarum (256,257), eruptive vellus hair cysts (258), multiple military osteomas of the face (259), colloid milium (260), periungual warts (261), rhinophyma (262), Darier's disease and Hailey–Hailey disease (263), Dowling–Degos disease (264), and Zoon's balanitis (265).

Dyspigmentation
Superficial (epidermal) and deep (dermal) pigmentation problems can be addressed with Er:YAG laser resurfacing. Photo-induced dyspigmentation responds well to Er:YAG laser resurfacing. Melasma, on the other hand, tends to recur after Er:YAG resurfacing. Adjunctive therapy with topical bleaching agents (e.g., hydroquinone, azelaic acid, tretinoin, and glycolic acid peel) and daily sunscreen is typically necessary when treating melasma. Additionally, the Er:YAG laser has been found useful for the preparation of recipient site prior to epidermal grafting in patients with vitiligo (266).

Contraindications to Er:YAG Laser Resurfacing
The contraindications to Er:YAG laser resurfacing are the same as for CO_2 laser resurfacing and are listed in Box 6.2.

Clinical Situations Where the Er:YAG Laser Confers a Definite Technical Advantage
Given its relative lack of adnexal structures and delayed healing when compared with facial skin (15,267), resurfacing of nonfacial skin in areas such as the neck, arms, and hands must be approached with caution. Previous experience with CO_2 laser resurfacing of nonfacial skin has been plagued by a host of complications including permanent scarring and hypopigmentation. Kilmer and colleagues have published a protocol for CO_2 laser resurfacing of the neck, but it should only be attempted by those who are experienced and have a mastery of laser–tissue interaction (40). Fitzpatrick et al. noted no improvement in wrinkling and four cases of permanent hypopigmentation (one with scarring) after single-pass

resurfacing of the neck with the UltraPulse CO_2 laser (268). Another study by Rosenberg also reported scarring of the lower neck after resurfacing with the UltraPulse laser (269).

Given the high rate of complications found in previous studies, resurfacing of the neck with the CO_2 laser is considered relatively contraindicated by most experts today. In contrast, resurfacing of the neck, arms, and hands has been safely and effectively accomplished with Er:YAG laser systems (Fig. 6.37). Goldberg et al. resurfaced the neck skin of 10 patients with four passes of a short-pulsed Er:YAG laser at a fluence of 3–4.5 J/cm^2. At the 6-month follow-up, they noted at least a 25% improvement in wrinkling and 50% improvement in mottled dyspigmentation. No scarring or pigmentary complications occurred (14). Goldman et al. evaluated the results of neck resurfacing with an Er:YAG laser (Derma-20, ESC Medical Systems, Needham, Massachusetts, USA. This is now made by Lumenis) in 20 patients. Fluences of 8.7–13.5 J/cm^2 and spot sizes of 4–5 mm were used for the first pass and 2–9 J/cm^2 and 5- to 10-mm spot diameters for the second pass. In total, 51% of patients were satisfied with their results, and 39% improvement in texture and 37% improvement in skin color were noted. All patients healed within 7–10 days and no permanent adverse side effects occurred (15). Jimenez and Spencer resurfaced the skin of the neck, hands, and forearms of 12 patients with a 300-μs pulsed Er:YAG laser with a 5-mm spot size at a fluence of 5 J/cm^2. Two to three passes were performed on the arm and forearms and one or two passes were performed on the neck. Overall, they reported a mild improvement in photodamage and the majority of patients were pleased with their results. Healing took 2–3 weeks and two of seven patients who underwent resurfacing of the hands and forearms developed infections that were successfully treated. No scarring or permanent pigmentary alterations were observed (270).

Pigmentary disturbances in patients with Fitzpatrick skin phototypes III and higher have been a frequent complication of CO_2 laser skin resurfacing (16–18,101). The reported incidence of pigmentary alterations after Er:YAG laser skin resurfacing of patients with darker skin phototypes (Fitzpatrick skin phototype III or higher) is significantly lower than that reported after CO_2 laser skin resurfacing. The Er:YAG laser has shown a clear advantage over the CO_2 laser in the resurfacing of patients with darker (III–VI) Fitzpatrick skin phototypes (2). Polnikorn et al. utilized the Er:YAG laser to treat 50 Asian patients (Fitzpatrick skin phototypes III and IV) with rhytides, photodamage, acne, and varicella scars. Significant improvement was noted in all patients. Although 30% of patients experienced transient hyperpigmentation, only one patient developed transient hypopigmentation (271).

The Er:YAG laser has also proven useful for removal of part of the zone of thermal damage left behind after CO_2 laser resurfacing, a technique that has been shown to decrease the duration of postoperative erythema and healing time. Several studies have documented the positive impact of Er:YAG laser resurfacing on postoperative recovery when performed immediately after CO_2 laser resurfacing. Goldman and colleagues randomized 10 patients to receive three passes with the CO_2 laser alone (300 mJ, CPG settings of 596, 595, and 584) to one side of the face and two CO_2 laser passes (300 mJ, CPG settings of 596 and 595) followed immediately by two passes with the Er:YAG laser (Derma-20 or Derma-K, ESC Medical systems; 4-mm spot, 14 J cm^2 now made by Lumenis). They noted faster reepithelialization (1–2 days faster) and decreased duration of postoperative erythema (2–3 weeks vs. more than 8 weeks) in those areas treated with the CO_2–Er:YAG laser combination (Fig. 6.38). This beneficial effect was accomplished without compromising clinical outcome (31). McDaniel et al. randomized 40 treatment

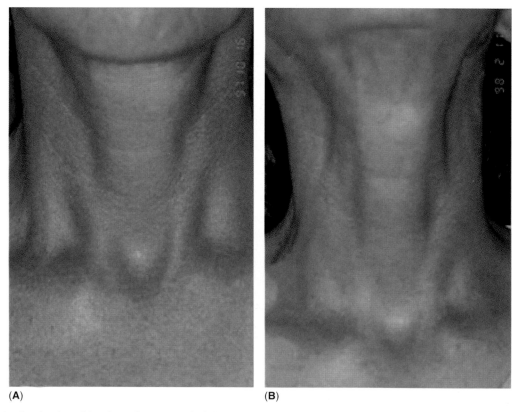

(A)   (B)

Figure 6.37 Treatment of neck using erbium laser allows removal of photodamaged epidermis without dermal injury. Improvement of skin texture and blending of color are reasonable goals. Improvement of 40–50% has been observed. (**A**) Before treatment; (**B**) 4 months postoperatively.

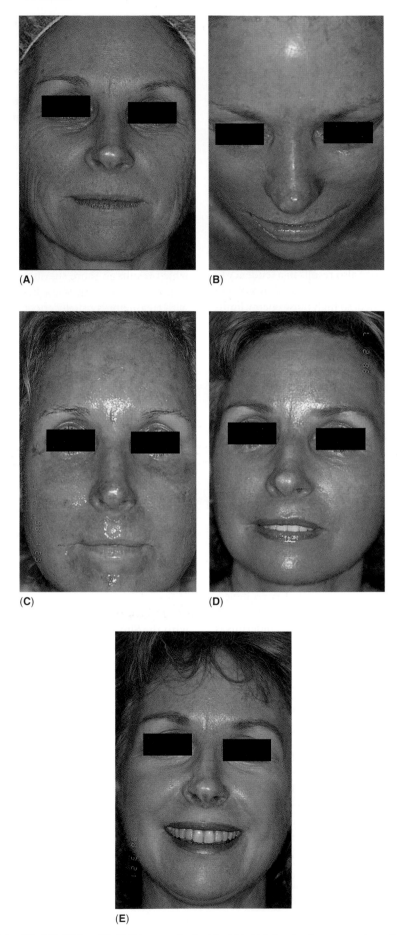

Figure 6.38 Combination UltraPulse CO$_2$ (UP CO$_2$) and Er:YAG laser use (patients's right side) showing improvement equal to the left side treated with the UP CO$_2$ laser alone. (**A**) Before treatment. (**B**) Immediately after treatment (as described in the text). (**C**) 7 days after laser resurfacing. (**D**) 3 weeks after resurfacing. (**E**) 2 months after resurfacing. *Source*: From Ref. 304.

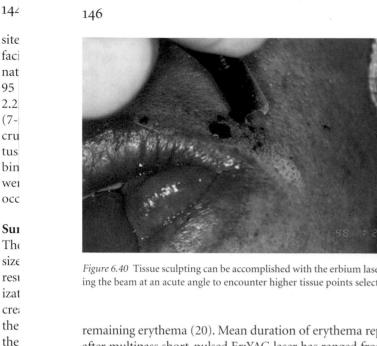

Figure 6.40 Tissue sculpting can be accomplished with the erbium laser, holding the beam at an acute angle to encounter higher tissue points selectively.

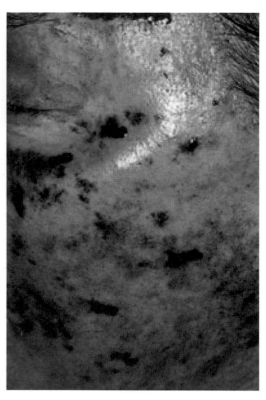

Figure 6.41 Because the erbium laser does not leave enough residual thermal necrosis to cauterize dermal vessels, bleeding will be encountered. Pinpoint bleeding is first seen in the upper papillary dermis and becomes more significant as the upper reticular dermis is reached.

remaining erythema (20). Mean duration of erythema reported after multipass short-pulsed Er:YAG laser has ranged from 1 to 4 weeks in most studies as compared with 1–3 months for most patients after multipass treatment with CO_2 lasers (2,5,12).

Hyperpigmentation

Transient hyperpigmentation has been reported in up to 37% of patients after CO_2 laser resurfacing, with a higher frequency in patients with Fitzpatrick skin types IV and above. Transient hyperpigmentation in patients with darker skin phototypes also occurs frequently 4–6 weeks after treatment with the short-pulsed Er:YAG laser.

In their large series of 625 patients treated with multiple passes of a short-pulsed Er:YAG laser, Weinstein et al. observed a transient hyperpigmentation rate of 3.4% (10). Ziering et al. reported a 12% incidence of transient hyperpigmentation in his series of 50 patients resurfaced with multipass short-pulsed Er:YAG laser (7). Three additional studies that treated with multiple passes of the short-pulsed Er:YAG reported transient hyperpigmentation rates of 24% (13,20) and 25%, respectively (5). Kye treated 30 patients with pitted facial scars and Fitzpatrick skin phototypes III and IV with multiple passes of a short-pulsed Er:YAG and noted only two cases of hyperpigmentation at the 3-month follow-up. All of his patients, however, were treated preoperatively for 2–4 weeks with tretinoin 0.05% and postoperatively for 2–4 weeks with a combination of hydroquinone 4%, tretinoin 0.05%, and hydrocortisone 1% (250). In their series of 22 patients with Fitzpatrick skin phototype IV, Sriprachya-Anunt et al. found no statistically significant difference in the rate of transient hyperpigmentation induced by treatment with either the CO_2 or the short-pulsed Er:YAG laser alone, or a combination of both (273). Moreover, Kim et al. resurfaced 190 patients with facial scars and Fitzpatrick skin phototypes III and above with either the short-pulsed Er:YAG laser or a modulated Er:YAG laser. They observed transient hyperpigmentation rates of 24.7%, 42.3%, and 65.9% for the short-pulsed, variable-pulsed (CO_3, Cynosure, Chelmsford, Massachusetts, USA), and the dual-mode (Contour, Sciton Corporation, Palo Alto, California, USA) lasers, respectively (274). Although hyperpigmentation in darker skin phototypes appears to occur just as frequently with both the CO_2 and

Er:YAG lasers, it is often less severe and of shorter duration after Er:YAG laser resurfacing (275).

Hypopigmentation

Delayed-onset permanent hypopigmentation is thought to be related to depth of ablation and the degree of residual thermal damage. Reported in up to 16% of patients after CO_2 laser resurfacing, hypopigmentation has a significantly lower incidence after short-pulsed Er:YAG laser resurfacing.

Alster resurfaced the face of 12 patients with Fitzpatrick skin phototypes I–IV with multiple passes of six different short-pulsed Er:YAG lasers and noted no instances of hypopigmentation (5) Weinstein observed a 4% incidence of delayed-onset permanent hypopigmentation in a series of 625 patients resurfaced with a short-pulsed Er:YAG laser (10). In their series of 21 patients treated with multipass short-pulsed Er:YAG laser, Khatri et al. noted a 5% incidence of hypopigmentation at the 6-month follow-up (20). Bass et al. reported a 12% rate of hypopigmentation in their series of 25 patients treated with multipass short-pulsed Er:YAG laser (13). In their series of 190 patients with Fitzpatrick skin phototypes III and above, Kim et al. found hypopigmentation rates of 8.0%, 15.3%, and 24.4% after resurfacing with the short-pulsed Er:YAG, variable-pulsed Er:YAG (CO_3, Cynosure), and dual-mode (Contour®, Sciton Corp.) Er:YAG lasers, respectively. The mean onset and duration of hypopigmentation in their patient populations were 2 and 5.1 months, respectively. Only 15% of their patients had remaining hypopigmentation at the 12-month follow-up.

Scarring

In contrast to CO_2 laser resurfacing, most series utilizing the short-pulsed Er:YAG for facial resurfacing have reported negligible rates of scarring (5,7,11,13). In her large series of 625 patients, Weinstein observed a 0.8% incidence of scarring. In her study, scarring developed on the chest, lower eyelid, and upper lip. All of these scars responded well to a 50/50 mixture of intralesional triamcinolone (10 mg/kg) and 5-fluorouracil.

Resurfacing of the neck and other nonfacial areas with the CO_2 laser has resulted in a high incidence of scarring and hypopigmentation in a number of studies. A study by Fitzpatrick and Goldman reported a 33% incidence of hypertrophic scarring after resurfacing of the lower neck with a single pass of the UltraPulse CO_2 laser. Another study by Rosenberg et al. also reported scarring of the lower neck after single-pass resurfacing with the UltraPulse CO_2 laser. The increased risk of scarring of nonfacial skin is thought to be due to the relative lack of pilosebaceous units in nonfacial skin as compared with facial skin (269,275).

In contrast to CO_2, skin resurfacing of nonfacial areas including the neck, arms, and hands with the Er:YAG laser has been demonstrated to be safe and moderately effective in several studies.

McDaniel et al. used the short-pulsed Er:YAG with a 5-mm spot diameter and a fluence of 2.5 J/cm^2 to resurface the dorsal hands of three patients and the neck of one patient (two or three passes) and observed an improvement in the appearance of 48% and 44%, respectively, and no cases of scarring or hypopigmentation (236). Goldberg et al. treated 11 necks and 4 dorsal hands with multiple passes of the short-pulsed Er:YAG laser at fluences of 4–5 J/cm^2 and reported significant clinical improvement of photodamage (25%–100%) and no adverse sequelae (14). Goldman et al. treated the neck of 20 patients with two passes of the short-pulsed Er:YAG at higher fluences (up to 13.5 J/cm^2) and reported an overall patient satisfaction of 51%, an average improvement in the skin texture of 39%, and an average improvement in the skin color of 37%. All their patients healed within 7–10 days had resolution of their erythema within 2 weeks (except for one patient who developed an infection) and reported no permanent adverse effects (15). Jimenez et al. treated seven patients with photodamage of the forearms and hands and five patients with photodamage of the neck with one to three passes of the short-pulsed Er:YAG laser using a 5-mm spot size and a fluence of 5 J/cm^2. They reported no permanent adverse side effects with these laser parameters. However, they noted that the cosmetic improvement achieved was only mild, the healing time was significantly longer (2–3 weeks) than for Er:YAG facial resurfacing, topical anesthesia was inadequate, and two of the seven patients who underwent hand and forearm resurfacing experienced infections that required oral antibiotics (270).

Infection

As with any other cutaneous resurfacing method, infection is a potential risk of Er:YAG laser resurfacing. However, the reported infection rates have generally been low. Most infections occur during the first week, prior to reepithelialization. *S. aureus* and *P. aeruginosa* are the most common bacterial pathogens and *Candida* is responsible for most of the fungal infections. Weinstein et al. reported only one case of bacterial infection (on the neck) in their large series of 625 patients resurfaced with a short-pulsed Er:YAG laser. Alster et al. reported one instance of herpes simplex reactivation in a series of 12 patients who underwent facial cutaneous resurfacing with short-pulsed Er:YAG lasers. Teikemeier et al., Khatri et al., Ziering et al., and Bass et al. observed no infections in their respective series of 20, 21, 25, and 50 patients resurfaced with the short-pulsed Er:YAG laser (5,7,10,11,13). A detailed discussion of the treatment of the complications described above is provided in the section "Complications of CO_2 Laser Resurfacing."

Modulated (Coagulative and Ablative) Er:YAG Laser Systems

Despite the initial enthusiasm for the Er:YAG laser, clinicians quickly came to realize that clinical results achieved with the conventional short-pulsed Er:YAG lasers were considerably less impressive than those attained with CO_2 lasers. The hopes of those who had envisioned the Er:YAG laser as the resurfacing tool that would entirely replace the CO_2 laser were swiftly shattered.

There were a number of factors that limited the resurfacing potential of early generation Er:YAG lasers. First, early short-pulsed Er:YAG lasers were slow and underpowered. They had low repetition rates of only 1–2 Hz, produced modest fluences no greater than 10 J/cm^2, and had small beam diameters of 1–2 mm. Multiple passes were required to achieve epidermal ablation with these systems (244,276,277). Alster et al. tested six different early generation short-pulsed Er:YAG lasers in skin resurfacing and found that with all of them, three passes were needed for complete epidermal ablation (5).

The low ablation rates of early generation Er:YAG lasers, which typically hovered at around 20 mm per second, represented a significant disadvantage when compared with the high peak power, short-pulsed CO_2 lasers (276). Second, although early Er:YAG lasers proved efficacious for superficial ablation, their limited coagulative effect precluded good hemostasis and significantly limited depth of ablation (23,24,278).

However, early Er:YAG lasers proved to be excellent tools for resurfacing of mild-to-moderate rhytides. Furthermore, postoperative erythema and reepithelialization time after Er:YAG resurfacing turned out to be significantly less than seen after CO_2 resurfacing (11). Despite its advantageous side effect profile, clinicians quickly came to realize that skin resurfacing with the Er:YAG laser produced results that were considerably inferior to those attained with the CO_2 laser (11,19–22,236,279).

A number of studies suggested that thermally induced effects on the dermal collagen contributed to the beneficial effects of CO_2 lasers in the treatment of facial rhytides and perhaps underlie the superior results achieved after CO_2 laser skin resurfacing. Tissue contraction, tightening of facial skin, synthesis of new collagen, and collagen remodeling were demonstrated after CO_2 laser skin resurfacing in several studies (2,6,280,281).

Therefore, a number of authors hypothesized that the relative lack of efficacy of traditional short-pulsed Er:YAG laser skin resurfacing was related to a relative lack of thermally mediated coagulative effects in the upper dermis (6, 19–22, 54,279). Several studies demonstrated less coagulative effect and thermal residual damage after Er:YAG laser skin resurfacing as compared with CO_2 laser skin resurfacing (32,280,281). Adrian et al. compared the short-pulsed Er:YAG with a pulsed CO_2 laser in a bilateral comparison study and found that the Er:YAG was able to improve fine rhytides but showed less efficacy treating moderate-to-deep rhytides than the CO_2. In all instances, except for mild rhytides, the CO_2 laser produced superior and longer lasting results (19).

With the notion that immediate tissue contraction and induction of thermally mediated changes in dermal collagen were important for long-term laser skin resurfacing results, investigators began exploring ways to "modulate" the Er:YAG laser to endow it with enhanced coagulative power while maintaining its powerful ablative capacity and extremely favorable side effect profile (282).

Traditional Er:YAG lasers operated with pulse durations of 350 μs and typically produced 10–20 μm of residual thermal damage. In 1998, Adrian et al. studied the effect of increasing the pulse of the Er:YAG at a fluence of 5 J/cm^2 during skin resurfacing procedures to 10 ms (CO_3, Cynosure, no longer made) (21). Histology revealed a 60-μm residual thermal damage zone after multiple passes with this long-pulsed (10 ms) Er:YAG laser. More significantly, this increased zone of residual thermal damage correlated well with increased tissue contraction when compared with the 350-μs Er:YAG laser and the clinical results achieved were similar to those attained with the high peak power, short-pulsed CO_2 laser. This and other subsequent studies (282) showed that as the pulse width increased, both the zone of residual thermal damage and the clinical effect approached the magnitudes seen after short-pulsed CO_2 laser resurfacing (21,100,283).

In an attempt to overcome the shortcomings of the conventional short-pulsed (350 μs) Er:YAG laser, namely poor hemostasis, which limited depth of ablation and its inability to resurface deep rhytides effectively, modulated Er:YAG laser systems that conveniently combine long pulse (coagulative) and short pulse (ablative) capabilities in the same device were introduced in the late 1990s.

Currently there is one commercially available modulated Er:YAG laser system with combined ablative and coagulative capabilities: a dual-mode (ablation and subablative/coagulation modes) pulsed Er:YAG laser (Contour TRL, Sciton Corp.). Additionally, there are devices that are no longer made but are of historical interest, including a variable-pulsed Er:YAG laser (CO_3, Cynosure), which can deliver single pulses of variable widths, and a modulated Er:YAG laser system that is a hybrid CO_2–Er:YAG laser (Derma-K, ESC Medical Systems, now part of Lumenis), which is no longer commercially available but, given that these may still be in use by some clinicians, will be briefly reviewed next.

The dual-mode Contour TRL Er:YAG laser (Sciton Corp.) uses a process called optical multiplexing that stacks together groups of individual Er:YAG laser pulses to create either short (200–300 μs) ablative pulses of high fluence or long-duration pulses of low fluence (subablative and coagulative). These pulses can be delivered as purely ablative, purely coagulative, or a combination of both. Ablation depths of up to 200 μm can be achieved with a single pulse. At 50% overlap, high fluences of up to 100 J/cm^2 can be generated and the entire epidermis can be removed in a single pass. The coagulative component can produce thermal damage in the dermis and

tissue contraction that approaches that seen with CO_2 laser skin resurfacing (244,284). The Contour's touch screen control panel allows the surgeon to "dial in" the desired depths of ablation and coagulation and to choose the corresponding clinically appropriate laser parameters. The Contour has a built-in safety feature that automatically adjusts the displayed fluence to reflect the effect of changes in the degree of overlap. For example, an increase from 10% to 30% overlap will alert the surgeon to the fact that the delivered fluence has increased by approximately 65%. At 45 W, the Contour Er:YAG is a powerful laser that makes the use of a pulse scanner quite feasible and advantageous (285). Several studies have investigated the histologic effects of dual-mode Er:YAG Contour laser resurfacing. A close correlation was found between the programed and actual measured depths of ablation for single and multiple passes. It is clinically important to note that the chosen depth of coagulation correlates well with the histologic changes for the first pass, but this correlation deteriorates with subsequent passes (286–288).

Zachary et al. achieved significant tissue contraction and good-to-excellent control of bleeding with the dual-mode Contour Er:YAG laser using 50% overlap, 84 μm of ablation (21 J/cm^2), and 50–100 μm of coagulation. A "CO_2-like" tissue contraction was observed during the second and subsequent passes with this laser (284). Grekin and Zachary reported their experience resurfacing over 100 patients with the dual-mode Contour Er:YAG laser (285,289). Average reepithelialization time for their patients was 3–5 days and they noted significant improvement in rhytides and acne scars. Full-face and regional resurfacing was accomplished in patients with all skin types. In comparison with the CO_2 laser, postoperative erythema cleared more rapidly and there were no cases of scarring. Transient hyperpigmentation was seen in most patients with darker skin phototypes, but it resolved in every case with the use of topical bleaching agents and sun protection. Of note, these authors reported two cases of delayed hypopigmentation that occurred in patients with lighter skin phototypes.

In another study, Tanzi and Alster utilized the dual-mode Contour Er:YAG laser to treat 25 patients with moderate-to-severe atrophic facial acne scars. Their laser parameters were 90 mm of ablation (22.5 J/cm^2) with 50% spot overlap and 50 mm of coagulation delivered with a rapid pulse scanner. Two to three passes were performed. The average clinical improvement score at the 12-month follow-up was 2.16 (25–50% improvement). Side-effects were limited to transient erythema in all patients (mean duration of 3 weeks), one case of prolonged erythema, hyperpigmentation (44%), and acne flare-up that responded well to oral minocycline (32%). No cases of hypopigmentation or scarring occurred (28).

Kwon et al. evaluated the efficacy and safety of scar resurfacing with the dual-mode Contour Er:YAG laser. Nine of 12 hypertrophic scars, 17 of 20 depressed scars, and 2 of 4 burn scars improved more than 50%. Side effects were minimal and included one case of postinflammatory hyperpigmentation and mild persistent erythema in all patients with burn scars (29).

The variable-pulsed CO_3–Er:YAG laser system can deliver pulse durations ranging from 500 μs to 10 ms. Short pulses are used for ablation, whereas longer pulses produce thermal effects mimicking the CO_2 laser–tissue response. With the longer pulse mode of 10 ms and a fluence of 5 J/cm^2, thermal damage zones of 30–40 µm have been reported.

The CO_3 laser is no longer made by Cynosure but may be in use by some practitioners. Rostan et al. performed a split-face study comparing resurfacing with the variable-pulsed (CO_3, Cynosure) Er:YAG laser versus the 950-µs UltraPulse CO_2 laser. Sixteen patients were randomized to receive resurfacing with either UltraPulse CO_2 or CO_3 laser with a 10-ms pulse on one side of the face, followed immediately by a pass with the short-pulsed Er:YAG laser. Two passes with the CO_3 parameters set at 2 J, 10–10.5 J/cm^2, 10-ms pulse, 4–10 Hz, 5-mm spot were performed. One additional pass with the CO_3 laser (same settings) over the areas of greatest scarring and photodamage was followed by a single pass with a 500-µs Er:YAG at 1.5 J, 7.7 J/cm^2, 5- to 7-mm spot, and a repetition rate of 10 Hz. UltraPulse CO_2 treatment was performed utilizing the CPG for two or three passes at settings of 596, 595, and 584 followed by a single pass with a short-pulsed Er:YAG at 14–16 J/cm^2 with a 4-mm spot size and up to 50% overlap. Overall clinical improvement was found to be equal for both the sides treated with UltraPulse CO_2 and variable-pulsed Er:YAG (CO_3) lasers, with an average improvement in photoaging scores of 57%. Moreover, decreased erythema and edema and faster healing were observed on the side treated with the variable-pulsed (CO_3) Er:YAG laser (26).

Newman et al. performed a side-by-side comparison study of the histologic and clinical effects of the variable-pulsed CO_3–Er:YAG versus the UltraPulse CO_2 laser after perioral resurfacing. Four ablative-mode passes with the CO_3 laser (5-mm spot size, fluence of 5.2 J/cm^2, and a 500 µs pulse width) were followed by a single coagulative mode pass (5-mm spot, fluence of 2.6 J/cm^2, and a 10-ms pulse width). A final pass, designed to remove the thermally damaged tissue partially, used parameters identical to the initial ablative passes. Histology showed a 90-µm layer of ablation and a 10-µm layer of residual thermal damage. The authors postulated that the final ablative pass partly removed the zone of thermal necrosis generated by the 10-ms coagulative pulse. Two months after treatment, there was a 54% improvement in rhytides treated with the variable-pulsed CO_3–Er:YAG laser, compared with 63% improvement with the CO_2 laser. Reduced duration of crusting (3.5 vs. 7.8 days) was observed on the sides treated with the variable-pulsed CO_3–Er:YAG laser. They observed no cases of permanent hyperpigmentation, hypopigmentation, or scarring (27).

Christian et al. conducted a six-patient, split-face study that evaluated the impact of single-pass resurfacing ("micro-resurfacing peel") at two different pulse durations (500 µs vs. 4 ms) of the variable-pulsed (CO_3) modulated Er:YAG laser. Six of eight peels were performed at a fluence of 7.1 J/cm^2. Erythema was found to be significantly greater on the 4-ms side at postoperative days 3–4, but this difference was no longer significant at postoperative day 7. Average time to reepithelialization was found to be 3.6 days (290).

Finally, the Derma-K (ESC Medical Systems, now Lumenis) hybrid Er:YAG–CO_2 laser was available commercially in the USA. Given that some clinicians continue to utilize the Derma-K system for skin resurfacing and reports of its efficacy continue to appear in the literature (291), we will briefly review this laser system as well.

The Derma-K laser is a hybrid laser system that delivers ablative Er:YAG laser pulses followed immediately by coagulative CO_2 laser pulses. The Er:YAG component produces a fluence of up to 28 J/cm^2 with a 350-µs pulse. The CO_2 component can deliver a subablative/coagulative pulse varying from 1 to 100 ms at 1- to 10-W power, providing excellent hemostasis. The CO_2 coagulative component can be programed to be delivered during a fraction or all of the time between the ablative Er:YAG laser pulses.

Energy can be delivered using either a CPG with a 3-mm spot or a noncollimated 0.2- to 8-mm spot. Zones of thermal necrosis of up to 50 mm in depth have been observed after resurfacing with this laser system (30,292).

Goldman et al. performed full-face resurfacing of 10 patients with the Derma-K hybrid laser. They performed four passes with a 4-mm spot, Er:YAG laser parameters of 350 µs, 1.7 J/cm^2, and the CO_2 component set at 5 W, 50 ms with a frequency of 10 Hz. Their patients experienced a 44% and 38% improvement in perioral and periorbital rhytides at their 3-month follow-up and an overall improvement of 39% in their facial photoaging score. Histology revealed a 20-µm zone of thermal damage immediately after treatment and an average depth of collagen of 54-µm (86% increase from baseline) 3 months postoperatively. Weinstein et al. have also reported good-to-excellent results after facial resurfacing with the Derma-K Er:YAG–CO_2 hybrid laser. They noted a mean reepithelialization time of 11.3 days and postoperative erythema that lasted an average of 8.3 weeks, in their study (30).

Trelles et al. performed single-pass resurfacing of 102 patients with skin phototypes I–V with the Derma-K hybrid laser. They used an ablative Er:YAG laser pulse (350 µs, 28 J/cm^2) followed immediately by a coagulative CW CO_2 laser shot (4–6 W, 50 ms) through a 3-mm collimated handpiece (3-mm spot) with 50% overlapping and a repetition rate of 10 Hz. In total, 67 patients scored their results as very good, 25 as good, and 10 as fair and the patient's rating correlated well with those of the treating physician and three independent observers. Mean duration of follow-up in their study was 1.76 years. Mild, transient side effects were seen in only four of their 102 patients. Histology 2 months postoperatively demonstrated a band of well-oriented newly synthesized collagen underneath a healthy epidermis (293).

As previously described, one of the main benefits of cutaneous resurfacing with a CO_2 laser is tissue contraction, which is believed by a number of authors to underlie the superior resurfacing results achieved with the CO_2 laser. All of the new modulated Er:YAG laser systems have demonstrated the capability to produce "CO_2-like" tissue contraction not only clinically but also histologically. Kist et al. studied collagen contraction after CO_3 laser treatment in a bovine tendon collagen model. The depth of irreversible and reversible collagen fibril changes (measures of collagen contraction) was assessed by electron microscopy. With a constant fluence of 6.1 J/cm^2, the maximum irreversible collagen fibril change was achieved at the highest pulse duration (10 ms) and it measured 3.25 µm. The maximum depth of reversible collagen change at the same fluence was found to be 9.52 µm and it was attained at the 7-ms pulse duration. Their study showed that when pulse duration or fluence was increased while the other variable was held constant, there was a steady increase in the mean maximum tissue contraction and collagen fibril diameter. Remarkably, the degree of collagen contraction achieved in their study was consistent with that achieved with a pulsed CO_2 laser in a previous study using the same bovine tendon collagen model (294).

Fitzpatrick et al. compared the collagen tightening induced by a pulsed CO_2 laser and the modulated Derma-K laser. One eyelid, treated with three passes of a pulsed CO_2 (UltraPulse, Coherent Medical Group, Santa Clara, CA now Lumenis), was compared with the contralateral eyelid, treated with the Derma-K laser (ESC, now Lumenis), to an endpoint of early pinpoint bleeding. Intraoperative contraction of 43% after CO_2 resurfacing versus 12% after Derma-K laser resurfacing was measured. However, at 1 month and beyond, the degree of CO_2-induced skin tightening and that of modulated Er:YAG-induced skin tightening was found to be identical (25).

Modulated Er:YAG Lasers: Clinical Considerations

Their capability to produce precise ablation at highly efficient rates, provide excellent hemostasis with their coagulative pulses, and generate "CO_2-like" thermally induced changes in dermal collagen and their superior side effect profile have made these powerful modulated Er:YAG lasers a true alternative to the CO_2 laser.

In contrast to CO_2 laser resurfacing, treatment with the modulated Er:YAG lasers can often be performed using local anesthesia. Topical anesthesia, nerve blocks, and local infiltration typically are supplemented with a benzodiazepine (i.e., midazolam or diazepam) and/or an analgesic such as fentanyl or meperidine.

Currently available modulated Er:YAG lasers are powerful systems with efficient ablation rates that make the use of a scanner feasible. Alternatively, freehand ablation can be performed efficiently at a repetition rate of 5 Hz and with an overlap of 50% that produces the equivalent of two-pass ablation in a single pass. Single passes are typically performed with a 20–30% overlap to prevent irregularities inherent to their Gaussian beam. Up to 40 μm of tissue per pass can be ablated at a fluence of 10 J/cm^2 with both, the Contour and CO_2 lasers (272,284,289).

Long pulse durations with the currently available modulated Er:YAG laser system, Contour TRL (Sciton Corp.), produce clinically evident, "CO_2-like" intraoperative tissue contraction during and after the second pass. As a general rule, deeper rhytides and severe photodamage are optimally treated with the longest pulse durations available, whereas superficial rhytides and minimal photodamage are treated with short pulse durations. Wiping between passes, although not necessary, can afford a better view of rhytide effacement and depth of vaporization (Fig. 6.42).

The short-pulsed mode of the modulated lasers can be used for purely ablative functions such as fine tissue sculpting and to remove the residual zone of thermal necrosis left behind by the coagulative mode of these lasers. Removal of this zone of residual thermal damage after CO_2 laser resurfacing has been shown to improve postoperative healing.

The clinical endpoint during modulated Er:YAG laser skin resurfacing is not obvious. The long pulses (coagulative) of the modulated Er:YAG lasers produce excellent control of intraoperative hemostasis. Thus, punctate bleeding, which helps to signal the clinical endpoint during conventional short-pulsed Er:YAG resurfacing, does not occur when resurfacing with the modulated Er:YAG lasers. Furthermore, the

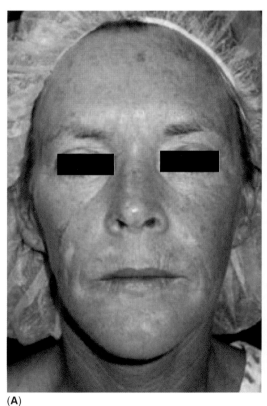

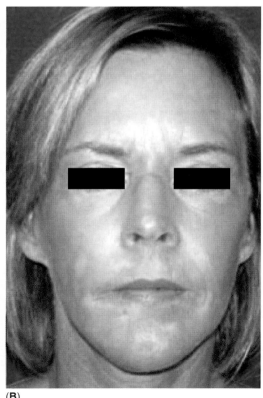

(A)　　　　　　　　　　　　　　　　　　　(B)

Figure 6.42 Treatment with the Cynosure CO_2 laser. (**A**) Before treatment; (**B**) 6 months after treatment with two passes at 10 J/cm^2 and 10 ms followed by two passes with 10 J/cm^2 and 0.5 ms.

typical depth-related color changes seen during CO_2 resurfacing also do not occur during modulated Er:YAG resurfacing. Therefore, when resurfacing with the modulated Er:YAG lasers, the surgeon must carefully choose clinically appropriate laser parameters based on anatomic considerations and the desired depth of tissue ablation. For example, the epidermal thickness of the eyelid is approximately 60 μm. Using the modulated Er:YAG lasers at a fluence of 15 J/cm² and 30% overlap, the entire epidermis of the eyelid can efficiently be removed in a single pass.

Modulated Er:YAG Lasers: Complications
Overall, the side effect profile of the modulated Er:YAG lasers has been reported to be slightly more than that of the short-pulsed Er:YAG laser but considerably more favorable than that of the CO_2 laser. As with the CO_2 laser, potential complications include prolonged postoperative erythema, pigmentary disturbances, scarring, and infection.

Prolonged Erythema
Prolonged postoperative erythema, thought to be related to the degree of thermal damage and depth of ablation, can occur in up to 20% of patients treated with the CO_2 laser. Most studies have reported a decreased duration of postoperative erythema and a shortened recovery period after resurfacing with the modulated (coagulative and ablative) Er:YAG lasers as compared with CO_2 laser resurfacing. Alster et al. resurfaced 50 patients with a dual-mode Er:YAG laser (Contour, Sciton Corp.) and found that reepithelialization was complete in an average of 5 days, and only three patients (6%) experienced prolonged postoperative erythema (295). In a split-face comparison of 16 patients following pulsed CO_2 and variable-pulsed Er:YAG laser skin resurfacing, Rostan et al. reported decreased erythema, less edema, and faster reepithelialization on the side treated with the variable-pulsed (CO_3, Cynosure) Er:YAG laser (26).

Postoperative Hyperpigmentation
Transient postinflammatory hyperpigmentation is not uncommon following modulated (coagulative and ablative) Er:YAG laser skin resurfacing. However, the reported duration of hyperpigmentation after modulated Er:YAG resurfacing has been shorter than that observed after CO_2 laser resurfacing (16,296).

Jeong et al. reported hyperpigmentation in 8 of 35 (29%) patients (Fitzpatrick skin types III–V) treated with a variable-pulsed Er:YAG laser for pitted acne scars. Similarly, Alster et al. reported a 40% incidence of hyperpigmentation in their series of 50 patients resurfaced with a variable-pulsed Er:YAG laser. In both series, the hyperpigmentation was transient and responded well to topical agents. In their series of 20 patients with pitted acne scars, Jeong et al. reported an incidence of hyperpigmentation of 60% and an incidence of hypopigmentation of 5%, following resurfacing with the dual-mode Contour Er:YAG laser (Sciton Corp.). In all cases, the hyperpigmentation was transient and resolved within 3 months postoperatively (297).

Delayed Permanent Hypopigmentation
Delayed permanent hypopigmentation, a common side effect after CO_2 laser resurfacing (15–20% reported incidence), has not been reported in most series that utilized a modulated (coagulative and ablative) Er:YAG laser. One year postoperatively, Tanzi and Alster noted no cases of delayed hypopigmentation in their series of 50 patients resurfaced with the Contour Er:YAG laser (295).

Sapijaszko and Zachary, however, reported two cases of hypopigmentation in their series of over 100 patients resurfaced with a modulated Er:YAG laser (Contour) (285). Kim et al. resurfaced 190 patients of Fitzpatrick skin type III–V with Er:YAG lasers and observed an incidence and mean duration of hyperpigmentation of 24.7% (6.5 weeks), 42.3% (7.3 weeks), and 65.9% (7.8 days) with the short-pulsed, variable-pulsed (CO_3, Cynosure), and dual-mode (Contour, Sciton) lasers, respectively. The incidence and mean duration of hypopigmentation observed were 8.0% (4.4 months), 15.3% (5.3 months), and 24.4% (5.7 months) for the short-pulsed, variable-pulsed (CO_3, Cynosure), and dual-mode (Contour, Sciton) Er:YAG lasers (274). Goldman and Fitzpatrick have resurfaced over 1000 patients with the variable-pulsed Er:YAG laser (CO_3, Cynosure) and have not yet seen a case of prolonged hypopigmentation resulting from treatment with this particular laser (personal communication).

Topical photochemotherapy and the excimer laser have both been reported to be efficacious in the treatment of laser resurfacing-induced hypopigmentation. Grimes et al. reported moderate-to-excellent repigmentation in five of seven patients (71%) treated biweekly with a mean number of 25 sessions of topical photochemotherapy with 0.001% methoxypsoralen (55). Friedman and Geronemus reported 75% improvement of laser resurfacing-induced hypopigmentation in two patients treated with the 308-nm excimer laser for 8–10 treatment sessions. Initial treatment was performed at the minimal erythema dose minus 50 J/cm². If erythema was not seen 24 hours after the first treatment, the dose was increased by 50 mJ/cm² until erythema occurred. The average cumulative UVB dose was 1750 mJ/cm². They observed no complications and good retention of pigment at 1-month follow-up (56).

In summary, the modulated (coagulative and ablative modes) Er:YAG lasers have been able to produce "CO_2-like" clinical results with a side-effect profile that has turned out to be considerably more favorable than that of the CO_2 lasers.

COMBINATION CO_2 AND Er:YAG LASER TREATMENT
Necrotic tissue directly dysregulates wound healing and induces proteases and inflammation. Many experts believe that the thermally induced zone of necrosis left behind by the CO_2 laser is one of the main factors contributing to its adverse sequelae including prolonged postoperative erythema, pain, delayed healing, and scarring. Therefore, some authors have investigated the effect of removal of this residual zone of thermally damaged tissue after CO_2 laser resurfacing.

Goldman and colleagues studied the effect of Er:YAG laser resurfacing aimed to remove the residual zone of thermal damage left behind after CO_2 laser resurfacing (31). They randomized 10 patients to receive resurfacing to one-half of the face with a 950-μs pulsed CO_2 laser (three passes, 300 mJ, CPG settings of 596, 595, and 584) and resurfaced the other side of the face with two passes of the same CO_2 laser at the same settings followed by two passes with a short-pulsed Er:YAG laser (4-mm spot, 1.7 J, 14 J/cm²). They found that both the reepithelialization time and the duration of

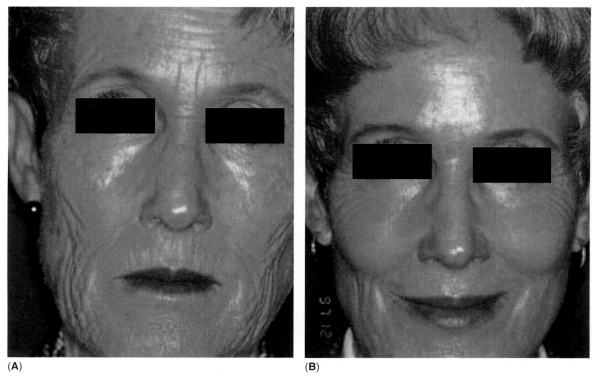

(A)   **(B)**

Figure 6.43 (**A**) With more advanced photodamage, full treatment with CO_2 laser is performed (two or three passes) and then erbium laser is used to remove layer of thermal necrosis and selectively sculpt tissue. (**B**) This technique reduces residual erythema, quickens healing, and results in enhanced clinical results, as seen 2 months postoperatively. CO_2 laser provides tissue tightening periorbitally and on cheeks, whereas erbium laser sculpts deep lines of upper lip, glabella, and forehead.

erythema were significantly less for the side treated with the combination CO_2–Er:YAG as compared with the side treated with CO_2 laser alone (Figs 6.43 and 6.44). Moreover, this beneficial effect on postoperative healing was accomplished without compromising clinical efficacy. Biopsies taken at 2–3 days, 1 week, and 4–8 weeks showed that thermal necrosis was greatly reduced by adding the erbium laser treatment, speeding healing by 2–3 days without compromising new collagen production. In addition, inflammation was reduced at 1 week, and angiogenesis was decreased at 1–8 weeks, reflecting the decreased erythema that was seen clinically (Figs 6.45 and 6.46).

McDaniel et al. compared resurfacing of the upper lip using a CO_2 laser alone (UltraPulse 5000-C, two passes, 300 mJ, 95 W, CPG density 6, spot diameter 2.25 mm, 7.5 J/cm²) with the combination of the same CO_2 laser treatment followed by three passes with a short-pulsed Er:YAG laser (7-mm spot, 2 J, 5.2 J/cm²). Medium-to-deep (class III) rhytides were improved with both techniques. However, the duration of postoperative crusting, swelling, and pruritus was significantly reduced at the sites treated with the CO_2–Er:YAG laser combination (32).

PROTOCOLS FOR COMBINATION CO_2–Er:YAG LASER TREATMENT

Both the CO_2 laser and the Er:YAG laser have unique qualities that can be exploited during resurfacing. The CO_2 laser is unique in the following ways:

- Hemostasis is achieved.
- A plateau of ablation is reached, limiting resurfacing depth if proper treatment protocols are followed.

- Collagen (skin) tightening occurs as a heat-related phenomenon, resulting in correction of loose tissue and atrophic scars.
- The first pass causes an epidermal–dermal split that allows easy and complete removal of the epidermis with a single pass.

The Er:YAG laser is unique in the following ways:

- Minimal residual thermal damage or tissue heating occurs.
- This pure-ablation laser continues to ablate with each pass and does not reach an ablation plateau with depth.
- Only minimal tissue water is required for laser–tissue interaction.

The most successful use of lasers for resurfacing would utilize each laser to take advantage of its unique benefit and to eliminate the disadvantages of each as much as possible. Accordingly, the following protocols are followed for early photodamage and for moderate to advanced photodamage.

Early Photodamage and Superficial Scars

When treating early photodamage or when patients desire a more superficial treatment allowing early return to work and as little healing time as possible (Fig. 6.47), the laser surgeon performs the following steps:

1. The epidermis is removed with a single pass of the CO_2 laser, usually with a density overlap of 20–30%. This can be accomplished very efficiently with the CO_2 laser, and biopsy studies have shown 0–10 μm of residual thermal necrosis with this single pass.

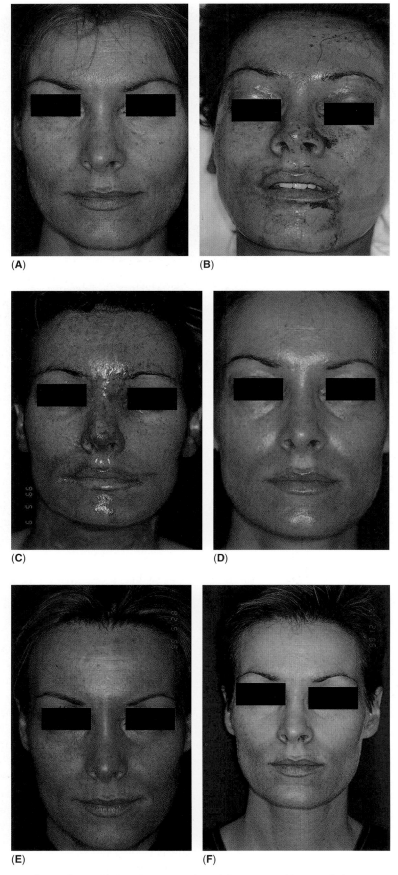

Figure 6.44 Laser resurfacing comparing the CO_2 laser with the Sciton Er:YAG laser. (**A**) A 38-year-old woman before treatment. (**B**) Immediately after treatment with two passes of the UP CO_2 laser on the right side of the face at a setting of 300 mJ, computer pattern generator with a density of 5 followed by two passes with the Er:YAG at 5 J/cm². The left side was treated with the Sciton laser using a 50 μm of ablation and 100% coagulation for two passes followed by two passes with 0% coagulation and 5 J/cm². (**C**) 2 days after treatment, the CO_2 laser-treated side is more swollen and erythematous. (**D**) 1 week after treatment, the CO_2 laser-treated side is more swollen and erythematous. (**E**) 3 weeks after treatment, the CO_2 laser side is more erythematous. (**F**) 30 weeks after treatment, there is no appreciable difference between both sides of the face.

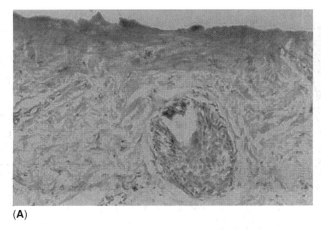
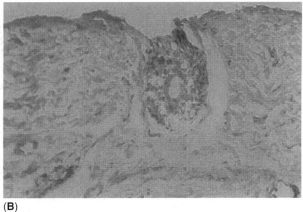

(A)   **(B)**

Figure 6.45 (**A**) Two passes of CO_2 laser at 7 J/cm² leaves approximately 70 µm of residual thermal necrosis. (**B**) Two passes of erbium laser at 10 J/cm² result in removal of approximately 50 µm of this necrotic tissue, resulting in faster wound healing.

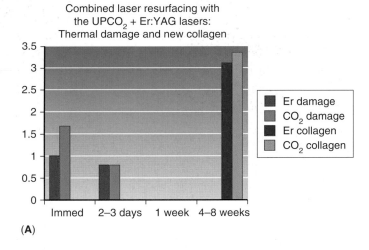

(A)

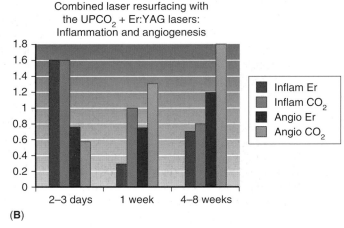

(B)

Figure 6.46 (**A**) Initial thermal necrosis was shown to be reduced significantly by adding erbium laser passes after the use of ultrapulsed CO_2 (UP CO_2) laser, without compromising new collagen formation at 4–8 weeks. (**B**) Inflammation was greatly reduced at 1 week postoperatively by removing thermal necrosis with erbium laser. Angiogenesis was also reduced at 1–8 weeks compared with the use of UP CO_2 laser alone.

If only epidermal removal is desirable, treatment is completed by using the Er:YAG laser to clean up any epidermal remnants and to feather the periphery. If dermal treatment of acne scars or photodamage is required, the areas of treatment are assessed with consideration of step 2.

2a. The CO_2 laser may be used with either the 3-mm spot or the CPG in small areas that will benefit from collagen tightening, such as the lower eyelids or medial cheeks and areas of atrophic acne scarring.

2b. The Er:YAG laser may be used uniformly in one or two passes to remove superficial photodamage and fine wrinkles and to feather the periphery.

Significant Photodamage and Scars

When treating patients who desire the maximal improvement in a single treatment and who have significant photodamage or acne scarring, the laser surgeon performs the following steps:

1. The epidermis is removed with a single pass of the CO_2 laser, usually with a density overlap of 30%.
2. A second pass of the CO_2 laser is done uniformly across the entire face, usually with a density overlap of 20–30%.
3. A third pass of the CO_2 laser is done in areas still having visible photodamage or scarring, generally the glabella and nose, middle lower forehead, middle-to-lateral cheeks and upper lip, and lateral chin areas, usually with a density overlap of 20–30%.
4. The 3-mm spot of the CO_2 laser is used to vaporize or induce thermal necrosis in areas of distinct photodamage or selectively to tighten loose photodamaged tissue, such as the eyelids, lateral cheeks, and atrophic scars. When used to induce thermal necrosis, the handpiece is moved slowly across the shoulder of a deep wrinkle line, the sharp edges of a scar crater, along the elevated portions of a linear scar, or over any dermal or epidermal growth, such as rhinophyma, syringoma, or seborrheic keratosis. The intent is to cause some superficial brownish char that will subsequently be ablated with the erbium laser.
5. The Er:YAG laser is used in a uniform manner, as in step 2b for early photodamage, removing the superficial portion of the 50–70 µm of residual thermal damage left by the CO_2 laser, thereby enhancing the reepithelialization process. This requires two passes at 1.7 J and a 4-mm pulse.

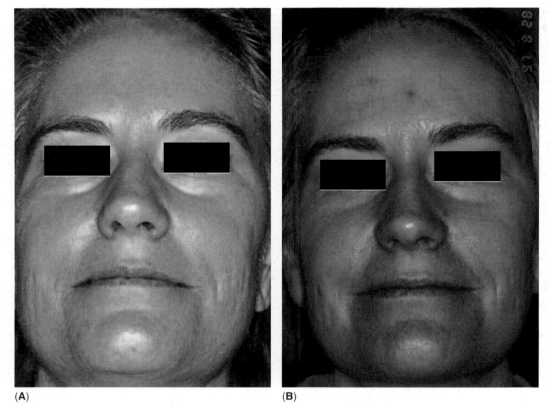

(A)   **(B)**

Figure 6.47 When treating early photodamage (**A**) especially if the patient desires to return to work with as little healing time as possible, epidermis is removed with CO_2 laser and superficial dermal resurfacing performed with erbium laser. (**B**) Although moderate improvement is seen, tissue tightening of cheeks and removal of deeper lines are not accomplished.

6. The Er:YAG laser is used with a small, focused spot size to sculpt tissue previously treated with the 3-mm CO_2 spot to smooth the tissue as uniformly as possible by ablating the necrotic tissue.
7. The periphery is feathered with the Er:YAG laser using a defocused energy of 1.0–1.7 J and a 5- to 8-mm diameter spot. This treatment protocol maximizes the benefit that can be achieved with each laser (Fig. 6.41).

THE Er:YSGG LASER
Er:YSGG Laser–Tissue Interactions
The Er:YSGG that emits laser energy at a wavelength of 2790 nm and has a water absorption coefficient of 5000/cm², roughly midway between Er:YAG (12,500/cm²) and CO_2 (1000/cm²) (58). This corresponds to an ablative threshold of about 3 J/cm² when deployed with a pulse duration between 200 and 800 μs. Interest in the Er:YSGG laser, much like the "modulated" Er:YAG, stems from its potential to impart a balance of depth and thermal impact not easily achievable with either of the other ablative wavelengths. Additionally, Ross and colleagues (58) suggested that tissue ablation can occur without removal of the ablative tissue, thereby allowing it to serve as a "biological dressing," thereby increasing the rate of healing following the procedure. The recovery time for Er:YSGG laser resurfacing based on limited current literature is about 3–5 days and is considerably shorter than traditional CO_2 resurfacing. The Er:YSGG 2790-nm laser is produced by Cutera (Brisbane, California, USA).

Currently, there are limited published data on ablative resurfacing with the Er:YSGG laser and hence a full discussion of indications, potential side effects, and recommendations for treatment are not possible until larger studies are completed (58–62,298). Ross et al. found statistically significant improvements in pigmentation, wrinkles, and skin tone following two treatments spaced 1 month apart in a small case series of eight patients (58). There were no noted cases of postinflammatory hyperpigmentation, infections, or scarring. Then, longer-term efficacy was demonstrated by Zelickson and colleagues (298), who evaluated 11 subjects with the Er:YSGG laser using a fluence of 3.5 J/cm², pulse duration of 0.4 ms, and 20% overlap. Two treatments were performed 6 weeks apart. Ninety-one percent of subjects showed improvement in tone/texture, 82% of subjects showed improvement in dyschromia and fine lines, and 54% showed improvement in wrinkles 6 weeks after the final treatment. At the 2-year follow-up visit, 57% of the overall improvement achieved at 6 weeks was maintained. No adverse events were reported throughout the study. The role of Er:YSGG resurfacing appears to be promising, although more data are needed before its role in facial rejuvenation gains clarity.

FUTURE TRENDS
A wealth of clinical literature has established the ablative resurfacing lasers as reliable, effective, and versatile tools for cutaneous rejuvenation. Patient satisfaction from cutaneous laser resurfacing remains high. A prospective survey of patients who underwent full-face resurfacing 30 months before reported that 88% of these patients felt that their appearance had improved, 75% would recommend the procedure, and 71% of them would undergo laser skin resurfacing again (57).

Newer and more versatile technologies like the modulated (coagulative and ablative mode) Er:YAG lasers and improvements in treatment protocols and postoperative care regimens have improved clinical outcomes and increased the safety of laser skin resurfacing. This added margin of safety has made it appealing for cosmetic surgeons to begin exploring the potential benefits of simultaneously combining laser resurfacing with other surgical rejuvenation techniques.

Laser skin resurfacing has been regularly, safely, and effectively combined with nonablative laser treatments in the same session. Pigmented lesions, tattoos, and periorbital hyperpigmentation can be treated safely and more effectively when a Q-switched laser (i.e., ruby, alexandrite, or Nd:YAG) is used following ablative laser resurfacing. A 100% improvement of facial telangiectasiae has been reported in patients treated with the pulsed dye laser (PDL) prior to ablative facial skin resurfacing (33).

Moreover, in both of these clinical situations, combination treatment achieves cosmetic results that are superior to those attainable with either laser alone. By combining ablative laser skin resurfacing with other problem-specific nonablative laser technologies, cosmetic surgeons are now more effectively addressing multiple cosmetic concerns for their patient in a single-treatment session.

Facial aging involves both gravity-induced ptosis of soft tissue elements and photodamage of the overlying skin. Simultaneous rhytidectomy and full-face laser resurfacing address both of these components of facial aging and theoretically should produce superior cosmetic outcome than can be achieved with either treatment modality alone. Unfortunately, early reports of skin necrosis (34–36), after simultaneous undermining and chemical peeling, initially discouraged surgeons from exploring the benefits of this therapeutic combination.

However, as rhytidectomy and laser resurfacing techniques have improved, the combination of both of these techniques has become increasingly more popular. Cosmetic surgeons are now regularly combining laser resurfacing with transconjunctival blepharoplasty, endoscopic brow lifting, and endoscopic face-lifts (39,299–302). A meta-analysis by Koch et al. of 10 series (493 patients) in which simultaneous treatment with rhytidectomy and full-face CO_2 laser resurfacing was performed found the complication rates to be no greater than those previously reported for rhytidectomy or CO_2 laser resurfacing alone (37).

The precise depth of ablation and significantly smaller zone of thermal damage produced by the Er:YAG laser as compared with the CO_2 laser are considerably advantageous when resurfacing the skin of face-lift flaps that may have compromised vascular supply. Weinstein and colleagues reported excellent results in 98% of their 257 patients who underwent combined face-lifting and full-face Er:YAG laser skin resurfacing. Two of their patients, who were heavy smokers, developed small areas of skin necrosis that healed with residual pigmentary changes. They observed no additional cases of scarring, infection, or pigmentary alterations in their large series (38). In another large series of 242 patients treated with combined face-lift and full-face resurfacing with a short-pulsed Er:YAG laser, no flap complications were observed (39). A later retrospective study of 34 patients who underwent combination CO_2 or Er:YAG laser skin resurfacing and surgical lifting, including S-lift rhytidectomy, blepharoplasty, and brow lift, reported a side effect profile that was similar to that reported after laser skin resurfacing alone (303).

Given their improved efficacy, favorable side effect profile, and remarkable versatility, resurfacing lasers will no doubt continue to have a place in the armamentarium of cosmetic surgeons striving for a comprehensive approach to facial rejuvenation.

New Resurfacing Laser Technologies

While ablative resurfacing in experienced hands has been shown to be safe and effective, the postprocedure recovery time and side effects of hypopigmentation are unacceptable to many patients. To overcome some of the morbidity and complications associated with ablative skin resurfacing, a new concept of skin rejuvenation called fractional photothermolysis was developed several years ago. In contrast to ablative skin resurfacing, which produces homogeneous thermal damage at a particular depth within the skin, fractional photothermolysis creates microscopic columns of thermal damage or tissue ablation and specifically spares the intervening tissue. A detailed review of the current state-of-the-art practices for ablative and nonablative fractional resurfacing is covered in detail in chapters 7 and 8, respectively.

ACKNOWLEDGMENTS
Portions of this chapter were updated from the chapter by Alex Carcoma and Mitchel P. Goldman in Goldman MP, ed. Cutaneous and Cosmetic Laser Surgery. St. Louis: Mosby, 2006.

REFERENCES
1. Welch AJ. The thermal response of laser irradiated tissue. IEEEJ Quantum Electron 1984; 20: 1471.
2. Alster TS. Cutaneous resurfacing with CO_2 and erbium:YAG lasers: preoperative, intraoperative and postoperative considerations. Plast Reconstr Surg 1999; 103: 619.
3. Weinstein C. Ultrapulse CO_2 laser removal of periocular wrinkles in association with laser blepharoplasty. J Clin Laser Med Surg 1994; 12: 205.
4. Lowe NJ, Lask G, Griffin ME, et al. Skin resurfacing with the UltraPulse CO_2 laser: observations on 100 patients. Dermatol Surg 1995; 21: 1025.
5. Alster TS. Clinical and histologic evaluation of six Er:YAG lasers for cutaneous resurfacing. Lasers Surg Med 1999; 24: 87.
6. Ross VE, McKinlay JR, Anderson RR. Why does CO_2 resurfacing work: a review. Arch Dermatol 1999; 135: 444.
7. Ziering CL. Cutaneous laser resurfacing with the Er:YAG laser and the char-free CO_2 laser: a clinical comparison of 100 patients. Int J Aesthetic Rest Surg 1997; 5: 29.
8. Alster TS, Lupton JR. Erbium:YAG cutaneous laser resurfacing. Dermatol Clin 2001; 19: 453.
9. Kauvar ANB, Waldorf HA, Geronemus RG. A histolopathological comparison of 'char-free' CO_2 lasers. Dermatol Surg 1996; 22: 343.
10. Weinstein C. Erbium laser resurfacing: current concepts. Plast Reconstr Surg 1999; 103: 602.
11. Teikemeier G, Goldberg DJ. Skin resurfacing with the Er:YAG laser. Dermatol Surg 1997; 23: 685.
12. Papadavid E, Katsambas A. Lasers for facial rejuvenation: a review. Int J Dermatol 2003; 42: 480.
13. Bass LS. Erbium:YAG laser skin resurfacing: preliminary clinical evaluation. Ann Plast Surg 1998; 40: 328.
14. Goldberg DJ, Meine JG. Treatment of photoaged neck skin with the pulsed erbium:YAG laser. Dermatol Surg 1998; 24: 619.
15. Goldman MP, Fitzpatrick RE, Manuskiatti W. Laser resurfacing of the neck with the Er:YAG laser. Dermatol Surg 1999; 25: 164.

16. Nanni CA, Alster TS. Complications of CO_2 laser resurfacing. An evaluation of 500 patients. Dermatol Surg 1998; 24: 315.

17. Nanni CA, Alster TS. Complications of cutaneous laser surgery: a review. Dermatol Surg 1998; 24: 209.

18. Alster TS, West TB. Resurfacing of atrophic facial acne scars with a high-energy, pulsed CO_2 laser. Dermatol Surg 1996; 22: 151.

19. Adrian RM. Pulsed CO_2 and erbium-YAG laser resurfacing: a comparative clinical and histologic study. J Cutan Laser Ther 1999; 1: 29.

20. Khatri KA, Ross V, Grevelink J, Magro C, Anderson RR. Comparison of Er:YAG and CO_2 lasers in resurfacing of facial rhytides. Arch Dermatol 1999; 135: 391.

21. Adrian RM. Pulsed CO_2 and long-pulsed 10-ms erbium-YAG laser resurfacing: a comparative clinical and histologic study. J Cutan Laser Ther 1999; 1: 197.

22. Khatri KA, Ross V, Grevelink JM, Magro CM, Anderson RR. Comparison of erbium:YAG and CO_2 lasers in resurfacing of facial rhytides. Arch Dermatol 1999; 135: 391.

23. Kaufmann R, Hibst R. Pulsed 2.94 mm Er:YAG laser skin ablation: experimental results and first clinical application. Clin Exp Dermatol 1990; 15: 389.

24. Kaufmann R, Hibst R. Pulsed Er:YAG and 308 nm UVexcimer laser: an in vitro and in vivo study of skin ablative effects. Lasers Surg Med 1989; 9: 132.

25. Fitzpatrick RE, Rostan EF, Marchell N. Collagen tightening induced by CO_2 laser versus Er:YAG laser. Lasers Surg Med 2000; 27: 395.

26. Rostan EF, Fitzpatrick RE, Goldman MP. Laser resurfacing with a long pulse Er:YAG laser compared to the 950 ms pulsed CO_2 laser. Lasers Surg Med 2001; 29: 136.

27. Newman JB, Lord JL, Ash K, McDaniel DH. Variable pulse Er:YAG laser skin resurfacing of perioral rhytides and side-by-side comparison with CO_2 laser. Lasers Surg Med 2000; 26: 208.

28. Tanzi EL, Alster TS. Treatment of atrophic facial acne scars with a dual-mode Er : YAG laser. Dermatol Surg 2002; 28: 551.

29. Kwon SD, Kye YC. Treatment of scars with a pulsed Er:YAG laser. J Cutan Laser Ther 2000; 2: 27.

30. Weinstein C, Scheflan M. Simultaneously combined Er:YAG and CO_2 laser (Derma K) for skin resurfacing. Clin Plast Surg 2000; 27: 273.

31. Goldman MP, Manuskiatti W. Combined laser resurfacing with the 950 msec pulsed CO_2 + Er:YAG lasers. Dermatol Surg 1999; 25: 160.

32. McDaniel DH, Lord J, Ash K, Newman J. Combined CO_2/Erbium:YAG laser resurfacing of peri-oral rhytides and side-by-side comparison with CO_2 laser alone. Dermatol Surg 1999; 25: 285–93.

33. Manuskiatti W, Fitzpatrick RE, Goldman MP. Treatment of facial skin using combinations of CO_2, Q-switched alexandrite, flashlamp-pumped pulsed dye and Er:YAG lasers in the same treatment session. Dermatol Surg 2000; 26: 114–20.

34. Spira M, Gerow FJ, Hardy SB. Complications of chemical face peeling. Plast Reconstr Surg 1974; 54: 397.

35. Litton C. Chemical face lifting. Plast Reconstr Surg 1962; 29: 371.

36. Baker TL, Gordon HL. Chemical face peeling: an adjunct to surgical facelifting. South Med J 1963; 56: 412.

37. Koch BB, Perkins SW. Simultaneous rhytidectomy and full-face CO_2 laser resurfacing: a case series and meta-analysis. Arch Facial Plast Surg 2002; 4: 227.

38. Weinstein C, Poszner J, Scheflan M. Combined Er:YAG laser resurfacing and face lifting. Plast Reconstr Surg 2001; 107: 586.

39. Roberts TL III, Pozner JN. Lasers, facelifting and the future. Clin Plast Surg 2000; 2: 293.

40. Kilmer SL, Chotzen VA, Silva SK, McClaren ML. Safe and effective carbon dioxide laser skin resurfacing of the neck. Lasers Surg Med 2006; 38: 653–7.

41. Kilmer SL, Chotzen V, Zelickson BD, et al. Full-face laser resurfacing using a supplemented topical anesthesia protocol. Arch Dermatol 2003; 139: 1279–83.

42. Weinstein C, Ramirez OM, Pozner JN. Postoperative care following CO_2 laser resurfacing: avoiding pitfalls. Plast Reconstr Surg 1997; 100: 1855.

43. Sriprachya-Anunt S, Fitzpatrick RE, Goldman MP, et al. Infections complicating CO_2 laser resurfacing. Dermatol Surg 1997; 23: 527.

44. Monheit GD. Facial resurfacing may trigger the herpes simplex virus. Cosmet Dermatol 1995; 8: 9.

45. Manuskiatti W, Fitzpatrick RE, Goldman MP, Krejci-Papa N. Prophylactic antibiotics in patients undergoing laser resurfacing of the skin. J Am Acad Dermatol 1999; 40: 77.

46. Ross VE, Amesbury EC, Barile A, et al. Incidence of postoperative infection or positive culture after facial laser resurfacing: a pilot study, a case report, and a proposal for a rational approach to antibiotic prophylaxis. J Am Acad Dermatol 1998; 39: 975.

47. Alster TS, Nanni CA. Famciclovir prophylaxis of herpes simplex virus reactivation after laser skin resurfacing. Dermatol Surg 1999; 25: 242.

48. Batra RS, Ort RJ, Jacob C, et al. Evaluation of a silicone occlusive dressing after laser skin resurfacing. Arch Dermatol 2001; 137: 1317.

49. Goldman MP, Roberts TL III, Skover G, et al. Optimizing wound healing in the face after laser ablation. J Am Acad Dermatol 2002; 46: 399.

50. Newman JP, Fitzgerald P, Koch RJ. Review of closed dressings after laser resurfacing. Dermatol Surg 2000; 26: 562.

51. Newman JP, Koch RJ, Goode RL. Closed dressings after laser skin resurfacing. Arch Otolaryngol Head Neck Surg 1998; 124: 751.

52. Eaglstein WH. Occlusive dressings. J Dermatol Surg Oncol 1993; 19: 716.

53. Horton S, Alster TS. Preoperative and postoperative considerations for CO_2 laser resurfacing. Cutis 1999; 64: 399.

54. West TB, Alster TS. Effect of pretreatment on the incidence of hyperpigmentation following cutaneous CO_2 laser resurfacing. Dermatol Surg 1999; 25: 15.

55. Grimes PE, Bhawan J, Kim J, et al. Laser resurfacing-induced hypopigmentation: histologic alterations and repigmentation with topical photochemotherapy. Dermatol Surg 2001; 27: 515.

56. Friedman PM, Geronemus RG. Use of the 308-nm laser for postresurfacing leukoderma. Arch Dermatol 2001; 137: 824.

57. Batra RS, Jacob C, Hobbs L, et al. A prospective survey of patient experiences after laser skin resurfacing. Results from 2.5 years of follow up. Arch Dermatol 2003; 139: 1295.

58. Ross EV, Swann M, Soon S, et al. Full-face treatments with the 2790-nm Erbium:YSGG laser system. J Drugs Dermatol 2009; 8: 248–52.

59. DiBernardo B. Assessment of the impact of high-fluence, high-overlap settings on full face treatments with the 2,790 nm Pearl YSGG laser. Laser Surg Med 2008; 40: 91.

60. Munavalli GS, Turley A, Silapunt S, Biesman B. Combining confluent and fractionally ablative modalities of a novel 2790 nm YSGG laser for facial resurfacing. Lasers Surg Med 2011; 43: 273–82.

61. Campo-Voegeli A, Arboles MP. Multi-wavelength single treatment rejuvenation program. Laser Surg Med 2009; 41: 599.

62. Perez M, Lupo M. Improvement after minimally ablative resurfacing with the confluent 2,790 nm YSGG laser: A survey of 44 fee-for-service patients and their treating physicians. Laser Surg Med 2009; 41: 603.

63. Manstein D, Herron GS, Kink RK, et al. Fractional photothermolysis: a new concept for cutaneous remodeling using microscopic patterns of thermal injury. Lasers Surg Med 2004; 34: 426.

64. Dover JS, Smoller BR, Stern RS, et al. Low-fluence CO_2 laser irradiation of lentigines. Arch Dermatol 1988; 124: 1219.

65. Kamat BR, Tang SV, Arndt KA, et al. Low-fluence CO_2 laser irradiation: selected epidermal damage to human skin. J Invest Dermatol 1985; 85: 274.

66. Wheeland RG. Revision of full-thickness skin grafts using the CO_2 laser. J Dermatol Surg Oncol 1988; 14: 130.

67. Garrett AB, Dufresne RG, Ratz JL, Berlin AJ. CO_2 laser treatment of pitted acne scarring. J Dermatol Surg Oncol 1990; 16: 737.

68. Goldman L, Shumrick DA, Rockwell J. The laser in maxillofacial surgery: preliminary investigative surgery. Arch Surg 1968; 96: 397.

69. David LM. Laser vermilion ablation for actinic cheilitis. J Dermatol Surg Oncol 1985; 11: 605.

70. Brauner G, Schliftman A. Laser surgery in children. J Dermatol Surg Oncol 1987; 13: 178.

71. David LM, Lask GP, Glassberg E, et al. Laser ablation for cosmetic and medical treatment of facial actinic damage. Cutis 1989; 43: 583.

72. Walsh JJ, Deutsch TF. Pulsed CO_2 laser tissue ablation: measurement of the ablation rate. Lasers Surg Med 1988; 8: 264.

73. Fitzpatrick RE, Goldman MP, Ruiz-Esparza JR. Clinical advantage of the CO_2 laser superpulsed mode: treatment of verruca vulgaris, sebor-

rheic keratoses, lentigines and actinic cheilitis. J Dermatol Surg Oncol 1994; 20: 449.

74. Olbricht SM. Use of the CO_2 laser in dermatologic surgery: a clinical relevant update for 1993. J Dermatol Surg Oncol 1993; 93: 364.

75. Fitzpatrick RE, Goldman MP. CO2 laser surgery. In: Cutaneous Laser Surgery: The Art and Science of Selective Photothermolysis. St Louis: CV Mosby, 1994.

76. Anderson RR, Parrish JA. Selective photothermolysis: precise microsurgery by selective absorption of pulsed radiation. Science 1983; 220: 524.

77. Green HA, Burd E, Nishioka NS. Pulsed CO_2 laser ablation of burned skin: in vitro and in vivo analysis. Lasers Surg Med 1990; 10: 476.

78. Green HA, Burd E, Nishioka NS, et al. Mid-dermal wound healing: a comparison between dermatomal excision and pulsed CO_2 ablation. Arch Dermatol 1992; 128: 639.

79. Fitzpatrick RE, Tope WD, Goldman MP, Satur NM. Pulsed CO_2 laser, tricholoroacetic acid, Baker-Gordon phenol, and dermabrasion: a comparative clinical and histological study of cutaneous resurfacing in a porcine model. Arch Dermatol 1996; 132: 469.

80. Kauver ANB, Waldorf HA, Geronemus RG. A histopathological comparison of 'char-free' CO_2 lasers. Dermatol Surg 1996; 22: 343.

81. Cotton J, Hood AF, Gonin R, et al. Histologic evaluation of preauricular and postauricular human skin after high-energy, short pulse CO_2 laser. Arch Dermatol 1996; 132: 425.

82. Stuzin JM, Baker TJ, Baker TM, Kligman AM. Histologic effects of the high energy pulsed CO_2 laser on photoaged facial skin. Plast Reconstr Surg 1997; 97: 2036.

83. Alster TS. Histology of CO_2 resurfacing. Semin Cutan Med Surg 1996; 15: 189.

84. Ross EV, Domankevitz Y, Skrobal M, Anderson RR. Effects of CO_2 laser pulse duration in ablation and residual thermal damage: implications for skin resurfacing. Lasers Surg Med 1996; 19: 123.

85. Venugopalan V, Nishioka N, Mikic B. The effect of laser parameters on the zone of thermal injury produced by laser ablation of biological tissue. ASME Biomech Eng 1994; 116: 62.

86. Gardner ES, Reinisch L, Stricklin GP, et al. In vitro changes in non-facial human skin following laser resurfacing: a comparison study. Lasers Surg Med 1996; 19: 379.

87. Schomacker K, Walsh J, Flott T, Deutsch T. Thermal damage produced by high-irradiance continuous wave CO_2 laser cutting of tissue. Lasers Surg Med 1990; 10: 74.

88. McKenzie A. How far does thermal damage extend beneath the surface of CO_2 laser incisions? Phys Med Biol 1983; 28: 905.

89. Walsh J, Flotte T, Anderson R, Deutsch T. Pulsed CO_2 laser tissue ablation: effects of tissue type and pulse duration on thermal damage. Lasers Surg Med 1988; 8: 108.

90. Hobbs E, Bailin P, Wheeland R, Ratz J. Superpulsed lasers: minimizing thermal damage with short duration, high irradiance pulses. J Dermatol Surg Oncol 1987; 13: 955.

91. Apfelberg DB. The UltraPulse CO_2 laser with computer pattern generator automatic scanner for facial cosmetic surgery and resurfacing. Ann Plast Surg 1996; 36: 522.

92. Rubach BW, Schoenrock LD. Histological and clinical evaluation of facial resurfacing using a CO_2 laser with the computer pattern generator. Arch Otolaryncol Head Neck Surg 1997; 123: 929.

93. Apfelberg DB. UltraPulse CO_2 laser with CPG scanner for full-face resurfacing for rhytids, photoaging, and acne scars. Plast Reconstr Surg 1997; 99: 1817.

94. Apfelberg DB, Smoller B. UltraPulse CO_2 laser with CPG scanner for deepithelialization: clinical and histologic study. Plast Reconstr Surg 1997; 99: 2089.

95. Hruza GJ, Fitzpatrick RE, Dover JS. Laser skin resurfacing. In: Arndt KA, Olbricht SM, Dover JS, eds. Cutaneous Laser Surgery. Philadelphia: Lippincott-Raven, 1997.

96. Stuzin JM, Baker TJ, Baker TM, Kligman AM. Histologic effects of the high-energy pulsed CO_2 laser on photoaged facial skin. Plast Reconstr Surg 1997; 99: 2036.

97. Waldorf HA, Kauvar ANB, Geronemus RG. Skin resurfacing of fine to deep rhytides using char-free CO_2 laser in 47 patients. Dermatol Surg 1995; 21: 940.

98. Rein R. Physical and surgical principles governing CO_2 laser surgery on the skin. Dermatol Clin 1991; 9: 297.

99. Chernoff G, Shoenrock L, Cramer H, et al. Cutaneous laser resurfacing. Int J Aesthetic Rest Surg 1995; 3: 57.

100. Fitzpatrick RE, Smith SR, Sriprachya-Anunt S. Depth of vaporization and the effect of pulse stacking with a high energy, pulsed CO_2 laser. J Am Acad Dermatol 1999; 40: 615.

101. Fitzpatrick RE, Goldman MP, Satur NM, Tope WD. Pulsed CO_2 laser resurfacing of photoaged skin. Arch Dermatol 1996; 132: 395.

102. Ross EV, Naseef M, Skrobal JM, et al. In vivo dermal collagen shrinkage and remodeling following CO_2 laser resurfacing. Lasers Surg Med 1996; 19: 38.

103. Brugmans MJP, Kemper J, Gijsbers GHM, et al. Temperature response of biological materials to pulsed non-ablative CO_2 laser irradiation. Lasers Surg Med 1991; 11: 587.

104. Alster TS. Comparison of two high-energy pulsed CO_2 lasers in the treatment of periorbital rhytides. Dermatol Surg 1996; 22: 541.

105. Manuskiatti W, Fitzpatrick RE, Goldman MP. Long-term effectiveness and side effects of CO_2 laser resurfacing for photoaged facial skin. Am Acad Dermatol 1999; 40: 401–11.

106. Ross EV, Grossman MC, Duke D, Grevelink JM. Long-term results after CO_2 laser skin resurfacing: a comparison of scanned and pulsed systems. J Am Acad Dermatol 1997; 37: 709.

107. Weinstein C. CO_2 laser resurfacing: long-term follow-up in 2123 patients. Clin Plast Surg 1998; 25: 109.

108. Abergel RP, Dahlman CM. The CO_2 laser approach to the treatment of acne scarring. Cosmet Dermatol 1995; 8: 33.

109. Hruza JG. Skin resurfacing with lasers. Fitzpatrick's J Clin Dermatol 1995; 3: 38.

110. Alamillos-Granados FJ, Naval-Gias L, Dean-Ferrer A, et al. CO_2 laser vermilionectomy for actinic cheilitis. J Oral Maxillofac Surg 1993; 51: 118.

111. Stanley RJ, Roenigk RK. Actinic cheilitis: treatment with the CO_2 laser. Mayo Clin Proc 1988; 63: 230.

112. Robinson JK. Actinic cheilitis: a prospective study comparing four treatment methods. Arch Otolaryngol Head Neck Surg 1989; 115: 848.

113. Zelickson BD, Roenigk RK. Actinic cheilitis: treatment with the CO_2 laser. Cancer 1990; 65: 1307.

114. Dufresne RJ, Garrett AB, Bailin PL, et al. CO_2 laser treatment of chronic actinic cheilitis. J Am Acad Dermatol 1988; 19: 876.

115. Johnson TM, Sebastien TS, Lowe L, et al. CO_2 laser treatment of actinic cheilitis: clinicohistopathologic correlation to determine the optimal depth of destruction. J Am Acad Dermatol 1992; 27: 737.

116. Ries WR, Duncavage JA, Ossoff RH. CO_2 laser treatment of actinic cheilitis. Mayo Clin Proc 1988; 63: 294.

117. Scheinberg RS. CO_2 laser treatment of actinic cheilitis. West J Med 1992; 156: 192.

118. Whitaker DC. Microscopically proven cure of actinic cheilitis by CO_2 laser. Lasers Surg Med 1987; 7: 520.

119. Frankel DH. CO_2 laser vermilionectomy for chronic actinic cheilitis. Facial Plast Surg 1989; 6: 158.

120. Goldman MP, Fitzpatrick RE, Smith SS. Resurfacing complications and their management. In: Coleman WP, Lawrence N, eds. Laser Resurfacing. Baltimore, MD: Williams & Wilkins, 1997.

121. Lowe NJ, Lask G, Griffin ME. Laser skin resurfacing: pre- and post-treatment guidelines. Dermatol Surg 1995; 21: 1017.

122. Fitzpatrick RE, Goldman MP. Laser treatment of benign pigmented lesions using a 300 nanosecond pulse and 510 nm wavelength. J Dermatol Surg Oncol 1993; 19: 341.

123. Goldberg D. Benign pigmented lesions of the skin: treatment with the Q-switched ruby laser. J Dermatol Surg Oncol 1993; 19: 376.

124. Brauner GJ, Schliftman AB. Treatment of pigmented lesions of the skin with the alexandrite laser. Lasers Surg Med 1992; 4: 72.

125. Monheit GD. The Jessner's TCA peel: a medium-depth chemical peel. J Dermatol Surg Oncol 1989; 15: 945.

126. Brody HJ, Hailey CW. Medium-depth chemical peeling of the skin: a variation of superficial chemosurgery. J Dermatol Surg Oncol 1986; 12: 1268.

127. Taylor CR, Anderson RR. Ineffective treatment of refractory melasma and post-inflammatory hyperpigmentation by Q-switched ruby laser. J Dermatol Surg Oncol 1994; 20: 592.

128. Greenbaum SS, Krull EA, Watnich K. Comparison of CO_2 laser and electrosurgery in the treatment of rhinophyma. J Am Acad Dermatol 1988; 18: 363.

129. Wheeland RG, Bailin PL, Ratz JL. Combined CO_2 laser excision and vaporization in the treatment of rhinophyma. J Dermatol Surg Oncol 1987; 13: 172.

130. Apfelberg DB, Maser MR, Lash H, et al. Superpulse CO_2 laser treatment of facial syringomata. Lasers Surg Med 1987; 7: 533.

131. Wheeland RG, Bailin PL, Kronberg E. Carbon dioxide (CO_2) laser vaporization for the treatment of multiple trichoepithelioma. J Dermatol Surg Oncol 1984; 10: 470.

132. Apfelberg DB, Maser MR, Lash H, et al. Treatment of xanthelasma palpebrum with the CO_2 laser. J Dermatol Surg Oncol 1987; 13: 149.

133. Wheeland RG, Bailin PL, Kantor GR, et al. Treatment of adenoma sebaceum with CO_2 laser vaporization. J Dermatol Surg Oncol 1985; 11: 861.

134. Ratz JL, Bailin PL, Wheeland RG. CO_2 laser treatment of epidermal nevi. J Dermatol Surg Oncol 1986; 12: 567.

135. Hohenleutner U, Landthaler M. Laser therapy of verrucous epidermal nevi. Clin Exp Dermatol 1993; 18: 124.

136. Lask G, Keller G, Lowe N, Gormley D. Laser skin resurfacing with the SilkTouch flashscanner for facial rhytides. Dermatol Surg 1995; 21: 1021.

137. Blitzer A, Brin MF, Keen MS, et al. Botulinum toxin for the treatment of hyperfunctional lines of the face. Arch Otolaryngol Head Neck Surg 1993; 119: 1018.

138. Carruthers JDA, Carruthers JA. Treatment of glabellar frown lines with C. botulinum-A exotoxin. J Dermatol Surg Oncol 1992; 18: 17.

139. Garcia A, Fulton JE. Cosmetic denervation of the muscles of facial expression with botulinum toxin: a dose-response study. Dermatol Surg 1996; 22: 39.

140. Keen M, Blitzer A, Aviv J, et al. Botulinum toxin-A for hyper-kinetic facial lines: results of a double-blind, placebo-controlled study. Plast Reconstr Surg 1994; 94: 94.

141. Bhawan J, Gonzales-Serva A, Nehal K, et al. Effects of tretinoin on photodamaged skin: a histologic study. Arch Dermatol 1991; 127: 666.

142. Orringer JS, Kang S, Johnson TM, et al. Tretinoin treatment before carbon-dioxide laser resurfacing: a clinical and biochemical analysis. J Am Acad Dermatol 2004; 51: 940.

143. Ruiz-Esparza J, Barba Gomez JM. Labastida Gomez de la Torre O. Erythema after laser skin resurfacing. Dermatol Surg 1998; 24: 79.

144. Ruiz-Esparza J, Lupton JR. Laser resurfacing of darkly pigmented patients. Dermatol Clin 2002; 20: 113.

145. Alster TS. Combined laser resurfacing and tretinoin treatment of facial rhytides. Cosmet Dermatol 1997; 10: 39–42.

146. Bernstein LJ, Kauvar ANB, Grossman MC, Geronemus RG. The short- and long-term side effects of carbon dioxide laser resurfacing. Dermatol Surg 1997; 23: 519–25.

147. Nanni CA, Alster TS. Complications of carbon dioxide laser resurfacing. Dermatol Surg 1998; 24: 315–20.

148. Waldorf HA, Kauvar ANB, Geronemus RG. Skin resurfacing of fine to deep rhytides using a char-free carbon dioxide laser in 47 patients. Dermatol Surg 1995; 21: 940–6.

149. Gaspar ZE, Vincuillo C, Elliott T. Antibiotic prophylaxis for full-face laser resurfacing: is it necessary? Arch Dermatol 2001; 137: 313–15.

150. Friedman PM, Geronemus RG. Antibiotic prophylaxis in laser resurfacing patients. Dermatol Surg 2000; 26: 695.

151. Walia S, Alster TS. Cutaneous CO_2 laser resurfacing infection rate with and without prophylactic antibiotics. Dermatol Surg 1999; 25: 857.

152. Grekin RC. Cutaneous CO_2 laser resurfacing infection rate with and without prophylactic antibiotics. Dermatol Surg 1999; 25: 51.

153. Raz R, Miron D, Colodner R, et al. A 1-year trial of nasal mupirocin in the prevention of recurrent staphylococcal nasal colonization and skin infection. Arch Intern Med 1996; 156: 1109.

154. Russell SW, Dinehart SM, Davis I, Flock ST. Efficacy of corneal shields in protecting patients' eyes from laser irradiation. Dermatol Surg 1996; 22: 613.

155. Fitzpatrick RE, Williams B, Goldman MP. Preoperative anesthesia and postoperative considerations in laser resurfacing. Semin Cutan Med Surg 1996; 15: 170.

156. Dvork HF. Tumors: wounds that do not heal: similarities between tumor stroma generation and wound healing. N Engl J Med 1986; 315: 1650.

157. Peacock EE Jr. Inflammation and the cellular response to injury. In: Peacock EE Jr, ed. Wound Repair. Philadelphia: WB Saunders, 1984.

158. Peacock EE Jr. Biological and pharmacological control of scar tissue. In: Peacock EE Jr, ed. Wound Repair. Philadelphia: WB Saunders, 1984.

159. Kanzler MH, Gorsulowsky DC, Swanson NA. Basic mechanisms in the healing cutaneous wound. J Dermatol Surg Oncol 1986; 12: 1156.

160. Goslen JB. Wound healing for the dermatologic surgeon. J Dermatol Surg Oncol 1988; 14: 959.

161. Stenn KS, Malhotra R. Epithelialization. In: Cohen IK, Diegelmann RF, Lindblad WJ, eds. Wound Healing: Biochemical and Clinical Aspects. Philadelphia: WB Saunders, 1992.

162. Waldorf H, Fewkes J. Wound healing. Adv Dermatol 1995; 10: 77.

163. Bach R, Nemerson Y, Konigsberg W. Purification and characterization of bovine tissue factor. J Biol Chem 1981; 256: 8324.

164. Leibovich SJ, Ross R. A macrophage-dependent factor that stimulates the proliferation of fibroblasts in vitro. Am J Pathol 1976; 84: 501.

165. Leibovich SJ, Ross R. The role of the macrophage in wound repair: a study with hydrocortisone and antimacrophage serum. Am J Pathol 1975; 78: 71.

166. Shavit ZB, Ray A, Goldman R. Complement and Fc receptor-mediated phagocytosis of normal and stimulated mouse peritoneal macrophages. Eur J Immunol 1979; 9: 385.

167. Littman BH, Ruddy S. Production of the second component of complement by human monocytes: stimulation by antigen-activated lymphocytes or lymphokines. J Exp Med 1979; 145: 1344.

168. Clark RAF. Cutaneous tissue repair: basic biologic considerations. J Am Acad Dermatol 1985; 13: 701.

169. Clark RAF. Basics of cutaneous wound repair. J Dermatol Surg Oncol 1993; 19: 693.

170. Bailey AJ, Bazin S, Sims TJ, et al. Characterization of the collagen of human hypertrophic and normal scars. Biochim Biophys Acta 1974; 21: 404.

171. Oliver N, Baba M, Diegelmann R. Fibronectin gene transcription is enhanced in abnormal wound healing. J Invest Dermatol 1992; 99: 579.

172. Skuta GL, Parrish RK II. Wound healing in glaucoma filtering surgery. Surv Ophthalmol 1987; 32: 149.

173. Ross R, Raines EW, Bowen-Pope DR. The biology of platelet-derived growth factor. Cell 1986; 46: 155.

174. Ross R. Fibroblast proliferation induced by blood cells. Agents Actions Suppl 1980; 7: 81.

175. Bijrkedal-Hansen H. Catabolism and turnover of collagens: collagenases. Methods Enzymol 1987; 144: 140.

176. Liu X, Wu H, Byrne M, et al. A targeted mutation at the known collagenase cleavage site in mouse type I collagen impairs tissue remodeling. J Cell Biol 1995; 130: 227.

177. Matrisian LM, Hogan BL. Growth factor-regulated proteases and extracellular matrix remodeling during mammalian development. Curr Top Dev Biol 1990; 24: 219.

178. Prockop D, Kivirikko K. Heritable diseases of collagen. N Engl J Med 1984; 311: 376.

179. Mast BA. The skin. In: Cohen IK, Diegelmann RF, Lindblad WJ, eds. Wound Healing: Biochemical and Clinical Aspects. Philadelphia: WB Saunders, 1992.

180. Lamberg SI, Stoolmiller AC. Glycosaminoglycans: a biochemical and clinical review. J Invest Dermatol 1974; 63: 433.

181. VanLis JM, Kalsbeek GL. Glycosaminoglycans in human skin. Br J Dermatol 1973; 88: 355.

182. Levensen SM, Geever EG, Crowley LV, et al. The healing of rat skin wounds. Ann Surg 1965; 161: 293.

183. Rudolph R. Contraction and the control of contraction. World J Surg 1980; 4: 279.

184. Gabbiani G, Ryan GB, Majne G. Presence of modified fibroblasts in granulation tissue and their possible role in wound contraction. Experientia 1971; 27: 549.

185. Majno G. Contraction of granulation tissue in vitro: similarity to smooth muscle. Science 1971; 173: 543.

186. Rudolph R, Berg JV, Ehrlich HP. Wound contraction and scar contracture. In: Cohen IK, Diegelmann RF, Linblad WJ, eds. Wound Healing: Biochemical and Clinical Aspects. Philadelphia: WB Saunders, 1992.

187. Bourne G, ed. The Biochemistry and Physiology of Bone. New York: Academic Press, 1956.

188. Fisher AA. Lasers and allergic contact dermatitis to topical antibiotics, with particular reference to bacitracin. Cutis 1996; 58: 252.

189. Dooms-Goossens A, Degreef H. Contact allergy to petrolatums. II. Attempts to identify the nature of allergens. Contact Dermat 1983; 9: 247.

190. Hinman CC, Maibach H, Winter GD. Effect of air exposure and occlusion on experimental human skin wounds. Nature 1963; 200: 377.

191. Schilling RSF, Roberts M, Goodman N. Clinical trial of occlusive plastic dressings. Lancet 1950; 1: 293.

192. Hunter GR, Change FC. Outpatient burns: a prospective study. J Trauma 1976; 16: 191.

193. Eaglstein WH, Mertz PM. 'Inert' vehicles do affect wound healing. J Invest Dermatol 1980; 74: 90.

194. Martin A. The Use of antioxidants in healing. Dermatol Surg 1996; 22: 156.

195. O'Donnell-Torney J, Nathan CF, Lanks K. Secretion of pyruvate: an antioxidant defense of mammalian cells. J Exp Med 1987; 165: 500.

196. Shacter E. Serum-free medium for growth factor-dependent and independent plastocytomas and hybridomas. J Immunol Meth 1987; 99: 259.

197. Winter GD. Formation of scab and rate of epithelialization of superficial wounds in the skin of the domestic pig. Nature 1962; 193: 293.

198. Rovee DY, Kurowsky CA, Lobun J, et al. Effect of local wound environment on epidermal healing. In: Maibach HL, Rovee DT, eds. Epidermal Wound Healing. Chicago: Year Book, 1972.

199. Geronemus RG, Robins P. The effect of two new dressings on epidermal wound healing. J Dermatol Surg Oncol 1982; 8: 850.

200. Mandy S. A new primary wound dressing made of polyethylene oxide gel. J Dermatol Surg Oncol 1983; 9: 153.

201. May SR. Physiology, immunology and clinical efficacy of an adherent polyurethane wound dressing: Op-Site. In: Wise DL, ed. Burn Wound Coverings. vol 2 Boca Raton, FL: CRC, 1984.

202. Eaglstein WH, Mertz PM. New methods for assessing epidermal wound healing: the effects of triamcinolone acetonide and polyethylene film occlusion. J Invest Dermatol 1978; 71: 382.

203. Barnett A, Berkowitz RL, Mius R, et al. Comparison of synthetic adhesive moisture vapor permeable and fine mesh gauze dressings for split-thickness skin graft donor sites. Am J Surg 1983; 145: 379.

204. Van Rijswijk L, Brown D, Friedman S, et al. Multicenter clinical evaluation of hydrocolloid dressing for leg ulcers. Cutis 1985; 35: 173.

205. Eaton AC. A controlled trial to evaluate and compare a sutureless skin closure technique (Op-Site skin closure) with conventional skin suturing and clipping in abdominal surgery. Br J Surg 1980; 67: 857.

206. Kannon GA, Garrett AB. Moist wound healing with occlusive dressings: a clinical review. Dermatol Surg 1995; 21: 583.

207. Eaglstein WH. Experiences with biosynthetic dressings. J Am Acad Dermatol 1985; 12: 434.

208. Bolton LL, Johnson CL, Rijswijk LV. Occlusive dressings: therapeutic agents and effects on drug delivery. Clin Dermatol 1992; 9: 573.

209. Winter GD. Epidermal regeneration studied in the domestic pig. In: Maibach HL, Rovee DT, eds. Epidermal Wound Healing. Chicago: Year Book, 1972.

210. Alvarez OM, Mertz PM, Eaglstein WH. The effect of occlusive dressings on collagen synthesis and re-epithelialization in superficial wounds. J Surg Res 1983; 35: 142.

211. Brown GL, Curtsinger L III, Brightwell JR, et al. Enhancement of epidermal regeneration by biosynthetic epidermal growth factor. J Exp Med 1986; 163: 1319.

212. Eaglstein WH, Davis SC, Mehle AL, Mertz PM. Optimal use of an occlusive dressing to enhance healing: effect of delayed application and early removal on wound healing. Arch Dermatol 1988; 124: 392.

213. Mertz PM, Eaglstein WH. The effect of semi-occlusive dressing on the microbial population in superficial wounds. Arch Surg 1984; 119: 287.

214. Geronemus RG, Mertz PM, Eaglstein WH. The effects of topical antimicrobial agents. Arch Dermatol 1979; 115: 1311.

215. Linsky CB, Rovee DT, Dow T. Effect of dressing on wound inflammation and scar tissue. In: Dineen P, Hildick-Smith G, eds. The Surgical Wound. Philadelphia: Lea & Febiger, 1981.

216. Marples RR. The effect of hydration on the bacterial flora of the skin. In: Maibach HI, Hildick-Smith G, eds. Skin Bacteria and Their Role in Infection. New York: McGraw-Hill, 1963.

217. Buchan IA, Andrews JK, Lang SM. Laboratory investigation of the composition and properties of pig skin wound exudate under Op-Site. Burns 1981; 8: 39.

218. Buchan IA, Andrews JK, Lang SM. Clinical and laboratory investigation of the composition and properties of human skin wound exudate under semi-permeable dressing. Burns 1981; 7: 326.

219. Oliveria-Gandia M, Davis SC, Mertz PM. Can occlusive dressing composition influence proliferation of bacterial wound pathogens? Wounds 1998; 10: 4.

220. Hutchison JJ, McGuckin M. Occlusive dressings: a microbiologic and clinical review. Am J Infect Control 1990; 18: 257.

221. Handfield-Jones SE, Grattan CEH, Simpson RA, et al. Comparison of a hydrocolloid dressing and paraffin gauze in the treatment of venous ulcers. Br J Dermatol 1988; 118: 425.

222. Gilchrist B, Reed C. The bacteriology of chronic venous ulcers treated with occlusive hydrocolloid dressings. Br J Dermatol 1989; 121: 337.

223. Leydon JL, Steward R, Kligman AM. Updated in vivo methods for evaluating topical antimicrobial agent on human skin. J Invest Dermatol 1979; 72: 165.

224. Mertz PM, Ovington LG. Wound healing microbiology. Dermatol Clin 1993; 11: 739.

225. Christian MM, Behroozan DS, Moy RI. Delayed infections following full-face CO_2 laser resurfacing and occlusive dressing use. Dermatol Surg 2000; 26: 32.

226. Fitzpatrick RE, Geronemus RG, Grevelink JM, et al. The incidence of adverse healing reactions occurring with UltraPulse CO_2 resurfacing during a multicenter study. Lasers Surg Med Suppl 1996; 8: 34.

227. Yurt RW. Burns. In: Mandell GL, Bennett JE, Dolin R, eds. Mandell, Douglas and Bennett's Principles and Practice of Infectious Diseases. New York: Churchill Livingstone, 1995.

228. Phillips LG, Heggers JP, Robson MC, et al. The effect of endogenous skin bacteria on burn wound infection. Ann Plast Surg 1989; 23: 35.

229. Husain MT, Karim QN, Tajuri S. Analysis of infection in a burn ward. Burns 1989; 15: 299.

230. Shalita A. Personal communication. Int J Dermatol 1997; 36: 783–7.

231. Roberts TL, Lettieri JT, Ellis LB. CO_2 laser resurfacing: recognizing and minimizing complications. Aesth Surg Q 1996; 16: 141.

232. Coates J. Basic physics of erbium laser resurfacing. J Cutan Laser Ther 1999; 1: 71.

233. Walsh JT, Deutsch TF. Er:YAG laser ablation of tissue: measurement of ablation rates. Lasers Surg Med 1989; 9: 327.

234. Hibst R, Kaufmann R. Fundamentals of pulsed UV and mid-infrared laser skin ablation. In: Steiner R, Kaufmann R, Landthaler M, Braun-Falco O, eds. Lasers in Dermatology. Berlin: Springer-Verlag, 1991.

235. Hohenleutner U, Hohenleutner S, Bäumler Landthaler M. Fast and effective skin ablation with an Er:YAG laser: determination of ablation rates and thermal damage zones. Lasers Surg Med 1997; 20: 242.

236. McDaniel DH, Ash K, Lord J, et al. The Er : YAG laser: a review and preliminary report on resurfacing of the face, neck and hands. Aesthetic Surg J 1997; 17: 157.

237. Hibst R, Kaufmann R. Effects of laser parameters on pulsed Er : YAG laser skin ablation. Lasers Med Sci 1991; 6: 391.

238. Kaufmann R, Hartmann A, Hibst R. Cutting and skin ablative properties of pulsed mid-infrared laser surgery. J Dermatol Surg Oncol 1994; 20: 112.

239. Walsh JT, Flotte TJ, Deutsch TF. Er:YAG laser ablation tissue: effect of pulse duration and tissue type on thermal damage. Lasers Surg Med 1989; 9: 314.

240. Kaufmann R, Hibst R. Vergleich verschildener Mittelin-frafot: Laser für die ablation der Hauset. Lasermedizin 1995; 11: 19.

241. Walsh JT. Pulsed Laser Ablation Of Tissue: Analysis of the Removal Process and Tissue Healing. Cambridge, MA: PhD thesis, MIT archives, 1988.

242. Wolbarsht ML. Laser surgery: CO_2 or HF.IEEE. J Quantum Electronics 1984; 20: 1427.

243. Kaufmann R, Hibst R. Pulsed UV and mid-infrared laser skin ablation: experimental and first clinical results. In: Steiner R, Kaufmann R, Landthaler M, Braun-Falco O, eds. Lasers in Dermatology. Berlin: Springer-Verlag, 1991.

244. Hughes PS. Skin contraction following Er:YAG laser resurfacing. Dermatol Surg 1998; 24: 109.

245. Goldberg DJ, Cutler KB. The use of the Er:YAG laser for the treatment of class III rhytids. Dermatol Surg 1999; 25: 713.

246. Weinstein C. Computerized scanning Er:YAG laser for skin resurfacing. Dermatol Surg 1998; 24: 83.

247. Ymauchi PS, Lask G, Lowe NJ. Botulinum toxin type A gives adjunctive benefit to periorbital laser resurfacing. J Cosmet Laser Ther 2004; 6: 145.

248. Rostan EF, Goldman MP, Fitzpatrick RE. Laser resurfacing with a dual mode, long-pulse Erbium : YAG laser compared to the 950 ms pulsed CO_2 laser. Am J Cos Surg 2000; 17: 227.

249. Jeong JT, Kye YC. Resurfacing of pitted facial acne scars with a long-pulsed Er:YAG laser. Dermatol Surg 2001; 27: 107.

250. Kye YC. Resurfacing of pitted facial scars with a pulsed Er:YAG laser. Dermatol Surg 1997; 23: 880.

251. Ammirati CT, Cottingham TJ, Hruza GJ. Immediate postoperative laser resurfacing improves second intention healing on the nose: 5-year experience. Dermatol Surg 2001; 27: 147.

252. Khatri KA. Ablation of cutaneous lesions using an Er:YAG laser. J Cosmet Laser Ther 2003; 5: 150.

253. Jiang SB, Levine VJ, Nehal KS, et al. Er:YAG laser for the treatment of actinic keratoses. Dermatol Surg 2000; 26: 437.

254. Park JH, Hwang ES, Kim SN, Kye YC. Er:YAG laser treatment of verrucous epidermal nevi. Dermatol Surg 2004; 30: 378.

255. Trelles MA, Moreno-Arias GA. Becker's nevus: erbium:YAG versus Q-switched neodinium : YAG? Lasers Surg Med 2004; 34: 295.

256. Borelli C, Kaudewitz P. Xanthelasma palpebrarum: treatment with the Er:YAG laser. Lasers Surg Med 2001; 29: 260.

257. Drnovsek-Olup B, Vedlin B. Use of Er:YAG laser for benign skin disorders. Lasers Surg Med 1997; 21: 13.

258. Kageyama N, Tope W. Treatment of multiple eruptive hair cysts with erbium:YAG laser. Dermatol Surg 1999; 25: 819.

259. Hughes PSH. Multiple military osteomas of the face ablated with the Er:YAG laser. Arch Dermatol 1999; 135: 378.

260. Ammirati CT, Giancola JM, Hruza GJ. Adult-onset facial colloid milium successfully treated with the long-pulsed Er:YAG laser. Dermatol Surg 2002; 28: 215.

261. Langdon R. Erbium : YAG laser enables complete ablation of periungual verrucae without the need for injected anesthetics. Dermatol Surg 1998; 24: 157.

262. Orenstein A, Haik J, Tamir J, et al. Treatment of rhynophyma with Er:YAG laser. Lasers Surg Med 2001; 29: 230.

263. Beier C, Kaufmann R. Efficacy of Er:YAG laser ablation in Darier's disease and Hailey–Hailey disease. Arch Dermatol 1999; 135: 423.

264. Wenzel J, Petrow W, Tappe K, Gerdsen R. Treatment of Dowling–Degos disease with Er:YAG laser: results after 2.5 years. Dermatol Surg 2003; 29: 1161.

265. Albertini JG, Holck DEE, Farley MF. Zoon's balanitis treated with Er:YAG laser ablation. Lasers Surg Med 2002; 30: 123.

266. Yang JS, Kye YC. Treatment of vitiligo with autologous epidermal grafting by means of pulsed Er : YAG laser. J Am Acad Dermatol 1999; 38: 280.

267. Brody HJ. Complications of chemical peels. In: Brody HM, ed. Chemical Peeling. St Louis: Mosby Yearbook, 1992.

268. Fitzpatrick RE, Goldman MP, Sriprachya-Anunt S. Resurfacing of photodamaged skin on the neck with an UltraPulse® CO_2 laser. Lasers Surg Med 2001; 28: 145.

269. Rosenberg JR. Full-face and neck laser skin resurfacing. Plast Reconstr Surg 1997; 100: 1846.

270. Jimenez G, Spencer J. Erbium:YAG laser resurfacing of the hands, arms and neck. Dermatol Surg 1999; 25: 831.

271. Polnikorn N, Goldberg DJ, Suwanchinda A, Ng SW. Erbium : YAG laser resurfacing in Asians. Dermatol Surg 1998; 24: 1303.

272. Airan LE, Hruza G. Current lasers in resurfacing. Facial Plast Surg Clin North Am 2005; 13: 127.

273. Sriprachya-Anunt S, Marchell NL, Fitzpatrick RE, et al. Facial resurfacing in patients with Fitzpatrick skin type IV. Lasers Surg Med 2002; 30: 86.

274. Kim YJ, Lee HS, Son SW, et al. Analysis of hyperpigmentation and hypopigmentation after Er:YAG laser skin resurfacing. Lasers Surg Med 2005; 36: 47.

275. Fitzpatrick RE, Goldman MP. Resurfacing of photodamage on the neck with an Ultrapulse CO_2 laser. Lasers Surg Med 1997; 20: 33.

276. Walsh JT Jr, Deutsch TF. Erbium:YAG laser ablation of tissue: measurement of ablation rates. Lasers Surg Med 1989; 9: 327.

277. Perez MI, Bank DE, Silvers D. Skin resurfacing of the face with the erbium:YAG laser. Dermatol Surg 1998; 24: 653.

278. Kaufmann R, Hibst R. Vergleich verschildener Mittelinfrafot: Laser für die ablation der Hauset. Lasermedizin 1995; 11: 19; abstract.

279. Venugopalan V, Nishioka NS, Mikic BB. Thermodynamic response of soft biological tissues to pulsed infrared-laser irradiation. Biophys J 1996; 70: 2981.

280. Ross EV, Naseef GS, McKinlay JR, et al. Comparison of CO_2 laser, Er:YAG laser, dermabrasion and dermatome: a study of thermal damage, wound contraction and wound healing in a live pig model: implications for skin resurfacing. J Am Acad Dermatol 2000; 42: 92.

281. Smith KJ, Skelton HG, Graham JS, et al. Depth of morphologic skin damage and viability after one, two and three passes of a high-energy, short pulse CO_2 laser (TruPulse) in pig skin. J Am Acad Dermatol 1997; 37: 204.

282. Zelickson R, Kist D. Effect of varied pulse duration and fluence of the CO_3 laser on coagulation and depth of collagen contraction. Lasers Surg Med 2000; 12: 14.

283. Woo SH, Park JH, Kye YC. Resurfacing of different types of facial acne scar with short pulsed, variable-pulsed and dual-mode Er:YAG laser. Dermatol Surg 2004; 30: 488.

284. Zachary CB. Modulating the Er:YAG laser. Lasers Surg Med 2000; 26: 223.

285. Sapijaszko MJ, Zachary CB. Er:YAG laser skin resurfacing. Dermatol Clin 2002; 20: 87.

286. Pozner JM, Goldberg DJ. Histologic effect of a variable pulsed Er:YAG laser. Dermatol Surg 2000; 26: 733.

287. Pozner JN, Roberts TL III. Variable-pulsed width ER:YAG laser resurfacing. Clin Plast Surg 2000; 27: 263.

288. Ross EV, McKinlay JR, Sajben FP, et al. Use of a novel erbium laser in a Yucatan minipig: a study of residual thermal damage (RTD), ablation, and wound healing as a function of pulse duration. Lasers Surg Med 2002; 30: 93.

289. Zachary CB, Grekin RC. Dual mode Er : YAG laser systems for skin resurfacing. Available from: http://www.LaserNews.Net].

290. Christian MM. Microresurfacing using the variable pulse erbium:YAG laser: a comparison of the 0.5 and 4-ms pulse durations. Dermatol Surg 2003; 29: 605.

291. Mueller DF, Zimmermann A, Borelli C. The efficiency of laser for the treatment of Ehlers–Danlos syndrome. Lasers Surg Med 2005; 36: 76.

292. Goldman MP, Marchell N, Fitzpatrick RE. Laser skin resurfacing of the face with a combined CO_2/Er:YAG laser. Dermatol Surg 2000; 26: 102.

293. Trelles MA, Allones I, Luna R. One-pass resurfacing with a combined-mode Er:YAG/CO_2 laser system: a study of 102 patients. Br J Dermatol 2002; 146: 473.

294. Kist DA, Sierra R, Sherr E, Zelickson BD. Collagen fibril contraction in bovine tendon and poultry skin after CO_3 laser exposure. Available from: http://www.LaserNews.net] [accessed March 2000].

295. Tanzi EL, Alster TS. Side effects and complications of variable pulsed erbium: yttrium-aluminum-garnet laser skin resurfacing: extended experience with 50 patients. Plast Reconstr Surg 2003; 111: 1524.

296. Tanzi EL, Alster TS. Treatment of atrophic facial acne scars with dual mode Er:YAG laser. Dermatol Surg 2002; 28: 551. Skin Resurfacing with Ablative Lasers 247.

297. Jeong JT, Park JH, Kye YC. Resurfacing of pitted facial acne scars using Er:YAG laser with ablation and coagulation mode. Aesthetic Plast Surg 2003; 27: 130.

298. Walgrave SE, Kist DA, Noyaner-Turley A, Zelickson BD. Minimally ablative resurfacing with the confluent 2,790 nm erbium:YSGG laser: a pilot study on safety and efficacy. Lasers Surg Med 2012; 44: 103–11.

299. Roberts TL III. Laser blepharoplasty and laser resurfacing of the periorbital area. Clin Plast Surg 1998; 25: 95.

300. Roberts TL III. In pursuit of optimal rejuvenation of the forehead: endoscopic browlift with CO_2 laser resurfacing. Plast Reconstr Surg 1998; 101: 1075.

301. Ramirez OM, Pozner JN. Laser resurfacing as an adjunct to endo-forehead lift, endofacelift and biplanar facelift. Ann Plast Surg 1997; 38: 315.

302. Ramirez OM, Pozner JN. Subperiosteal minimally invasive laser endoscopic rhytidectomy: the SMILE facelift. Aesthetic Plast Surg 1996; 20: 463.

303. Alster TS, Doshi SN, Hopping SB. Combination surgical lifting with ablative laser skin resurfacing of facial skin: a retrospective analysis. Dermatol Surg 2004; 30: 1191.

304. Fitzpatrick RE, Goldman M. Cosmetic Laser Surgery. St Louis: Mosby, 2000.

305. Avram DV, Goldman MP. The safety and effectiveness of single-pass Er: YAG laser in the treatment of mild to moderate photodamage. Dermatol Surg 2004; 30: 1073–6.

7 Ablative fractional lasers

Douglas A. Winstanley and E. Victor Ross

BACKGROUND

The popularity of laser treatment for curing photoaging has increased within the past decade. Although the results of fully ablative (confluent) resurfacing are predictable and substantive, there are significant risks and an obligatory period of downtime. This limited the procedure to a select group of patients.

Ablative fractional technology has revolutionized the field of laser dermatology. Since its introduction by Manstein et al. in 2004 (1), a variety of nonablative and ablative fractional lasers have become available. Decreased healing times and a lower incidence of adverse outcomes make the use of fractional technology appealing to physicians and patients. Fractionated lasers are being used in a wider variety of applications, including treatment of photoaging, acne scars, and surgical scars. More recent applications include the treatment of pigmentation disorders, removal of tattoos, and destruction of premalignancies.

Traditional ablative devices operate in the infrared spectrum, using water as the primary chromophore. These lasers have been used for many years to address rhytides and photoaging. However, the downtime and associated risks of scarring and dyspigmentation limited their application to those patients who could accommodate 1–2 weeks of minimal social interaction. The distinction of ablative fractional devices from fully ablative lasers is pixilation of the laser beam. These devices achieve epidermal and dermal injury without damaging the entire skin surface. The islands of undamaged skin serve as reservoirs for rapid healing. Coupled with a shortened healing time is a decrease in the overall risks of the procedure, including infection, scarring, and dyspigmentation (2). Together, these properties make ablative fractional treatments safer while still achieving significant improvement in tone, texture, and pigmentation of the skin. However, the lack of confluent laser ablation usually results in the lack of permanent resolution of dyspigmentation, cutaneous carcinoma, or premalignant skin disease. This chapter addresses the current state of ablative fractional laser technology. A brief review of the technology, molecular effects, applications, and complications is discussed.

CHARACTERISTICS OF ABLATIVE FRACTIONAL LASERS

Although the specifics of laser–tissue interactions are discussed elsewhere in this text, a review of some of the specific components of ablative fractional injury is imperative to understanding the differences in these devices and how settings can be optimized for maximum cosmetic enhancement and minimum downtime.

The primary characteristic among ablative lasers that distinguishes one wavelength from another is the degree of water absorption. The absorption of water is relatively low throughout the visible wavelengths and near-infrared spectrum. Beyond approximately 1200 nm, the absorption of water increases, with the peak absorption at 2935 nm. There are currently three available wavelengths among the ablative fractional lasers (with respective tissue absorption coefficients, assuming 70% water content): 2790-nm erbium-doped:yttrium-scandium-gallium-garnet laser (Er:YSGG), with an absorption coefficient of 4000 cm^{-1}; 2940-nm erbium-doped:yttrium-aluminum-garnet (Er:YAG) laser, with an absorption coefficient of 10,000 cm^{-1}, nearly 16 times that of CO_2; and 10,600-nm CO_2 laser, with an absorption coefficient over 800 cm^{-1} (Fig. 7.1).

With water serving as the chromophore for these devices, several skin components are targeted. In general, the affected structures are keratinocytes, collagen, and blood vessels (3). A recent article examined the definition of the terms "ablation" (4) and "fractional." In this article, the authors confined "nonablative" treatments to those where the epidermis is not "structurally breached," and where erosions and other changes associated with ablation do not occur. Also they confine "fractional" treatments to those where less than 50% of the surface area is damaged and where microinjuries are no greater than 500 μm in diameter. We respectfully disagree on this point and would prefer that fractional injuries be divided into *macrospot* (wounds >500 μm in diameter), small-depth (<200-μm deep) lesions, and *microspot* (<500 μm in diameter), higher-depth (>200-μm depth) lesions. Although the "spirit" of the descriptions in the article by Alam et al. (4) is correct, formally "ablation" should be defined in terms of "removal" or vaporization (5). Where the term "ablation" becomes more ambiguous is in cases where water is "vaporized" within a skin structure, but the gross structural (skin framework) change is not immediately observed. An example is conventional pulsed CO_2 laser with fluences in the range of 3–5 J/cm^2 (applications with larger spots). In this case, the epidermis, although irreparably damaged and denatured, remains on this skin as a skeleton (the water having been vaporized with the keratin skeleton remaining) (Fig. 7.2). Within days this layer "sloughs" off and the dermis is exposed. In this case, although the epidermis is not grossly removed in the immediate lasing session, the vaporization of water satisfies the criteria of ablation. Visible light technologies and wavelengths with small water absorption coefficients, on the other hand, do not result in vaporization and therefore are termed nonablative.

Because the chromophore is water, fractional lasers from 2.79 to 10.6 μm with larger absorption coefficients will ablate

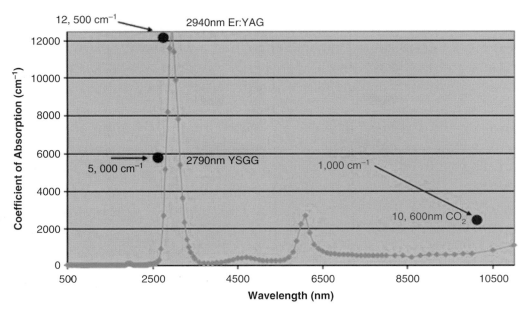

Figure 7.1 Absorption of energy by water as a function of wavelength. A 10,600-nm (CO_2) laser has a low coefficient of absorption of approximately 1000 cm^{-1}, which produces a relatively high amount of coagulation in proportion to ablation. A 2790-nm (YSGG) laser has an intermediate coefficient of absorption of approximately 5000 cm^{-1}, which produces a relatively balanced amount of ablation in proportion to coagulation. A 2940-nm (Er:YAG) laser has a high coefficient of absorption of approximately 12,500 cm^{-1}, which produces a relatively higher amount of ablation in proportion to coagulation. *Abbreviations*: CO_2, carbon dioxide; Er:YAG, erbium-doped:yttrium-aluminum-garnet; YSGG, yttrium-scandium-gallium-garnet laser.

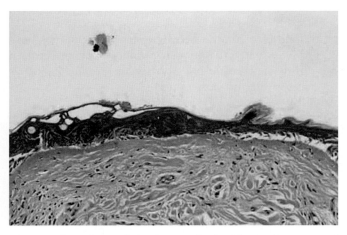

Figure 7.2 Photomicrograph showing coagulated epidermis after one pass of confluent carbon dioxide laser (7 J/cm^2, 1 ms, 3-mm spot); note that water in epidermis has been "vaporized" but epidermal skeleton remains.

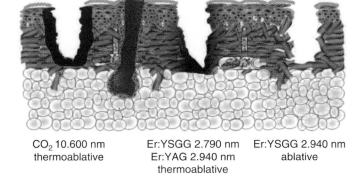

| CO_2 10.600 nm thermoablative | Er:YSGG 2.790 nm Er:YAG 2.940 nm thermoablative | Er:YSGG 2.940 nm ablative |

Figure 7.3 In the variants of ablative fractional laser therapy, a wavelength- and parameter-dependent coagulation zone (microscopic coagulation zone, red margin) of differing extent develops. *Abbreviations*: CO_2, carbon dioxide; Er:YAG, erbium-doped:yttrium-aluminum-garnet; YSGG, yttrium-scandium-gallium-garnet laser. *Source*: From Ref. 53.

epidermis and dermis to variable depths depending on the energy, wavelength, and beam dimensions (Fig. 7.3) (6). Most devices produce vertical columns of damage in the skin that have been termed microscopic treatment zones (MTZs). One exception (Palomar 2940 nm "groove" optic, Palomar Medical Technologies, Burlington, Massachusetts, USA) creates linear "grooves" in the skin (Fig. 7.4). Within an MTZ, there are areas of ablation (microscopic ablation zones) and areas of thermal damage (microscopic coagulation zones) (Fig. 7.3) (7).

Although there are differences in each ablative wavelength, parameters can be adjusted to produce somewhat comparable injury and effects within the skin. The most important determinants of wound healing and clinical efficacy are (*i*) the percentage (cross-sectional area) of skin ablated (a.k.a. density), (*ii*) the diameter of the individual microwounds, and (*iii*) the depths of the individual injuries. The ratio of ablation to coagulation in the microwounds might also play an important role in wound

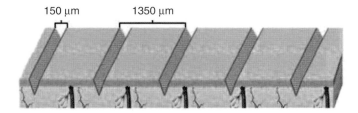

Figure 7.4 Grooves in skin formed by ablation and coagulation created by the Groove Optic. *Source*: From Palomar Medical Technologies.

healing and cosmetic outcomes. No study has examined the role of thermal damage as an independent parameter. In other words, the total volume of injury (ablative plus coagulative) might be similar, but if the volumes comprise different ratios of ablation to coagulation, wound healing and cosmetic improvement might vary. Also, although ablation appears to achieve

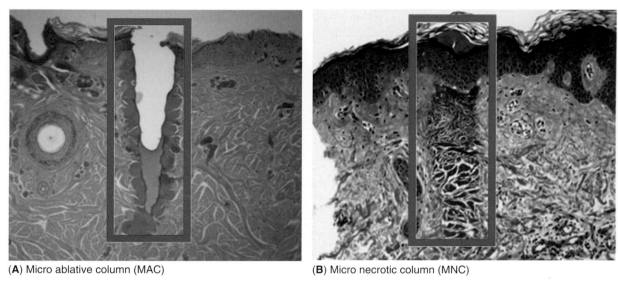

(A) Micro ablative column (MAC) **(B)** Micro necrotic column (MNC)

Figure 7.5 (**A**) Ablative and (**B**) nonablative fractional wounds with same "wounded" volumes and dimensions.

greater cosmetic outcomes than 100% coagulative injuries (nonablative fractional) with the same geometries (Fig. 7.5), the counterpoint would be that microwounds that are about 70:30 ratios of ablation:coagulation seem to create longer healing times but possibly better cosmetic outcomes than those where either (*i*) the ratio of ablation to coagulation might be 90:10 (i.e., fractional Er:YAG) or (*ii*) only coagulative microinjuries (also known as nonablative fractional wounds) are created. There is considerable variation in parameters between different devices, making comparisons difficult (8).

FRACTIONATED ER:YSGG LASERS (2790 nm)
The fractionated 2790-nm device achieves more thermal damage than the 2940-nm laser without the depth and extent of thermal injury of the 10,600-nm laser (9,10). Because of dynamic changes in water absorption in this wavelength range, the ablation dynamics are more "Er:YAG-like" than "CO_2-like." The currently available platform (Pearl and Pearl Fractional, Cutera, Brisbane, California, USA) has both confluent and ablative fractional settings, which can be used in the same treatment session (11). The depth of ablation is controlled by adjusting the microbeam pulse energy of the fractional laser and the macrofluence (1–3.5 J/cm^2) of the confluent handpiece. The laser assembly in this device fits inside the handpiece, and although this design adds some weight to the handpiece, an advantage is that beam alignment issues are mitigated and reliability increases.

FRACTIONATED ER:YAG LASERS (2940 nm)
The characteristic that distinguishes the Er:YAG laser most from CO_2 laser is the stronger water absorption at the 2940-nm wavelength (12,000 cm^{-1} for Er:YAG vs. 800 cm^{-1} for CO_2). Because the laser beam is so highly absorbed by water, the effect is almost pure ablation with very little heating of the surrounding skin. The lack of coagulation is evident by the postoperative pinpoint bleeding observed usually after exceeding a 200-µm depth of ablation (12). Some fractional Er:YAG lasers scan a raster pattern, whereas others emit a larger beam that is broken up into smaller beamlets by a microlens array. A recent study showed that unlike the CO_2 fractional lasers [where

change in the pulse duration alters the residual thermal damage (RTD)], changes in fractional Er:YAG pulse duration over a range of 0.25–60 ms, at least for deeper ablation (>500 µm), did not make a great impact on RTD (or immediate postoperative hemorrhage) (13,14). On the other hand, another study by Dierickx et al. showed an increase in RTD from about 15 to 25 µm when increasing pulse duration from 0.25 to 5 ms when the same 5 mJ/mb were applied over a 180-µm-diameter microspot. Ablation, on the other hand, was 25% deeper with the shorter pulse.

FRACTIONATED CO_2 LASERS (10,600 nm)
There are a number of commercially available fractional CO_2 devices. The various designs cover a range of deployment types, microspot sizes, densities, and pulse durations (Table 7.1 and Fig. 7.6).

Scanning handpieces are commonly used. There are two broad types of scanners. In one case (Fraxel Re:Pair, Solta, Santa Clara, California, USA), the microbeam is emitted via a rolling tip and multiple passes are made (usually four) at a certain percent coverage per pass. The multipass approach tends to create a random distribution of microbeams that prevents unwanted patterning or hot or cold spots within the scanned areas. The primary advantage to using a random scanning delivery system is to avoid the potential issues of bulk heating as well as avoid patterning of the microbeams. One popular CO_2 fractional laser (Deep FX, Lumenis, San Jose, California, USA) scans a "pattern" of microbeams over a certain area after which the operator moves the handpiece to an adjacent spot and repeats the process. These fixed scanners can deliver a range of patterns, including sequential, linear, hexagonal, and square footprints. With these devices, there is a sharp demarcation between the areas that are treated and those that remain untouched. The advantage of this particular fixed scanner laser is very short pulses (on the order of 20–200 µs vs. >1 ms for most competitor fractional CO_2 lasers). The shorter pulses result in faster healing times and less posttreatment erythema.

A potential advantage of random distributions of microbeams is to provide a more "feathered" margin between treated and untreated areas, resulting in a more natural appearing

Table 7.1 Commercially Available Ablative Fractional Devices

Manufacturer/Device	Type/Wavelength	Energy Output	Pulse Duration	Features/Comments
Alma Lasers				
Harmony	Fractional Er:YAG Pixel/2940 nm	200–2500 mJ/macropulse P		Fractional Er:YAG handpiece for use with Harmony XL platform
Pixel CO_2	Fractional CO_2/10,600 nm	70 W	50–1000 μs	Three tip options: 7 mm × 7 mm, 9 mm × 9 mm, 1 mm × 7 mm pixel array
Pixel Omnifit	Handpiece for CO_2 platforms	30–100 W	N/A	Fits Coherent, Lumenis and Sharplan CO_2 lasers
Cutera				
Xeo Pearl Fractional	Fractional Er:YSGG/ 2790 nm	60–320 mJ/microspot	600 μs	Real-time calibration. Deep ablation >1 mm. Connector for smoke evacuator
Cynosure				
Smart Skin	Fractional CO_2/10,600 nm	30 W	1–20 ms	Variable scanning patterns. Adjustable power, depth of ablation, dwell time, spot pitch, and scan shapes
DEKA				
SmartXide DOT 30/50 W	Fractional CO_2 scanner/ 10,600 nm	30 W	200–2000 μs	Adjustable ablation and dwell time. Variable scanning modes
Ellman				
Ellumine Fractional CO_2 Laser System	CO_2 fractional scanner/ flexible fiber/10,600 nm	Up to 105 mJ	2–7 ms	Adjustable scan density and pulse duration
Focus Medical				
NaturaLase CO_2	Fractional CO_2/10,600 nm	50 W	10 ms	Pending FDA approval
Hironic Co.				
MIXEL	Fractional CO_2/10,600 nm	60 mJ	Up to 5000 μs	Adjustable scan size and beam size
ILOODA Co.				
Fraxis	Fractional CO_2/10,600 nm	Up to 30 W	0.1–5 ms	Fast scanning mode
LASERING				
MiXto SX	Fractional CO_2/10,600 nm	0.5–30 W	2.5–16 ms	Variable spot sizes with focusing handpieces

(*Continued*)

Table 7.1 Commercially Available Ablative Fractional Devices (Continued)

Manufacturer/Device	Type/Wavelength	Energy Output	Pulse Duration	Features/Comments
Lumenis				
UltraPulse Active FX	Fractional CO_2/10,600 nm	1–225 mJ	<1 ms	9 mm × 9 mm scanner with CoolScan handpiece
UltraPulse Deep FX	Fractional CO_2/10,600 nm	2.5–50 mJ	<2 ms	120-μm spot size scanning handpiece with penetration depth up to 2 mm
UltraPulse Total FX	Fractional CO_2/10,600 nm	1–225 mJ	<2 ms	Combination of active/deep Fx
Ultrapulse SCAAR Fx	Fractional CO_2/10,600 nm	2.5–150 mJ	<2 ms	Increased depth of ablation to treat thicker scars
Acupulse Multimode	Fractional CO_2/10,600 nm	1–170 mJ	<2 ms	
Lutronic				
eCO₂	Fractional CO_2/10,600 nm	2–240 mJ	Variable	Multiple tip sizes and shapes. Handpiece available for continuous wave
Palomar				
Starlux 500 Platform Lux 2490 Fx	Fractional 2940 nm	2–9 mJ/microbeam	0.25–5 ms	IPL platform with multiple handpieces for different applications
Sandstone Medical Technologies				
Matrix LS-40 with Ultrafine-FS Fractional Scanner	Fractional CO_2/10,600 nm	Up to 40 W	Adjustable to 100 ms	Fractional scanner with 150 mm focusing handpiece
Cortex Resurfacing Work Station	CO_2 and Er:YAG/10,600 and 2940 nm		Adjustable to 100 ms	Fractional CO_2 combined with Er:YAG and fractionated erbium
Sciton				
Joule/ProFractional	Er:YAG/2940 nm	Up to 400 J/cm²	Variable	20 mm × 20 mm scanner with 250-μm spot size
Solta Medical				
Fraxel DUAL 1927	Thulium fiber laser/1927 nm	Up to 20 mJ/MTZ	N/A	IOTS, adjusts to hand speed to provide uniform delivery of laser energy
Fraxel Re:Pair	Fractional CO_2 laser/10,600 nm	5–70 mJ/MTZ	N/A	Integrated smoke evacuation system. Also with IOTS
Syneron & Candela				
CO₂RE	Fractional CO_2/10,600 nm	60 W		Multiple patterns allow for simultaneous superficial/deep treatment

Abbreviations: CO₂, carbon dioxide; Er:YAG, erbium-doped:yttrium–aluminum–garnet; Er:YSGG, erbium-doped:yttrium-scandium-gallium-garnet laser; FDA, Food and Drug Administration; IOTS, intelligent optical tracking system; IPL, intense pulsed light; MTZ, microscopic treatment zone; N/A, not available.

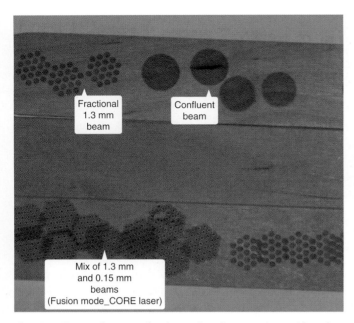

Figure 7.6 Tongue depressor showing various beam patterns with carbon dioxide lasers.

transition between treated and untreated skin (15). In the case of lasers that scan a fixed pattern and where the density per pass can be set by the user (i.e., between 5% and 25% per pass), greater pass numbers at smaller densities will allow for a more random distribution of microbeams (better case) versus fewer passes with greater density per pass. For example, if one applies 25% density with some overlap (OL), the density in the OL area will be 50% versus only increasing from 5% to 10% when overlapping in the lower density case. The drawback to multiple passes is the extra time requirement to complete the procedure. More recent developments include handpieces that use a "dynamic" mode in which the distribution of individual microbeams is randomized partly by the deliberate motion of the handpiece during the scan completion. Some companies incorporate both a dynamic and a "static" mode for their CO_2 scanners (Lutronic, Korea or Active FX, Lumenis), the former deployed by the physician in a constantly moving pattern, the latter in a more conventional "let the scanner complete the scan" and then move the handpiece fashion.

With equivalent fluences at 10.6 μm, longer pulse durations deliver more heat to tissue. Histologically, longer pulse durations (and therefore lower power densities) transform a cylinder of ablation and coagulation into a more triangular defect. This prolonged heating can result in subepidermal clefting at the edge of the crater and nonspecific thermal damage, which may be responsible for increased rates of postinflammatory erythema and hyperpigmentation (15). Microspot size is generally fixed for a particular device—an exception is the Lumenis Encore system, where two handpieces allow for 120- and 1300-μm spot sizes, respectively.

Alma Lasers (Buffalo, Grove IL, USA) has created a roller type scanner microspot Er:YAG and CO_2 system. The Er laser is driven by its base intense pulsed light (IPL) platform, whereas the CO_2 laser is a stand-alone product.

In addition, a radiofrequency (RF) pixel device (Pixel RF, Alma Lasers) is available and is being evaluated for several applications, including acne scarring, striae, and hyperpigmentation (Fig. 11.23).

MECHANISMS OF ACTION

The mechanisms by which ablative fractional lasers affect the skin are unclear. Both microscopic and biochemical studies suggest that the efficacy of ablative fractional treatments is related to molecular level effects. Several investigations have examined the wound healing process. Clinical observations suggest that fractional lasers increase collagen and/or elastin. Initial work by Orringer et al. examined the molecular effects on the skin of a fully ablative device. They found that laser treatment created a proinflammatory cascade that induced the expression of matrix metalloproteinases (MMPs). This wound healing sequence allowed for the breakdown of damaged collagen with replacement by new, well-structured collagen bundles (16).

More recent work has explored the underlying processes specific to fractional treatments. Xu et al. (17) demonstrated the expression of heat shock protein 70 within hours after laser treatment with persistence of these proteins for 3 months following the procedure. HSP 47 was detected 3 months following the procedure and persisted for an additional 3 months, suggesting the underlying mechanism for continuous improvement by serving as a "procollagen chaperone promoting neocollagenesis."

Reilly et al. studied ablative fractional lasers through assays of proteins in treated and normal skin. In their study, the levels of expression of MMPs were evaluated and compared with untreated skin at various times. RNA production for MMPs was specifically evaluated. It was discovered that interleukin-1β and tumor necrosis factor are induced quickly after laser treatment. Subsequently, MMPs in various concentrations were produced. MMP-1 and MMP-3, both collagenases, appeared in higher proportions along with MMP-9 (gelatinase). MMP-13 was also elevated posttreatment. MMP-13 seems to be a key protein in the reorganization of collagen and may play a primary role in the structuring of newly formed collagen after laser resurfacing (18). The role of coagulation as an independent factor in neocollagenesis and elastogenesis is unclear, that is, if one creates the same volumetric injury with a higher ratio of coagulation to ablation in individual craters, is there a tendency toward a more robust response with increasing degrees of coagulation?

Orringer et al. (19) has studied confluent and ablative fractional wounds and found that fractional wounds created less collagen than their confluent counterparts. This observation might explain the superior results achieved with confluent resurfacing versus fractional resurfacing in perioral rhytides, a region where fractional systems have "underperformed" (Fig. 7.7). They have also estimated that for ablative and nonablative *equivalent* wounds (i.e., when the same total cellular volume has been damaged, Fig. 7.5), the ablative fractional wound should create about 3× the collagen of the nonablative wound some 3 months after irradiation (personal communication).

Another study showed that for nonablative wounds (fractional), the total wound volume was more likely to determine the degree of neocollagenesis versus individual parameters of depth or density, that is, a low-density high-depth pattern created about the same degree of new collagen as one with high density and small depths (20).

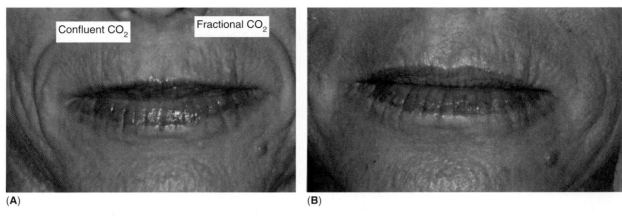

Figure 7.7 (**A**) Pretreatment perioral wrinkles. (**B**) Note greater improvement on confluent treated side. *Abbreviation*: CO_2, carbon dioxide.

CLINICAL CONSIDERATIONS

Although ablative fractional lasers have an improved safety profile versus their nonfractional counterparts, excessive heating (too large a depth or density) can create scarring, dyspigmentation, and infection. Accordingly, the surgeon must be familiar with the treatment device, the mechanisms underlying the treatment, and the appropriate parameters for the desired effects. It is also important that the patient's expectations are realistic, that they are tempered by the knowledge and experience of the treating physician and that they understand the inherent risks in undertaking such a procedure.

CONTRAINDICATIONS

Absolute contraindications to the procedure include a history of keloid scarring (of the face). Relative contraindications include a history of vitiligo and psoriasis (due to koebnerization), vasculitis, active skin infection in the area to be treated, use of oral retinoid within 6 to 12 months prior to the procedure (21), immunosuppression, and a history of radiation treatment to the target area (15).

PATIENT PREPARATION

The patient must acknowledge indications, the expected benefits, potential risks, complications, and adverse effects for the procedure. Pre- and posttreatment clinical photos should be taken and cataloged. Eye protection must be provided at all times during the procedure. If working around the periocular skin, metal corneal eye shields should be placed.

Analgesia may be provided by a number of methods. Most patients can tolerate a mild to moderately aggressive treatment with the use of topical anesthetic, local infiltration, refrigerated air, nerve blocks, tumescent anesthesia, or a combination thereof. Oral anxiolytics can be of great benefit. Patients having treatment of the face should be advised to have a driver transport them from the office after the procedure. In situations where the treatment will be very aggressive or the level of anxiety of the patient prohibits safe execution of the procedure, consideration can be given to conscious sedation or even general anesthesia.

Skin cooling before, during, and after the procedure can be invaluable. The use of an air chiller can provide a significant reduction in procedure-related pain and should be available for use.

Intraoperative hemorrhage is usually mild and transient, particularly with CO_2 lasers, and is associated with increasing depths of injury. Typically injury depths 400 μm or greater with CO_2 wounds and 200 μm or greater with Er:YAG wounds are associated with some intraoperative hemorrhage. Consideration should be given to the administration of antiviral and antibacterial prophylaxis. This is discussed in detail in the section on "Complications" associated with ablative fractional treatment.

APPLICATIONS

There is an ever-expanding group of applications for fractionated devices. Initial studies were focused on photoaging, including dyspigmentation and rhytides (Fig. 7.8). However, more recent investigations have revealed possible utility in other arenas.

Photoaging

The first studies using fractional devices were conducted by Manstein et al. using a nonablative laser in 2004 (1). Since that time, there have been many studies supporting the role of ablative fractional devices in the reversal of photoaging. Specifically, dyspigmentation in the form of lentigines and seborrheic keratoses, telangiectasia, and rhytides have all improved. The greatest advantage of fractional lasers is the lower risk of infection and long-term hypopigmentation. In cases of microspot ablative fractional remodeling, there have been no reports of delayed hypopigmentation (at least in the absence of any scarring or textural changes). On the other hand, fractional lasers have not achieved as durable responses in wrinkle reduction in the cheeks as traditional deeper CO_2 laser procedures (Fig. 7.9). Also, without a same session tool that addresses pigment (i.e., IPL, Q-switched laser), incomplete and only temporary dyschromia reduction is observed. One advantage of fractional lasers is the capacity for safety and efficacy *off* the face (Fig. 7.10). With the exception of very conservative confluent CO_2 and Er:YAG lasers (wounds confined to the upper half of the epidermis), extrafacial rejuvenation shows an unfavorable risk-to-benefit ratio (22).

Striae

Lee et al. treated 27 patients with white striae with a fractional CO_2 laser. Pulse energy was 10 mJ and density was 10%. Only one treatment was applied and improvement was assessed 3 months later. They found that about 60% of the participants showed 50% or greater improvement in the appearance of the

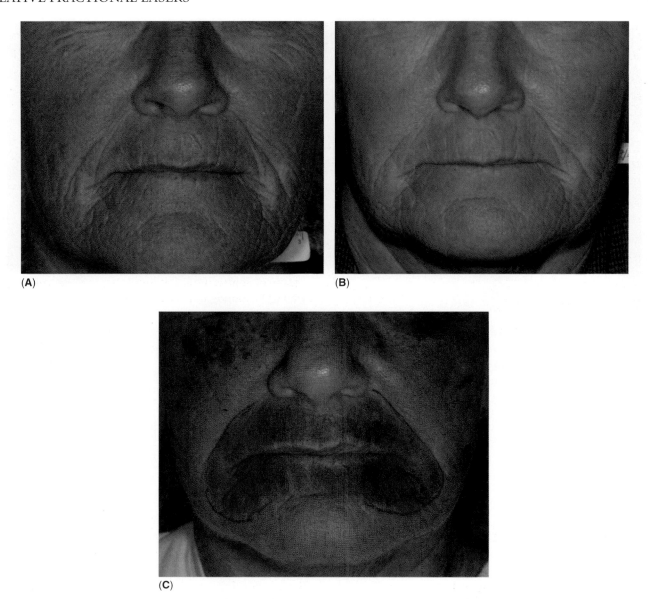

Figure 7.8 Erbium-doped:yttrium-aluminum-garnet fractional laser (**A**) before and (**B**) 3 months after three treatments 1 month apart (60% coverage and 250-μm depth per treatment; microwounds were 150 μm in diameter); (**C**) immediately after treatment.

striae. Side effects were mild, the most common being postinflammatory hyperpigmentation (PIH), which resolved in 4 weeks (23). Another study compared nonablative fractional resurfacing and ablative fractional resurfacing (AFR) in striae and found both to be effective, where about 35% and 50% of patients, respectively, were observed to have at least 26% global improvement in the appearance of the lesions (24). The ablative laser used in the study was a CO_2 laser (eCO_2, Lutronic) that deployed 100 pixels/cm² at 40–50 mJ over three treatment sessions 1 month apart. PIH was observed in the majority of AFR patients, and overall the ablative-treated side showed greater erosions and oozing.

The authors have studied an RF pixel device (Alma Lasers, Buffalo Grove, Illinois, USA) that creates 150-μm-diameter "plasmas" with a rolling mechanism. The plasma energy was applied in five patients with striae alba and showed a mean of about 50% improvement with follow-up at 3 months after 4 monthly treatments. The plasma generated by the RF device creates microwounds across the skin over eight passes (Fig. 7.11).

One of the editors (MPG) has not found an acceptable degree of efficacy with using the Active or Deep FX CO_2 laser due to minimal improvement associated with 3–9 months of PIH in treated patients even with a Fitzpatrick skin type II. Additional work with other wavelengths and/or energies will be necessary to achieve reproducible improvement with minimal adverse events.

Syringomas

Syringomas present a challenge in attempting to treat effectively without recurrence and without leaving a conspicuous scar. Cho et al. investigated the application of fractional CO_2 to these lesions. His group treated 35 patients with a fractional CO_2 laser with two sessions at 1-month intervals. The laser delivered 100 mb/cm² with two to three passes equivalent to about 20% density. Seventy percent of the patients were reported by the rating physicians to have between 25% and 75% improvement in the global severity of the syringomas. They also found that the maximum depth of the wounds was near the mean depth of the syringomas via biopsy (25).

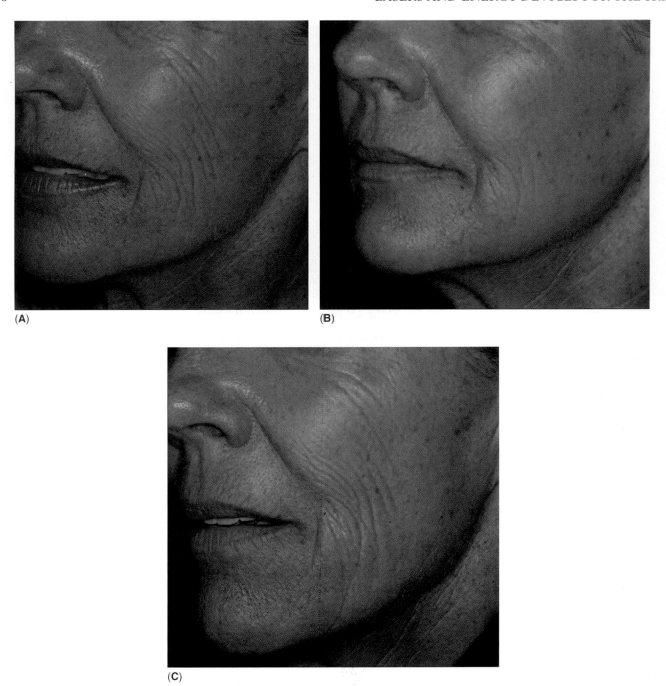

Figure 7.9 (**A**) Before and (**B**) 3 months after one treatment (fractional carbon dioxide) 30% coverage, 800-μm depth; (**C**) note relapse in wrinkles after 1 year.

Acne Scarring

Acne scarring presents a challenge to the dermatologic surgeon. There are a wide variety of scar morphologies, some being more amenable to ablative treatment than others (26). Large rolling types of scars require interventions in addition to fractional lasers—subcision, fillers, autologous transplanted fibroblasts, and neurotoxins can augment the laser's effects (26). We have found that small box car scars and even some ice pick scars respond well to ablative fractional lasers. The micro-injury depth required for optimal scar effacement is unknown. Conventional wisdom teaches that low density (<30%) and high depths (>500 μm) would be best to reverse the histology associated with acne scarring. However, no controlled study has corroborated this principle. The CROSS trichloroacetic acid (TCA) technique can be used in conjunction with ablative fractional lasers for focal ice pick scars. For optimal results, the TCA is applied very precisely first and allowed to "set" prior to laser. If the TCA is applied after the laser procedure, localization of the scar can prove difficult secondary to edema; moreover, the acid tends to leech into the surrounding damaged oozing skin. We have also combined nonfractional lasers in the same session, effacing individual boxcar scars with a small spot (1–2 mm) Er:YAG laser just prior to full-face fractional treatment. In our most commonly applied sequence for boxcar scars, we apply the Er laser for individual scars followed by CO_2 fractional treatment at about 25–30 mJ and 10%

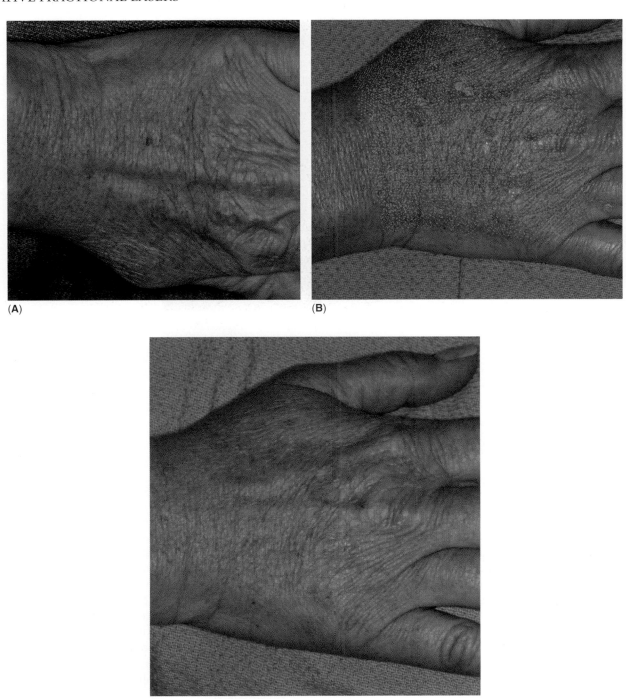

Figure 7.10 Hand (**A**) before, (**B**) immediately after one treatment (fractional carbon dioxide, 20% coverage, 150-µm depth), and (**C**) 1 month later.

coverage per pass for two passes with 120-µm spot Deep FX system. Healing requires about 10 days (Fig. 7.12).

The variable density of scarring, issues with dyspigmentation, and ongoing acne eruptions conspire to produce outcomes that may prove to be less than optimal. Also, many acne scarring patients are young adults who are unable to tolerate the prolonged downtime after an ablative procedure. Unlike photoaging, especially wrinkles, where ablative fractional lasers show a clear advantage over nonablative lasers, acne scarring (boxcar type) appears to respond almost as well to a series of four to five nonablative sessions as one to two ablative fractional treatments. One study compared CO_2 and 1550 nm in acne scars in type IV skin and found similar efficacy in the two systems (27).

Melasma/Hyperpigmentation/Hori's Nevus

Although disorders of pigmentation have traditionally been treated by either selective or nonselective destructive methods, fractional lasers can be applied as an adjunct therapy or used in a series of treatments to achieve at least partial pigment improvement. When used alone, ablative fractional lasers only produce temporary resolution of pigmented lesions since the majority of the pigmented cells are not vaporized; pigmentary dyschromia is often reestablished after a few months. Ideally one can combine a deep small spot, low-density technique with a larger spot more confluent technique (i.e., total FX). Alternatively, one can pretreat the skin with an IPL or Q-switched alexandrite laser for pigment followed by ablative fractional treatment on the same day.

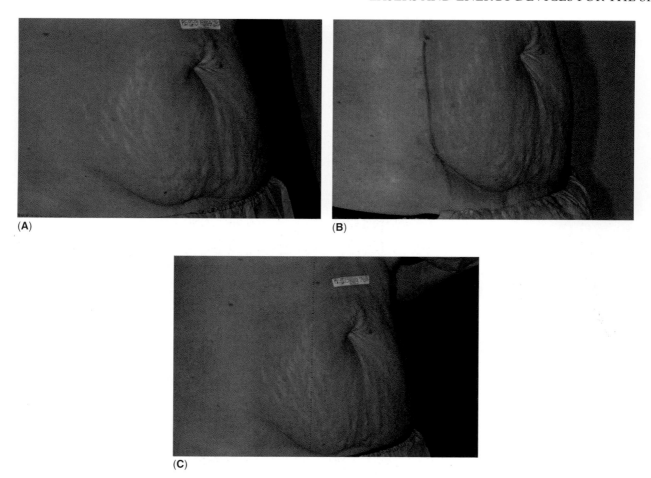

Figure 7.11 Striae (**A**) before, (**B**) immediately after, and (**C**) 3 months after three treatments with fractional radiofrequency device (wounds are 150 µm in diameter, 120-µm depth, and about 20% total coverage per treatment).

One challenge is the patient who presents with seborrheic keratoses. We normally treat the seborrheic keratoses at the beginning of the session with a 1- to 3-mm spot-pulsed CO_2 laser followed by the fractional laser.

Vitiligo
The use of lasers in vitiligo has been mostly confined to the 308-nm excimer laser. Other modalities to improve repigmentation in vitiligo include fully ablative lasers and dermabrasion in conjunction with ultraviolet B phototherapy (28). A small case series of 10 patients by Shin et al. suggest a possible adjunct role for fractional laser in increasing the rates of repigmentation of nonsegmental vitiligo in resistant location (29). Studies on a much larger scale would need to be undertaken to confirm efficacy and propose an underlying mechanism of effect if this treatment is indeed substantiated. On the other hand, Kilmer (personal communication) has reported the appearance of vitiligo 2 months after ablative fractional treatment for acne scarring. In this patient, there was a family history of vitiligo and presumably the side effect was a koebnorization phenomenon.

Tattoos
Traditionally, tattoo removal has been accomplished with the use of Q-switched lasers in the visible and near-infrared spectrum. Ablative fractional lasers have recently been studied as an adjunct strategy. A case report by Ibrahimi et al. describes two cases of tattoos that resulted in an allergic reaction treated

with ablative CO_2 laser. Each of the patients had significant improvement in the appearance of the tattoos as well as nearly complete resolution of symptoms associated with the allergic reaction to the tattoo ink over the course of three to four treatments (30). The proposed mechanism is transepidermal elimination of the tattoo ink through damaged dermis and epidermis. These results, although not yet carried out in a randomized prospective study, suggest a new avenue for approaching tattoo inks that are difficult to treat with currently available Q-switched lasers.

Surgical and Traumatic Scarring
One of the primary roles for ablative fractional technology has been in the treatment of scars. In contrast to thinking of the scar as being "treated," recent work has focused on the scar as a defect to be "rehabilitated" (Dr. Daniel Driscoll, Shriner's Hospital, Boston, Massachusetts, USA). In military dermatology, much work has been done in the treatment of contracture scars among wounded veterans. Preliminary data indicate a role for ablative lasers in improving skin pliability and increasing range of motion (13). Other data suggest a role in reducing chronic ulceration. The molecular mechanisms by which this may occur are unclear but may be associated with the deposition of type 3 nascent collagen in conjunction with a change in the therapeutic milieu of the scarred tissue. Clinically we usually apply two to three sessions 2–3 months apart. Regardless of the wavelength, normal total densities in any session range

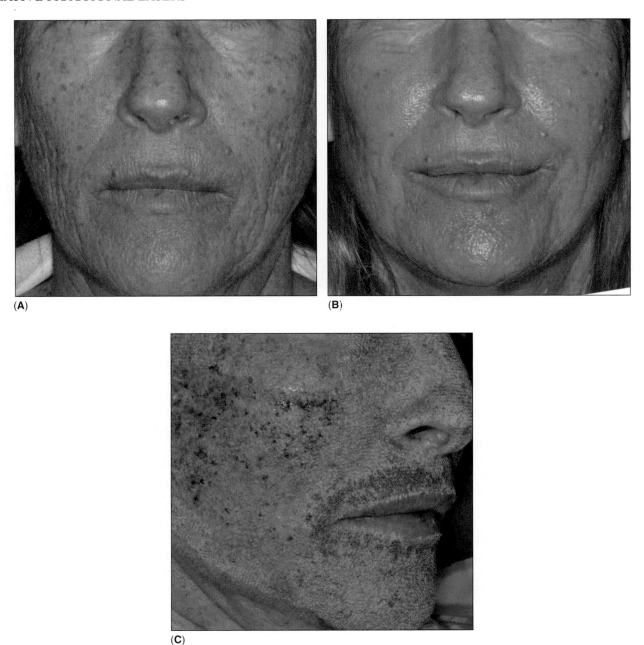

Figure 7.12 Fractional carbon dioxide for acne scars. (**A**) Before, (**B**) 3 months after one treatment, and (**C**) immediately posttreatment. (Cheek treated with 120-μm diameter beams, 20% total coverage, and about 700-μm depth.)

between 10% and 35% with microwound depths of 400–800 μm. A recent case report in improving the pliability and range of motion in a patient with scleroderma also attests to the utility of fractional lasers in improving scars (13).

Premalignancies

Although ablative lasers have been used to treat premalignant lesions (actinic keratoses), the use of ablative fractional devices to treat premalignant and malignant lesions of the skin is limited because less than 100% of the surface area of the skin is treated. Another potential issue is variability of the absorption characteristics of normal versus premalignant or malignant skin. Work examining the laser absorption characteristics of skin with nonmelanoma skin cancer and actinic keratoses (AKs) relative to normal skin was initiated by Togsverd-Bo et al. to address this question. A small sampling of patients with AKs, Bowen's disease, or superficial and nodular basal cell carcinomas

suggested that there is not a significant difference in the characteristics of the ablative profile of a CO_2 laser in diseased versus undamaged adjacent skin (31). However, a more promising use of a ablative fractional device is enhanced delivery of a drug, such as aminolevulinic acid (ALA) for photodynamic therapy (32), topical chemotherapeutic agents, or immunomodulators.

MISCELLANEOUS APPLICATIONS

Tuberous sclerosis lesions have been reduced by ablative fractional techniques. In case series of three patients, the authors combined pulse dye laser (PDL) and fractional CO_2 lasers (20–40 mJ, 40% coverage) (33). Individual larger lesions were "pre"-treated with pinpoint electrosurgery. The goal was to reduce the entire field of lesion density and volume. However, no one lesion would be likely to respond 100% with this approach. On the other hand, risks of hypopigmentation and scarring are reduced versus deep conventional laser treatment with a 1-mm spot directed toward individual lesions. A reasonable approach with a maximum benefit-to-risk ratio is treating individual larger lesions with a directed therapy followed immediately by fractional laser.

Becker's nevus (BN) has been treated with fractional CO_2 laser in a recent study of 11 patients. The authors performed three treatments 6 weeks apart at 10 mJ with a 120-μm spot microbeam and 35–45% coverage with only moderate success: the risk of PIH was high and only 4 of 10 patients who completed the study would recommend it to fellow BN patients (34).

COMPLICATIONS

The nature of fractional devices leads to a lower complication rate than that observed with fully ablative lasers. Most complications have occurred on the neck and chest and included scarring and infection. Facial complications with microspot treatment have usually been associated with too high a density and/or depth. It follows that the wounds mimicked "punch" biopsy-type wounds and resulted in thick scars. With the larger 1.3-mm macrospot applications (broad superficial injuries with only 100–200 μm total depth), wounds covering greater than 90% surface area have been associated with prolonged healing and greater infection risks.

One drawback of fractional treatments is the lack of clear clinical endpoints. Once a series of passes is applied, the cumulative number of pixels and therefore percent surface coverage must be followed closely by the provider. Most devices can display the total energy applied but cannot record exactly *where* that energy was delivered. Accordingly, the operator is treating by recipe rather than clinical endpoints.

Prolonged Erythema

Erythema posttreatment is normal. However, it is expected that most erythema will resolve after an ablative treatment within 4 weeks (12,34). Various treatments have been reported to reduce the duration of the erythema, including exposure to 590-nm light emitting diode (LED) light (36) and the application of ascorbic acid posttreatment (37). Patients should be advised to avoid potential irritants or sensitizers and to limit the degree of sun exposure through the use of protective clothing and sunscreens. We recommend that any topical preparations applied to the face have a minimal number of ingredients. Plain petrolatum serves this function well. Transition to a bland moisturizer after reepithelialization occurs (generally 5 to 7 days posttreatment depending on the aggressiveness of the treatment) and tends to maintain patient comfort and expedite healing without prolonging erythema. One of the editors (MPG) has found the nightly application of 0.1% fluocinolone in white petrolatum starting at postoperative day 2 and continuing to day 7 to be helpful in minimizing erythema secondary to inflammation. In addition, the use of a lower density setting and/or shorter pulses minimizes the degree of nonspecific thermal damage and resulting erythema.

Infection

One of the most common infections is cutaneous herpes simplex virus (HSV). In general, these infections will present within the first week posttreatment. It is imperative that these infections be recognized and treated expeditiously to avoid potential long-term sequelae, such as delayed wound healing and scarring. Although the rates of infection after ablative

fractional treatments are less than that reported with fully ablative treatments, they are still reported at between 0.3% and 2% of cases (38,39). The risk can be mitigated by beginning prophylaxis 1 day prior to the procedure and continuing treatment for a total of 7 days. Patients who present the day of treatment with an active herpes infection should not be treated due to the risk of HSV exacerbation (40).

Rates of bacterial infection are generally low with a reported incidence of 0.1% of cases. Patients with infection will generally present 1–4 days postoperatively with complaints of increasing pain, erythema, erosions, and crusting. Wound occlusion can increase the likelihood of infection, primarily with *Staphylococcus aureus* and *Pseudomonas aeruginosa*. Although there are no clear guidelines for the use of prophylactic antibiotics, strong consideration should be given in situations where the patient is immunocompromised. Where wound infection is suspected, cultures should be performed and antibiotic therapy initiated. Candidal infections occasionally occur and may manifest primarily as an increase in pruritus and/or erythema. A small case series by Alam et al. examined the relationship between posttreatment pruritus and positive fungal cultures. They found a significant relationship between positive culture and the development of significant pruritus but not with physician ratings of clinical signs (41). Fungal infections will generally present later than viral and bacterial infections—most often 1 to 2 weeks after the procedure with complaints of increased pruritus. Antifungal therapy should be initiated to mitigate any risk of scarring (42,43). An atypical mycobacterial infection has also been reported after AFR (44).

Scarring

Although hypertrophic scarring and keloid formation are less common in ablative fractional treatment versus conventional laser interventions, there have been reports of posttreatment scar formation. Infection is the most prevalent cause, as discussed in the previous section. The majority of primary scarring in fractional cases has occurred on the neck, likely due to the relatively poorer vascular supply and lower density of pilosebaceous units in the skin of the neck (Fig. 7.13). For this

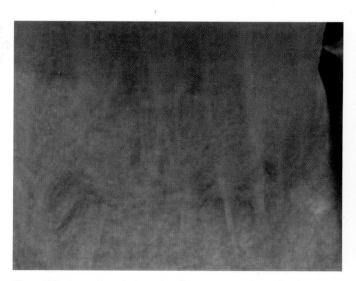

Figure 7.13 Approximately 3 weeks after treatment, the neck of a patient treated with carbon dioxide ablative fractional resurfacing (treated at a pulse energy of 20 mJ (630-μm depth) with 30% coverage of the exposed skin and a total treatment energy for the neck of 5.0 kJ) displays firm linear bands over the treated area consistent with multiple vertical and horizontal hypertrophic scars. *Source*: From Ref. 43.

reason, it is recommended that conservative energies and densities are used when treating the neck (45). Patients with a history of scarring or postoperative wound infection are at greater risk for scarring complications (46,47). Early intervention when scarring occurs may involve the use of PDL, topical and intralesional steroids, and/or 5% 5-fluorouracil injections and topical silicone gels (Hybrasil, Crescendo Therapeutics, Inc., San Diego, California, USA) or silicone sheeting (46,47).

Pigmentation

Postinflammatory hyperpigmentation with ablative fractional treatment is more common among patients with darker skin phototypes. Darker-skinned patients should be advised of the potential risk for PIH (Fig. 7.14). In addition, they should be counseled to avoid sun exposure for several weeks before and after treatment (48). Sun avoidance and protection measures should be implemented and consideration given to topical peeling (e.g., retinoids) or skin-lightening preparations (e.g., hydroquinone). Minimizing postoperative inflammation

with a decreased density of ablative spots and/or the use of postoperative topical corticosteroids has also been found to be helpful, especially in the Asian population. One advantage of fractional lasers is the absence of long-term hypopigmentation (so long as no skin textural change associated with overtreatment has occurred). This side effect was a major drawback of confluent resurfacing, was frequently observed particularly after multiple pass treatments, and was the primary reason for the CO_2 laser's waning popularity in the late 1990s.

Acne

Milia, papules, and pustules occur not uncommonly after ablative fractional treatment. Occlusive moisturizers play a significant role in the appearance of acne lesions, so ointments should be discontinued once reepithelialization occurs and crusting resolves. Transition to a nonocclusive bland moisturizer will lessen the occurrence of acne lesions. Significant acne eruptions can generally be well controlled with oral antibiotics, typically of the tetracycline class or alternatives as deemed appropriate (49).

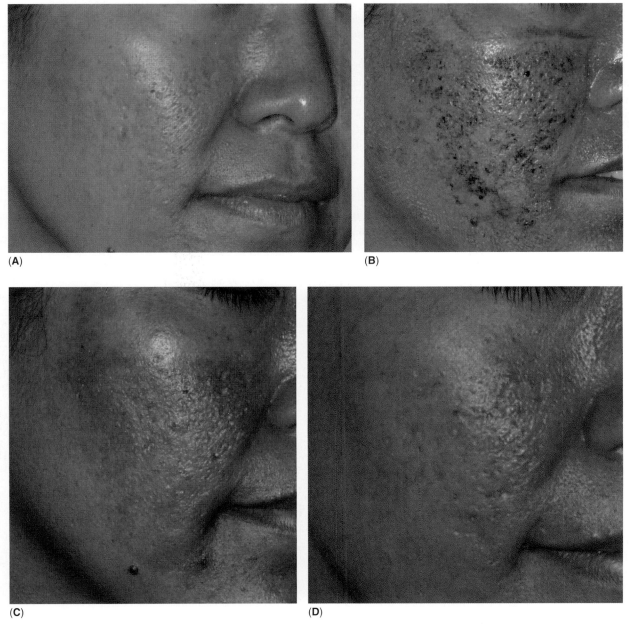

(A) (B)

(C) (D)

Figure 7.14 Asian female (**A**) before, (**B**) immediately postfractional carbon dioxide laser, (**C**) 6 weeks after treatment, and (**D**) 3 months after treatment. Note postinflammatory hyperpigmentation and slow resolution. Acne scarring continues to improve.

LONG-TERM EFFICACY OF ABLATIVE FRACTIONAL LASER TREATMENT

The durability of fractional results is highly variable and dependent on a number of factors. These include age, degree of preexisting photodamage, presence of other medical conditions, amount of posttreatment ultraviolet exposure, and the depth and density of lesions. In a study by Ortiz et al., a group of 10 patients was evaluated at 1 and 2 years after their 3-month follow-up postoperatively. Each was evaluated for overall skin texture, laxity, rhytides, and acne scars. Within this small group, it was found that subjects maintained 74% of their overall improvement (50). Patients should be advised of the durability of their treatment and measures that can be taken to prolong the benefits of the procedure.

HORIZONS OF ABLATIVE FRACTIONAL TECHNOLOGY

There have been many modifications to ablative fractional devices to optimize the efficacy of treatment while minimizing adverse effects or associated downtime. Creative combinations of NFR and AFR have been reported to enhance recovery and efficacy. Also, AFR can be confined with fillers and neurotoxins to enhance cosmetic outcomes. Fillers can be injected at the same session (just before lasing) as the filler depths extend beyond the reach of the ablative cylinders (51). The injection of neurotoxins should precede AFR, but the minimum interval is unclear. As the neurotoxin should be set by 30 minutes after injection, this time might be the minimum interval. If injected just before or just after AFR, edema might cause diffusion and unwanted facial asymmetry after injection.

DRUG DELIVERY

Because fractional ablation produces microscopic holes in the skin, the compromise in epidermal integrity accelerates the absorption of topical medications. In work done by Hadersdal et al., increased uptake of methyl-aminolevulinic acid relative to untreated skin was demonstrated in two Yorkshire pigs. Additional work by Letada et al. demonstrated the absorption of aminolevulinic acid after fractionated laser treatment to the palms of five human subjects. Absorption was demonstrated using Wood's lamp fluorescence (52). It has yet to be determined how well-increased absorption will translate into increased therapeutic effect, but the theoretical underpinnings appear sound. This could certainly have practical implications in the treatment of many skin conditions, including premalignant and malignant entities.

CONCLUSIONS

The advent of ablative fractional technology has revolutionized the application of lasers to a variety of dermatologic conditions. The lower incidence of side effects and decreased recovery time compensates for a small decrease in overall efficacy. Their utility has been proved in a variety of skin conditions. As a greater understanding of the underlying mechanisms of ablative fractional technology come to light, improvements in current treatment will undoubtedly occur. Additional applications of fractional ablation are in the process of being investigated and hold promise for treating conditions of the skin in novel ways.

REFERENCES

1. Manstein D, Herron GS, Sink RK, Tanner H, Anderson RR. Fractional photothermolysis: a new concept for cutaneous remodeling using microscopic patterns of thermal injury. Lasers Surg Med 2004; 34: 426–38.
2. Tierney EP, Kouba DJ, Hanke CW. Review of fractional photothermolysis: treatment indications and efficacy. Dermatol Surg 2009; 35: 1445–61.
3. Khan MH, Sink RK, Manstein D, Eimerl D, Anderson RR. Intradermally focused infrared laser pulses: thermal effects at defined tissue depths. Lasers Surg Med 2005; 36: 270–80.
4. Alam M, Dover JS, Arndt KA. To ablate or not: a proposal regarding nomenclature. J Am Acad Dermatol 2011; 64: 1170–4.
5. Venugopalan V, Nishioka NS, Mikić BB. The effect of laser parameters on the zone of thermal injury produced by laser ablation of biological tissue. J Biomech Eng 1994; 116: 62–70.
6. Laubach H, Chan HH, Rius F, Anderson RR, Manstein D. Effects of skin temperature on lesion size in fractional photothermolysis. Lasers Surg Med 2007; 39: 14–18.
7. Hantash BM, Bedi VP, Kapadia B, et al. In vivo histological evaluation of a novel ablative fractional resurfacing device. Lasers Surg Med 2007; 39: 96–107.
8. Bogdan Allemann I, Kaufman J. Fractional photothermolysis—an update. Lasers Med Sci 2009; 25: 137–44.
9. Ciocon DH, Engelman DE, Hussain M, Goldberg DJ. A split-face comparison of two ablative fractional carbon dioxide lasers for the treatment of photodamaged facial skin. Dermatol Surg 2011; 37: 784–90.
10. Munavalli GS, Turley A, Silapunt S, Biesman B. Combining confluent and fractionally ablative modalities of a novel 2790 nm YSGG laser for facial resurfacing. Lasers Surg Med 2011; 43: 273–82.
11. Dierickx CC, Khatri KA, Tannous ZS, et al. Micro-fractional ablative skin resurfacing with two novel erbium laser systems. Lasers Surg Med 2008; 40: 113–23.
12. Rahman Z, MacFalls H, Jiang K, et al. Fractional deep dermal ablation induces tissue tightening. Lasers Surg Med 2009; 41: 78–86.
13. Kineston D, Kwan JM, Uebelhoer NS, Shumaker PR. Use of a fractional ablative 10.6-µm carbon dioxide laser in the treatment of a morphea-related contracture. Arch Dermatol 2011; 147: 1148–50.
14. Kist DA, Elm CM, Eleftheriou LI, et al. Histologic analysis of a 2940 nm fractional device. Lasers Surg Med 2011; 43: 79–91.
15. Paasch U, Haedersdal M. Laser systems for ablative fractional resurfacing. Expert Rev Med Dev 2011; 8: 67–83.
16. Orringer JS, Kang S, Johnson TM, et al. Connective tissue remodeling induced by carbon dioxide laser resurfacing of photodamaged human skin. Arch Dermatol 2004; 140: 1326.
17. Xu XG, Luo YJ, Wu Y, et al. Immunohistological evaluation of skin responses after treatment using a fractional ultrapulse carbon dioxide laser on back skin. Dermatol Surg 2011; 37: 1141–9.
18. Reilly MJ, Cohen M, Hokugo A, Keller GS. Molecular effects of fractional carbon dioxide laser resurfacing on photodamaged human skin. Arch Facial Plast Surg 2010; 12: 321–5.
19. Orringer JS, Sachs DL, Shao Y, et al. Direct quantitative comparison of molecular responses in photodamaged human skin to fractionated and fully ablative carbon dioxide laser resurfacing. Dermatol Surg 2012; 38: 1668–77.
20. Orringer JS, Rittié L, Baker D, Voorhees JJ, Fisher G. Molecular mechanisms of nonablative fractionated laser resurfacing. Br J Dermatol 2010; 163: 757–68.
21. Rubenstein R, Roenigk HH, Stegman SJ, Hanke CW. Atypical keloids after dermabrasion of patients taking isotretinoin. J Am Dermatol 1986; 15: 280–5.
22. Fitzpatrick RE. CO_2 laser resurfacing. Dermatol Clin 2001; 19: 443–51; viii.
23. Lee SE, Kim JH, Lee SJ, et al. Treatment of striae distensae using an ablative 10,600-nm carbon dioxide fractional laser: a retrospective review of 27 participants. Dermatol Surg 2010; 36: 1683–90.
24. Yang YJ, Lee G-Y. Treatment of striae distensae with nonablative fractional laser versus ablative CO(2) fractional laser: a randomized controlled trial. Ann Dermatol 2011; 23: 481–9.
25. Cho SB, Kim HJ, Noh S, et al. Treatment of syringoma using an ablative 10,600-nm carbon dioxide fractional laser: a prospective analysis of 35 patients. Dermatol Surg 2011; 37: 433–8.
26. Goodman G. Post acne scarring: a review. J Cosmet Laser Ther 2003; 5: 77–95.

27. Alajlan AM, Alsuwaidan SN. Acne scars in ethnic skin treated with both non-ablative fractional 1,550 nm and ablative fractional CO_2 lasers: comparative retrospective analysis with recommended guidelines. Lasers Surg Med 2011; 43: 787–91.

28. Bayoumi W, Fontas E, Sillard L, et al. Effect of a preceding laser dermabrasion on the outcome of combined therapy with narrowband ultraviolet B and potent topical steroids for treating nonsegmental vitiligo in resistant localizations. Br J Dermatol 2011; 166: 208–11.

29. Shin J, Lee JS, Hann S-K, Oh SH. Combination treatment of 10,600 nm ablative carbon dioxide fractional laser and narrow band UVB in refractory non-segmental vitiligo: A prospective, randomized half-body comparative study. Br J Dermatol 2011; 166: 658–61.

30. Ibrahimi OA, Syed Z, Sakamoto FH, Avram MM, Anderson RR. Treatment of tattoo allergy with ablative fractional resurfacing: a novel paradigm for tattoo removal. J Am Acad Dermatol 2011; 64: 1111–14.

31. Togsverd-Bo K, Paasch U, Haak CS, Haedersdal M. Lesion dimensions following ablative fractional laser treatment in non-melanoma skin cancer and premalignant lesions. Lasers Med Sci 2011; 27: 675–79.

32. Haedersdal M, Sakamoto FH, Farinelli WA, et al. Fractional CO_2 laser-assisted drug delivery. Lasers Surg Med 2010; 42: 113–22.

33. Weiss ET, Geronemus RG. Combining fractional resurfacing and Q-switched ruby laser for tattoo removal. Dermatol Surg 2011; 37: 97–9.

34. Meesters AA, Wind BS, Kroon MW, et al. Ablative fractional laser therapy as treatment for Becker nevus: a randomized controlled pilot study. J Am Dermatol 2011; 65: 1173–9.

35. Chapas AM, Brightman L, Sukal S, et al. Successful treatment of acneiform scarring with CO_2 ablative fractional resurfacing. Lasers Surg Med 2008; 40: 381–6.

36. Alster TS, Wanitphakdeedecha R. Improvement of postfractional laser erythema with light-emitting diode photomodulation. Dermatol Surg 2009; 35: 813–15.

37. Alster TS, West TB. Effect of topical vitamin C on postoperative carbon dioxide laser resurfacing erythema. Dermatol Surg 1998; 24: 331–4.

38. Graber EM, Tanzi EL, Alster TS. Side effects and complications of fractional laser photothermolysis: experience with 961 treatments. Dermatol Surg 2008; 34: 301–5; discussion 305–7.

39. Setyadi HG, Jacobs AA, Markus RF. Infectious complications after nonablative fractional resurfacing treatment. Dermatol Surg 2008; 34: 1595–8.

40. Rokhsar CK, Fitzpatrick RE. The treatment of melasma with fractional photothermolysis: a pilot study. Dermatol Surg 2005; 31: 1645–50.

41. Alam M, Pantanowitz L, Harton AM, Arndt KA, Dover JS. A prospective trial of fungal colonization after laser resurfacing of the face: correlation between culture positivity and symptoms of pruritus. Dermatol Surg 2003; 29: 255–60.

42. Fife DJ, Fitzpatrick RE, Zachary CB. Complications of fractional CO_2 laser resurfacing: four cases. Lasers Surg Med 2009; 41: 179–84.

43. Avram MM, Tope WD, Yu T, Szachowicz E, Nelson JS. Hypertrophic scarring of the neck following ablative fractional carbon dioxide laser resurfacing. Lasers Surg Med 2009; 41: 185–8.

44. Palm MD, Butterwick KJ, Goldman MP. *Mycobacterium chelonae* infection after fractionated carbon dioxide facial resurfacing (presenting as an atypical acneiform eruption): case report and literature review. Dermatol Surg 2010; 36: 1473–81.

45. Goldman MP, Fitzpatrick RE, Manuskiatti W. Laser resurfacing of the neck with the erbium:YAG laser. Dermatol Surg 1999; 25: 164–7; discussion 167–8.

46. Alster T, Zaulyanov L, Zaulyanov-Scanlon L. Laser scar revision: a review. Dermatol Surg 2007; 33: 131–40.

47. Alster TS, Tanzi EL. Hypertrophic scars and keloids: etiology and management. Am J Clin Dermatol 2003; 4: 235–43.

48. Chan HHL, Manstein D, Yu CS, et al. The prevalence and risk factors of post-inflammatory hyperpigmentation after fractional resurfacing in Asians. Lasers Surg Med 2007; 39: 381–5.

49. Alster TS, Tanzi EL, Lazarus M. The use of fractional laser photothermolysis for the treatment of atrophic scars. Dermatol Surg 2007; 33: 295–9.

50. Ortiz AE, Tremaine AM, Zachary CB. Long-term efficacy of a fractional resurfacing device. Lasers Surg Med 2010; 42: 168–70.

51. Farkas JP, Richardson JA, Brown S, Hoopman JE, Kenkel JM. Effects of common laser treatments on hyaluronic acid fillers in a porcine model. Aesthet Surg J 2008; 28: 503–11.

52. Letada PR, Shumaker PR, Uebelhoer NS. Demonstration of protoporphyrin IX (PpIX) localized to areas of palmar skin injected with 5-aminolevulinic acid (ALA) and pre-treated with a fractionated CO_2 laser prior to topically applied ALA. Photodiagnosis Photodyn Ther 2010; 7: 120–2.

53. Grunewald S, Bodendorf MO, Simon JC, Paasch U. Update dermatologic laser therapy. J Dtsch Dermatol Ges 2011; 9: 146–59.

8 Nonablative fractional lasers

Karen L. Beasley and Robert A. Weiss

BACKGROUND

The development of fractional photothermolysis is one of the most important discoveries in the field of laser medicine and surgery. Fractional photothermolysis, first described by Manstein (1), refers to laser generated zones of microscopic thermal injury of the skin. This concept revolutionized laser skin resurfacing and the practice of esthetic dermatology, dermatologic surgery, and laser medicine. Previously patients could only significantly enhance their skin through fully ablative lasers, like the 10,600-nm carbon dioxide (CO_2) laser or the 2940-nm erbium-doped yttrium aluminum garnet (Er:YAG) laser. These laser treatments required at least 1–2 weeks of recovery depending on the depth of resurfacing and the type of laser utilized. With deeper resurfacing procedures, patients could experience considerable discomfort and side effects. Results could be exceptional but patients soon became aware of the potential disadvantages of aggressive procedures. Besides the potential side effects of infection or permanent scarring, many patients who were treated with deep CO_2 laser resurfacing experienced prolonged redness or erythema of the skin for 6 months to a year. Many also developed unexpected permanent hypopigmentation of their treated skin (2,3). In addition, patients also became aware of the stark contrast as their beautiful resurfaced facial skin lay adjacent to their severely sun damaged neck and chest. Fully ablative laser resurfacing was fraught with severe complications when used off the face. Darker skin types were not candidates for the procedure. With these limitations, traditional deep ablative resurfacing began to decrease in popularity.

Nonablative infrared lasers were developed in hopes of remodeling and rejuvenating the skin with fewer side effects. Infrared lasers such as the 1320-nm Nd:YAG, 1450-nm diode, and 1540-nm erbium: glass lasers were developed. These lasers demonstrated modest improvements in fine rhytides and acne scars (4–6). More importantly, these lasers were able to produce results in patients with darker skin types (7). But the results from these nonablative lasers paled in comparison with the traditional ablative procedures, leading patients and physicians to seek more efficacious treatments. A comparison of types of ablative and nonablative lasers is shown diagrammatically in Figure 8.1.

In addition to efficacy, it is important to consider the risk–benefit ratio of a laser procedure and its potential for post-procedure downtime. In our current culture, many patients do not want to take the risk of a serious side effect in exchange for a cosmetic improvement. Alternatively, many patients have busy work or social schedules that do not allow for extended recovery times. Nonablative fractional laser (NAFL) resurfacing allows for real results with fewer side effects and less downtime. This technology also allows for the treatment of darker skin types and can successfully treat a multitude of skin conditions and body areas. The disadvantages, compared with ablative resurfacing, are the need to return for multiple treatments and decreased efficacy.

FRACTIONAL PHOTOTHERMOLYSIS

During fractional photothermolysis, the laser creates microscopic noncontiguous columns of thermal injury in the dermis, referred to as microthermal zones (MTZs) (Fig. 8.2) (1). Each MTZ is surrounded by a limited zone of heat shocked tissue which is surrounded by a larger zone of healthy unaffected tissue. The MTZ allows for transport and extrusion of necrotic dermal content through the compromised dermal epidermal junction (8). The precise nature of the coagulated tissue allows for quicker healing and recovery (1,8,9). Immunohistochemical studies have shown increased collagen III production around treated MTZs by 7 days and replacement of damaged collagen in the MTZs by 3 months after treatment (9). In addition, histology also reveals that there is a localized, well-controlled melanin release and a transport mechanism that uses microscopic exudative necrotic debris (MEND) as the vehicle for pigmentary redistribution (9). In other words, NAFL resurfacing improves pigmentation by shuttling the melanin through the MENDs where it is exfoliated off the skin. The initial paper by Manstein et al. also reported that there was little to no pigmentary alteration in dark skinned patients when using lasers with low to medium MTZ densities per treatment (1). This essential combination of creating a precise injury that has an enhanced healing rate coupled with the ability to build collagen and redistribute pigment is the hallmark of fractional photothermolysis.

NONABLATIVE FRACTIONAL LASERS

Two main NAFL families currently dominate the world laser market; the Solta family of NAFLs (Solta Medical, Hayward, California, USA) and the Palomar family of NAFLs (Palomar Medical Technologies, Inc., Burlington, Massachusetts, USA). Both families contain a variety of effective nonablative resurfacing lasers. The laser wavelengths used in both families are in the infrared region of the light spectrum and utilize water as their tissue target or chromophore. The families differ by using slightly different wavelengths in their respective lasers. But the most striking difference between the two families is the manner in which the laser energy is delivered to the skin. Besides these two main families, there is also a multi-wavelength NAFL

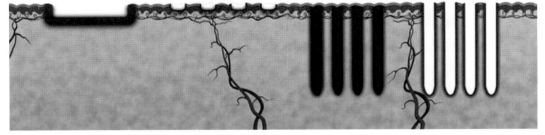

Ablative resurfacing (CO₂ & 2.94 Erb:YAG) 10–200 μm **Superficial ablative fractional resurfacing** (CO₂ & 2.94 Erb:YAG) 10–70 μm **Nonablative fractional resurfacing** 600–1000 μm **Ablative fractional resurfacing** 600–1000 μm

Figure 8.1 Schematic representation of laser impact from several lasers. NAFL is thermal only without vaporization.

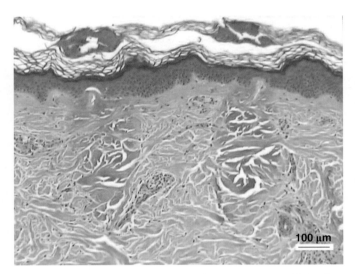

Figure 8.2 Microthermal zones of damage from 1550-nm fractional laser.

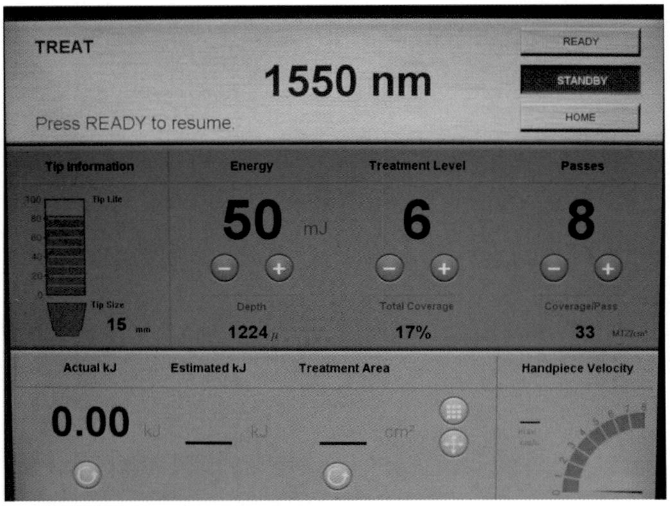

Figure 8.3 Treatment screen of 1550-nm nonablative fractional laser. Fluence, density, and number of passes with rolling handpiece to achieve that density. For these settings it takes eight passes to achieve 17% surface coverage.

by Cynosure, Inc. (Westford, Massachusetts, USA), a fractional 910-nm laser by Syneron Medical Ltd (Irvine, California, USA), and the fractional Q-Switched 1064 nm by Alma Lasers (Buffalo Grove, Illinois, USA). There are also other NAFLs that are marketed outside the USA or that are currently in development.

THE SOLTA FAMILY OF NAFL

The Solta family consists of the Fraxel division of laser devices and the Clear and Brilliant™ laser system (10). The Fraxel division includes the Fraxel 1550-nm laser, the Fraxel DUAL 1550/1927-nm laser, a stand alone Fraxel 1927-nm laser, and the Fraxel re:fine 1410-nm laser, which is mostly marketed outside the USA. All of the Fraxel laser systems have an interface which allows for a customized treatment by controlling the pulse energy, TL, and the number of passes (Fig. 8.3). The pulse energy is delivered in microjoules and it controls the depth of penetration or the depth of the MTZ. Different depths of the skin can be treated for different indications (Fig. 8.4). The treatment level is the percentage of skin treated or covered by MTZs during one treatment session and it controls the aggressiveness of treatment. The number of passes is also set during the procedure. A pass is defined as a single

unidirectional motion over the skin that lays down one row of MTZs. On an average, eight passes are performed. Additional passes can be applied to individual areas of scarring or deep lines. The total energy delivered per treatment session is constant regardless of the number of passes. For example, the quantity of energy per pass decreases as the number of passes increase. Alternately, the quantity of energy per pass increases as the number of passes decrease. To increase patient comfort, a higher number of passes with less density of MTZ per each pass can be performed. Typically, passes are delivered by alternating horizontal and perpendicular passes within one cosmetic unit at a time. Before a laser treatment series begins, the skin surface can be measured and an estimated energy in total kilojoules of the treatment will be computed by the laser treatment screen according to the set treatment parameters.

All of the Solta lasers have a continuous motion handpiece, which is equipped with rollers. The Fraxel laser treatment tip comes in two different sizes, 15 mm and 7 mm. Smaller cosmetic units like the eyelid, nose, or lip can be treated with the smaller tip (Fig. 8.5A). The Clear + Brilliant™ system is a nonablative fractional 1440-nm laser. It is based on the technology of the Fraxel lasers and has a similar, yet more simplified interface. In all the NAFL devices by Solta Medical, the

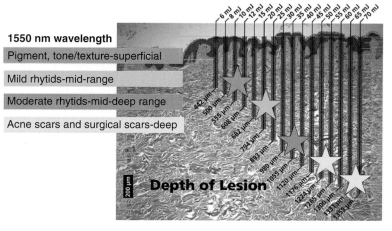

1550 nm wavelength

Pigment, tone/texture-superficial

Mild rhytids-mid-range

Moderate rhytids-mid-deep range

Acne scars and surgical scars-deep

Depth of Lesion

Figure 8.4 Approximate depths of thermal impact by fluence.

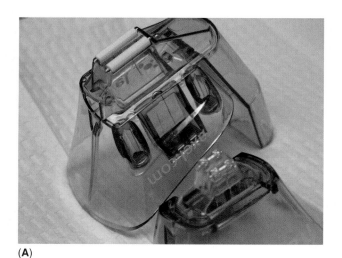

(A)

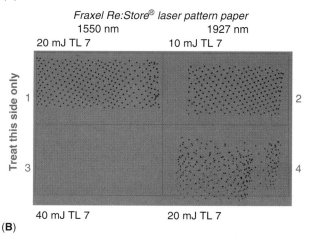

Fraxel Re:Store® laser pattern paper

1550 nm   1927 nm

20 mJ TL 7   10 mJ TL 7

Treat this side only

40 mJ TL 7   20 mJ TL 7

(B)

Figure 8.5 (**A**) Tip for rolling device. This must be replaced approximately every 5–10 treatments. (**B**) Rolling patterns for rolling devices (1550 and 1927 nm).

handpieces should be positioned perpendicular to the skin and it should not be lifted while the foot switch is depressed. Handpiece velocity is also measured on the laser during treatment. Passes should be smooth and controlled and stay within the recommended velocity levels. If the treatment passes are delivered too fast, the laser microdots become oval rather than round and therefore the energy delivered may be reduced by up to 50% which leads to undertreatment. Pulses delivered by the rolling technique may not be uniformly distributed. Some pulses overlap while others are adjacent and some are farther apart (Fig. 8.5B).

Fractional 1550-nm Laser

The Fraxel 1550-nm laser, which is the most extensively studied nonablative resurfacing laser, was introduced in 2006. It is indicated for moderate skin damage resurfacing for periorbital wrinkles, pigmented lesions, dyschromia, scars, melasma, and actinic keratosis. It can deliver laser energy ranging from 4 to 70 mJ. Its TLs range from 5% to 48% coverage. Maximum absorption depth into the skin is estimated to be 1400–1500 μm deep. As discussed previously, different depths of the skin can be treated for different indications and TLs can be adjusted to determine the aggressiveness of treatment. For example, to target a deep scar with the Fraxel 1550-nm laser, a higher energy like 50–70 mJ will be selected. An example of an aggressive TL will be 12 and cover 35% of the facial skin in one treatment. In patients with darker skin types (Fitzpatrick types IV–VI), the density must be delivered at a lower TL like 4–6 or 11–17% coverage to reduce the chances of post-inflammatory hyperpigmentation (PIH) (Table 8.1).

Fractional 1550-nm and 1927-nm Lasers

Fraxel DUAL 1550/1927 (Solta Medical) was introduced in October 2009. Both lasers are housed in the same platform and function independently of each other. A fully 1550-nm treatment or a fully 1927-nm treatment may be performed. The lasers may also be used in combination with a different wavelength used in different cosmetic units/body areas or both lasers can be layered on top of each other for a combination treatment. The thulium 1927-nm wavelength has a higher absorption coefficient for water than the 1550-nm wavelength so it has a greater ability to target the epidermis. See Figure 8.6 that illustrates the absorption of the two wavelengths. Energy fluences for the 1927-nm laser range from 5 to 20 mJ and the TL ranges from 20% to 70% coverage. It has a maximum depth of penetration of 200 μm into the skin. Therefore, this wavelength is more effective in treating epidermal processes like actinic keratoses. An average energy and TL for a patient with a Fitzpatrick skin type (I–III) will be 10–20 mJ and a TL of 3–6 that corresponds to 30–45% coverage (Table 8.2). In 2011, the

Fraxel 1927-nm laser became available in a stand alone laser platform. The 1927-nm wavelength is currently FDA approved in the treatment of actinic keratosis.

The 1550-nm and 1927-nm lasers can be combined for a "DUAL" resurfacing treatment. When combining the 1550-nm and 1927-nm wavelengths, four passes of 1550-nm laser are performed over the treatment area to target the dermis and then four passes of 1927-nm laser are performed to provide an epidermal treatment. Laser energies and TLs are set at a level lower than if the lasers were used separately. Our experience has taught us to use caution when treating with both wavelengths on the same day. Recovery times and discomfort may be greater than if the lasers were used individually (Table 8.3).

Fractional 1440-nm Laser

The Clear and Brilliant system is a fractional diode 1440-nm laser launched in May 2011. It is indicated for general skin resurfacing. The laser has a fixed spot size of 140 μm. Energy can be delivered on a low (4 mJ), medium (7 mJ), or high level (9 mJ). The depth of penetration ranges from 280 to 390 μm depending on the energy level used. The low level setting corresponds to 4% coverage, the medium level to 7% coverage,

Table 8.1 Fraxel 1550-nm Laser Treatment Settings

| Indication | **Mild to Moderate Parameters** | |
	Pulse Energy (Depth)	Treatment Level (Coverage)
Fitzpatrick Skin Phototype I–III		
General Resurfacing (Pigmented lesions, textural irregularities, fine lines)		
Face	10–25 mJ	4–8 (11–23%)
Eyelids (within orbital rim)	10–20 mJ	4–7 (11–20%)
Off-Face	10–25 mJ	4–7 (11–20%)
Deep Wrinkles, Acne Scars		
Face	25–70 mJ	5–9 (14–26%)
Off-Face	25–40 mJ	4–8 (11–23%)
Melasma (Evaluate patient after each treatment. 2–3 treatments)		
Face	6–15 mJ	5–8 (14–23%)
Surgical Scars	40–70 mJ	5–8 (14–23%)
Fitzpatrick Skin Phototype IV–VI		
General Resurfacing (Pigmented lesions, textural irregularities, fine lines)		
Face	10–25 mJ	3–7 (9–20%)
Eyelids (within orbital rim)	10–20 mJ	3–6 (9–17%)
Off-Face	10–25 mJ	3–6 (9–17%)
Deep Wrinkles, Acne Scars		
Face	25–70 mJ	4–7 (11–20%)
Off-Face	25–40 mJ	4–6 (11–17%)
Melasma		
Face	6–15 mJ	3–7 (9–20%)
Surgical Scars	40–70 mJ	4–7 (11–20%)

Source: Adapted from Solta Laser Systems Operator Manual.

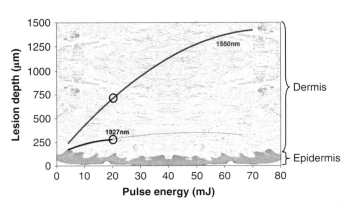

Figure 8.6 Comparison of depths of 1550 nm vs. 1927 nm for depth of thermal impact.

Table 8.2 Fraxel 1927-nm Laser Treatment Settings

| Indication | **Moderate Parameters** | |
	Pulse Energy (Depth)	Treatment Level (Coverage)
Fitzpatrick Skin Phototype I–VI		
General Resurfacing		
Face	5–20 mJ	1–5 (20–40%)
Eyelids (within orbital rim)	5–20 mJ	1–4 (20–35%)
Off-Face	5–15 mJ	1–4 (20–35%)
Fitzpatrick Skin Phototype I–III		
Actinic Keratosis		
Face	10–20 mJ	3–5 (30–40%)
Off-Face	10–20 mJ	2–4 (25–35%)

Source: Adapted from Solta Laser Systems Operator Manual.

Table 8.3 Fraxel 1550-nm/1927-nm Dual Laser Treatment Settings

| Indication | **Moderate Parameters: 1550 nm** | | **Moderate Parameters: 1927-nm** | | |
	Pulse Energy (Depth)	Treatment Level (Coverage)	Pulse Energy (Depth)	Treatment Level (Coverage)	Total Coverage
Fitzpatrick Skin Phototype I–III					
General Resurfacing					
Face	10–25 mJ	3–5 (9–14%)	5–20 mJ	1–3 (20–30%)	(30–40%)
Eyelids (within orbital rim)	10–20 mJ	2–4 (7–11%)	5–20 mJ	1–3 (20–30%)	(30–35%)
Off-Face	10–25 mJ	1–3 (5–9%)	5–20 mJ	1–2 (20–25%)	(25–35%)
Fitzpatrick Skin Phototype IV–VI					
General Resurfacing					
Face	10–25 mJ	1–4 (5–11%)	5–20 mJ	1–3 (20–30%)	(25–35%)
Eyelids (within orbital rim)	10–20 mJ	1–3 (5–9%)	5–20 mJ	1–3 (20–30%)	(25–35%)
Off-Face	10–25 mJ	1–3 (5–9%)	5–20 mJ	1–3 (20–25%)	(20–30%)

Source: Adapted from Solta Laser Systems Operator Manual.

and the high level to 9% coverage. It utilizes a disposable treatment tip per treatment. It can be used in all skin types, although we have experience with other 1440-nm devices and find that the risk of PIH is higher with 1440-nm than with 1540- to 1500-nm devices. It is marketed as a preventive laser treatment and provides a superficial treatment with minimal down time. It is marketed to medical spas primarily.

THE PALOMAR FAMILY OF NAFL

The Palomar family of NAFLs (Palomar Medical Technologies, Inc.) includes a 1540-nm erbium: glass laser, a 1440-nm Nd:YAG laser, and a 1410-nm diode home use laser. With the exception of the 1410-nm diode home use laser, these wavelengths are delivered through a variety of microlenses, which can be used in three different laser/pulsed light platforms: the StarLux, Artisan, and Icon. These devices, like the Cynosure Affirm laser, are based on the stamping mode of delivering fractional energy with the microdots of energy coming through microlens arrays. The latest generation of Palomar's NAFL is available through the Icon™ Aesthetic system platform which has four unique 1540-nm handpiece microlenses; the original 10-mm and 15-mm microlenses, the 15-mm XF Microlens, and the XD Microlens. See Figure 8.7 that illustrates the ICON 1540-nm interface. Furthermore, the new XD Microlens can be used on any of the previous generation 1440-nm and 1540-nm fractional handpieces with the appropriate software and factory calibration.

The original fractional microlenses are composed of a microlens array that delivers a lattice of optical microbeams that create microdenatured columns in the skin. The microlens is responsible for taking a single beam of laser energy and separating it out into smaller lasers beams at a predetermined pitch. See Figure 8.8A,B for photos of the original microlens. The XD Microlens is a chilled 12×12 mm^2 sapphire contact window that is composed of 49 microcompression pins each coaligned with a microbeam. Figure 8.9 depicts the XD microlens tip, which allows for much deeper (XD = extra deep) penetration of energy by compression water from the upper layers of dermis. This new microlens is used with manual compression into the skin to achieve deeper penetration of laser energy into the dermis. A footprint of the XD is seen after 30 seconds of manual pressure (Fig. 8.10). The act of compression displaces water

into interstitial spaces of the skin. With less water to absorb, the scattering of laser light is reduced which enables increased absorption of light by deeper targets. The compression into the skin not only enhances beam penetration, it enhances the skin cooling effect due to loss in heating in the epidermis. Better cooling means decreased epidermal temperature and injury. Clinically, this translates into fewer side effects, less downtime, and a more comfortable treatment. The XF optic provides higher coverage per pulse, compared with the original optics, allowing faster treatments times, similar to 1440 nm but with the added benefit of increased depth due to the increased penetration of the 1540-nm wavelength.

These laser treatments are customized by controlling the microbeam energy, the amount of overlap between pulses and the number of passes. The pulse energy is delivered in millijoules per microbeam (mJ/mb) and it controls the depth of penetration or the depth of the MTZ. Energies should be adjusted for the skin condition being treated. Lower energies are utilized for more superficial conditions and higher energies, which penetrate deeper, are used for deeper indications. The percentage of skin treated or covered by MTZs during one treatment session is determined by the amount of overlapping

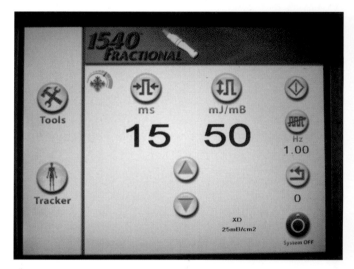

Figure 8.7 Treatment screen for 1540-nm fractional. Here each pulse is 15 ms and each thermal zone is 50 mJ/cm^2. Coverage is determined by percent overlap of each stamp.

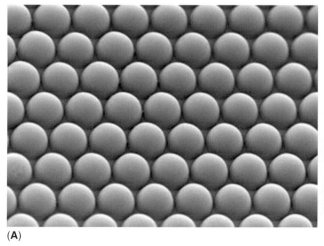

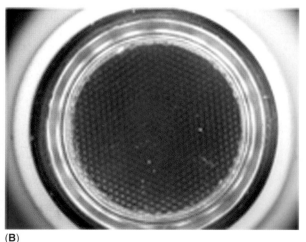

(**A**)   (**B**)

Figure 8.8 (**A**) Microlens array for stamped 1540-nm nonablative fractional laser and (**B**) 15-mm handpiece lens array.

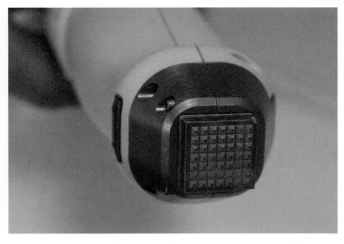

Figure 8.9 XD optic showing optical prongs to press water out of tissue.

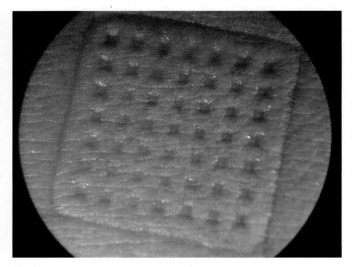

Figure 8.10 Prong pattern of 1540 XD after 30 seconds of compression on the skin.

passes performed with the stamping technique of the microlens. More overlapping and passes increase the aggressiveness of treatment (total surface coverage). Additionally, use of manual compression with the standard and XD Microlens is suspected to increase penetration of laser energy into the skin.

Regardless of the tip or wavelength used, the laser procedure is delivered in a stamped method. Multiple stamps are delivered into the skin with varying amounts of overlap. The amount of overlap between the stamps usually varies from 20% to 50%. Rows of stamps are performed in a single cosmetic unit at a time. The rows may be overlapped from 0% to 50% depending on the wavelength, the microlens used, and the desired total coverage and rate at which the coverage is administered. One pass is completed when the entire cosmetic unit is covered by the stamps. Passes are then alternated between perpendicular and horizontal directions. This is also known as the tile cascade method (Fig. 8.11). One to five passes are typically performed, depending on the total desired coverage. It is important to keep the treatment tip in full continuous contact with the skin during each laser pulse. As with the roller technique for delivering fractionated laser pulses, when there are overlapping stamped pulses, they also produce laser impact sites, which are not evenly distributed on the skin surface.

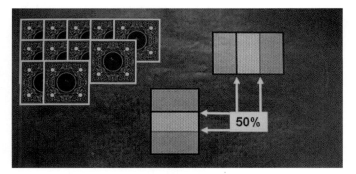

Figure 8.11 Tile cascade for stamping nonablative fractional laser showing 50% overlap pulse to pulse.

Fractional 1540-nm Laser

The 1540-nm original microlenses from the Palomar Starlux™ and Artisan™ Fractional laser platforms are available in two sizes. A flat circular 10-mm tip has a microbeam density of 100 mb/cm² and a flat circular 15-mm tip has a microbeam density of 320 mb/cm². The pulse durations are adjustable to 10 or 15 ms. The 10-mm tip can deliver energies between 14 and 70 mJ/mb. The 10-mm tip delivers a smaller number of higher energy beams of laser light that can penetrate deeper with a wider coagulation column diameter in one pulse when compared with the 15-mm tip. The 15-mm tip can deliver energies between 3 and 15 mJ/mb. The standard 10-mm tip averages a 725 μm depth of penetration while the 15-mm tip averages a 600 μm depth of penetration (Table 8.4).

The Palomar Icon™ Aesthetic System can use a standard 10-mm or 15-mm handpiece, but additionally has the 12 × 12-mm XD Microlens (25 mb/cm²) and the 15-mm XF Microlens (115 mb/cm²). The XD Microlens delivers laser energies from 20 to 70 mJ/mb. The XF Microlens emits energies from 6 to 60 mJ/mb. The XF Microlens provides a higher coverage per pulse compared with the original optics allowing fast treatment coverage comparable to the 1440 with the added benefit of increased depth. Average depth of penetration of the microbeam is approximately 750 μm for the XF and 1060 μm for the XD Microlens. Pulse stacking has been studied with the XD Microlens. For example, three stacked pulses with the LUX 1540 XD tip have reached a depth of 1900 μm into the dermis. Settings for the XD microlens are typically from 40 to 70 mJ/mb and three to seven passes with overlap ranging from 10% to 50% depending on the desired total coverage and clinical condition treated (Table 8.5).

Palomar Fractional Laser for Home Use

PaloVia® Skin Renewing Laser was cleared by the FDA in 2009. It is the first FDA-cleared at-home laser treatment delivering nonablative fractional treatment. The wavelength is specified as 1410 (±20) nm. It delivers a pulse duration of 10 ms with a maximum of 15 mJ of energy. The PaloVia® Skin Renewing Laser has been FDA cleared to reduce fine lines and wrinkles in the periorbital area. In a study of 124 subjects who used the device daily for 4 weeks, blinded evaluations revealed improvement in the Fitzpatrick Wrinkle Score by one or more grades in 90% of the subjects. Post-treatment erythema was graded as trace in the majority of test subjects.

Table 8.4 Starlux 1540-nm Laser Treatment Settings

	Superficial/ Moderate Corrections	Deep Corrections
Handpiece (mm)	15	10
Millijoules per microbeam	6–15	25–50
Pulse width (ms)	5–10	5–10
Passes (20–50% overlap)	2–5	2–4
Number of treatments	3–5	3–5
Treatment intervals (wk)	3–4	3–4

Source: Adapted from Palomar Laser Systems Operator Manual.

Table 8.5 Icon 1540-nm Laser Treatment Settings

	15-mm tip	10-mm tip	XD Microlens	XF Microlens
Millijoules per microbeam	10–15	40–70	40–70	30–50
Pulse width (ms)	10–15	10–15	15	10–15
Number of passes (20–50% overlap)	3–4	3–6	3–6	1–2
Number of treatments	2–5	2–5	2–5	1–2
Treatment interval	3–4 wk	3–4 wk	3–4 wk	1–3 mo

Source: Adapted from Palomar Laser Systems Operator Manual.

THE MULTI-WAVELENGTH FRACTIONAL 1440-nm/1320-nm LASER

The Affirm™ Multiplex laser (Cynosure Inc.) is a fractional laser the emits a combination of 1440-nm and 1320-nm wavelengths of Nd:YAG laser. The Multiplex technology is defined as the sequential emission of two laser wavelengths using one laser fiber. It has a diffractive lens array that consists of 1000 diffractive elements per cm^2 to affect more surface area per single pulse. The laser uses combined apex pulse (CAP) technology. CAP technology reportedly delivers apex pulses of high-fluence regions for collagen remodeling and low-fluence regions to stimulate collagen growth. The 1440-nm wavelength heats a column of tissue to a depth of 300 μm and the 1320-nm wavelength penetrates deeper (12). Cynosure's Smart Cool™ air cooling system van be attached to the handpiece to protect and cool the skin. Usually, topical anesthesia is not necessary. A 14-mm spot size is used; usually two passes are suggested with a 15–20% overlap. Four to six treatments spaced 3–6 weeks apart are necessary for improvement in superficial scars and photodamage. The 1440-nm laser has a maximum energy of 8 J and the 1320-nm laser has a maximum energy of 14 J. Typical treatment parameters for skin rejuvenation would be 2–3 J/cm^2 for the 1440-nm component and 6–10 J/cm^2 for the 1320-nm component (13).

OTHER FRACTIONAL LASERS

A fractional Q-switched ruby laser (TattooStar FRx, Asclepion, Jena, Germany) has been reported to improve melasma in Korean patients (14). A 1540-nm fractional erbium glass laser (Mosaic, Lutronic Co. Ltd, Seoul, South Korea) has been studied in the treatment of male and female pattern hair loss and in skin rejuvenation (15–17). The 1540-nm and 1340-nm fractional lasers are available through the DEKA Dot platform (DEKA laser, Firenze, Italy). In the USA, there is a also a fractional 910-nm laser by Syneron Medical Ltd. and a fractional Q-Switched 1064 nm by Alma Lasers. Prototypes of a fractional 1940-nm and a 1208 nm laser have also been studied.

CLINICAL CONSIDERATIONS

Before initiating an NAFL treatment series, several clinical considerations need to be carefully examined. Specifically, the treating physician and support staff should carefully consult with each patient about the indications for treatment and expected results of treatment, and review the treatment process in detail.

Also, a medical history and physical examination must be performed to identify contraindications for or impediments to treatment. Patient selection for NAFL resurfacing is very important. The ideal candidate has mild to moderate skin damage or discoloration. Those with severely damaged skin with deep acne scars/wrinkles or extreme laxity will benefit more from an ablative fractional/fully ablative or surgical procedure. Patients must also be counseled to have realistic expectation of the treatment results. NAFL resurfacing yields slow gradual improvement over a series of treatments. Fine lines and scars do decrease but they are not completely removed. Definitive improvement in brown pigmentation and actinic keratoses can be seen but patients must be counseled that they may recur with continued sun exposure and time. Daily sun protection is necessary for all patients after treatment. Also, the final results from treatment may take 3–6 months after the last treatment. This time is necessary to achieve the full effect of collagen remodeling from the NAFL. During the consultation, the treatment experience is also discussed in detail. Patients are instructed that a series of treatments will be necessary. Usually, the treatment can be accomplished over 2–5 sessions spaced 4–6 weeks apart, depending on the clinical indication. Topical anesthetic will be applied to the treatment area for approximately 60 minutes before the laser treatment and the treatment itself will take 20–40 minutes depending on surface area treated. Cool air and cold ice rollers can be used to increase comfort during the treatment. A prickly heat sensation or a zap of heat can be felt on the skin depending on which NAFL system is used during the treatment. After treatment, patients may feel like they have a sun burn. Redness and swelling should be expected initially. Skin dryness with a flaky dot appearance can last a few days up to 2 weeks depending on the intensity of the problem and the body area treated. During the consultation, side effects are discussed, a medical history is reviewed, and physical examination of the treatment area is performed. Contraindications include oral retinoid use within the last 6 months, predisposition to keloid formation or excessive scarring, and lesions that appear to be suspicious for malignancy in the treatment area. Recent sun exposure or tanned skin, pregnancy, an active infection in the treatment area, or a medical condition that compromises healing time or predisposes to infection also can be added to the list. History of herpes simplex virus infection is a mandatory portion of the medical history as reactivation of the virus can occur with NAFL treatment. Pretreatment with an oral antiviral is recommended. For darker skins types or patients prone to hyperpigmentation, pre- and post-treatment with a hydroquinone bleaching cream are recommended and strict sun protection is discussed with all patients.

TREATMENT PREPARATION

To prepare for NAFL treatment, patients are asked to remove all jewelry and makeup and cleanse their skin with a mild cleanser. Consents are reviewed and signed. Premedication with an oral antiviral for patients with a history of herpes simplex virus is documented. Pretreatment standardized photographs are taken. Our practice uses the Canfield Omnia system and the Vectra 3D system (Canfield Scientific Inc., Fairfield, New Jersey, USA). The Visia™ system (Canfield Scientific Inc.) can be used for finer textural changes and wrinkle assessment. The treatment area is wiped with 70% isopropyl alcohol and allowed to dry. A moderately thick (a quarter inch) application of a topical anesthetic is made. We use compounded topical anesthetic with 15% lidocaine and 5% prilocaine in an ointment base for the treatment of the face or localized body area. A two-treatment area restriction should be considered when using these stronger, compounded topical anesthetic agents. Lidocaine overdose is possible and lidocaine toxicity has been reported during NAFL treatment (18). The fractional laser consensus panel recommends to limit the area to 300–400 cm² to minimize potential lidocaine toxicity (19). If larger skin surfaces are to be treated, a standard topical anesthetic cream can be used like lidocaine 5% cream (L.M.X. 5, Ferndale Healthcare Inc., Ferndale, Michigan, USA). The topical anesthetic should be blended into the perimeter of the anticipated treatment area to ensure comfort. After 60 minutes, the topical anesthetic is removed with a dry gauze pad. Chapter 16 details topical anesthesia. Use of eye protection for the patient, practitioner, and support staff is mandatory during the NAFL treatment. If the eyelid skin inside the orbital rim is to be treated, intraocular metal eye shields should be inserted. Handpieces are sanitized with Sani-Cloth® (Professional Disposables International, Inc., Orangeburg, New York, USA) before each treatment. Laser system tests are performed to ensure a properly performing laser. A paper test strip is available for use with the Fraxel laser systems (Fig. 8.5B).

When treating the patient with any NAFL, divide the treatment area into smaller cosmetic units. For example, the cosmetic units of forehead, cheeks, nose, lip, and chin are treated as separate areas. These units can be customized to the preferences of the individual practitioner. Completely treat one cosmetic unit at a time. Be careful not to overlap treatment between the individual cosmetic units that could cause overtreatment. In our practice, we use forced cold air during the treatment, which has been shown to reduce pain but can also affect the thermal laser injury (20). After the NAFL treatment is concluded, patients are treated with a light-emitting diode treatment (Gentlewaves, LLC., Virginia Beach, Virginia, USA) to reduce the intensity and duration of post-treatment erythema (21). They are also treated with topical thermal water gel and spray (Avene Thermal Water, Pierre Fabre Dermo Cosmétique USA, Parsippany, New Jersey, USA) to alleviate discomfort and a physical sunblock is applied before they leave the office. The next treatment is scheduled in 3–6 weeks.

POST-CARE ROUTINE

Gentle post-care is of paramount importance. In our practice, we supply our patients with a skin care kit to be used during their laser treatment series. It consists of a gentle cleanser, non-occlusive moisturizer, thermal water spray, and a physical sunblock. Post-care instructions are reviewed verbally with the patient after treatment and they are also sent home with written instructions. The patient is instructed to cleanse the treated area twice a day with the cleanser and immediately apply the moisturizer. The broad spectrum sun protection must be applied before exposure to sunlight and reapplied as necessary. Patients can also apply cool compresses or cold packs and spray their face with the thermal water spray as needed to help reduce swelling and discomfort. Narcotic pain medication is rarely necessary, but over-the-counter acetaminophen can be taken if needed. Patients should sleep with their head elevated for the first few nights to help diminish swelling. They should avoid vigorous exercise or activity while swollen or red. They should avoid smoking and excessive alcohol consumption. Strict sun protection must be observed using a broad spectrum SPF of 30 or greater. Direct sun exposure should be avoided for 3 months after treatment. Topical products and medications can usually be restarted 3–7 days after treatment depending on the level of treatment and sensitivity of the patient. Those patients prone to PIH or who are being treated for melasma will restart a topical hydroquinone cream 1–4 days post-procedure.

COMPLICATIONS

Complications are a possibility with any NAFL treatment, even though the potential for and the incidence of serious side effects are exponentially less than with traditional and ablative resurfacing. Nonablative skin resurfacing has a low complication rate. Most side effects are transient in nature. Possible side effects include erythema, swelling, blistering, scarring, infection, pigmentary changes, herpes reactivation, and acne flare-up. Transient erythema and swelling are to be expected and the patient should be instructed to expect these. In a review of short-term adverse effects from 1550-nm NAFL treatment by Fisher et al., all patients displayed post-treatment erythema and edema was present in 82% of patients (22). Prolonged erythema, massive swelling, blistering, and subsequent scarring can occur if aggressive treatment parameters were used and overheating of the skin occurs. These side effects can be easily avoided with a prudent selection of treatment parameters. Infection is rarely seen with nonablative fractional resurfacing. Hyperpigmentation definitely occurs and is more prevalent with darker skin types (IV–V). This can be reduced with pre- and post-treatment with hydroquinone bleaching agents and strict sun protection. Also, treatment densities and fluencies must be lowered to reduce this side effect. Reactivation of herpes simplex is a real side effect. Patients who are prone to herpes simplex should be pretreated with oral antivirals. There have also been three cases of herpes zoster along the trigeminal nerve, which have been reported after NAFL (23). Acneiform eruptions can also occur. If patients are prone to acne, they can be treated with oral antibiotics, like minocycline or doxycycline and/ or a topical antibiotics, such as clindamycin. The nonablative resurfacing complication rate has been studied over several years (24–26). A retrospective study of 961 nonablative 1550-nm laser treatments recorded a 7.6%

complication rate (26). The two most common complications encountered were acneiform eruption and herpes simplex reactivation. However, these were only encountered at a 1.87% and 1.77% rate respectively. Overall, NAFL is a very safe treatment and has minimal side effects at the recommended settings.

CLINICAL APPLICATIONS

Nonablative lasers have been used to treat an expansive range of conditions. Numerous clinical studies have shown its effectiveness in a variety of treatments (19,27,28). The main areas of treatment include photodamage and wrinkling, scars, stretch marks, pigmentary disorders, and actinic keratosis. Evolving applications include the enhancement of drug and topical product delivery through NAFL resurfacing which takes advantage of increased permeability of the epidermis and dermis after treatment. Case reports have also shown NAFL treatment to be useful in miscellaneous other applications that include improving residual hemangiomas, minocycline-induced pigmentation, nevus of Ota, granuloma annulare, and male and female pattern hair loss (15,16,29–32).

Photodamage

Many studies have examined nonablative fractional resurfacing of the face and non-facial skin for improvement in sun induced discoloration and wrinkles. In 2007, Wanner et al. examined 50 patients with mild to moderate photodamage, rhytides, and dyspigmentation who received three successive treatments with a 1550-nm erbium-doped laser (Fraxel SR750, Reliant Technologies, Inc.,[1] Mountain View, CA) (33). At least 51–75% improvement in photodamage was observed in 73% and 55% of facial and non-facial (chest and neck) treated skin at the 9-month follow-up. Fractional laser photothermolysis for photoaging of the hands was examined specifically in a small cohort of patients by Jih et al. (34). Ten patients were randomized to either receive five NAFL treatments with a 1550-nm laser (Fraxel SR, Reliant Technologies, Inc.) to their left or right hand. Statistically significant improvements in skin pigmentation and skin texture were noted at the 1- and 3-month follow-up. Skin biopsies were also taken at baseline, 1- and 3-month follow-ups. The post-treatment biopsies showed thickening of the epidermis and notably increased collagen density in the papillary and upper reticular dermis. Moreover, the study was safe and showed limited side effects. A 1550-nm laser consensus panel also convened to discuss their recommended treatment settings for photoaging (19). The panel recommended settings of 10–20 mJ of energy with a TL of 7–11 to improve dyschromia in patients with Fitzpatrick skin types I–III. For rhytides, specifically in the periorbital region, the consensus recommended settings of 30–70 mJ of energy using a TL of 7–11 with 8 passes. For dyschromia of the neck and chest the panel recommended 10–40 mJ of energy using a TL of 7–11 and 8 passes for Fitzpatrick skin types I–III. Newer versions of the 1550-nm laser, as well as other NAFLs of other wavelengths, have been developed since the consensus meeting. Hopefully, another consensus meeting will be planned that will include recommended treatment guidelines for all NAFL systems. A clinical example of results with 1927 nm are shown in Figure 8.12. Results using a 1550 nm laser are shown in Figures 8.13 and 8.14.

Scars

Improvement in scars may significantly improve the patient's self-esteem and quality of life. Common causes of scars include surgery, trauma, and acne. Two main categories of scars include atrophic and hypertrophic scars. They can vary in color from white to red to brown. In 2007, an initial pilot study by Vasily studied 31 subjects with 13 surgical and 18 traumatic scars using the Lux 1540-nm 10-mm handpiece (35). Treatments using laser energies in the range of 30–60 mJ/mb, a 10-ms pulse duration, 3–5 passes, and a series of 1–8 treatments were performed. A blinded observer saw 51–75% improvement in scars at 1 month after treatment in 59% of patients. The most improvement was seen after the first three treatments. NAFL treatment of surgical scars was also compared with and outperformed the standard scar treatment of pulsed dye laser (PDL) (36). A randomized blinded split-scar study was performed in 12 patients comparing the Fraxel RS (Reliant Technologies) against the 595-nm V-Beam PDL (Candela Corporation, Inc., Wayland, Massachusetts, USA). Treatment with a fluence of 70 mJ, TL 8, and 16 passes was performed on the NAFL side and with 7.5 J/cm², pulse duration of 0.45 ms, and a spot size of 10 × 3 mm was performed on the PDL side. After a series of four treatments, greater overall mean improvement was seen on the NAFL side (75.6%) compared with the PDL side (53.9%). Also, hypopigmented scars, hypertrophic scars, and traumatic thermal burn scars were studied in small cohorts and demonstrated improvement with NAFL (37–39). The 1550-nm NAFL consensus panel recommended the settings of 50–70 mJ of energy with a TL of 7–11 for skin types I–III in the treatment of surgical scars (19). Like surgical scars, acne scars can be cosmetically and psychologically disturbing to patients. NAFL has been proven successful in the treatment of acne scars. In 2008, Weiss et al. presented a retrospective analysis of over 500 acne scar treatments with the Lux 1540-nm laser (40). The fluences used were 50–70 mJ/mb with a minimum of three passes. Results assessed by blinded photographic evaluation showed a median of 50–75% improvement in acne scars; 85% of patients rated their skin as improved. Acne scars were also studied with the Fraxel 1550 nm SR750 (Reliant Technologies) by Alster et al. (41). Fifty-three patients with acne scarring received three laser treatments. Ninety percent of patients were found to have 51–75% improvement by an independent observer. The 1550-nm laser consensus panel meeting recommended selection of treatment settings of acne scars based on skin types (19). They recommended settings of 30–70 mJ at TL 7–11 for 8–12 passes for skin types I–III and 30–70 mJ, TL 4–5 and 8 passes for skin types IV–V. We presently employ the Icon system with the 1540-nm XD handpiece for scars and anecdotally have seen responses for scars resistant to all other NAFL devices. Flattening of a scar after IPL tattoo removal is shown in Figure 8.15.

Striae

Striae are disrupted areas of collagen in the skin that can occur during growth spurts, topical and oral steroid use, and conditions of hormonal change like pregnancy. It is estimated that 75–90% of women form some degree of stretch marks during

---

[1]Reliant Technologies, Inc. was acquired by Solta Medical, Inc. in 2008.

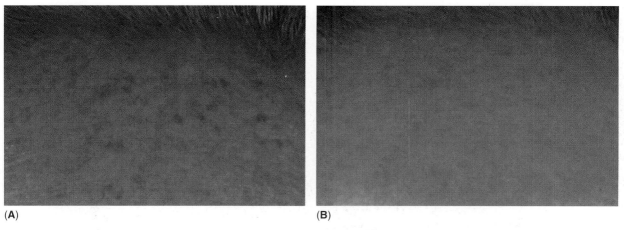

Figure 8.12 Pigmentation clinical results (**A**) before and (**B**) after using 1927 nm after one treatment.

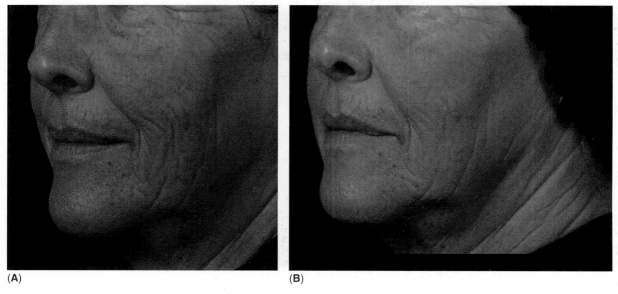

Figure 8.13 Clinical results (**A**) Before and (**B**) after two treatments using 1550 nm.

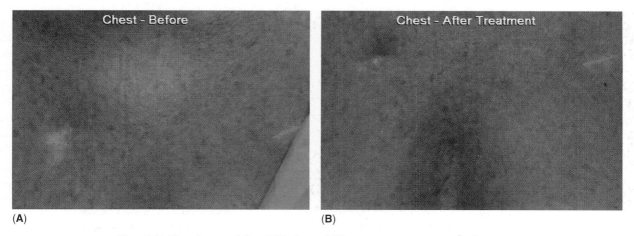

Figure 8.14 Photodamage of chest (**A**) before and (**B**) response to two treatments of 1550 nm.

pregnancy. Previous treatments have been ineffective or inconsistent and not suitable for all skin types (42). Histology of striae is very similar to that of atrophic scars, so treatment with NAFL is attempted. The Palomar 1540-nm NAFL is currently the only laser to gain FDA clearance for the treatment of striae. One of the first studies with the LUX 1540-nm laser evaluated

51 subjects with striae of the abdomen, legs, buttocks, arms and flanks (43). Fluences of 35–55 mJ/mb with a 10-mm tip or 12–14 mJ/mb with the 15-mm tip were performed. Two to four treatments were performed. Patient and independent observer evaluations noted improvements of 50% or greater in all patients at 6 months past the last treatment. Fraxel 1550-nm

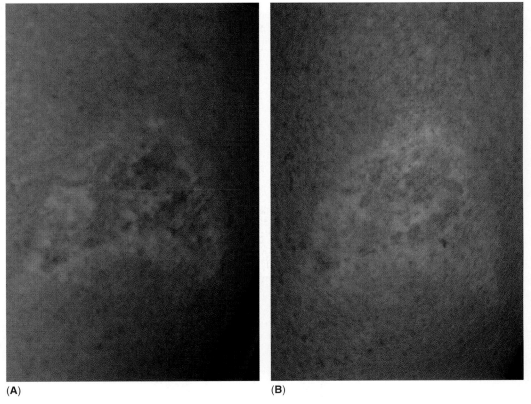

(A)   **(B)**

Figure 8.15 Flattening and improvement in hypopigmentation of a scar (**A**) before and (**B**) after several treatments of 1550 nm laser.

NAFL has also been studied in the treatment of striae even though it is not approved by the FDA for this indication. Twenty patients with striae were studied over six laser treatments. Randomly chosen photos of eight patients were chosen from the study and an independent observer rated a 26–50% level of overall improvement in five out of eight patients (44). The 1550-nm NAFL Consensus panel recommended the settings of 40 mJ, TL 10 for 8 passes in skin types I–III and TL 4–7 in darker skin types (19). When treating striae, a laser test area is always suggested. Pre- and post-treatment with a hydroquinone bleaching cream is suggested in darker skin types and areas prone to prolonged PIH, like the legs. A clinical example of striae response to 1540 nm is shown in Figure 8.16.

Pigmentary Disorders

Increased pigmentation of the skin, as seen in photodamage and melasma, has shown improvement through NAFL treatment. Melasma can be quite distressing to patients and is notoriously difficult to treat. It is a chronic skin condition seen primarily in female patients. It presents as a brown patchy discoloration over sun-exposed areas like the cheeks, forehead, upper lip and sometimes arms. Contributing factors include sun exposure, hormones, pregnancy, and genetics (45). Many therapeutic modalities have been investigated over the years but none have been shown to be uniformly successful (46,47). When the first 1550-nm laser was released, several melasma studies were initiated. The first pilot study was by Rokhsar et al. using 1550-nm laser on 10 patients (48). It showed some success with 60% of patients demonstrating excellent clearing and 30% of patients demonstrating mild improvement. Vasily used the Starlux 1540-nm laser with a 15-mm handpiece and delivered 4 passes with 50% overlap in the treatment of

6 patients with melasma (49). After 4 treatments, patients showed 40–50% lightening of melasma and improvement was maintained at 3-month follow-up. Another study compared 1550-nm laser resurfacing with a topical bleaching cream through a split face study (50). The patients in the study showed preference to the topical bleaching cream side over the 1550-nm NAFL side. The 1927-nm laser is not approved for melasma but initial reports seem promising. An initial pilot study by Polder et al. used the Fraxel 1927 nm in the treatment of 18 patients with melasma (51). They performed 3–4 treatments using 10–20 mJ of energy, a TL corresponding to 20–45% coverage, and 8 passes. Using the standard Melasma Area and Severity Index (MASI) and blinded independent photographic review of standardized photos, they reported a 51% reduction in the MASI scores at 1-month follow-up. There was still a 33% and a 34% reduction of MASI score at 3- and 6-month follow-ups respectively. Although NAFL treatment has shown success in the treatment of melasma, its long-term efficacy is still limited by the inherent recurrence rate of melasma. In some patients with melasma, we have also noted increased hyperpigmentation and prolonged erythema after NAFL treatment. Most NAFL and other laser treatments for melasma work best when combined with topical depigmenting skin care and aggressive sun protection.

Actinic keratoses

An actinic keratosis (AK) is a precancerous, epidermal, scaly macule or papule that occurs on sun damaged skin. Treatment of these lesions is indicated, as there is potential for them to progress into invasive squamous cell carcinoma. The 1550-nm and the 1927-nm wavelengths have been studied and have shown success in the treatment of these precancerous growths.

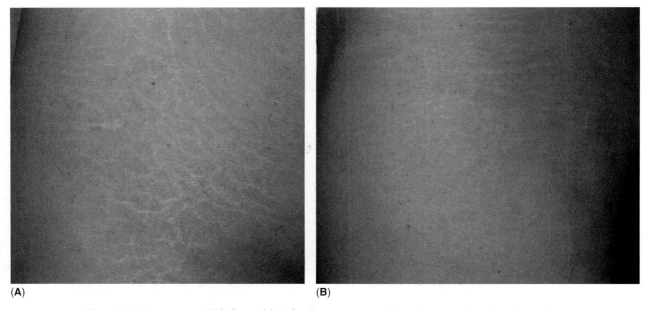

(A)   **(B)**

Figure 8.16 Striae response (**A**) before and (**B**) after three treatments with 1540 nm stamping using 50% overlap.

Initially, the 1550-nm fractional laser (Fraxel re:store, Solta Medical) was investigated in a small group of men with AKs (52). These men underwent 5 nonablative resurfacing laser treatments every 2 to 4 weeks. Energies ranged from 20 to 70 mJ during the treatment but the majority of treatments were performed at 70 mJ. TL was 11 and 8–10 passes were performed. A baseline biopsy was performed and then repeated at the 3-month follow-up immediately adjacent to the initial biopsy site. AKs were counted at 1-, 3-, and 6-month follow-up visits. There was clinical improvement after each session, although histologically, precancerous changes were still evident. At the 1-, 3-, and 6-month visits; actinic keratosis reduction from baseline was 73.1%, 66.2%, and 55.6% respectively. With the introduction of the 1927-nm thulium fiber fractional laser (Fraxel Dual, Solta Medical), more AK treatment studies began. This superficial wavelength selectively targets the epidermis and upper dermis and was postulated to have greater efficacy in the treatment of the mostly epidermal AKs. Weiss et al. studied 25 subjects with facial AKs receiving up to 4 treatments with a 1927-nm fractional laser (Fraxel Dual, Solta Medical) (53). One month after the final treatment, average AK clearance was 88.9%. At 6 months after treatment, it was 75%. They found this treatment to be effective and well tolerated by patients. Friedman et al. performed a split face laser treatment of AKs using the 1550 nm in combination with the 1927-nm laser versus the 1927-nm laser alone (54). They found that the side treated with 1927 nm alone had greater clinical reduction in AKs as well as improvement in sun-induced pigmentation. Furthermore, the 1927-nm laser was also applied to the treatment of AKs of the lip, otherwise known as actinic cheilitis (55). This condition is notoriously hard to treat, prone to recurrence, and can be quite painful for patients. Anolik et al. performed a retrospective chart analysis of a small group of actinic cheilitis patients and found that after 1–2 treatments patients were improved by 50–75% or 75–100% as rated by blinded, non-treating staff dermatologists (56). The procedure was well tolerated by patients and had much less side effects when compared with ablation, surgery, or treatment with topical chemotherapeutic agents or immune modulators. Unfortunately, whenever biopsies were performed on clinically improved AK treated with NAFL, persistent evidence of dystrophic epidermal cells was present. We therefore cannot recommend NAFL as a stand-alone treatment for AK at this time.

ENHANCEMENT IN DELIVERY OF TOPICAL DRUGS AND PRODUCTS

Research in this application of NAFL is still in its infancy. Enhancement of photodynamic therapy (PDT) has been studied with NAFL. In a study by Ruiz-Rodriguez et al., patients underwent a split treatment of perioral Fraxel 1550-nm resurfacing and resurfacing plus PDT (57). Immediately after NAFL treatment, methyl–5-aminolevulinate was applied to half of the perioral area for 3 hours and then activated by a red light source. After two treatment sessions, all patients noted greater improvement in the side treated with NAFL and PDT. In my practice, we often pretreat our PDT patients with 2–4 passes of NAFL, which allows for faster penetration of topical levulinic acid. This is especially helpful in areas like the arms and legs in which incubation time with levulinic acid would otherwise be hours. Enhancement of platelet-rich plasma (PRP) treatment of the skin has also been studied in NAFL (17). The study showed that when PRP was combined with NAFL with a 1550-nm laser (Mosaic, Lutronic Co. Ltd, Seoul, South Korea), patient satisfaction and skin elasticity increased while erythema index of the skin decreased. Histologically, patients who were treated with PRP plus NAFL demonstrated increased length of the dermal epidermal junction, amount of collagen, and number of fibroblasts compared with those treated with fractional laser alone.

CONCLUSIONS

Fractional photothermolysis, and its application of NAFL skin resurfacing, is still considered a leading groundbreaking technology. Both the stamping modes and the continuous motion handpiece with rollers are effective methods to deliver the energy. New understanding and advances in engineering have allowed the development of optics that drive energy more deeply and more safely to obtain better results on scars and other clinical problems. NAFL's proven efficacy in a multitude of skin conditions leads us to utilize NAFL as an integral part of our daily practice of dermatology and medicine. Clinical applications include among others photodamage, wrinkling, acne and surgical scars, stretch marks, pigmentary disorders, and actinic keratosis. Study after study demonstrates that fractional resurfacing is effective, safe, and has minimal side effects. NAFL continues to be further refined and ongoing studies will elucidate better settings and newer applications. Enhancement of penetration of topicals including levulinic acid for photodynamic therapy is among the many uses currently being developed.

REFERENCES

1. Manstein D, Herron G, Sink RK, et al. Fractional photothermolysis: a new concept for cutaneous remodeling using microscopic patterns of thermal injury. Lasers Surg Med 2004; 34: 426–38.
2. Bernstein L, Kauvar A, Grossman M, et al. The short and long term side effects of carbon dioxide laser resurfacing. Dermatol Surg 1997; 23: 519–25.
3. Helm T, Shatkin S Jr. Alabaster skin after CO_2 laser resurfacing: evidence for suppressed melanogenesis rather than just melanocytic destruction. Cutis 2006; 77: 15–17.
4. Bhatia A, Dover J, Arndt K, et al. Patient satisfaction and reported long-term therapeutic efficacy associated with 1,320 nm Nd:YAG laser treatment of acne scarring and photoaging. Dermatol Surg 2006; 32: 346–52.
5. Tanzi E, Alster T. Comparison of a 1450 nm diode laser and a 1320 nm Nd:YAG laser in the treatment of atrophic facial scars: a prospective clinical and histological study. Dermatol Surg 2004; 30: 152–7.
6. Lupton J, Williams C, Alster T. Non-ablative laser skin resurfacing using a 1540 nm erbium glass laser: A clinical and histologic analysis. Dermatol Surg 2002; 28: 833–5.
7. Chan H, Lam L, Wond D, et al. Use of 1,320 nm laser for wrinkle reduction and the treatment of acne scarring in Asians. Lasers Surg Med 2004; 34: 98–103.
8. Hantash B, Bedi V, Sudireddy V, et al. Laser-induced transepidermal elimination of dermal content by fractional photothermolysis. J Biomed Opt 2006; 11: 041115.
9. Laubach H, Tannous Z, Anderson R, et al. Skin responses to fractional photothermolysis. Lasers Surg Med 2006; 38: 142–9.
10. Data on file, Solta Medical, Hayward, CA. [Available from: http://www.solta.com/Technologies.cfm]
11. Data on file, Palomar Medical Technologies, Inc., Burlington, MA. [Available from: http://www.palomarmedical.com/resources.aspx]
12. Data on file, Cynosure Inc., Westford, MA. [Available from: http://www.cynosure.com/products/affirm/clinicals.php]
13. Peterson JD, Goldman MP. Rejuvenation of the aging chest: a review and our experience. Dermatol Surg 2011; 37: 555–71.
14. Jang WS, Lee CK, Kim BJ, et al. Efficacy of 694 nm Q-switched ruby fractional laser treatment of melasma in female Korean patients. Dermatol Surg 2011; 37: 1133–40.
15. Lee GY, Lee HI, Kim WS. The effect of a 1550 nm fractional erbium – glass laser in female pattern hair loss. J Eur Acad Venerol 2011; 25: 1450–4.
16. Kim WS, Lee HI, Lee JW, et al. Fractional photothermolysis laser treatment of male pattern hair loss. Dermatol Surg 2011; 37: 41–51.
17. Shin MK, Lee JH, Lee SJ, Kim NI. Platelet-rich plasma combined with fractional laser therapy for skin rejuvenation. Dermatol Surg 2012. doi: 10.1111/j.1524-4725.2011.02280.x. [Epub ahead of print] PubMed PMID: 22288389.
18. Marra DE, Yip D, Fincher EF, et al. Systemic toxicity from topically applied lidocaine in conjunction with fractional photothermolysis. Arch Dermatol 2006; 142: 1024.
19. Sherling M, Friedman PM, Adrian R, et al. Consensus recommendations on the use of an erbium-doped 1,550-nm fractional laser and its applications in dermatologic laser surgery. Dermatol Surg 2010; 36: 461–9.
20. Fisher GH, Kim KH, Bernstein LJ, et al. Concurrent use of a handheld forced cold air device minimizes patient discomfort during fractional photothermolysis. Dermatol Surg 2005; 31: 1242–3.
21. Alster TS, Wanitphakdeedecha R. Improvement of post-fractional laser erythema with light-emitting diode photomodulation. Dermatol Surg 2009; 35: 813–15.
22. Fisher GH, Geronemus RG. Short-term side effects of photothermolysis. Dermatol Surg 2005; 31: 1245–9.
23. Firoz B, Katz T, Goldberg L, et al. Herpes zoster in the distribution of the trigeminal nerve after nonablative fractional photothermolysis of the face: report of 3 cases. Dermatol Surg 2011; 37: 249–52.
24. Metelitsa AI, Alster TS. Fractionated laser skin resurfacing treatment complications: a review. Dermatol Surg 2010; 36: 299–306.
25. Vaiyavatjamai P, Wattanakrai P. Side effects and complications of fractional 1550-nm erbium fiber laser treatment among Asians. J Cosmet Dermatol 2011; 10: 313–16.
26. Graber EM, Tanzi EL, Alster TS. Side effects and complications of fractional laser thermolysis: experience with 961 treatments. Dermatol Surg 2008; 34: 305–7.
27. Tierney EP, Kouba DJ, Hanke CW. Review of fractional photothermolysis: treatment indications and efficacy. Dermatol Surg 2009; 35: 1445–61.
28. Alexiades-Armenakas MR, Dover JS, Arndt KA. The spectrum of laser skin resurfacing: nonablative, fractional and ablative laser resurfacing. J Am Acad Dermatol 2008; 58: 719–37.
29. Blankenship CM, Alster TS. Fractional photothermolysis of residual hemangioma. Dermatol Surg 2008; 34: 1112–14.
30. Izikson L, Anderson RR. Resolution of blue minocycline pigmentation of the face after fractional photothermolysis. Lasers Surg Med 2008; 40: 399–401.
31. Liu A, Hexsel CL, Moy RL, et al. Granuloma annulare successfully treated using fractional photothermolysis with a 1550-nm erbium doped yttrium aluminum garnet fractionated laser. Dermatol Surg 2011; 37: 712.
32. Kouba DJ, Fincher EF, Moy RL. Nevus of Ota successfully treated by fractional photothermolysis using a fractionated 1,440 nm ND:YAG laser. Arch Dermatol 2008; 144: 156–8.
33. Wanner M, Tanzi EL, Alster TS. Fractional photothermolysis: treatment of facial and nonfacial cutaneous photodamage with a 1,550-nm erbium-doped fiber laser. Dermatol Surg 2007; 33: 23–8.
34. Jih MH, Goldberg LH, Kimyai–Asadi A. Fractional photothermolysis for photoaging of hands. Dermatol Surg 2008; 34: 73–8.
35. Vasily DB, Cerino ME, Ziselman EM, et al. Non-ablative fractional resurfacing of surgical and post-traumatic scars. J Drugs Dermatol 2009; 11: 998–1005.
36. Tierney E, Mahmoud BH, Srivastava D, et al. Treatment of surgical scars with nonablative fractional laser versus pulsed dye laser: a randomized controlled trial. Dermatol Surg 2009; 35: 1172–80.
37. Haedersdal M, Moreau KE, Beyer DM, et al. Fractional nonablative 15450 nm resurfacing for thermal burn scars: a randomized controlled trial. Lasers Surg Med 2009; 41: 189–95.
38. Niwa AB, Mello AP, Torezan LA, et al. Fractional photothermolysis for the treatment of hypertrophic scar: clinical experience of eight cases. Dermatol Surg 2009; 35: 773–7.
39. Glaich AS, Rahman Z, Goldberg LH, et al. Fractional resurfacing for the treatment of hypopigmented scars: a pilot study. Dermatol Surg 2007; 33: 289–94.
40. Weiss RA, Weiss MA, Beasley KL. Long term experience with fixed array 1540 fractional erbium laser for acne scars. Lasers Surg Med 2008; 68: 27.
41. Alster TS, Tanzi EL, Lazarus M. The use of fractional laser photothermolysis for the treatment of atrophic scars. Dermatol Surg 2007; 33: 295–9.
42. Elsaie ML, Baumann LS, Elsaaiee LT. Striae distensae (stretch marks) and different modalities of therapy: an update. Dermatol Surg 2009; 35: 563–73.
43. De Angelis F, Kolesnikova L, Renato F, et al. Fractional nonablative 1540-nm laser treatment of striae distensae in Fitzpatrick skin types II-IV: clinical and histological results. Aesthet Surg J 2011; 31: 411–19.
44. Stotland M, Chapas AM, Brightman L, et al. The safety and efficacy of fractional photothermolysis for the correction of striae distensae. J Drugs Dermatol 2008; 7: 857–61.
45. Sheth VM, Pandya AG. Melasma: a comprehensive update, part I. J Am Acad Dermatol 2011; 65: 689–97.
46. Tierney EP, Hanke CW. Review of the literature: treatment of dyspigmentation with fractionated resurfacing. Dermatol Surg 2010; 36: 1499–508.
47. Sheth VM, Pandya AG. Melasma: a comprehensive update, part II. J Am Acad Dermatol 2011; 65: 699–714.
48. Rokhsar CK, Fitzpatrick RE. The treatment of melisma with fractional photothermolysis: a pilot study. Dermatol Surg 2005; 31: 1645–50.

49. David Vasily. Lasers Surg Med 2007.

50. Kroon MW, Wind BS, Beck JF, et al. Nonablative 1550-nm fractional laser therapy versus triple topical therapy for the treatment of melasma: a randomized controlled pilot study. J Am Acad Dermatol 2011; 64: 516–23.

51. Polder KD, Bruce S. Treatment of melasma using a novel 1,927 nm fractional thulium fiber laser: a pilot study. Dermatol Surg 2012; 38: 199–206.

52. Katz TM, Goldberg LH, Marquez D, et al. Nonablative fractional photothermolysis for facial actinic keratoses: 6-month follow up with histologic evaluation. J Am Acad Dermatol 2011; 65: 349–56.

53. Weiss ET, Anolik R, Brightman L, et al. Long term follow-up of 1927 nm fractional resurfacing for actinic keratoses of the face. Lasers Surg Med 2011; 43: 926.

54. Friedman PM, Landau JM, Moody MN, et al. 1550 nm and 1927 nm fractional laser resurfacing for the treatment of actinic keratosis and Photodamage: A comparative study. Surg Med 2011; 43: 926.

55. Ghasri P, Admani S, Petelin A, et al. Treatment of actinic cheilitis using a 1927 nm thulium fractional laser. Dermatol Surg 2012; 38: 504–7.

56. Anolik R, Friedman PM, Weiss ET, et al. Non-ablative fractional resurfacing with the 1927 nm thulium laser is an effective, well-tolerated treatment for actinic cheilitis. Lasers Surg Med 2011; 43: 927.

57. Ruiz-Rodriguez R, Lopez L, Candelas D, et al. Enhanced efficacy of photodynamic therapy after fractional resurfacing: fractional photodynamic rejuvenation. J Drugs Dermatol 2007; 6: 818–20.

9 Treatment of scars

Richard E. Fitzpatrick

It has been estimated that over 100 million people develop surgical scars each year in the developed world secondary to over 55 million elective surgeries and approximately 25 million operations after trauma (1). There are at least an equal number of various traumatic scars including burns. Acne occurs in approximately 50% of people and about 10% of these develop scarring of some type, so with a population of 311 million in the USA there will be about 15 million persons with acne scars. There are, at least, a comparable number of scars secondary to minor procedures, excisions, and biopsies performed in medical offices.

Treatment of scars to decrease pain, pruritus, and contracture with limitations of motion or to improve their cosmetic appearance has progressed significantly over the past decade. The visibility of a scar depends on its width, texture, color, and flatness. Some of these characteristics can be controlled during the wound healing process and they can all be altered with early intervention. Mature scars will respond to treatment as well. As will be discussed, the orientation toward treatment of scars has shifted to prevention of scarring preferably rather than improvement of scars after they have healed.

As pointed out by Tsao et al. (2), there are basically three types of scars: (*i*) atrophic (most commonly seen in acne and chickenpox scars), (*ii*) exophytic scars (hypertrophic scars and keloids), and (*iii*) flat scars, which are considered normal scars that gradually become imperceptible with time.

Abnormal wound healing results in hypertrophic scars and keloids. These were first described in the Smith Papyrus around 1700 BC (3). In 1802, Jean Louis Albert described abnormal scarring that invaded adjacent normal tissue with extensions similar to a crab's legs and coined the term "cheloide" to describe this entity (4). In 1962, Mancini differentiated keloids from hypertrophic scars by the observation that hypertrophic scars remain confined to the original borders of the injury, whereas keloids project beyond the original wound margins (5). Distinguishing keloids from hypertrophic scars can be difficult, particularly because the original wound margin may remain intact but expand as more scar tissue forms, especially with tension on the wound. This will result in a hypertrophic scar that appears to extend beyond the borders of the original wound, but really does not. As stated by Roseborough et al. (6), this definition leads to confusion because it implies that there is a continuum from normal scar to hypertrophic scar and then to keloid as the scar has exceeded a vaguely defined wound border. In reality, they are both unique entities.

Keloids tend to have a familial predisposition and are more common in dark-skinned individuals, with an incidence of 6–16% in African populations (7,8). They may develop without a known injury and do not regress spontaneously, whereas hypertrophic scars usually occur within 8 weeks of skin trauma and sometimes regress over a period of a few years (9).

Histologically, they both show an overabundance of collagen, but hypertrophic scars are characterized by fine wavy bundles parallel to the surface and nodules containing myofibroblasts, whereas in keloids the collagen bundles are thicker and disorganized without nodules of excess myofibroblasts (10,11). Keloid-derived fibroblasts produce increased amounts of collagen per cell and appear to function autonomously (12). Overall, collagen synthesis in keloids is approximately 20 times that of normal skin (13).

A genome-wide association study (GWAS) identified the enzyme NEDD4 and its encoding gene (neural precursor cell expressed developmentally downregulated protein 4) as one of possible genes associated with keloid susceptibility. A possible mechanism of NEDD4 involvement in keloid formation is through enhancement of proliferation and invasiveness of fibroblasts accompanied by upregulation of type I collagen expression (14). Furthermore, NEDD4 upregulates expressions of fi bronectin and also contributes to the excessive accumulation of extracellular matrix (ECM) also. Fibroblasts are considered to be the key cellular mediators of fibrogenesis in keloid scars. Fibroblast activation protein-alfa (FAP-α) and dipeptidyl peptidase IV (DPPIV) are proteases located at the plasma membrane promoting cell invasiveness and tumor growth and have been associated with keloid scars (15). A study that associates cell invasiveness and tumor-like activity found that FAP-α and DPPIV are found in increased levels in fibroblasts taken from punch biopsies of keloid scars (15). These proteases located at the plasma membrane promote cell invasiveness and tumor growth. FAP-α and DPPIV may increase the invasive capacity of keloid fibroblasts rather than by modulating inflammation or ECM production. Since FAP expression is restricted to reactive fibroblasts in wound healing and normal adult tissues are generally FAP-α negative, inhibiting FAP-α/DPPIV activity may be a novel treatment option to prevent keloid progression. Keloids may be best considered almost as "tumors" of scar tissue.

Knowledge of the wound healing process is necessary to understand when and how to intervene. There are three distinct phases: inflammation, which occurs during the initial 48–72 hours after wounding and is characterized by recruitment of various cells necessary for wound repair. The second stage of proliferation lasts 3–6 weeks and is the time period of deposition of the extracellular matrix as a structural framework; myofibroblasts initiate wound contracture. The maturation phase is the third stage that lasts as long as a year or more during which a balance is achieved between new tissue biosynthesis and degradation (16).

In patients with normal wound healing, investigators found persistent fibroblast activity similar to the proliferation phase at 4 months and that most scars fade at about 7 months, but a considerable proportion had persistent redness at 12 months (17,18).

As stated by Roseborough et al. (6), the most important factors that are known to contribute to the degree of scar formation are the extent and duration of inflammation, the degree of mechanical tension on the wound, and the genetic phenotype of the patient. Control of inflammation is paramount in the prevention of excessive scarring. That includes prevention of infection, removal of foreign bodies in the wound, prevention of mechanical abrasion or irritation of the wound, and maintenance of a moist environment. However, the failure of anti-inflammatory therapies to improve fibroproliferative diseases such as pulmonary fibrosis suggests that factors other than inflammation may be critical (17). Areas of investigation include direct inhibition of cytokine elaboration, fibroblast proliferation, and ECM deposition (19).

The complexity of the wound healing process dictates that a multifaceted approach is used in the prevention of scarring as well as in improving the cosmetic appearance of scars. Those facets include (*i*) surgical—use of appropriate surgical principles in primary procedures as well as in revisions of scars; (*ii*) medical—use of topical and intralesional (IL) medications that may influence the wound healing cascade or decrease inflammation; (*iii*) laser intervention—use of various lasers to improve the color, texture, and contours of scars.

The first report of treatment of hypertrophic scars and keloids with a laser was by Ginsbach and Kuhnel (20) about argon laser treatment of keloids in 1978. Hulsbergen-Henning et al. (21) reported temporary improvement in keloids treated with the argon laser, but Apfelberg et al. (22) reported no improvement in 13 keloids treated with the argon laser. Proposed mechanisms of action have been coagulation of capillaries leading to localized tissue anoxia (20) and heat conduction causing dermal shrinkage (21).

The CO_2 laser has also been reported as useful in the management of keloids. Used as a continuous wave beam for excision of keloids, Bailin (23) reported success in 1982, which he attributed to its nontraumatic and anti-inflammatory properties. However, others were not able to confirm his findings, and recurrences as high as 90% were reported (22,24,25).

The use of a high-energy, short-pulsed (<1 ms) CO_2 laser was much more successful. Bernstein et al. (26) reported in 1998 their results of using CO_2 lasers with these characteristics to treat 24 patients with postsurgical hypertrophic and keloidal scars as well as six patients with traumatic, acne, or varicella scars. All 30 patients showed greater than 50% improvement.

The erbium laser (Er:YAG, 2940 nm) has a coefficient of absorption for water that is 16 times greater than that of the CO_2 laser. This results in enhanced tissue vaporization and much less residual thermal damage (27,28). It is interesting that Bailin (23) considered the CO_2 laser to be nontraumatic and anti-inflammatory. It is the senior author's observation (REF) that thermal injury is very inflammatory and this needs to be carefully controlled. The ablative effects of the erbium laser are much less inflammatory but also do not result in hemostasis, which make its use problematic. However, the combined use of pulsed CO_2 followed by pulsed erbium can result in a much less inflammatory wound. Used in this manner a hypertrophic scar or sharply defined atrophic scar can be carefully sculpted to achieve a smoother surface (27,28).

The principles of selective photothermolysis (29) revolutionized the field of cutaneous laser surgery. By adhering to these principles, the short-pulsed CO_2 laser can be used with minimal residual thermal damage. It is this characteristic that makes the UltraPulse CO_2 laser appropriate for use in some cases of hypertrophic scarring and keloids.

The use of these same principles with the 585-nm pulsed dye laser (PDL) resulted in a successful treatment of atrophic, hypertrophic, and keloid scars. Alster et al. (30) reported improvement in erythema, skin texture, and flattening of hypertrophic portions of scars. Ten scars received five treatments over a 10-month period. These scars had been present for 15–120 months prior to treatment. PDL treatment of 14 erythematous hypertrophic scars present for a minimum of 2 years resulted in 57% and 83% improvement after one and two treatments (31). Treatment parameters were a pulse duration of 0.45 ms and a fluence of 6.5–7.25 J/cm^2 with a 5-mm spot size. Dierickx et al. (32) found similar results using the PDL to treat erythematous hypertrophic scars. Goldman and Fitzpatrick (33) treated 48 hypertrophic and erythematous scars. Thirty-seven were treated with PDL alone, while eleven received concomitant IL corticosteroid [triamcinolone acetonide (TAC), 5–10 mg/mL]. Those scars treated with both modalities achieved greater resolution than those receiving only PDL treatment. An average of 4.4 treatments was needed for objective clinical improvement. Alster and Williams (34) used 585-nm PDL treatment to one-half of median sternotomy hypertrophic scars, using the untreated half as a control. They compared optical profilometry, clinical, histological, and symptomatic responses. Significant improvement was seen in all parameters in the treated half versus the control half.

Manuskiatti and Fitzpatrick (35) reported that 585-nm PDL using a pulse width of 0.45 ms was more effective in decreasing scar size and improving scar pliability than a pulse of 40 ms.

Wittenberg et al. (36) and Alster (37) reported randomized controlled trials combining silicone gel sheeting (36) and IL steroid injections (37) with PDL versus PDL alone. Both trials found PDL to be effective, but no added benefit with combining the second modality (38). This conclusion has not been supported by other studies, which will be reviewed in other sections of this chapter.

Nonoverlapping laser pulses with fluences of 6.0–7.5 J/cm^2 using a 7-mm spot or 4.5–5.5 J/cm^2 with a 10-mm spot have been recommended for treatment of hypertrophic scars and keloids. In the experience of the senior author (REF), these parameters work well, when used with a 6- or 10-ms pulse width. Tanzi and Alster (39) found that two to six treatment sessions may be needed to successfully improve scar resolution, which includes scar color, height, pliability, and texture. Alster and McMeekin (40) reported improvement in facial acne scars after treatment with the 585-nm PDL and Alster and Nanni (41) reported improvement in hypertrophic burn scar using this same laser.

A review (42) of the use of the PDL for nonvascular lesions revealed several reports showing better clinical improvement using low-to-moderate fluences that do not cause purpura.

This fluence will vary depending on the pulse width and spot size.

In addition to improvement in erythema and flattening of scars, there is a clear reduction in itching and pain as well as optimization of skin texture (31).

Not all reports have been as positive. Allison et al. (43) found the PDL to be effective in alleviating the intense pruritus that often occurs during the healing of a burn injury but did not reveal significant reduction in scar redness or improvement in height and texture of the scars. In a similar manner, Chan et al. (44) treated one-half of each of 27 hypertrophic scars using 585 nm, 5-mm spot, 7–8 J/cm², and 2.5-ms pulse with three to six treatments. They found significant improvement in pain and touch sensitivity on the treated side, but no improvement in thickness or elasticity of the treated side. Perhaps the small spot site and relatively high fluence had some negative effects on their outcome. Karsai et al. (42) report that 5–10 PDL sessions lead to only a moderate reduction in hypertrophy but a significant decrease in pain and irritation.

The mechanism of action of the PDL on scars is unclear. The laser's specific targeting of vessels may damage the microvasculature directly, leading to hypoxia and an increase in collagen degradation. In addition, superheating of collagen fibers can result in the dissolution of disulfide bonds (45) and subsequent collagen fiber realignment with decreased fibroblast proliferation as well as release of histamine (13). It is interesting how similar this thesis is to the proposed mechanism of action of the argon laser, another vascular-targeting laser.

These hypotheses are supported by work done by Reiken et al. on hypertrophic scar implants in athymic mice (46). The degree of inhibition of scar growth was found to be proportional to PDL fluence that was used, ranging from 6 to 10 J/cm². They also found maximum effect at the lowest wavelength tested (585–600 nm). On histological examination, significant vessel wall necrosis was seen in the treated scars, confirming that the microvasculature is the primary target. A decrease in mast cells was also seen after treatment and this is thought to alter fibroblast proliferation and contribute to success as well (45).

Alster and Williams (34) reported that their biopsy studies showed a proliferation of mast cells. These mast cells could indirectly influence the proliferation of fibroblasts through the release of histamine, which may contribute to keloid development (47). Histamine would be released right after treatment and prolonged mast cell activity has been associated with increased scar "activity," because histamine is capable of enhancing collagen synthesis (48).

Biochemical studies performed by Kuo et al. (49,50) have shown a decrease in the induction of transforming growth factor-beta1 (TGF-β1) and upregulation of matrix metalloproteinase (MMP) expression in keloid tissue treated with a 585-nm PDL. This would favor collagen degradation and fibroblast apoptosis. They reported 50% improvement in 26 of 30 patients with keloids after five to six treatments using 585 nm, 0.45-ms pulse, 5-mm spot, and 10–18 J/cm² (51).

A study (52) has shown that PDL treatment of keloids downregulates the expression of connective tissue growth factor (CTGF) in greater than 80% of patients studied. CTGF is not found in normal skin but found only in pathological scar tissue, specifically keloids (53). Blocking TGF-β will affect both normal and pathologic scarring (54), whereas blocking CTGF will attenuate only pathologic scarring (55) and the PDL role in this regard is likely to be one of its mechanisms of action on keloids.

The optimum time for treatment has not been definitively determined, but most clinicians agree that early treatment is preferable. McCraw and colleagues (51) have promoted early postoperative initiation of PDL treatment in order to prevent excessive scar formation. They described scar prevention effects by treating surgical wounds either 2 weeks after surgery or 1–2 weeks after suture removal. Scar induration and redness were diminished as was the incidence of hypertrophic scarring. This concept is supported by Mancini et al. (5) who showed that keloid fibroblasts do not deviate from their normal pattern for at least 3 weeks after surgery. Therefore, initiating treatment at 2–3 weeks after surgery may be preventative. Nouri et al. (55) treated one-half of each surgical scar in 11 patients starting on the day of suture removal, twice more at monthly intervals using the PDL. A definite improvement in the treated half was seen using the Vancouver Scar Scale. They also recommend using a larger spot size.

The most common adverse side effect of 585-nm PDL treatment is purpura, which usually takes 7–10 days to resolve. Hyperpigmentation has been reported to occur in 1–24% of patients (56,57). Transient hypopigmentation and blistering have also been reported (37,44).

NONABLATIVE FRACTIONAL RESURFACING FOR SCARS

In 2004, Manstein and Anderson introduced a new concept of skin treatment called fractional photothermolysis (FP) that delivers an array of microscopic treatment zones (MTZs) of thermal damage of controlled depth, width, and density to the skin (58). These MTZs are surrounded by untreated areas of viable epidermis and dermis that allow for rapid repair of these small volumes of thermal heating and tissue damage.

Laubach and colleagues provided a detailed histologic study on the biologic response to nonablative fractional resurfacing (NAFR) using a prototype diode laser (59). Within 1 hour after laser irradiation, well-defined columns of epidermal and dermal thermal damage are evident, but the overlying stratum corneum remains intact. The importance of preserving the stratum corneum is that it protects against possible bacterial infection as it serves as a barrier function of the skin and also enhances hydration of the underlying wound. Within 24 hours, viable cells from the periphery of the MTZs migrate and proliferate rapidly to replace the thermally damaged epidermis (60). Exfoliation of coagulated tissue occurs from the formation of microepidermal necrotic debris (MENDs). Studies have shown that MENDs comprise thermally damaged epidermal and dermal cells along with melanin and elastin (61,62). MENDs undergo transepidermal extrusion between 3 and 7 days, and initiation of a biologic signaling cascade is seen by an increased expression of cellular markers of dermal wound healing and neocollagenesis such as heat shock protein 70, proliferating cell nuclear antigen, α-smooth muscle actin, collagen III, and TGF-β (58,59).

Clinically, fractional resurfacing with nonablative microscopic delivery of high energies to targeted depths in the dermis has allowed significant clinical improvement, including photodamage, scarring, and dyspigmentation. The fractional approach requires a series of two to six treatment sessions at 2- to 4-week intervals. The primary advantage has been greater safety, without any reports of scarring or permanent hypopigmentation (58,59,62). In addition, it has the ability to treat off-face areas in an effective and safe manner.

The first fractional resurfacing laser developed was the Fraxel SR 750® (Reliant Technologies, Mountain View, California, USA), which consisted of a diode-pumped erbium fiber laser, emitting light at 1550 nm to target water in the skin. Two different MTZ density settings (125 and 250 MTZ/cm²) were available for the first-generation Fraxel laser. The final treatment density was then determined by both MTZ setting and the number of laser passes, varying from 5% to 35% of the surface. MTZs of 81–180 μm in width and 300 μm to greater than 900 μm in depth are produced in the skin depending on the pulse energies used (63). An Intelligent Optical Tracking System monitors and adjusts for variable hand speed so that aids in the deposition of uniform MTZs.

The second-generation Fraxel SR 1500, or Fraxel Re:Store® introduced several changes including a telescoping zoom lens that allowed adjustment of the diameter of the treatment column depending on the treatment energy, resulting in more superficial columns and smaller in diameter with lower energy and more penetrating columns and larger in diameter with higher energy (64). The pulse energy ranges from 10 mJ, which penetrates approximately 200 μm, to a maximum energy of 70 mJ, which penetrates approximately 1.4 mm, whereas up to 60% of the skin's surface can be treated in one session. Competing fractional delivery devices including the Lux® 1540 fractional erbium (Er):Glass (Palomar Medical Technologies Inc., Burlington, Massachusetts, USA), Affirm® (Cynosure, Inc., Westford, Massachusetts, USA), Matrix® IR (Syneron Medical Ltd, Yokneam, Israel), and Mosaic (Lutronic, Inc., Ilsan, Korea) use a "stamping" approach to deliver the fractionated infrared laser beam. The main disadvantage of stamping a fixed pattern is the high likelihood of posttreatment skip areas and the production of Moire artifacts from inadvertent overlap of treatment sites. On the other hand, most stamping devices do not require consumables and are also often associated with less pain, even with equivalent total depths and densities, compared with their scanning counterparts.

The use of NAFR has been well studied for the treatment of scarring, including acne scars, surgical scars, and traumatic scars. Narurkar reported a retrospective review of 877 cases treated with the second-generation erbium-doped 1550-nm Fraxel and found that treatment of acne scars, surgical scars, and mild-to-moderate photodamage achieved the most consistent results, whereas the most variable results were seen in the treatment of melasma and deep rhytides (65). Noteworthy that although CO_2 and the Er:YAG ablative resurfacing with 100% coverage of the treated surface achieve exceptional results for facial rhytides, lesser degrees of improvement were seen for scarring with both lasers. One of the reasons might be that the depth of macroscopic tissue ablation is limited with those lasers because 100% of the surface area is treated, whereas NAFR can deliver the MTZs deeply (>1300 μm) into the dermis with great safety, particularly with regard to preservation of pigment (64). Treatment to the full depth of the scar appears to be an important factor in a successful treatment.

Rahman and colleagues treated 40 patients with a variety of scars (14 acne scars, 11 surgical scars, 13 traumatic scars, and 15 striae) and found that at 3 months, 22 of 49 scars (44.9%) were moderately to completely improved (66). Subjects reported moderate-to-complete improvement in 32 out of 52 scars (61.5%). Surgical scars and acne scars had the highest improvement scores, whereas traumatic scars had the lowest. Surgical scars showed the greatest improvement in surface texture and atrophy, whereas acne scars had the greatest improvement in color mismatch.

Several other studies have demonstrated the efficacy and safety of NAFR in the treatment of scars (67–70). Rokhsar and colleagues reported improvement in skin texture and decreased scar severity in all patients (67). Ten patients with atrophic acne scars and five with surgical scars were treated with an average of four sessions of Fraxel Re:Store at weekly or monthly intervals, at fluences of 8–20 mJ and density of 2000 MTZ/cm². Behroozan and colleagues reported greater than 75% improvement rated by both the patient and an independent physician evaluator in the degree of erythema, induration, and overall texture in a surgical hypertrophic scar (68). This patient had been treated once with the Fraxel SR 1500 at a pulse energy of 8 mJ and density of 2000 MTZ/cm² 1 month after a Mohs' surgery procedure.

Interestingly, fractional laser treatment has shown to be an effective treatment for different types of scars: hypertrophic, atrophic, erythematous, and dyschromic.

Treatment of both atrophic and hypertrophic surgical scars in 13 patients using Fraxel SR 1500 was reported by Kunishige and colleagues (69). Patients received one to eight laser sessions at 4-week intervals using energy levels from 6 to 70 mJ and densities of 312–2500 MTZ/cm² (12–87.5% density). At 2 weeks after the last treatment, nine patients had greater than 75% improvement, two patients had 51–75% improvement, and two patients had 25–50% improvement. The results were maintained for all subjects at 2 months of follow-up. Longer follow-up would be expected to show greater degrees of improvement as remodeling of scar tissue proceeds.

Treatment of hypertrophic scars with NAFR has been reported by Niwa and colleagues (70). Eight patients with hypertrophic scars (seven from surgical procedures and one from burn injury) received two to three treatments with Fraxel Re:Store at 4-week intervals, using fluences of 35–50 J/cm² and treatment densities of 20–26%. At 4 weeks after last treatment, three patients achieved 51–75% improvement and five patients achieved 26–50% improvement. Improvement in hyperpigmented scars occurred in all hyperpigmented scars and postinflammatory hyperpigmentation (PIH) was not observed in this small study even in patients with Fitzpatrick skin type IV. Clinical improvement of pigmented lesions with FP has been correlated histologically to the formation of microscopically small areas of epidermal necrotic debris and dermal contents containing melanin. Those necrotic contents are progressively eliminated through extrusion, releasing pigment and resulting in the improvement of pigmented lesions (71). In addition, Goldberg and colleagues showed histologic and ultrastructural evidence that FP decreases the number of melanocytes and the amount of melanin granules within the keratinocytes, which is consistent with this elimination process aforementioned (72).

The use of 1550-nm fractional resurfacing laser outperformed the use of the 595-nm PDL in a randomized split-scar study conducted by Tierney and colleagues (73). Fifteen scars of minimum 2 months after Mohs' surgery received four treatments at 2-week intervals and were evaluated regarding dyspigmentation, thickness, texture, and overall cosmetic appearance. Fluences of 70 mJ at treatment level 8 (coverage 23%) were used for the Fraxel SR 1500, whereas fluences of 7.5 J/cm² with a pulse duration of 0.45 ms were used for the PDL. The Fraxel Re:Store was superior in all categories of evaluation with a mean cosmetic improvement of 75.9% versus 53.9% of improvement on the PDL-treated half of the scar. In addition, the 1550-nm fractional resurfacing showed unique improvement in hypopigmented scars (65% vs. 0%) and atrophic scars (68% vs. 13%). The authors attribute the success of Fraxel® Re:Store to both hypertrophic and atrophic scars to the controlled delivery of high fluences to the deep dermis, which serves to maximize the tissue effects of normalization of neocollagenesis and collagenolysis. In addition, scars with significant erythematous component showed significant improvement with the nonablative fractional laser likely due to specific targeting of dermal blood vessels, which has been demonstrated histologically (Fig. 9.1) (59).

Repigmentation of hypopigmented scars with NAFR has been reported by previous studies in the literature (74,75). Mechanisms of partial repigmentation remain speculative but may be attributed to stimulation of melanocyte proliferation and migration from the periphery of the wound (76,77). The excimer laser has been effective in the repigmentation of hypopigmented scars; however, the results diminished over time and maintenance was required at 1–4 months (78). In 2007,

Glaich and colleagues conducted a pilot study with seven patients with hypopigmented facial scars (six from inflammatory acne and one from a gas fire) treated with a series of two to four Fraxel Re:Store treatments at 4-week intervals (74). Energy settings ranged from 7 to 20 mJ at a total density of 1000–2500 MTZ/cm² (35–87.5% total coverage). At 4 weeks after the last treatment, independent physician evaluation revealed 51–75% improvement in hypopigmentation in six of seven patients. All patients reported improvement in hypopigmentation lasting greater than 3 months after last treatment.

Massaki and colleagues combined the use of erbium-doped 1550-nm fractionated laser (Fraxel Re:Store) with topical bimatoprost and either topical tretinoin or pimecrolimus for the treatment of hypopigmented scars (79). Fourteen patients with hypopigmented scars from various causes were treated with an average of 4.5 sessions of Fraxel Re:Store at 4- to 8-week intervals and simultaneously started topical bimatoprost and tretinoin or pimecrolimus. At 4 weeks after the last laser treatment, 5 patients had more than 75% improvement in hypopigmentation and 12 had more than 50% improvement. Noteworthy is that after a mean follow-up of 20.1 months, all patients showed persistent clinical improvement. Although additional studies are required to compare the efficacies of these treatment modalities individually, this combination therapy appears to have a synergistic effect in the improvement of hypopigmented scars (Fig. 9.2).

Pham and colleagues investigated the efficacy of 1550-nm Fraxel in 13 patients with mostly atrophic and hypopigmented facial surgical scars (80). Four treatments were performed at intervals of 4 weeks at an initial setting of 40 mJ and treatment level 4 (11% density). Patients' assessments showed statistically

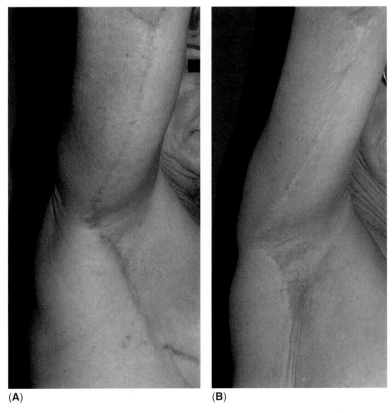

(A)   (B)

Figure 9.1 (**A**) Erythematous atrophic scar 6 months after brachioplasty. (**B**) Significant improvement is seen in the scar 6 months following four treatments with Fraxel Re:Store at monthly intervals using 20 mJ and 20% density.

significant improvement in color match, stiffness, thickness, and irregularity. The results were maintained at follow-up visits at 6 months after last treatment. The authors suggested that laser treatments may be more effective for earlier treatment of scars as two patients who had no improvement had scars for more than 2 years after surgery (Fig. 9.3).

As previously discussed with the PDL, earlier treatment with the 1550-nm fractional Er:Glass laser to prevent hypertrophic scar formation has been reported by Choe and colleagues (81). Twenty-seven Korean patients at 2–3 weeks postoperative of thyroidectomy received four sessions with the MOSAIC laser® (Lutronic Corp., Seoul, South Korea) using 10 mJ, 1500 spot/cm², and static mode at 1-month intervals. Subjects were compared with a cohort of untreated thyroidectomy scars at 6 months after the final treatment. The laser-treated scars achieved significantly better cosmetic results than the untreated control in the aspects of prevention of hypertrophic scar formation and the Vancouver Scar Scale, which is based on the grade of pigmentation, vascularity, pliability, and height of scars. The authors suggest that using low-energy, high-density parameters may avoid excessive stimulation of cytokines in the deep dermis that can result in a greater chance of scar formation and can be safely used in colored Asian skin. Although further practical experiences with diverse parameters are required to establish a standardized protocol for postsurgical scarring,

including the exact timing of scar treatment, earlier treatment with lasers and light devices, including fractional lasers, appears to optimize the wound healing process and possibly suppress the formation of hypertrophic scar (68,82).

Tierney et al. (73) hypothesize that the success of NAFR in treating scars is related to delivering high-energy pulses deep in the dermis, while Choe et al. (81) suggest that the prevention of scarring with the use of NAFR may be related to the use of high density, but low-energy pulses in order to avoid stimulation of the deep dermis. It is possible that these two different situations require different laser parameters for success (Figs. 9.4 and 9.5).

Kunishige and colleagues also confirmed that nonablative fractional laser treatment can be effective in different types of scars, including hypertrophic, atrophic, erythematous, and hyperpigmented (83). Thirteen patients with surgical scars were treated up to eight monthly sessions (average 3) with the Fraxel Re:Store laser using energy levels from 6 to 70 mJ and final densities from 312 to 2500 MTZ/cm² (about 17% to >100% coverage). At the 2-month follow-up visit, almost all patients achieved at least 50% improvement with more than half of the subjects achieving 75% improvement or greater. Differently from other studies, the authors found that scars older than 1 year improved as much as scars that were younger.

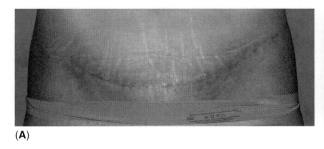
(A)

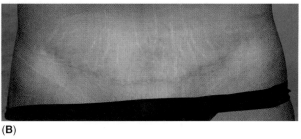
(B)

Figure 9.2 (**A**) Multiple flat scattered hypopigmented scars of nose are present 15 years following pulsed CO_2 laser resurfacing and 10 treatments of Fraxel Re:Store at 1- to 6-month intervals. (**B**) The addition of topical bimatoprost BID (Latisse) and tretinoin 0.025% qd resulted in >75% improvement in the hypopigmentation.

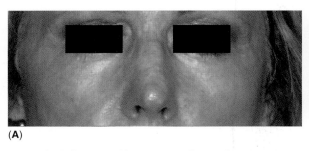
(A)

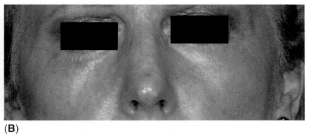
(B)

Figure 9.3 (**A**) Sharply defined atrophic hypopigmented scars are very visible 3 months after a brow lift positioned just superior to the eyebrows bilaterally. (**B**) Significant improvement in color and texture is seen after 4 treatments with Fraxel Re:Store performed at 2- to 4-week intervals using 40 mJ and 36% density.

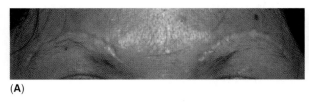
(A)

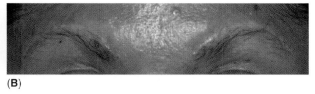
(B)

Figure 9.4 (**A**) Abdominoplasty scar 2 weeks following suture removal. (**B**) The scar is cosmetically improved by the use of Fraxel Re:Store starting 2 weeks after suture removal and repeated at 4-week intervals for four treatments using 30 mJ and 17% density.

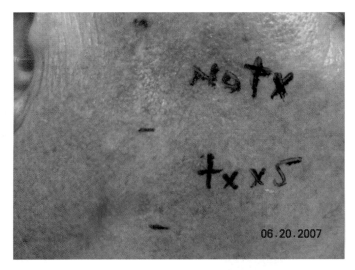

Figure 9.5 A series of surgical scars were divided into two sections: one untreated and one treated with Fraxel Re:Store starting on the day of suture removal and at 2-week intervals for a total of five treatments. The treated half was invariably less visible 3 months after the fifth session. *Source*: Photo courtesy of Cameron Rhoksar, MD.

Efficacy and safety using the 1540-nm Er:Glass fractional nonablative laser (Lux1540, Palomar Medical Technologies, Inc.) to treat 33 surgical and posttraumatic scars were demonstrated by Vasily and colleagues (84). Three to seven treatments with energies up to 60 mJ and 5 passes were performed at 3- to 6-week intervals. At 1 month of follow-up, 73% of treated scars improved 50% or more and 43% improved 75% or more. Investigators also found a modest inverse correlation between scar age and percent improvement with a mean improvement score of 69% ± 20% (s.d.) for scars up to 10 years old versus 41% ± 18% (s.d.) for scars older than 10 years ($p<0.001$). However, even older scars showed marked improvement.

The observations made in these two studies (85,86) showing that older scars do respond to NAFR are an important and significant observation that the senior author can confirm from his personal experience.

Burn scars often pose a therapeutic challenge with limited available treatments. New modalities of treatment are clearly needed as patients affected by these thermal scars frequently suffer from morbidities and psychological impairments.

Haedersdal and colleagues conducted a randomized controlled trial of 17 adult patients with burn scars of 1 year or older with side-by-side test areas of three monthly 1540-nm fractional laser (Lux1540, Palomar Medical Technologies) versus no treatment (85). Energy ranged from 70 to 100 mJ/mb and 15-ms pulse duration in 3–4 passes. At 12 weeks after the last treatment, laser-treated skin was significantly more even and smooth compared with adjacent untreated sides. Eight out of 17 patients evaluated the burn scars to be moderately or significantly improved, eight patients reported mild improvement, and one patient reported no benefit from the treatments. Superficial burn scars appeared to respond better than deeper possibly due to limited penetration depth of laser into the dermis. Moreover, skin grafted, meshed sites also responded better than non-meshed sites in this study suggesting that nonthermally damaged zones of transplant tissue might respond better than thermally damaged, fibrotic tissue.

Waibel and Beer published case reports in 2008 (86) and 2009 (87) on the use of fractional lasers (AFR and NAFR) for the treatment of burn scars, which showed improvement in hyperpigmentation, erythema, and texture.

Waibel and colleagues treated 10 patients with burn scars with five monthly sessions of Fraxel Re:Store (88,89). Pulse energies of 40–70 mJ and densities of 232–552 MTZ/cm² (level 7–13; densities of 20–38%) were used. At 3 months after final treatment, improvement in texture was seen in all patients and improvements in dyschromia, atrophy, or hypertrophy were seen in 96% of patients.

ABLATIVE FRACTIONAL RESURFACING FOR SCARS

Fractional delivery systems for both CO_2 and Er:YAG lasers emerged in an attempt to achieve the clinical results obtained with traditional ablative lasers. Unlike nonablative fractional lasers, which were previously discussed, these devices ablate epidermis and variable depths of the dermis, requiring downtime for healing, but often only a single treatment session. The combination of epidermal and dermal ablation seems to produce a more significant wound healing response and dermal neocollagenesis, which helps explain the more predictable and faster response in the treatment of wrinkle lines, skin tightening, scarring, and dyschromias compared with nonablative devices. Compared with conventional ablative lasers, ablative fractional resurfacing (AFR) has greater safety and diminished healing time, as normal skin is preserved in adjacent areas, as well as the ability to treat off-face in an effective and safe manner.

Several ablative fractional lasers are available on the market. The Fraxel Re:Pair system (Reliant Technologies, Mountain View, California, USA) is similar to the nonablative Fraxel lasers in operation with a continuous scanning mode with an optical tracking system in which each individual spot is precisely delivered in an even distribution. Other devices have a stamping handpiece from which all spots are delivered in a single pulse passing through a lens array; and a scanning stamp pattern delivered by a computer pattern generator such as the Lumenis Active FX and Deep FX, the Er:YSGG laser (Pearl®, Cutera, Brisbane, California, USA), and Er:YAG lasers including Alma Pixel®, Palomar Er:YAG, and Sciton Profractional®. Varying depths of ablation and coagulation with varying spot sizes and shapes are possible with these devices. Unlike conventional CO_2 or Er:YAG lasers, deeper coagulation of up to 1600 μm can be safely used because of the fractional delivery of laser irradiation (63).

Histological evaluation of wound healing with an ablative fractional CO_2 device from Reliant Technologies using increasing pulse energies *in vivo* showed a parallel column of epidermal and dermal ablation as deep as 1700 μm with a 70-mJ pulse. By 48 hours, adjacent epidermal cell migrate into the ablated areas and there is formation of MENDs as well as expression of heat shock protein 72, which diminishes by 3 months (90). Heat shock protein 47 is detected at 7 days and persists for 3 months, indicating persistent collagen remodeling. By 1 week after treatment, the re-epithelialization is complete with extrusion of the MENDs. At 3 months after treatment, newly formed compact collagen is observed throughout the dermis (64).

Hale and colleagues reported the use of the prototype Fraxel Re:Pair laser for the treatment of facial traumatic and surgical scars in 13 patients (91). One to three treatments were performed with energy levels of 20–70 mJ per pulse and 200–300 MTZ/cm^2 (densities of 10–17%). All patients reported significant improvement with no significant long-term sequelae.

A multicenter clinical study reported the use of fractional CO_2 laser (SmartXide® DOT, Deka) for the treatment of rhytides, photoaging, scar, and striae distensae in 52 patients (92). Subjects received one to five monthly treatments with 5–30 W, 200–2000 μs of dwell time, and 200- to 2000-μm DOT pitch. Significant improvement at 1 and 3 months of follow-up was seen in rhytides, photoaging, and scarring, and variable and inconsistent results were found for striae distensae. The mean grade improvement for scars was moderate at 2.25 (s.d. ± 0.5) on a 4-point improvement scale (0 = no improvement, 1 = minimal improvement, 2 = moderate improvement, 3 = advanced improvement; 4 = complete resolution of scars) and required multiple treatment sessions.

Two studies compared the use of fractional CO_2 laser with classic dermabrasion for the treatment of scars and both found that laser-treated scars showed quicker clinical recovery with superior or equivalent clinical efficacy (93,94). Cervelli and colleagues compared the fractionated ultrapulsed CO_2 laser (UltraPulse® Encore, Lumenis Ltd, Santa Clara, California, USA) with classic dermabrasion in 60 patients with posttraumatic and pathological scars (93). The Deep FX was used first with pulse energy ranging from 12.5 to 17.5 mJ followed by the Active FX with a pulse energy ranging from 90 to 130 mJ. Significant difference emerged between the laser and dermabrasion groups regarding the duration of the procedure (CO_2 laser; $p<0.05$), the postoperative pain (greater for dermabrasion $p = 0.03$). In addition, healing was complete in 7 days for the laser and 12 days for the dermabrasion group ($p<0.05$). Both physician and patients assessed that pigmentation, texture, and appearance of skin were slightly superior in the laser group versus the dermabrasion group ($p<0.05$). Christophel and colleagues used a split-scar method to compare fractionated CO_2 laser (Fraxel) Re:Pair and diamond fraise dermabrasion on 12 postsurgical scars of the face (94). Fluence of 40 mJ and treatment level 8 (23% density) with 4 passes were used for the fractionated CO_2 laser. Dermabrasion had significantly greater erythema, edema, and eschar formation than the matched section of fractionated laser at 1 week posttreatment and a trend toward greater erythema at 1 month of follow-up ($p = 0.06$). Three blinded physicians evaluated the cosmetic improvement at 3 months and found that both treatment modalities had equivalent cosmetic efficacy. However, it should be pointed out that diamond fraise dermabrasion is much more dependent on the skills of the operator, so it is difficult to reach any general conclusions from this study.

Atrophic postoperative and traumatic scars were successfully treated with three treatments of CO_2 AFR at 1- to 4-month intervals by Weiss and colleagues (95). Nineteen atrophic scars received treatment with the Fraxel Re:Pair with 70 mJ per pulse, 200 MTZ/cm^2 per pass, 2–3 passes (27–38% coverage) on facial scars and 40 mJ per pulse, 200 MTZ/cm^2, and 2–3 passes (20–30% coverage) on off-face scars. The authors noted prolonged erythema when using higher fluences and higher coverage levels on off-face scarring that often becomes a cosmetic concern for patients; therefore, lower settings were chosen for off-face scars even though the efficacy is possibly reduced with lower energy and lower levels of coverage. At the 6-month follow-up visit, both patient and investigator scores revealed improvement in skin texture, pigmentation, atrophy, and overall scar appearance for all scars. Image analysis with a 3D optical profiling system revealed a 38% mean reduction of volume and 35.6% mean reduction of maximum scar depth. No pigmentary changes or scarring were noted at the 3-month follow-up visit.

This prolonged healing and erythema, which have been reported with the use of higher fluences or higher densities of AFR used on the torso, arms, and legs, has also been seen by the senior author and is significant enough to advise that the use of AFR in these locations of scars needs careful consideration. Often NAFR is preferable because of avoidance of prolonged erythema.

Interestingly, not only NAFR, which has been shown to produce significant improvement in hypopigmentation of both acne and surgical scars (68,73,74), but also ablative fractional CO_2 laser appears to improve hypopigmentation. Tierney and colleagues reported a case of facial hypopigmentation after traditional ablative CO_2 laser successfully treated with a series of three treatments at 8-week intervals with a fractionated CO_2 laser (Dermal Optical Thermolysis, DOT laser, Eclipse Med, Dallas Texas, USA) (96). Treatment parameters were 30 W, 500-μm pitch 500 μs for the face and 20 W, 500-μm pitch, 500 μs for the neck. At 2 months after last treatment, the hypopigmentation and line of pigmentary demarcation between the face and the neck improved by 75%.

Waibel and colleagues reported the successful outcome in a patient with a third-degree burn scar that was more than 50 years old after a single session with an ablative fractional CO_2 laser (Lumenis, Santa Clara, California, USA) (87). The Deep FX mode was used first with 12.5 mJ/cm^2, density 3, and the Active FX was used for the second pass, with 80 mJ/cm^2, density of 1. According to the authors, who had previously described successful treatment of burn scars with NAFR (86), AFR may require fewer treatments and be a more cost-effective treatment option for patients. However, this will depend on the characteristics of the scar as well as its location (Figs. 9.6 and 9.7).

Haedersdal reported a case of a man with a 5-year-old thermal burn scar on his arm with skin grafting that left a "mesh-like" pattern, successfully treated with fractional CO_2 laser (MedArt, Hvidovre, Denmark) (97). A single pass was performed with 8 W, 24 mJ, 3 ms, and two different densities of 64 and 100 MTZ/cm^2 (13 and 20% coverage, respectively). Another area was left as untreated control. Three months after treatment, significant improvement in texture and color of the side treated with high-density coverage was seen, with skin texture appearing more even and smooth compared with that of the control side. Although less remarkable, slight improvement was seen in the area treated with lower-density coverage.

Previous reports had suggested that early treatment with the nonablative fractional Er:Glass lasers improves the appearance of postoperative scars, reducing the incidence of hypertrophic scarring (81). This same approach can be used with AFR. Jung and colleagues reported that early postoperative treatment of thyroidectomy scars using fractional CO_2 laser resulted in clinical improvement of more than 51% in 12 out of 23 subjects treated (98). Patients received a single session with the eCO$_2$® laser (Lutronic Corporation, Goyang, Korea) 2–3 weeks after

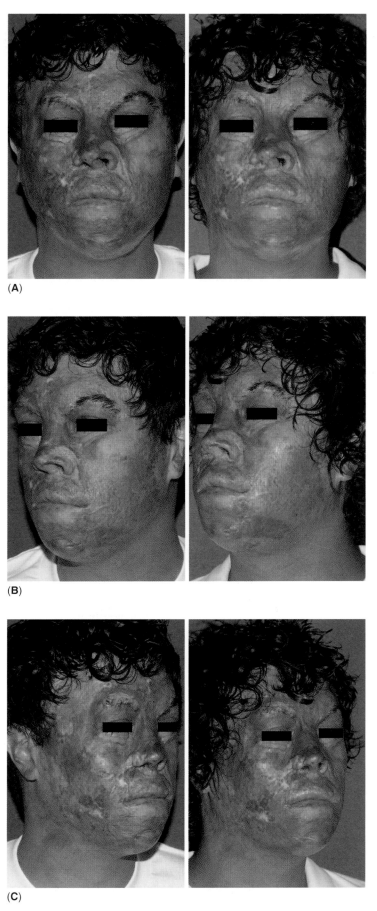

Figure 9.6 Before and 1 year following treatment with Fraxel Re:Pair 40 mJ and 30% density: perioral, bilateral cheeks and lower eyelids, in three different views (**A–C**).

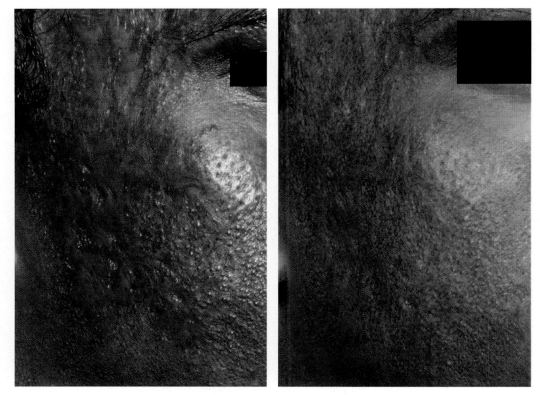

Figure 9.7 Improvement in facial burn scar following treatment with Fraxel Re:Pair. *Source*: Photo courtesy of William Groff, MD.

surgery using 50 mJ of pulse energy, density of 100 spots/cm^2, 2 passes in the static mode (coverage 12.7%). Follow-up results 3 months after treatment revealed that 4 of 23 patients had near total clinical improvement (>75%), 8 marked improvement (51–75%), and 9 moderate improvement (26–50%). Two patients had posttreatment hyperpigmentation that spontaneously resolved within 1 month (Fig. 9.8).

Ozog and Moy published a clinical trial showing that intraoperative treatment of surgical wounds using a fractional CO_2 laser improved the appearance and texture of the surgical scar (99).

ACNE SCARRING

One of the most common and difficult conditions to treat is acne scarring. It almost always requires more than one treatment session and more than one treatment modality to be successful.

The most comprehensive acne study performed, HANES-1 (100), studied 20,749 US citizens of age 1–74 years in 1978 and found the prevalence of acne vulgaris to be 68 per 1000. A more restricted study of 749 patients aged 25–58 years (101) determined overall acne prevalence as 58% for women and 40% for men. Scarring was noted in 14% of the women and 11% of the men (102). Even though there are very effective treatments for acne, only 16% seek appropriate treatment (103), which greatly increases the risks and incidence of scarring.

It is useful to classify acne scars morphologically in order to choose an appropriate treatment modality. A simple classification deals with tissue loss or excess. If there is excess tissue, we are dealing with a hypertrophic scar or keloid—most common along the jawline and glabellar areas.

Jacob et al. (104) describe a useful classification of acne scars with loss of tissue or damage to tissue. Ice-pick scars are small in diameter (<2 mm) but have sharply defined edges and

penetrate deep into the dermis. These scars are commonly seen on the mid-cheeks and chin. The second category, boxcar scars, may be shallow or deep, but generally measure 1.5–4.0 mm in diameter and have sharply defined, often vertical walls and the base may be very firmly bound down. The third category, rolling hills, have soft edges and may be circular or linear but generally >4 mm in diameter. A simple but very significant test regarding possible response to treatments that tighten the skin is to grasp the skin tightly and observe how much improvement results with simply stretching the skin. Rolling hills scars will usually improve 50–100% with this maneuver, whereas boxcar scars show minimal improvement (0–25%) and ice-pick scars show no change.

When treating rolling hills scars, full face or full areas are generally treated with procedures that peel the skin and stimulate new collagen. These will be discussed in greater detail. For the ice-pick and boxcar scars, a better result may be obtained by first performing a surgical procedure: punch or elliptical excision of the scar to convert it to a linear scar that can then be blended. Punch elevation of the base of the boxcar scar may also be considered (103). The sharply defined edges of a boxcar scar may also be improved by the use of ablative resurfacing precisely to convert the scar to a soft rolling hills scar that is much more responsive to treatment. Subcision was first described by Orentreich and Orentreich in 1995 (105), as a procedure using a tri-bevel needle to puncture the skin and then in arcs parallel to the surface of the skin to break up scar tissue that is binding the base of an atrophic scar. This procedure has been particularly promoted for rolling hills scars and is said to induce neocollagenesis over 6 months or more (106). Improvement of approximately 50% has been reported (107) and some consider it the surgical procedure of choice for rolling hills scars (103). However, this author's experience is more

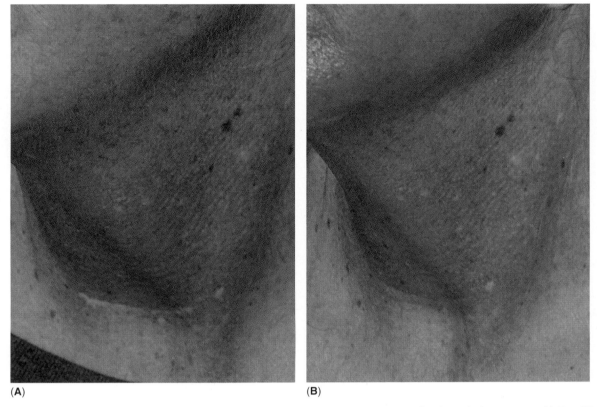

Figure 9.8 (**A**) Thyroidectomy scar at least 5 years after surgery. (**B**) Significant improvement is seen 6 weeks after a single treatment with Fraxel Re:Pair using 20 mJ and 15% density. Although early treatment is preferable, even older scars such as this may respond extremely well. Only the scar was treated, not the photodamaged neck.

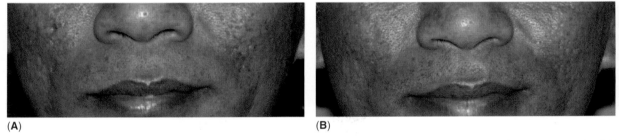

Figure 9.9 Sharply defined ice-pick and small crater scars are visible (**A**) prior to treatment. (**B**) Improvement in scars was achieved in a step-wise fashion using punch excision followed by AFR over the full cheeks and then NAFR using Fraxel Re:Store 50 mJ, 35% density in multiple sessions confined to the visible scars.

in line with that of the blinded evaluators who found minimal change with subcision at 3 and 6 months (108,109) in 20 patients. It would be unusual for subcision to result in significant improvement as an isolated single treatment as done in this study. Once of these adjunctive surgical procedures have been performed, then laser treatment should be more effective (Fig. 9.9).

In evaluating acne scarring, there are two types of dyspigmentation that are particularly bothersome to patients. Although they are not truly scars, they may persist for as long as a year or more and should be treated to hasten their resolution. These two macular dyspigmentations follow inflammatory acne and are postinflammatory erythema and PIH (107–110). PIH generally occurs in patients with Fitzpatrick skin types III and IV. Topical therapy with retinoids and hydroquinone is often effective, but at times it is necessary to treat with lasers. Generally, spot treatment is done with Q-switched alexandrite or ruby lasers or IPL. It is best to treat at low

fluences as too aggressive an approach is likely to result in the recurrence of PIH. Therefore, two to four sessions are planned at 2- to 4-week intervals.

When the patient has red macules that are secondary to the healing phase of inflammatory acne, there is usually some active acne as well. The PDL and the IPL have both been used in managing this condition. The mechanism of action is thought to be absorption of light energy by porphyrins produced by *Propionibacterium acnes*, which induces bacterial death (111).

There are conflicting reports in the literature regarding efficacy. One controlled study of 40 patients treated with one or two sessions of subpurpuric dosing using 585-nm PDL showed no benefit (112). However, a very similar study of 41 patients by a different group found significant improvement (113).

A study performed in 2006 (114) demonstrated a significant increase in TGF-β1 messenger RNA levels induced by 585-nm PDL treatment. This may be significant as far as promoting collagen synthesis. Prevention and treatment of various types of scars have been reported with the PDL (31,34,115,116).

Most practitioners have found elimination of unwanted erythema and vessels is more efficient with purpuric settings, but subpurpuric settings will work with additional treatment sessions. Treatment of acne as well as macular erythema has three potential benefits: improvement in the acne, elimination of postinflammatory erythema, and stimulation of new collagen that enhances wound healing and minimizes scarring.

NONABLATIVE FRACTIONAL PHOTOTHERMOLYSIS FOR ACNE SCARRING

Resurfacing procedures such as dermabrasion, medium-to-deep chemical peels, and ablative laser resurfacing have been traditionally used to treat patients with extensive, widespread acne scarring (117–120). These techniques remove the epidermis and upper dermis without affecting the skin appendages (sebaceous glands, hair follicles, and sweat ducts), which allow the regeneration of the skin and collagen production through skin's healing process (117–120). Particularly the CO_2 laser, which has been recognized as the gold standard resurfacing procedure (121–125), also heats the nonablated dermis, resulting in immediate thermally induced skin tightening.

Despite the dramatic results achieved with the CO_2 laser for the treatment of photoaged skin, wrinkle removal, skin tightening, and acne scars, it has been associated with prolonged erythema, extended recovery periods, hyper- and hypopigmentation, and in rare cases scarring (119,120). Because of these potential risks and significant downtime for healing (2–4 weeks), nonablative lasers using long-pulsed infrared wavelengths (1320, 1440, 1450, and 1540 nm) were developed as a safe alternative (126,127). These nonablative, nonfractional lasers create a controlled thermal injury to the dermis that initiates a cascade of wound healing and remodeling events, resulting in neocollagenesis (126). However, a series of treatments are often required, and the improvement in photodamage and acne scars, particularly atrophic or ice-pick scars, was significantly less noticeable than that achieved with the ablative CO_2 and Er:YAG devices (126,128,129). The reduced efficacy has been partially attributed to the lack of epidermal contribution to the wound healing process as well as the use of epidermal cooling (130). The degree of improvement correlates to some extent to the aggressiveness of treatment. In order to keep the treatments safe and without significant downtime, the treatments are delivered in a conservative manner because the devices deliver energy throughout the dermis. As a consequence, multiple treatment sessions are needed and results are generally subtle.

NAFR developed by Anderson and Manstein (58) resulted in a rather predictable improvement of photoaged skin, color, texture, and scars of all types compared with nonablative lasers with better side effect profiles and less downtime than with traditional ablative resurfacing devices (64).

NAFR has known effects on tissue tightening with clinical improvement of fine lines and rhytides, likely due to stimulation of collagen production (58). The mechanism of action of NAFR for improving acne scarring is thought to be analogous to its effects on tissue shrinkage; that these columns of thermally damaged tissue initiate a cascade of wound healing and remodeling events, resulting in neocollagenesis (131). In addition, the deep penetration of the MTZs (>1300 μm) and the fractional approach allow greater efficacy and much greater safety (64).

In 2006, Geronemus first reported the use of NAFR (original prototype Fraxel laser) for the treatment of acne scarring (60). Seventeen patients with ice-pick, boxcar, and rolling scars received a series of five treatments at 1- to 3-week intervals. Mean improvement levels evaluated by digital photography, high-resolution typographic imaging, and patient-completed questionnaires were in the range of 25–50%, 22–62%, and 29–67%, respectively. Posttreatment erythema, mild facial edema, and moisturizer-responsive xerosis were observed. No scarring or unwanted pigmentary changes were seen. Favorable results were seen in patients with darker skin phototypes and acne scars treated with NAFR.

Weinstein reported one of the largest series with 357 patients, Fitzpatrick skin types I–VI, with acne scarring treated with the Fraxel SR750 (132). One to five treatments with pulse energies of 25–35 mJ according to scar severity and depth and density of 125 MTZ/cm², 4–10 passes. At 3 months after last treatment, 12% achieved excellent improvement (>75%), 73% had good improvement (50–75%), and 15% achieved fair improvement (25–50%). One patient developed transitory PIH and one subject had localized scarring that resolved with IL 5-fluorouracil (5-FU).

A study by Alster and colleagues found that the mean clinical improvement scores for atrophic acne scars after three monthly treatments with Fraxel SR750 were higher than those reported for facial rhytides in a study with similar design (133). Fifty-three patients with mild-to-moderate atrophic facial acne scars were treated with pulse energies of 8–16 J and densities of 125 and 250 MTZ/cm² for 8–10 passes. Thirty-eight patients (71%) received two or more treatments. In total, 48 patients (91%) had at least 25–50% improvement after a single treatment, whereas 87% of those receiving three treatments achieved greater than 50% improvement. Transient acneiform eruptions occurred after 5% of treatment sessions. One patient with skin phototype V developed transient PIH at a setting of 250 MTZ but not after subsequent treatment at 125 MTZ.

Weiss and colleagues reported their experience in over 500 treatment sessions for acne scarring using the Lux1540 (Palomar) (134). Three treatments were given at 4-week intervals using a fluence of 50–70 mJ/mb with a minimum of 3 passes for each treatment site. At 3 months after last treatment, blinded physician photographic analysis indicated a median improvement of 50–75%, whereas 85% of patients rated their skin as improved. Side effects were minimal and included mild posttreatment erythema and edema that resolved within 24 hours (Figs. 9.10 and 9.11).

Many reports and studies have shown the efficacy of NAFR in the treatment of acne scars (135–138). Weinstein and colleagues reported greater than 50% improvement in acne scars in 15 of 16 patients treated with two to four treatments with Fraxel at 2- to 4-week intervals using a pulse energy of 12–20 mJ and 125 MTZ/cm² (135). A final total density of 2500–2750 MTZ/cm² was achieved in each treatment.

Individuals with darker skin types and acne scarring, in whom previous ablative laser treatments carry the risk of permanent PIH, were successfully and safely treated with NAFR as

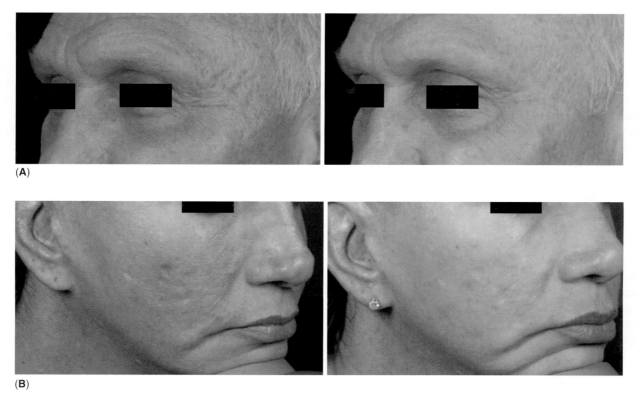

Figure 9.10 (**A**) Temples before and after seven treatments of resistant scars using Lux 1540-nm stamped NAFR using 50% overlap, 70 mJ/dot, 15 ms pulse. (**B**) Cheeks, excoriated acne, before and after three treatments using Lux 1540-nm stamped NAFR using 50% overlap, 60 mJ/dot, 15 ms pulse. *Source*: Photo courtesy of Robert Weiss, MD.

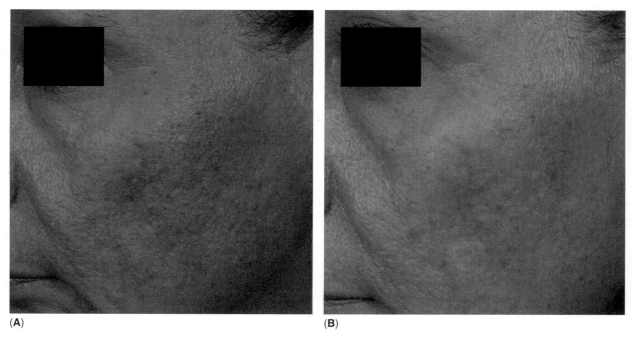

Figure 9.11 (**A**) Before and (**B**) after five treatments with LUX 1540-nm stamped NAFR using 50% overlap, 70 mJ/dot, 15 ms pulse: significant smoothing of acne scars is seen. *Source*: Photo courtesy of Robert Weiss, MD.

reported by several authors (139–143). Hasegawa and colleagues treated 10 Asian patients with acne scars using the Fraxel SR laser at 6 mJ of pulse energy and 1000–1500 MTZ/cm² of final density (139). The results after up to three treatments at 2- to 3-week intervals revealed that good-to-excellent improvement was reported in seven patients and fair improvement in three patients as assessed by physicians. No patients showed scarring or hyperpigmentation as a result of the treatment.

Lee and colleagues treated 27 Korean patients with moderate-to-severe atrophic acne scars, including ice-pick, boxcar, and rolling scars with the Fraxel SR750 (140). Three to five sessions were performed at 3- to 4-week intervals using 12–20 mJ and densities of 750–1500 MTZ/cm² (35–70%). At 3 months after last treatment, 8 patients (30%) reported excellent improvement, 16 patients (59%) significant improvement, and 3 patients (11%) moderate improvement in the appearance of acne scars.

Adverse events were transient pain, erythema, and edema with no incidence of PIH or scarring.

Chrastil and colleagues used the second-generation Fraxel SR1500 that allowed higher fluence to achieve deeper penetration into the dermis to treat 29 patients with Fitzpatrick skin types I–V and facial and back acne scarring of all types (ice-pick, boxcar, and rolling) (141). Two to six treatments at 1-month intervals were performed with pulse energies from 35 to 40 mJ and densities from 20% to 35%. At 1 month after last treatment, at least 50–75% improvement was seen in 23 of 29 patients. Five patients had greater than 75% improvement, five patients had 25–50% improvement, and one patient had less than a 25% response to treatment.

Cho and colleagues used the Mosaic 1550-µm Er:Glass laser (Lutronic Corporation, Gyeonggi, Korea) to treat 12 patients with mild-to-moderate acne scars and enlarged facial pores (142). Three sessions were performed at monthly intervals using pulse energies of 20–28 mJ and 400–900 spots/cm^2 in dynamic mode with a 10-mm handpiece. Results at 4 months after last treatment revealed that for acne scars, 5 of the 12 patients demonstrated clinical improvements of 51–75% and 3 had 76–100% improvement. Two patients had moderate improvements of 26–50% and two showed minimal to no improvements (<25%). As for enlarged facial pores, 5 of the 12 patients demonstrated 26–50% improvement, 3 had 76–100% improvement, 3 showed 51–75% improvement, and 1 showed minimal to no improvement (<25%).

Kim and colleagues compared the Mosaic laser to chemical reconstruction of skin scars (CROSS) using 100% trichloroacetic acid to ice-pick and rolling hills scars in a split-face study involving 20 patients (143). One side was treated with the 1550-nm Er:Glass fractional laser three times with a 6-week interval using a pulse energy of 30–32 mJ and density of 300–350 spots/cm^2 with a 6 mm × 6 mm handpiece. The other side was treated with CROSS method two times every 12 weeks. The fractional laser was found to be superior for treatment of rolling scars and equal to CROSS method for ice-pick scars. Although pain scores were significantly higher in the laser sides (4.49 vs. 3.33 on a 10-point scale), downtime (3.17 vs. 9.72 days), and lasting days of erythema (3.30 vs. 12.13 days) were significantly longer in the sides treated with the CROSS method.

Hu and colleagues reported similar improvement in 45 patients treated with a single treatment of Fraxel SR750 (first generation) or Fraxel SR1500 (second generation) for moderate-to-severe atrophic acne scars (144). Thirty-two patients received 15–20 mJ and densities of 1000–2000 MTZ/cm^2 with the first-generation laser and 13 received 30–40 mJ and densities of 392–520 MTZ/cm^2 with the second generation. There was no significant difference between the two groups. Physician evaluations revealed excellent results in 18%, good results in 31%, and fair results in 51%. Six patients (13%) developed PIH that lasted about 1 week.

Mahmoud and colleagues were the first to report the use of nonablative erbium 1550-nm fractional laser in the treatment of facial acne scars in patients with Fitzpatrick skin types IV–VI (145). Fifteen patients were randomized for treatment in two groups: one was treated with 10 mJ and the other with 40 mJ. Treatment level 6 (17% density) was used for both groups. Five monthly treatments were completed. Although there was significant improvement in acne scarring and overall appearance ($p<0.001$), there was no statistically significant difference between results of 10 and 40 mJ regarding acne scarring or overall appearance. Six patients developed moderate PIH even though patients had received the triple combination cream (fluocinolone 0.01%, hydroquinone 4%, and tretinoin 0.05%) before and after laser treatment. No significant difference was found in PIH induced by 10 mJ from that induced by 40 mJ, although the authors highlighted that the small number of subjects in the study may not have had enough power to conclude that the results from the two groups were the same. Overall patients were satisfied with the results, with 11 of 13 subjects rating 50% or greater improvement in their acne scars.

Glaich and colleagues reported marked improvement in postinflammatory erythema resulting from acne vulgaris in two patients who received a single treatment session with Fraxel laser (136). Pulse energies of 18 or 6 mJ with 125 (7–14% densities) or 250 MTZ/cm^2 and final densities of 1250 or 2000 MTZ/cm^2 were used for each of the patients, respectively. Moderate to marked clinical improvement in atrophic and ice-pick acne scars was noted 3 months after a series of five to six Fraxel treatments. The authors speculated that by targeting water, a major element of blood vessels, the 1550-nm wavelength may lead to photothermal destruction of dermal blood vessels, resulting in improvement of erythema. Previous reports have shown histological evidence of damage to dermal vasculature in patients undergoing FP; therefore, blood vessels located at various skin depths could be targeted for treatment by adjusting the pulse energy (146,147).

The use of the Affirm Laser (Cynosure) has shown to be effective for acne scars according to Kim and Lloyd (137,138). Kim and colleagues used the Affirm laser, which emits 1320- and 1440-nm wavelengths, for treatment of acne scars in 37 Korean patients (137). Three or four treatments were performed at monthly intervals with fluences of 3–4 J/cm^2 and 2 passes per treatment. Six of 18 patients and 13 of 19 patients had 51–75% improvement after three and four treatments, respectively (Fig. 9.12).

Lloyd and Tanghetti compared two treatment modalities with the Affirm laser for treatment of acne scars in 21 patients (138). The 1320-nm wavelength at 10 J/cm^2 was compared with the combination 1320 nm at 10 J/cm^2 plus 1440 nm at 2 J/cm^2 (Multiplex) after five treatments at 3-week intervals. All patients showed improvement in their scars, but both physicians and patients considered the Multiplex modality superior.

Skin tightening in 12 Asian patients with acne scarring after treatment with NAFR was reported by Dainichi and colleagues (148). A random half of the face was irradiated twice at 4-week intervals using a fractional 1540-nm Er:Glass (Lux 1540), 45 mJ/mb, and 3 passes. Statistical analysis of the facial images showed significant skin tightening effect 4 weeks after the first and second irradiation ($p<0.001$ after both treatments).

In 2010, consensus recommendations from experienced physicians on the use of Fraxel Re:Store were reported by Sherling and colleagues (149). The panel contended that NAFR improved the appearance of acne scars by as much as 50% after a series of four to five treatments, each spaced 1 month apart. Acne scarring associated with PIH also showed significant improvement with FP. The recommended treatments settings for acne scars depend on the skin type. For skin types I–III,

a nonablative laser (1064 Nd:YAG CoolGlide Vantage®, Cutera) in order to reduce complications and improve the efficacy (156). Twenty Asian subjects were divided into two groups that received three monthly treatments with an AFR using high energy (Group A) and low energy (Group B) on one half of the face and an AFR with low energy plus a nonablative laser on the other half. At 3 months after last treatment, the low-energy (15–35 mJ, 20% density) fractional CO_2 plus Nd:YAG (30 ms, 5-mm spot, and 40–50 J/cm²) group yielded slightly better results than the high-energy low-density fractional CO_2 group (50–70 mJ and 20% density). The average downtime decreased by 50% (3.6 vs. 7.5 days) with the dual treatment compared with the high-energy fractional CO_2. The average duration of erythema (2 vs. 6 days) and hyperpigmentation (1 vs. 3 weeks) was clearly reduced in the dual treatment group.

Cho and colleagues reported the use of combining two treatment modes of an ablative 10,600-nm CO_2 fractional laser system (UltraPulse Encore laser, Lumenis Inc., Santa Clara, California, USA) for the treatment of acne scars in Korean patients (157). Twenty patients with atrophic acne scars of all types received a single session of a CO_2 fractionated laser using the Deep FX mode to the scars (10–20 mJ, density 2, and 300 Hz) and the Active FX mode (50–100 mJ, 68% coverage, 75 Hz) over the entire face. At 3 months after the treatment, one patient had 76–100% improvement, nine had 51–75% improvement, seven had 26–50% improvement, and three had 25% improvement or less. One patient developed PIH that spontaneously resolved within 1 month. The authors advocated for the short-term use of systemic prednisolone to reduce the risk of post-therapy inflammatory reactions and subsequent pigmentary changes, particularly in Asian patients.

Shek and colleagues used the Active FX to evaluate the efficacy and the risk of PIH after the treatment of acne scars in Asian skin (158). Ten Chinese patients underwent a single treatment session using 100 mJ, 50 Hz, pattern 3, size 5, and density 2. At 3 months after treatment, 70% of patients reported moderate to significant improvement. Few instances of mild PIH were noted.

Cassuto and colleagues treated 30 patients with acne scarring, wrinkling, and tissue laxity with a microfractional CO_2 laser system (Mixto Sx Slim Evolution®, Lasering, Modena, Italy) (159). Subjects were divided into three groups to compare the use of higher energies with short pulse duration versus lower energies with longer pulse duration versus average energies and pulse duration. The settings were as follows: spot size 300 μm, energy 8–13 W, pulse duration 2.5–5 ms, and density 20% or 40%. The average improvement (71–85%) was similar in all three groups.

In 2010, Wang and colleagues confirmed the safety and efficacy of fractionated CO_2 laser (MiXto SX®; Lasering) in Asian skin (160). Five patients with moderate-to-severe atrophic acne scarring underwent two sessions, 6–8 weeks apart, with 28 J/cm², 2.5 ms, 300-μm spot size, 20% skin coverage, and single pass. At 2 months after last treatment, four patients had mild improvement and one had moderate improvement. No complications, including PIH, were observed. The authors attribute the modest results found in their patients to the conservative parameters used.

Cho and colleagues conducted a split-face study with blinded response evaluation to compare the efficacy of single-session treatments of nonablative 1550-nm Er:Glass and ablative

10,600-nm CO_2 fractional lasers for acne scars (161). Eight patients, Fitzpatrick skin type IV, with mild-to-severe atrophic acne scars had one side of the face treated with the Fraxel SR 1500 using 40 mJ and treatment level 6 (17% coverage). The other side of the face received the Deep FX mode on acne scars with 10–20 mJ, density 2 (10% coverage), and 300 Hz followed by the Active FX mode with 50–100 mJ, density 2 (68% coverage), 75 Hz. Three months after treatment, the mean grade of clinical improvement based on clinical assessment was 2.0 ± 0.5 for NAFL and 2.5 ± 0.8 for AFR ($p = 0.158$) on a 4-point scale. On each side treated using NAFR and AFR, the mean duration of post-therapy crusting and scaling was 2.3 ± 2.9 and 7.4 ± 2.4 days, respectively, and that of post-therapy erythema was 7.5 ± 5.7 and 11.5 ± 5.2 days, respectively. The mean visual analog scale pain score was 3.9 ± 2.0 for NAFR and 7.0 ± 2.0 for AFR. Only one patient developed PIH that spontaneously resolved within 2 weeks. The authors concluded that both NAFR and AFR were effective after a single session for acne scarring in Asian patients, but the AFR showed slightly greater efficacy while it caused more pain and more adverse effects.

Hedelund et al. (164) performed a single-blinded randomized controlled trial of treatment of moderate-to-severe atrophic acne scars using CO_2 AFR. Two facial areas of similar size representing similar scar morphology were compared at three and six monthly treatment sessions, using very conservative treatment parameters (topical anesthetic only and 2–3 days for healing). Statistically significant ($p<0.0001$) mild-to-moderate improvement in atrophy and texture were seen on the treated side.

Manuskiatti and colleagues reported higher incidence of PIH (92% of the subjects) noted after fractionated CO_2 laser for treatment of acne scars in Asian skin (162). Thirteen patients with mild-to-moderate atrophic facial acne scars underwent three sessions with a 15-W CO_2 laser (Ellipse Juvia, Ellipse A/S, Hørsholm, Denmark) on an average of 7-week interval. A single pass treatment was performed with pulse energies ranging from 75 to 105 mJ depending on the severity of the scars and density of 49 MTZ/cm² (9.6% coverage). At the 6-month follow-up, 85% of patients were rated as having at least 25–50% improvement of scars. At 1-month follow-up, image analysis evaluated by a UVA-light video camera (Visioscan VC 98, Courage-Khazaka, Köln, Germany) revealed that both surface smoothness ($p = 0.03$) and scar volume ($p<0.001$) had significant improvement compared with baseline measurements. Mild-to-moderate PIH was experienced by 12 of 13 subjects treated and lasted 2–16 weeks (average 5 weeks). All patients were successfully treated with hydroquinone 4% cream. The authors concluded that CO_2 AFR is an effective and well-tolerated treatment for dark-skinned patients with acne scarring that showed improved efficacy over nonablative dermal remodeling devices.

Fractionated resurfacing, including nonablative fractionated lasers and ablative fractionated lasers, represents a new treatment paradigm for acne scarring as well as scars overall as it combines the lesser risks of side effects such as delayed-onset hypopigmentation, PIH, scarring, and prolonged erythema compared with traditional ablative laser resurfacing with a more predictable clinical response compared with nonablative lasers. Another major advantage of fractional resurfacing is the possibility to treat off-face. In the senior author's experience, NAFR has a greater range in its spectrum of response than that of AFR and usually requires multiple treatment sessions (three to six) compared with one or two with AFR. However, the lack of downtime for healing and the potential of combining the two approaches make NAFR an interesting option. AFR has much greater ability to tighten the skin than NAFR devices, which correlates directly with the volume of tissue heated, or the depth and density of treatment. Therefore, deep tissue vaporization and coagulation associated with significant density of treatment correlate to better clinical outcome (64). However, it should be noted that the risk of adverse reactions with AFR is not absent, with a few reports of postoperative infection and scarring after AFL related to anatomical location as well as appropriate densities (Figs. 9.15 and 9.16) (165–167).

Finally, the use of this promising technology to prevent scarring postoperatively, particularly for cosmetic surgical procedures, should become a major area of concentration and success. Future studies with a longer follow-up and comparative efficacy of treatment parameters will result in an even greater margin of safety with better clinical outcomes (Figs. 9.17, 9.18, 9.19).

INTRALESIONAL CORTICOSTEROIDS

IL corticosteroid injections have been the primary treatment for keloids and hypertrophic scars for the past 50 years. These steroids are thought to decrease fibroblast proliferation, decrease collagen synthesis as well as glycosaminoglycan synthesis and to suppress proinflammatory mediators (168). Corticosteroids inhibit collagenase by inhibiting α2-macroglobulin. If this pathway is blocked, collagenase is elaborated, resulting in collagen breakdown (169,170).

TAC is the corticosteroid most commonly used (171) and was first reported in 1960 (172). It is generally used in concentrations of 10–20 mg/mL, but occasionally as high as 40 mg/mL. Injections are typically done at 3- to 4-week intervals. It is important to inject right into the center of the scar. Injecting too superficially can result in epidermal atrophy, and injecting too deep, especially subcutaneously, can result in long-lasting dermal/fat atrophy.

Various authors still affirm that IL corticosteroids are the treatment of choice for hypertrophic scars and keloids (173,174). Acknowledged side effects are pain with injection, atrophy, telangiectasia, and hypopigmentation at the injection site (175). Cushing's syndrome has been reported as a complication in pediatric patients (176–178). IL triamcinolone is generally successful in reducing the volume of a scar (179). Recurrence rates of 9–50% have been reported with the use of IL triamcinolone (180–186). A study using 3D imaging found mean scar volume to reduce from 0.73 ± 0.701 mL at baseline to 0.14 ± 0.302 mL following monthly IL triamcinolone (187).

However, success has not been uniform. Muneuchi et al. (179) reported the long-term outcome of 94 patients with keloids treated with 1–10 mg of TAC intralesionally at 4 weeks or longer intervals. Patients received 20–30 injections over 3–5 years. Thirty-one patients (33%) discontinued because of pain and lack of response. Fair or better results in decreasing the size of the keloid were seen in 40 patients (43%), but good or better results were seen in only 25 of this group of 40 responders (27%). This type of response is much more in line with the experience of the senior author (REF), not to mention the high rate of atrophy, telangiectasia, and hypopigmentation. The rate of

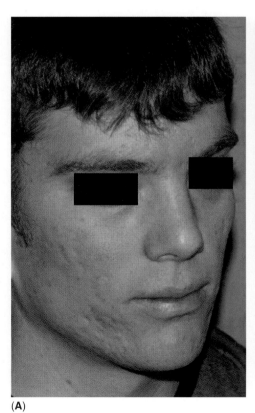
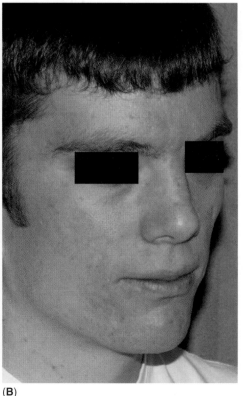

(A)   (B)

Figure 9.15 (**A**) Atrophic acne scars following a severe flare of nodular/cystic acne. (**B**) One year following a single treatment with Fraxel Re:Pair using 60 mJ and 50% density.

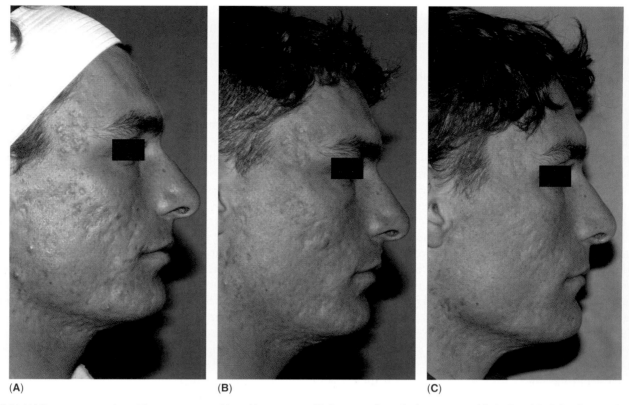

(A)   (B)   (C)

Figure 9.16 (**A**) Severe acne scarring with numerous atrophic and boxcar scars. (**B**) One year after a single treatment with the Fraxel Re:Pair using 70 mJ and 50% density. (**C**) One year after second treatment with Fraxel Re:Pair using 70 mJ and 50% density.

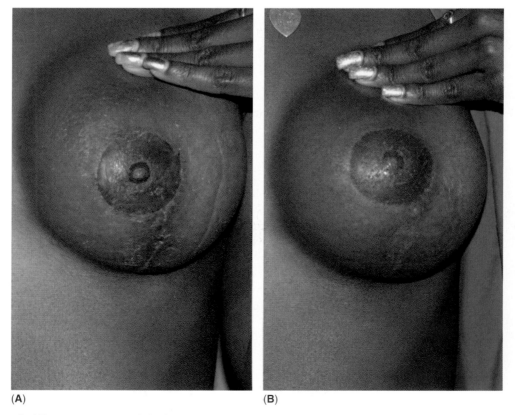

(A)   (B)

Figure 9.17 (**A**) Two weeks following suture removal after breast augmentation. (**B**) One month after two treatments at monthly intervals starting 2 weeks after suture removal. Fraxel Re:Store was used at 20 mJ and 20% density.

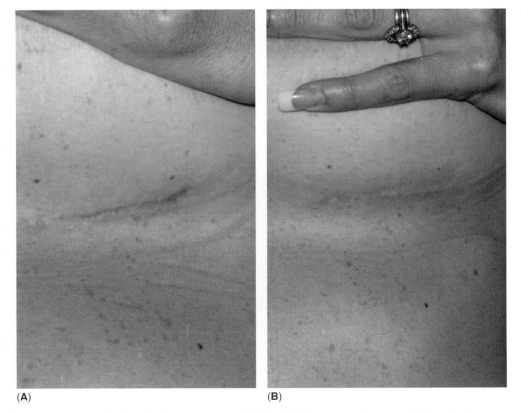

(A)   (B)

Figure 9.18 (**A**) Scar from breast augmentation 2 weeks after suture removal. (**B**) Fraxel Re:Store treatments were started 2 weeks after suture removal and repeated at 4-week intervals for four treatments using 30 mJ and 26% density.

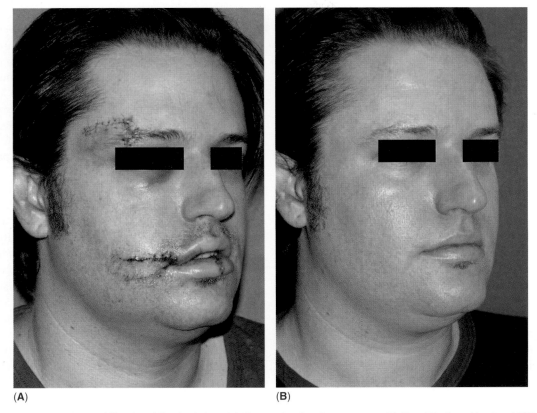

(A)   (B)

Figure 9.19 (**A**) Laceration secondary to fall; 3 days following injury. (**B**) Six months after six treatments with Fraxel Re:Store 20 mJ and 32% density at 2-week intervals starting 2 weeks after suture removal.

adverse reactions such as this has been around 40% as reported in two studies (35,170).

INTRALESIONAL 5-FU

Of all the various antimetabolites that have been studied for use as IL agents to treat keloids and hypertrophic scars, 5-FU stands out as a uniquely effective agent.

In 1989, the senior author (REF) began a clinical investigation of the use of IL 5-FU in the management of hypertrophic scars and keloids. Patients were initially treated with IL injections of 5-FU (50 mg/cc) in the range of 2–50 mg per treatment. Monthly treatment intervals were used at the onset, but this was found to be ineffective. Gradually, the intervals were decreased to as frequently as three times weekly until there was a clinical response. Once a significant response was seen, the treatment interval was gradually tapered to twice a week, once per week, and then once every 2 weeks. Follow-up treatments were resumed at the first signs of an inflammatory response. Generally an injection interval of once weekly was successful for most patients, but in general the more inflamed and indurated the scar is, the more frequent the injection interval needed to be. Through trial and error, it was found that the addition of 0.1 cc Kenalog 10 mg/cc alleviated some of the pain of injection as well as increased the clinical efficacy. A standard treatment protocol is to combine 0.1 cc of Kenalog 10 mg (1 mg Kenalog) with 0.9 cc 5-FU (45 mg) in the same syringe, making sure that the Kenalog is well dispersed in the 5-FU. The author's initial 9-year experience involving as many as 5000 injections in approximately 1000 scars was reported in 1999 (188).

Systemic administration of 5-FU can cause anemia, leucopenia, and thrombocytopenia. No systemic side effects have been reported even with doses of 90 mg 5-FU or higher per treatment session (35,170,188,189).

In the early 1980s, 5-FU was investigated as an adjunct to glaucoma filtering surgery to inhibit scarring after the surgical procedure (190–193) and has become a routine adjuvant as the safety and efficacy were demonstrated in a long-term multicenter study of 5-FU in trabeculectomy surgery (194).

It has an inhibitory effect on TGF-β-induced type I collagen gene expression in human fibroblasts (195) and subsequent collagen deposition. De Waard et al. (196) have shown inhibition of fibroblast proliferation and collagen synthesis by 5-FU. In vitro studies have shown a dose-related reduction by 5-FU in both keloid fibroblast proliferation and fibroblast-populated collagen lattice (197). It also inhibits proliferation and myofibroblast differentiation in dupuytren fibroblasts in vitro (198).

5-FU is an antimetabolite drug in the pyrimidine class. It interrupts both DNA and RNA synthesis at several levels, including the inhibition of thymidylate synthetase (199). This blocks the change of uridine to thymidine, which affects the biosynthesis of fibroblast DNA, which results in the inhibition of cell proliferation (200). 5-FU relies on thymidylate synthase activity to initiate apoptosis. Studies have shown pathologically low rates of apoptosis among keloid scars (201). Bulstrode et al. (202) have demonstrated that 5-FU selectively inhibits collagen synthesis. In animal studies, 5-FU has been shown to inhibit fibroblast proliferation and accelerate degradation of hypertrophic scar collagen (196).

Occleston et al. (203) have shown that type I collagen, fibronectin, and cell migration were inhibited by 5-FU for 48 days.

A similar time interval of the effects of a single dose of 5-FU was demonstrated in an in vivo study by Uppal et al. (204), which showed suppression of fibroblasts 4 weeks after 5-FU treatment. These studies suggest a treatment interval of 1 month might be appropriate. However, that has not been an effective treatment protocol in the author's experience. In fact, much more frequent injections (1–3 times per week) have proven to be much more successful.

Based on pharmacokinetic studies, Haurani et al. (205) report that 5-FU remains in the soft tissue for less than 10 days and in the bloodstream for less than 20 minutes. Perhaps these dynamics are more significant than the time of suppression of fibroblasts. It is metabolized and excreted by the kidney.

Uppal et al. (204) conducted a study of 11 patients with keloids using a single application of 5-FU (25 mg/cc) for 5 minutes to the open wound following excision of keloid. The wound was then flushed with saline prior to suturing with 5-0 nylon sutures. The patient served as its own control with a second keloid excision being soaked with saline for 5 minutes before suturing. Clinical assessment of the scars using a numerical scoring system showed 50% improvement at 6 months compared with the control scars. Biopsies of scars at 1 month showed significant reduction ($p<0.01$) in cellular markers for cell proliferation, inflammation, and TGF-β1.

In vivo studies have shown 5-FU to have a dose-dependent toxicity to fibroblasts (206). A dose of 25 mg/cc as used in this study was considered subtoxic, but an average loss of 5% of cells was found in tissue culture in this study. 5-FU has been shown to halt cell growth at any stage (207) of the cell, but no general toxicity was seen as wounds healed normally. Macrophage numbers were not altered.

Costa et al. (208) reported 50% improvement in 85% of patients at 1 year after treatment with 5-FU. A recurrence rate of 4.7% was seen at 1 year (209).

Davison et al. (199) performed a retrospective review of patient charts having 102 keloids treated from 1999 to 2006. There were 52 patients who were treated with 5-FU (37 mg) combined with TAC (2.5 or 10 mg) in the same syringe without excision and 4-week intervals. This group had an average of 81% reduction in lesion volume. Those treated using the same regimen without excision averaged 92% improvement and those treated with excision followed by TAC averaged 73% improvement. Symptoms resolved in 93% of patients treated with 5-FU.

Apikian and Goodman (210) demonstrated improvement in keloids in two patients treated with IL 5-FU.

Gupta and Kalra (211) have shown safety and efficacy in using 5-FU as an individual agent in the treatment of small symptomatic keloids in 24 patients. Weekly treatments of 50–150 mg of 5-FU were used. Symptoms resolved completely in over 70% of their patients and one-third had greater than 75% flattening of the treated keloid. Keloids ≤5 years in duration had a greater tendency to flatten (55%). Kontochristopoulos et al. (212) also studied 5-FU as monotherapy in 20 patients having more than 75 keloids. Injections of 5-FU (50 mg/cc) were performed at weekly intervals for an average of seven treatments. Maximum volume was 2.0 cc and average was 0.3 cc. A reduction in keloid volume was seen in 95% of patients, with 8 having more than 50% reduction and 8 having greater than 75% reduction and 1 having 100%. Recurrences were seen in nine patients (47%), 1–6 months after the last treatment. Keloids present for >2 years were more likely to recur. Biopsies before and after treatment (6 months) documented a diminution or elimination of collagenous fiber whorls and of thick hyalinized collagen bands. Ki-67, a cell proliferation marker, showed marked reduction ($p = 0.0001$). Liver function tests, renal function tests, and CBC were normal before and after treatment.

Manuskiatti and Fitzpatrick (35) studied the response of hypertrophic sternotomy scars to IL corticosteroids, IL 5-FU, and flashlamp-pumped PDL treatments. They found all three treatments to be roughly equivalent in efficacy, but that corticosteroids had a much higher incidence of long-term sequelae (atrophy, telangiectasia, and hypopigmentation), that is, 40% versus 0%. The combined use of 5-FU with the V-beam Perfecta and the Fraxel Re:Store has become standard therapy for scars in the practice of the senior author (Fig. 9.20).

Nanda and Reddy (189) reported a prospective uncontrolled trial of IL 5-FU (50 mg/cc) given at weekly intervals for 12 weeks (0.5–2 cc per treatment) and then having follow-up after an additional 24 weeks. Twenty-eight patients having 1–6 keloids were treated. Lesions ranged from 2 to 15 cm in size and 6 months to 15 years in duration. Eight patients had previously failed to respond to IL TAC 40 mg/cc every 3 weeks. All patients responded to treatment, with 71% having good response (>50% improvement) and 7% having excellent response (>75% improvement). Flattening of the keloid and peripheral regression were noted in all lesions. They noted no difference in response of older keloids (15 years) and younger lesions (6 months). Total and differential leukocyte counts were normal at baseline, 12 weeks, and 24 weeks.

Asilian et al. (170) performed a 12-week single-blinded clinical trial in which 69 patients with hypertrophic scars or keloids were assigned to one of three groups. A single lesion >10 mm in length was treated in each patient. All patients had CBC, liver, and renal function tests at baseline and 12 weeks—these were all normal. In Group 1, IL TAC (10 mg/cc) was injected at weekly intervals for 8 weeks. In Group 2, TAC plus 5-FU (0.1 cc of 40 mg/cc TAC added to 0.9 cc of 5-FU 50 mg/cc) was injected weekly for 8 weeks. Group 3 had TAC plus 5-FU as in Group 2, but also added 585-nm pulsed dye laser (5–7.5 J/cm²) at weeks 1, 4, and 8. Improvement was evaluated regarding length, width, height of scars, erythema (visual scale), pliability (5-point scale regarding induration), itching (4-point scale), and patient self-assessment and overall improvement graded by photos. Improvement in all areas was seen in each Group, but TAC + 5-FU as well as TAC + 5-FU + PDL showed greater improvement than TAC alone ($p<0.05$). Patient self-assessment regarding >50% improvement was 20% in Group 1, 55% in Group 2, and 75% in Group 3. Blinded observers rated >50% improvement as 15% in Group 1, 40% in Group 2, 70% in Group 3. Atrophy and telangiectasia were seen in 37% of those treated with TAC alone, that is, Group 1.

Darougheh et al. (213) studied 40 patients with keloids in a randomized double-blind clinical trial. Group 1 received TAC 10 mg/cc intralesionally, weekly for 8 weeks. Group 2 received 0.1 cc of TAC 4 mg mixed with 0.9 cc 5-FU 45 mg weekly for 8 weeks. Greater than 50% improvement at 12 weeks was reported in 20% of Group 1 and 55% of Group 2, while trained graders scored 15% in Group 1 and 40% of Group 2 as having >50% improvement. Liver and renal function tests as well as CBC were normal before and after 12 weeks.

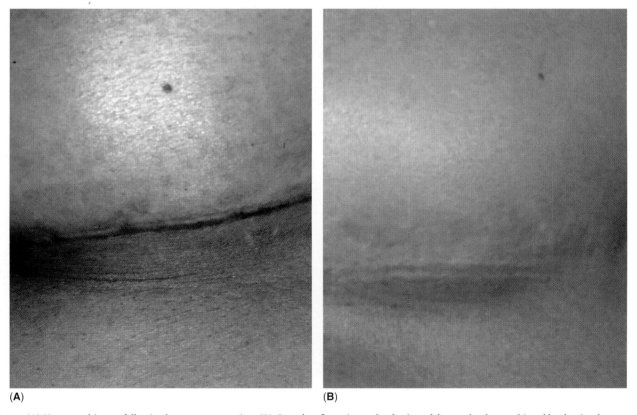

(A)   **(B)**

Figure 9.20 (**A**) Hypertrophic scar following breast augmentation. (**B**) Complete flattening and softening of the scar has been achieved by the simultaneous use of intralesional 5-FU, the V-beam Perfecta, and the Fraxel Re:Store.

Goldan et al. (214) reported successful treatment of hypertrophic scars occurring after facial dermabrasion in a 67-year-old woman. The scars were very painful and pruritic and involved the nasolabial folds and chin. Treatment with IL steroids was not successful. She received six treatments of IL 5-FU (50 mg/cc) at 2-week intervals. There was marked improvement in size, color, and texture of the scars as well as total elimination of her symptoms of pain and itching. Seven months after treatment all scars remained stable.

Mutalik and Patwardhan (215) reported a series of 24 patients with keloids that were treated with IL 5-FU (50 mg/cc) at 4-week intervals. Sixteen patients (67%) showed complete flattening of their keloids after an average of four treatment sessions. Twelve of these patients (75%) had no recurrence after 1 year. Some patients also had additional injections of triamcinolone 40 mg/cc, but no further information is provided except that two patients developed post-steroid hypopigmentation.

A prospective study of treatment of keloids and hypertrophic scars with IL 5-FU following excision of keloids and hypertrophic scars without excision revealed a 19% recurrence rate of keloids and a 50% median decrease in scar volume in hypertrophic scars (216).

Haurani et al. (205) performed a prospective case series study of 32 patients with keloids and 21 patients with hypertrophic scars, all of whom had failed to respond to IL steroid therapy. Those with keloids were treated with excision followed 2 weeks later with IL 5-FU (50 mg/cc). This was repeated at monthly intervals for 10 treatments with a follow-up of 1 year after the 10th treatment. Hypertrophic scars were treated with IL 5-FU (50 mg/cc) at monthly intervals without excision. A maximum dose of 50 mg per treatment was used. In the keloid group, the measured volume of the lesion after excision remained stable with only a 0.06 cm^3 increase in volume at the 1-year follow-up. Six patients were noted to have recurrence of scar growth (19%). In addition, 90% of patients had partial or complete relief of symptoms of pruritus or pain. In the hypertrophic scar group 86% had improvement in symptoms and a 40% reduction in scar volume after the 1-year follow-up.

A double-blind randomized clinical study of 50 patients with keloids (2–6 cm in size and 2–5 years in duration) involved two groups of 25 patients. In each group, keloids were excised, followed by application of silicon sheets for 6–12 months. The study group also received IL 5-FU (50 mg/cc) at days 7, 14, and 28 and at 2 and 3 months postoperatively. At 1 year, the study group showed 18 (75%) were keloid free and five (21%) had improvement in size, thickness, and texture. In the control group, 10 (43%) were keloid free, 8 (35%) had improvement, and 7 (22%) failed to respond (217).

Katz et al. (218) report a successful treatment of perioral scarring following phenol peel in a 75-year-old woman, using 595-nm PDL, 1450-nm diode laser in combination with 5-FU (45 mg/cc), and triamcinolone (0.1 cc of Kenalog 10 mg/cc) mixed in the same syringe. Treatments were performed at 1- to 2-month intervals with a total of 10 treatments over 1 year. After 1 month, greater than 25% improvement was noted; after five treatments, 90% improvement was noted; and after 2.5 years, the noted improvement persisted.

In a review of medical evidence levels A, B, and C, Gupta and Sharma (219) conclude that IL 5-FU is considered a safe and effective treatment of keloids and hypertrophic scars when used alone or in combination with IL steroids and surgical excision (Figs. 9.21 and 9.22).

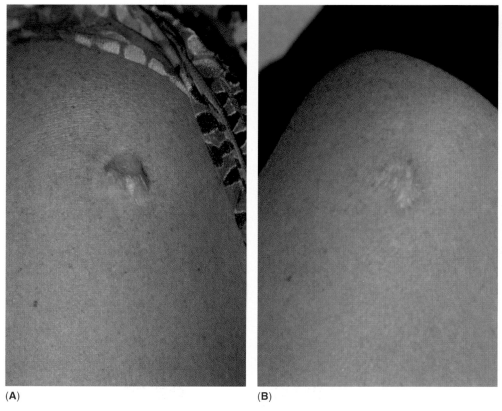

(A) (B)

Figure 9.21 (**A**) Hypertrophic scar of deltoid area. (**B**) Flattening of scar is seen after treatment with intralesional 5-FU (45 mg/cc) and triamcinolone (1 mg/cc) performed at 1- to 4-week intervals. Average volume injected was 0.2 cc and there were a total of 10 treatment sessions.

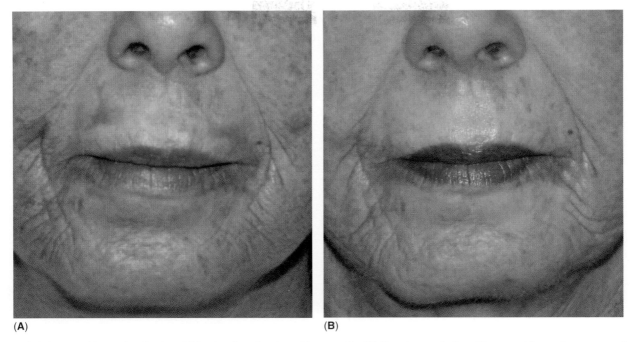

(A)   **(B)**

Figure 9.22 (**A**) Hypertrophic scarring developed following dermabrasion of the upper lip. (**B**) Complete resolution of hypertrophic scarring was seen after treatment with intralesional 5-FU (45 mg/cc) and triamcinolone (1 mg/cc) in conjunction with treatment of wrinkling with Fraxel Re:Pair.

Three publications from China reported the clinical success of low-dose (<10 mg/cc) IL 5-FU. Two publications (220,221) were published in the Chinese literature. The first article (220) reported 35 patients with 51 keloids treated with 5-FU (2–5 mg/cc) biweekly followed after 3–6 injections with IL steroid. After 6 months, 45.7% had complete remission, 48.6 had a great remission, and 2.9% had partial remission—a 97% response rate.

The second article (221) reported 83 patients with bilateral ear keloids. The keloids were excised and then treated with IL low-dose 5-FU (not defined) and corticosteroid (not defined) every 3–4 weeks. The mean treatment time was 7 months and the mean follow-up after treatment was 9 months. There was a 100% response rate, with 47% having complete resolution and 53% having "effective" response.

The third study is a case report (222) of a 53-year-old woman with a 28-year history of a chest keloid having 4+ pain, 4+ itching, 4+ erythema, and 2+ induration and measuring 10 cm × 7 cm × 0.3 cm thickness. The lesion had failed steroid therapy and cryotherapy. IL 5-FU was used in dosages of 3.45–1.42 mg/cc given at 2-week intervals. TAC was also used intralesionally at doses of 8.3–3.77 mg/cc. Fourteen months after treatment, there was dramatic improvement in the scar that had regressed to normal looking skin and was asymptomatic.

As a consequence of the success of these low-dose studies and publications in the Chinese literature, Huang et al. from Hong Kong proposed to alter the focus from cell destruction to the promotion of apoptosis and inhibition of fibroblast proliferation with 5-FU (223). They studied the cellular response of keloid fibroblasts at a range of doses as low as 1 mg/cc. At a dose of 25 mg/cc, there was complete inhibition of cell proliferation and 80% cell mortality. In contrast, lower doses (1–10 mg/cc) induced significant inhibition of proliferation and cell apoptosis in a dose-dependent fashion but did not cause immediate cell death. They found that 5-FU causes G2/M cell cycle arrest and induces dramatic p53 and p21

accumulation together with a decrease in cyclin B1 and Bcl-2 levels. Both p53 and p21 are associated with cellular apoptosis.

After reading these studies, the senior author (REF) has treated a small number of scars with low dose 5-FU (5 mg/cc) successfully (Fig. 9.23).

CONCLUSION

The treatment of scarring is very complex and cannot be accomplished successfully by the use of a single modality. It is a constant reality that each case must be analyzed carefully and a specific approach is developed for that individual and for each scar treated.

The availability of various vascular lasers, such as the V-beam Perfecta, has definitely enhanced our ability to successfully treat scars, particularly those with significant erythema. In a similar fashion, the advent of fractional lasers, such as the Fraxel lasers, has added a new dimension to the treatment of scars using both NAFR and AFR.

As far as dyspigmentation is concerned, the use of pigment lasers such as the alexandrite laser to remove excessive pigment and the use of the bimatoprost to stimulate pigment in areas of hypopigmentation give us greater control over these issues.

There are numerous studies documenting the superiority of IL 5-FU over corticosteroids in the treatment of hypertrophic scarring and keloids. Greater efficacy and dramatically lower incidence of side effects have been seen. It is hoped that the use of this drug in both prevention and treatment of scars becomes more widespread.

By combining these modalities for use simultaneously, we can achieve tremendous success (Figs. 9.24 and 9.25).

Early intervention has also been found to be critical and has the potential to prevent scarring when done properly. The optimum time for treatment has not been firmly established, but various studies as well as the clinical experience of the senior author are convincing that the earlier the better. It appears clear that treatment at the first signs of potential hypertrophic scarring is critical in preventing and minimizing scarring.

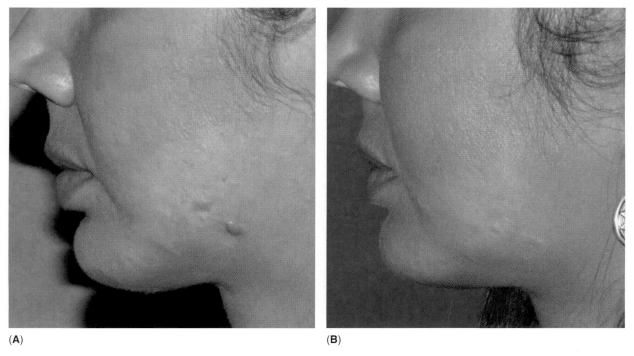

(A)   **(B)**

Figure 9.23 (**A**) Hypertrophic scarring of the left cheek following dermabrasion. (**B**) Flattening of the hypertrophic scars is seen after 12 treatments with intralesional 5-FU (5 mg/cc) performed at 1- to 4-week intervals.

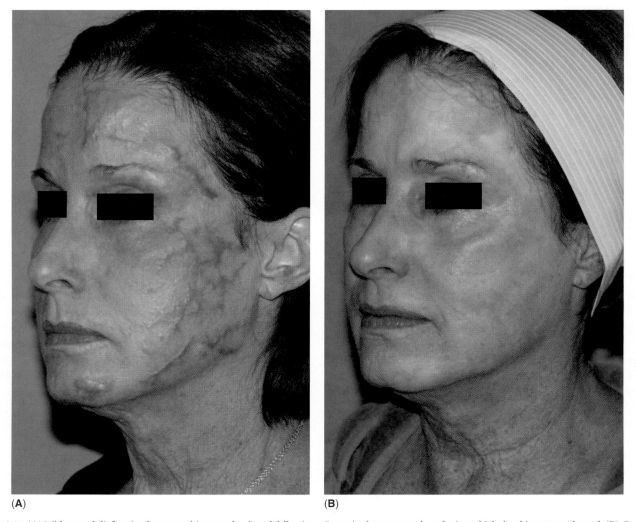

(A)   **(B)**

Figure 9.24 (**A**) Widespread disfiguring hypertrophic scars developed following a Portrait plasma procedure during which the skin was overheated. (**B**) Complete resolution of the hypertrophic nature of the scars has been achieved through the use of intralesional 5-FU, the V-beam Perfecta and Fraxel Re:Store.

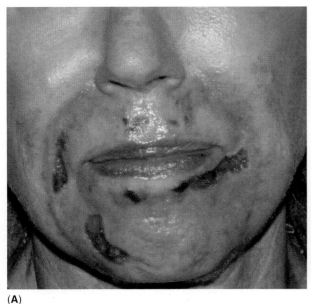

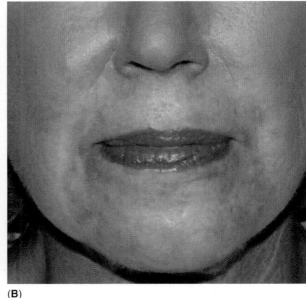

(A) **(B)**

Figure 9.25 (**A**) Full-thickness ulceration and deep erosions are seen following trichloroacetic acid peeling that penetrated too deeply. (**B**) Treatment was initially begun with oral antibiotics and ultrathin Duoderm. Once the ulcerations had healed, intralesional 5-FU (45 mg/cc) and triamcinolone (1 mg/cc) were used to control hypertrophic scars that developed. The V-beam Perfecta and Fraxel Re:Store were used to normalize the scar tissue.

REFERENCES

1. Sund B. New Developments in Wound Care. London: PJB Publications, 2000: 1–255.
2. Tsao SS, Dover JS, Arndt KA, Kaminer MS. Scar management: keloid, hypertrophic, atrophic, and acne scars. Sem Cut Med Surg 2002; 21: 46–75.
3. Breasted JH. The Edwin Smith Surgical Papyrus: Hieroglyphic Transaction and Commentary. Chicago: University of Chicago Press, 1970: 403–6.
4. Addison T. On the keloid of alibert and on true keloids. Med Chir Trans 1835; 19: 19.
5. Mancini RE, Quaife JV. Histogenesis of experimentally produced keloids. J Invest Dermatol 1962; 38: 143–81.
6. Roseborough IE, Grevious MA, Lee RC. Prevention and treatment of excessive dermal scarring. J Nat Med Assoc 2004; 96: 108–16.
7. Niessen FB, Sapuwen PH, Schalkwijk J, Kon M. On the nature of hypertrophic scars and keloids: a review. Plast Reconstr Surg 1999; 104: 1435–58.
8. Murray CJ, Pinnel SR. Keloids and excessive dermal scarring. In: Cohen IK, Diegelmann RF, Lindblad WJ, eds. Woundhealing, Biochemical and Clinical Aspects. Philadelphia: Saunders Elsevier, 1992: 500–9.
9. Murray JC. Keloids and hypertrophic scars. Clin Dermatol 1994; 12: 27–37.
10. Slemp AE, Kirschner RE. Keloids and scars: a review of keloids and scars, their pathogenesis, risk factors, and management. Curr Opin Pediatr 2006; 18: 396–402.
11. Sephel GC, Woodward SC. Repair, regeneration, and fibrosis. In: Rubin E, ed. Rubin's Pathology. Baltimore: Lippincott, Williams & Wilkins, 2001: 84–117.
12. Diegelmann RF, Cohen IK, McCoy B. Growth kinetics and collagen synthesis of normal skin, scar and keloid fibroblasts in vitro. J Cell Physiol 1979; 98: 341–6.
13. Cohen IK, Keiser HR, Sjoerdsmo A. Collagen synthesis in human keloid and hypertrophic scars. Surg Forum 1971; 22: 488.
14. Chung S, Nakashima M, Zembutsu H, Nakamura Y. Possible involvement of NEDD4 in keloid formation; its critical role in fibroblast proliferation and collagen production. Proc Jpn Acad Ser B Phys Biol Sci 2011; 87: 563–73.
15. Dienus K, Bayat A, Gilmore BF, Seifert O. Increased expression of fibroblast activation protein-alpha in keloid fibroblasts: Implications for development of a novel treatment option. Arch Dermatol Res 2010; 302: 725–31.
16. Gauglitz GG, Korting HC, Pavicic T, Ruzicka T, Jeschke MG. Hypertrophic scarring and keloids: pathomechanisms and current and emerging treatment strategies. Mol Med 2011; 17: 113–25.
17. Bond JS, Duncan JA, Sattar A, et al. Maturation of the human scar: an observational study. Plast Reconstr Surg 2008; 121: 1650–8.
18. Bond JS, Duncan JA, Mason T, et al. Scar redness in humans: how long does it persist after incisional and excisional wounding? Plast Reconstr Surg 2008; 121: 487–96.
19. Ladak A, Tredget EE. Pathophysiology and management of the burn scar. Clin Plast Surg 2009; 36: 661–74.
20. Ginsbach G, Kuhnel W. The treatment of hypertrophic scars and keloids by argon laser: Clinical data and morphological findings. Plast Surg Forum 1979; 1: 61–7.
21. Hulsbergen-Henning JP, Roskann Y, vanGemert M. Treatment of keloids and hypertrophic scars with an argon laser. Lasers Surg Med 1986; 6: 72–5.
22. Apfelberg DB, Maser MR, Lash H, et al. Preliminary results of argon and carbon dioxide laser treatment of keloid scars. Lasers Surg Med 1984; 4: 283–90.
23. Bailin P. Use of the CO_2 laser for non-PWS cutaneous lesions. In: Arndt KA, Noe JM, Rosen S, eds. Cutaneous Laser Therapy: Principles and Methods. New York, NY: John Wiley, 1983: 187–200.
24. Norris TE. The effect of carbon dioxide laser surgery on the recurrence of keloids. Plast Reconstr Surg 1991; 87: 44–9.
25. Olbricht SM, Arndt KA. Lasers in cutaneous surgery. In: Fuller T, ed. Surgical Lasers: A Clinical Guide. New York, NY: MacMillan, 1987: 113–46.
26. Bernstein LJ, Kauvar ANG, Grossman MC, et al. Scar resurfacing and high-energy, short-pulsed and flashscanning carbon dioxide lasers. Dermatol Surg 1998; 24: 101–7.
27. Goldman MP, Fitzpatrick RE. Cutaneous Laser Surgery: The Art and Science of Selective Photothermolysis, 2nd edn. St. Louis, MO: Mosby, Inc, 1999.
28. Nouri K, Laser treatment of scars. In: Elston D, ed. Drugs, Diseases and Procedures. New York: Medscape.com, 2010.
29. Anderson RR, Parrish JA. Selective photothermolysis: precise microsurgery by selective absorption of pulsed radiation. Science 1983; 22: 524–7.
30. Alster TS, Kurban AK, Grove GL, et al. Alteration of argon laser-induced scars by the pulsed dye laser. Lasers Surg Med 1993; 13: 368–73.
31. Alster TS. Improvement of erythematous and hypertrophic scars by the 585 nm pulsed dye laser. Ann Plast Surg 1994; 32: 186–90.
32. Dierickx C, Goldman MP, Fitzpatrick RE. Laser treatment of erythematous /hypertrophic and pigmented scars in 26 patients. Plast Reconstr Surg 1995; 95: 84–90.
33. Goldman M, Fitzpatrick RE. Laser treatment of scars. Dermatol Surg 1995; 21: 685–7.

34. Alster TS, Williams CM. Treatment of keloid sternotomy scars with 585 nm flashlamp-pumped pulsed dye laser. Lancet 1995; 345: 1198.

35. Manuskiatti W, Fitzpatrick RE. Treatment response of keloidal and hypertrophic sternotomy scars: Comparison among intralesional corticosteroid, 5-fluorouracil, and 585-nm flashlamp-pumped pulsed-dye laser treatments. Arch Dermatol 2002; 138: 1149–54.

36. Wittenberg GP, Fabian BG, Bogomilsky JL, et al. Prospective, single-blind, randomized, controlled study to assess the efficacy of the 585-nm flashlamp-pumped pulsed-dye laser and silicone gel sheeting in hypertrophic scar treatment. Arch Dermatol 1999; 135: 1049–55.

37. Alster T. Laser scar revision: comparison study of 585-nm pulsed dye laser with and without intralesional corticosteroids. Dermatol Surg 2003; 29: 25–9.

38. Alster TS, Handrick C. Laser treatment of hypertrophic scars, keloids, and striae. Semin Cutan Med Surg 2000; 19: 287–92.

39. Tanzi EL, Alster TS. Laser treatment of scars. Skin Therapy Lett 2004; 9: 4–7.

40. Alster TS, McMeekin TO. Improvement of facial acne scars by the 585 nm flashlamp-pumped pulsed dye laser. J Am Acad Dermatol 1996; 35: 79–81.

41. Alster TS, Nanni CA. Pulse dye laser treatment of hypertrophic burn scars. Plast Reconstr Surg 1998; 102: 2190–5.

42. Karsai S, Roos S, Hammes S, Raulin C. Pulsed dye laser: what's new in non-vascular lesions? J Eur Acad Dermatol Venerol 2007; 21: 877–90.

43. Allison KP, Kiernan MN, Waters RA, Clement RM. Pulsed dye laser treatment of burn scars: alleviation or irritation? Burns 2003; 29: 207–13.

44. Chan HH, Wong DS, Ho WS, et al. The use of pulsed dye laser for the prevention and treatment of hypertrophic scars in Chinese persons. Dermatol Surg 2004; 30: 987–94.

45. Urioste SS, Arndt KA, Dover JS. Keloids and hypertrophic scars: Review and treatment strategies. Sem Cut Med Surg 1999; 18: 159–71.

46. Reiken SR, Wolfort SF, Berthiaume F, et al. Control of hypertrophic scar growth using selective photothermolysis. Lasers Surg Med 1997; 21: 7–12.

47. Topol BM, Lewis VL Jr, Benveniste K. The use of antihistamine to retard the growth of fibroblasts derived from human skin, scar and keloid. Plast Reconstr Surg 1981; 68: 231–2.

48. Sandberg N. Accelerated collagen formation and histamine. Nature 1962; 194: 183.

49. Kuo YR, Wu WS, Jeng SF, Nicolini J, Zubillaga M. Activation of ERK and p38 kinase mediated keloid fibroblast apoptosis after flashlamp pulsed dye laser treatment. Lasers Surg Med 2005; 36: 31–7; LEVEL C.

50. Kuo YR, Jeng SF, Wang FS, et al. Flashlamp pulsed dye lasers (PDL) suppression of keloid proliferation through down-regulation of TGF-beta1 expression and extracellular matrix expression. Lasers Surg Med 2004; 34: 104–8; LEVEL C.

51. McCraw JB, McCraw JA, McMellin A, et al. Prevention of unfavorable scars using early pulsed dye laser treatments: A preliminary report. Ann Plast Surg 1999; 42: 7–14.

52. Yang Q, Ma Y, Zhu R, et al. The effect of flashlamp pulsed dye laser on the expression of connective tissue growth factor in keloids. Lasers Surg Med 2012; 44: 377–83.

53. Holmes A, Abraham DJ, Sa S. CTGF and SMADs, maintenance of scleroderma phenotype is independent of SMAD signaling. J Biol Chem 2001; 276: 10594–1601.

54. Colwell AS, Phan TT. Hypertrophic scar fibroblasts have increased connective tissue growth factor expression after transforming growth factor-beta stimulation. Plast Reconstr Surg 2005; 116: 1387–90.

55. Nouri K, Jimenez GP, Harrison-Balestra C, Elgart GW. 585-nm pulsed dye laser in the treatment of surgical scars starting on the suture removal day. Dermatol Surg 2003; 29: 65–73.

56. Fiskerstrand EJ, Svaasand LO, Volden G. Pigmentary changes after pulsed dye laser treatment in 125 northern European patients with port wine stains. Br J Dermatol 1998; 138: 477–9.

57. Hermanns JF, Petit L, Hermanns-Le T, Pierard GE. Analytic quantification of phototype-related regional skin complexion. Skin Res Technol 2001; 7: 168–71.

58. Manstein D, Herron S, Sink RK, Tanner H, Anderson RR. Fractional photothermolysis: a new concept for cutaneous remodeling using microscopic patterns of thermal injury. Lasers Surg Med 2004; 34: 426–38.

59. Laubach H-J, Tannous Z, Anderson RR, et al. Skin responses to fractional photothermolysis. Lasers Surg Med 2006; 38: 142–9.

60. Geronemus RG. Fractional photothermolysis: current and future applications. Lasers Surg Med 2006; 38: 169–76.

61. Hantash BM, Bedi VP, Sudireddy V, et al. Laser-induced transepidermal elimination of dermal content by fractional photothermolysis. J Biomed Opt 2006; 11: 041115.

62. Khan MH, Sink RK, Manstein D, et al. Intradermally focused infrared laser pulses: thermal effects at defined tissue depths. Lasers Surg Med 2005; 36: 270–80.

63. Jih MH, Kimyai-Asadi A. Fractional photothermolysis: a review and update. Semin Cutan Med Surg 2008; 27: 63–71.

64. Fitzpatrick RE. Fractional resurfacing. Expert Rev Dermatol 2010; 5: 269–91.

65. Narurkar VA. Retrospective analysis of 877 cases of nonablative fractional resurfacing with a second generation erbium doped 1550 nm laser. Lasers Surg Med 2008; 67: 27.

66. Rahman Z, Tanner H, Jiang K. Atrophic scar revision using fractional photothermolysis. Cosmet Dermatol 2007; 20: 593–602.

67. Rokhsar C, Rahman Z, Fitzpatrick RE. Fractional photothermolysis in the treatment of scars. Lasers Surg Med 2005; 36: 30.

68. Behroozan DS, Goldberg LH, Dai T, Geronemus RG, Friedman PM. Fractional photothermolysis for the treatment of surgical scars: a case report. J Cosmet Laser Ther 2006; 8: 35–8.

69. Kunishige J, Goldberg L, Geronemus R, Friedman P. Fractional photothermolysis for surgical scars. Lasers Surg Med 2008; 69: 28.

70. Niwa AB, Mello AP, Torezan LA, Osório N. Fractional photothermolysis for the treatment of hypertrophic scars: clinical experience of eight cases. Dermatol Surg 2009; 35: 773–7; discussion 777-8.

71. Tannous Z, Laubach HJ, Anderson RR, Manstein D. Changes of epidermal pigment distribution after fractional resurfacing: clinicopathologic correlation. Lasers Surg Med 2005; 36: 32.

72. Goldberg DJ, Berlin AL, Phelps R. Histological and ultrastructural analysis of melasma after fractional resurfacing. Lasers Surg Med 2008; 40: 134–8.

73. Tierney E, Mahmoud BH, Srivastava D, Ozog D, Kouba DJ. Treatment of surgical scars with nonablative fractional laser versus pulsed dye laser: a randomized controlled trial. Dermatol Surg 2009; 45: 1172–80.

74. Glaich AS, Rahman Z, Goldberg LH, Friedman PM. Fractional resurfacing for the treatment of hypopigmented scars: a pilot study. Dermatol Surg 2007; 33: 289–94; discussion 293-4.

75. Narukar VA. Nonablative fractional laser resurfacing. Dermatol Clin 2009; 27: 473–8.

76. Hirobe T. Proliferation of epidermal melanocytes during the healing of skin wounds in newborn mice. J Exp Zool 1983; 227: 423–31.

77. Bergamaschi O, Kon S, Doine A, et al. Melanin repigmentation after gingivectomy: a 5-year clinical and transmission electron microscopic study in humans. Int J Periodontics Restorative Dent 1993; 13: 85–92.

78. Alexiades-Armenakas MR, Bernstein LJ, Friedman PM, et al. The safety and efficacy of the 308-nm excimer laser for pigment correction of hypopigmented scars and striae alba. Arch Dermatol 2004; 140: 955–60.

79. Massaki AB, Fabi SG, Fitzpatrick R. Repigmentation of hypopigmented scars using an erbium-doped 1,550-nm fractionated laser and topical bimatoprost. Dermatol Surg 2012; 38: 995–1001.

80. Pham AM, Greene RM, Woolery-Lloyd H, Kaufman J, Grunebaum LD. 1550-nm nonablative laser resurfacing for facial surgical scars. Arch Facial Plast Surg 2011; 13: 203–10.

81. Choe JH, Park YL, Kim BJ, et al. Prevention of thyroidectomy scar using a new 1,550-nm fractional erbium-glass laser. Dermatol Surg 2009; 35: 1199–205.

82. Cartier H. Use of intense pulsed light in the treatment of scars. J Cosmet Dermatol 2005; 4: 34–40.

83. Kunishige JH, Katz TM, Goldberg LH, Friedman PM. Fractional photothermolysis for the treatment of surgical scars. Dermatol Surg 2010; 36: 538–41.

84. Vasily DB, Cerino ME, Ziselman EM, Tannous ZS. Non-ablative fractional resurfacing of surgical and post-traumatic scars. J Drugs Dermatol 2009; 8: 998–1005.

85. Haedersdal M, Moreau KE, Beyer DM, Nymann P, Alsbjørn B. Fractional nonablative 1540 nm laser resurfacing for thermal burn scars: a randomized controlled trial. Lasers Surg Med 2009; 41: 189–95.

86. Waibel J, Beer KR. Fractional laser resurfacing for thermal burns. J Drugs Dermatol 2008; 7: 12–14.

87. Waibel J, Beer K. Ablative fractional laser resurfacing for the treatment of a third-degree burn. J Drugs Dermatol 2009; 8: 294–7.

88. Waibel J, Lupo M, Beer K, Anderson RR. Treatment of burn scars with 1550 nm nonablative fractional erbium laser. Lasers Surg Med 2009; 101: 35.

89. Waibel J, Wulkan AJ, Lupo M, Beer K, Anderson RR. Treatment of burn scars with the 1,550 nm nonablative fractional erbium laser. Lasers Surg Med 2012; 44: 441–6.

90. Hantash BM, Bedi VP, Kapadia B, et al. In vivo histological evaluation of a novel ablative fractional resurfacing device. Lasers Surg Med 2007; 39: 96–107.

91. Hale EK, Bernstein L, Brightman L, Chapas AM, Geronemus RG. Ablative fractional resurfacing of the treatment of non-acne scarring. Lasers Surg Med 2008; 287: 86.

92. Alexiades-Armenakas M, Sarnoff D, Gotkin R, Sadick N. Multi-center clinical study and review of fractional ablative CO_2 laser resurfacing for the treatment of rhytides, photoaging, scars and striae. J Drugs Dermatol 2011; 10: 352–62.

93. Cervelli V, Gentile P, Spallone D, et al. Ultrapulsed fractional CO_2 laser for the treatment of post-traumatic and pathological scars. J Drugs Dermatol 2010; 9: 1328–31.

94. Christophel JJ, Elm C, Endrizzi BT, Hilger PA, Zelickson B. A randomized controlled trial of fractional laser therapy and dermabrasion for scar resurfacing. Dermatol Surg 2012; 38: 595–602.

95. Weiss ET, Chapas A, Brightman L, et al. Successful treatment of atrophic postoperative and traumatic scarring with carbon dioxide ablative fractional resurfacing: quantitative volumetric scar improvement. Arch Dermatol 2010; 146: 133–40.

96. Tierney EP, Hanke CW. Treatment of CO_2 laser induced hypopigmentation with ablative fractionated laser resurfacing: case report and review of literature. J Drugs Dermatol 2010; 9: 1420–6.

97. Haedersdal M. Fractional ablative CO(2) laser resurfacing improves a thermal burn scar. J Eur Acad Dermatol Venereol 2009; 23: 1340–1; 52ap.

98. Jung JY, Jeong JJ, Roh HJ, et al. Early postoperative treatment of thyroidectomy scars using a fractional carbon dioxide laser. Dermatol Surg 2011; 37: 217–23.

99. Ozog DM, Moy RL. A randomized split-scar study of intraoperative treatment of surgical wound edges to minimize scarring. Arch Dermatol 2011; 147: 1108–10.

100. Johnson MT, Roberts J. Skin conditions and related need for medical care among persons 1–74 years, United States, 1971–1974. Washington, DC: US Department of Health, Education and Welfare, Vital and Health Statistics, Series 11 No. 212, 1978.

101. Burke B M, Cunliffe WJC. The assessment of acne vulgaris: the Leeds grading technique. Br J Dermatol 1984; 111: 82–93.

102. Goulden V, Stables GI, Cunliffe WJ. Prevalence of facial acne in adults. J Am Acad Dermatol 1999; 41: 577–80.

103. Rivera AE. Acne scarring: A review and current treatment modalities. J Am Acad Dermatol 2008; 59: 659–76.

104. Jacob CI, Dover JS, Kaminer MS. Acne scarring: A classification system and review of treatment options. J AM Acad Dermatol 2001; 45: 109–17.

105. Orentreich DS, Orentreich N. Subcutaneous incision (subcision) surgery for the correction of depressed scars and wrinkles. Dermatol Surg 1995; 21: 543–9.

106. Vaishnani JB. Subcision in rolling acne scars with 24G needle. Indian J Dermatol Venereol Leprol 2008; 74: 677–9.

107. Alam M, Omura N, Kaminer MS. Subcision for acne scarring: technique and outcomes in 40 patients. Dermatol Surg 2005; 31: 310–17.

108. Sage RJ, Lopiccolo MC, Liu A, et al. Subcuticular incision versus naturally sourced porcine collagen filler for acne scars: A randomized split-face comparison. Dermatol Surg 2011; 37: 426–31.

109. Wasserman DI, Monheit GD. Subcision versus dermal collagen filler for acne scars. Dermatol Surg 2011; 37: 432.

110. Goodman GJ. Subcision versus 100% trichloroacetic acid in the treatment of rolling acne scars. Dermatol Surg 2011; 37: 634–6.

111. Liu A, Moy RL, Ross EV, Hamzavi I, Ozog DM. Pulsed dye laser and pulsed dye laser-mediated photodynamic therapy in the treatment of dermatologic disorders. Dermatol Surg 2012; 38: 351–66.

112. Orringer JS, Kang S, Hamilton T, et al. Treatment of acne vulgaris with a pulsed dye laser: a randomized controlled trial. JAMA 2004; 291: 2834–9.

113. Seaton ED, Charakida A, Mouser PE, et al. Pulsed-dye laser treatment for inflammation acne vulgaris: randomized controlled trial. Lancet 2003; 362: 1347–52.

114. Seaton ED, Mouser PE, Charakida A, et al. Investigation of the mechanism of action of nonablative pulsed-dye laser therapy in photorejuvenation and inflammatory acne vulgaris. Br J Dermatol 2006; 155: 748–55.

115. Bowes LE, Alster TS. Treatment of facial scarring and ulceration resulting from acne excoriée with 585-nm pulsed dye laser irradiation and cognitive psychotherapy. Dermatol Surg 2004; 30: 934–8.

116. Nouri K, Rivas MP, Stevens M, et al. Comparison of the effectiveness of the pulsed dye laser 585 nm versus 595 nm in the treatment of new surgical scars. Lasers Med Sci 2009; 24: 801–10.

117. Jordan R, Cummins C, Burls A. Laser resurfacing of the skin for the improvement of facial acne scarring: a systematic review of the evidence. Br J Dermatol 2000; 142: 413–23.

118. Moritz DL. Surgical correction of acne scars. Dermatol Nurs 1992; 4: 291–9.

119. Alster TS. Cutaneous resurfacing with CO_2 and erbium:YAG lasers: preoperative, intraoperative, and postoperative considerations. Plast Reconstr Surg 1999; 103: 619–32; discussion 633-4.

120. Walia S, Alster TS. Prolonged clinical and histologic effects from CO_2 laser resurfacing of atrophic acne scars. Dermatol Surg 1992; 25: 926–30.

121. Fitzpatrick RE, Goldman MP, Satur NM, et al. Pulsed carbon dioxide laser resurfacing of photo-aged facial skin. Arch Dermatol 1996; 132: 395–402.

122. Schwartz RJ, Burns AJ, Rohrich RJ, et al. Long-term assessment of CO_2 facial laser resurfacing: aesthetic results and complications. Plast Reconstr Surg 1999; 103: 592–601.

123. Manuskiatti W, Fitzpatrick RE, Goldman MP. Long-term effectiveness and side effects of carbon dioxide laser resurfacing for photodamaged facial skin. J Am Acad Dermatol 1999; 40: 401–11.

124. Fitzpatrick RE. CO_2 laser resurfacing. Dermatol Clin 2001; 19: 443–51.

125. Hruza GJ, Dover JS. Laser skin resurfacing. Arch Dermatol 1996; 132: 451–5.

126. Tanzi EL, Alster TS. Comparison of a 1,450-nm diode laser and a 1,320-nm Nd:YAG laser in the treatment of atrophic facial scars: a prospective clinical and histological study. Dermatol Surg 2004; 30: 152–7.

127. Alexiades-Armenakas M, Dover JS, Arndt KA. The spectrum of laser skin resurfacing: nonablative, fractional, and ablative laser resurfacing. J Am Acad Dermatol 2008; 58: 719–37.

128. Saddick NS. Update on non-ablative light therapy for rejuvenation: a review. Lasers Surg Med 2003; 32: 120–8.

129. Williams EF III, Dahiva R. Review of nonablative laser resurfacing modalities. Facial Plast Surg Clin North Am 2004; 12: 305–10.

130. Hantash BM, Mahmood MB. Fractional photothermolysis: a novel aesthetic laser surgery modality. Dermatol Surg 2007; 33: 525–34.

131. Tierney EP. Treatment of acne scarring using a dual-spot size ablative fractional carbon dioxide laser: review of the literature. Dermatol Surg 2011; 37: 945–61.

132. Weinstein C, Bosnich R. High energy fractional resurfacing for acne scarring. Lasers Surg Med 2007; S19: 34.

133. Alster TS, Tanzi EL, Lazarus M. The use of fractional laser photothermolysis for the treatment of atrophic scars. Dermatol Surg 2007; 33: 295–9.

134. Weiss RA, Weiss MA, Beasley KL. Long-term experience with fixed array 1540 fractional erbium laser for acne scars. Lasers Surg Med 2008; 68: 27.

135. Weinstein C, Chu R, Bosnich R. Fractional resurfacing of acne scarring. Lasers Surg Med 2006; 38: 73.

136. Glaich AS, Goldberg LH, Friedman RH, Friedman PM. Fractional photothermolysis for the treatment of postinflammatory erythema resulting form acne vulgaris. Dermatol Surg 2007; 33: 842–6.

137. Kim B, Chang S, Cho M. Microthermal laser treatment of acne scars in Koreans. Lasers Surg Med 2008; 343: 76.

138. Lloyd J, Tanghetti E. Comparison of Affirm 1320/1440 nm versus 1320 nm for the treatment of acne scars- a clinical and histological study. Lasers Surg Med 2008; 66: 27.

139. Hasegawa T, Matsukura T, Mizuno Y, et al. Clinical trial of a laser device called fractional photothermolysis system for acne scars: case report. J Dermatol 2006; 33: 623–7.

140. Lee HS, Lee JH, Ahn GY, et al. Fractional photothermolysis for the treatment of acne scars: a report of 27 Korean patients. J Dermatol Treat 2008; 19: 45–9.

141. Chrastil B, Glaich AS, Goldberg LH, Friedman PM. Second-generation 1,500-nm fractional photothermolysis for the treatment of acne scars. Dermatol Surg 2008; 34: 1327–32.

142. Cho SB, Lee JH, Choi MJ, Lee KY, Oh SH. Efficacy of the fractional photothermolysis system with dynamic operating mode on acne scars and enlarged facial pores. Dermatol Surg 2009; 35: 108–14.

143. Kim HJ, Kim TJ, Kwon YS, Park JM, Lee JH. Comparison of a 1,550 nm erbium:glass fractional laser and a chemical reconstruction of skin scars (CROSS) method in the treatment of acne scars: a simultaneous split-face trial. Lasers Surg Med 2009; 41: 545–9.

144. Hu S, Chen MC, Lee MC, Yang LC, Keoprasom N. Fractional resurfacing for the treatment of atrophic facial acne scars in Asian skin. Dermatol Surg 2009; 35: 826–32.

145. Mahmoud BH, Srivastava D, Janiga JJ, et al. Safety and efficacy of erbium-doped yttrium aluminum garnet fractionated laser for treatment of acne scars in Type IV to VI skin. Dermatol Surg 2010; 36: 602–9.

146. Laubach HJ, Tannous Z, Anderson RR, Manstein D. A histological evaluation of the dermal effects after fractional photothermolysis treatment. Laser Surg Med 2005; 36(S17): 86.

147. Behroozan DS, Goldberg LH, Glaich AS, et al. Fractional photothermolysis for treatment of poikiloderma of Civatte. Dermatol Surg 2006; 32: 298–301.

148. Dainichi T, Kawaguchi A, Ueda S, et al. Skin tightening effect using fractional laser treatment: I. A randomized half-side pilot study on faces of patients with acne. Dermatol Surg 2010; 36: 66–70.

149. Sherling M, Friedman PM, Adrian R, et al. Consensus recommendations on the use of an erbium-doped 1,550-nm fractionated laser and its applications in dermatologic surgery. Dermatol Surg 2010; 36: 461–9.

150. Hantash BM, Bedi VP, Chan KF, Zachary CB. Ex vivo histological characterization of a novel ablative fractional resurfacing device. Lasers Surg Med 2007; 39: 87–95.

151. Deng H, Yuan D, Yan CL, et al. A 2,940 nm fractional photothermolysis laser in the treatment of acne scarring: a pilot study in China. J Drugs Dermatol 2009; 8: 978–80.

152. Walgrave SE, Ortiz AE, MacFalls HT, et al. Evaluation of a novel fractional resurfacing device for the treatment of acne scarring. Lasers Surg Med 2009; 41: 122–7.

153. Chapas AM, Brightman L, Sukal S, et al. Successful treatment of acneiform scarring with CO2 ablative fractional resurfacing. Lasers Surg Med 2008; 40: 381–6.

154. Ortiz A, Elkeeb L, Truitt A, Tournas J, Zachary C. Evaluation of a novel fractional resurfacing device for treatment of acne scarring. Lasers Surg Med 2008; 79: 31.

155. Hale EK, Sukal S, Bernstein L, Chapas A, Geronemus G. Ablative fractional resurfacings for the treatment of moderate to severe acne scarring. Lasers Surg Med 2008; 80: 31.

156. Kim S, Cho KH. Clinical trial of dual treatment with an ablative fractional laser and a nonablative laser for the treatment of acne scars in Asian patients. Dermatol Surg 2009; 35: 1089–98.

157. Cho SB, Lee SJ, Kang JM, et al. The efficacy and safety of 10,600-nm carbon dioxide fractional laser for acne scars in Asian patients. Dermatol Surg 2009; 35: 1955–61.

158. Shek SY, Ho SGY, Yu CS, et al. Fractional carbon dioxide laser (Active Fx) for the treatment of acne scar in Asian skin. Lasers Surg Med 2008; 280: 84.

159. Cassuto DA, Scrimali L, Sirago P. Energy, pulse width and density: the role of each parameter in microfractional CO2 laser resurfacing. Lasers Surg Med 2008; 75: 30.

160. Wang YS, Tay YK, Kwok C. Fractional ablative carbon dioxide laser in the treatment of atrophic acne scarring in Asian patients: a pilot study. J Cosmet Laser Ther 2010; 12: 61–4.

161. Cho SB, Lee SJ, Cho S, et al. Non-ablative 1,550-nm erbium-glass and ablative 10,600-nm carbon dioxide fractional laser for acne scars: a randomized split-face study with blinded response evaluation. J Eur Acad Dermatol Venereol 2010; 24: 921–5.

162. Manuskiatti W, Triwongwaranat D, Varothai S, Eimpunth S, Wanitphakdeedecha R. Efficacy and safety of a carbon-dioxide ablative fractional resurfacing device for treatment of atrophic acne scars in Asians. J Am Acad Dermatol 2010; 63: 274–83.

163. Kim S. Clinical trial of a pinpoint irradiation technique with the CO2 laser for the treatment of atrophic acne scars. J Cosmet Laser Ther 2008; 29: 1–4.

164. Hedelung L, Haak CS, Togsverd-Bo K, et al. Fractional CO2 laser resurfacing for atrophic acne scars: A randomized controlled trial with blinded response evaluation. Lasers Surg Med 2012; 44: 447–52.

165. Biesman B. Fractional ablative resurfacing: complications. Lasers Surg Med 2009; 41: 177–8.

166. Fife D, Fitzpatrick RE, Zachary CB. Complications of fractional CO2 laser resurfacing: four cases. Lasers Surg Med 2009; 41: 179–84.

167. Avram M, Tope W, Yu T, et al. Hypertrophic scarring of the neck following ablative fractional carbon dioxide laser resurfacing. Lasers Surg Med 2009; 41: 185–8.

168. Wolfram D, Tzankov A, Pulzl P, Riza-Katzer H. Hypertrophic scars and keloids. review of their pathophysiology. risk factors, and therapeutic management. Dermatol Surg 2009; 35: 171–81.

169. Kelly AP. Medical and surgical therapies for keloids. Dermatol Ther 2004; 17: 212–18.

170. Asilian A, Darougheh A, Shariati F. New combination of triamcinolone, 5-Flurouracil and Pulsed Dye Laser for Treatment of Keloid and Hypertrophic Scars. Dermatol Surg 2006; 32: 907–15.

171. Hochman B, Locali RF, Matsuoka PK, Ferreira LM. Intralesional triamcinolone acetonide for keloid treatment: a systemic review. Aesth Plast Surg 2008; 32: 705–9.

172. Sexton GB. Local injection of triamcinolone acetonide in the management of certain skin conditions. preliminary report. Can Med Assoc J 1960; 83: 1379–81.

173. Hussain MA, Kuruppu L, Sarhadi N. Step-by-step guide of a technique using dental cartridges for intra-lesional steroid injection to keloids. Eur J Plast Surg 2011; 34: 307–9.

174. Atiyeh BS. Nonsurgical management of hypertrophic scars: evidence-based therapies, standard practices, and emerging methods. Aesthetic Plast Surg 2007; 31: 468–92.

175. Butler PD, Longaker MT, Yang GP. Current progress in keloid research and treatment. J Am Coll Surg 2008; 206: 731–41.

176. Kumar S, Singh RJ, Reed AM, et al. Cushing's syndrome after intra-articular and intradermal administration of triamcinolone acetonide in three pediatric patients. Pediatrics 2004; 113: 1820–4.

177. Ritota PC, Lo AK. Cushing's syndrome in postburn children following intralesional triamcinolone injection. Ann Plast Surg 1996; 36: 508–11.

178. Teelucksingh S, Balkaran B, Ganeshmoorthi A, et al. Prolonged childhood Cushing's syndrome secondary to intralesional triamcinolone acetonide. Ann Trop Paediatr 2002; 22: 89–91.

179. Muneuchi G, Suzuki S, Onodera M, et al. Long-term outcome of intralesional injection of triamcinolone acetonide for the treatment of keloid scars in Asian patients. Scand J Plast Reconstr Surg Hand Surg 2006; 40: 111–16; LEVEL B.

180. Berman B, Bieley HC. Keloids. J Am Acad Dermatol 1995; 33: 117–23.

181. Darzi MA, Chowdri NA, Kaul SK, et al. Evaluation of various methods of treating keloids and hypertrophic scars: a 10-year follow-up study. Br J Plast Surg 1992; 45: 374–9.

182. Sherris DA, Larrabee WF Jr, Murakami CS. Management of scar contractures, hypertrophic scars, and keloids. Otolaryngol Clin North Am 1995; 28: 1057–68.

183. Lawrence WT. In search of the optimal treatment of keloids: report of a series and a review of the literature. Ann Plast Surg 1998; 40: 490–3.

184. Boyadjiev C, Popchristova E, Mazgalova J. Histomorphologic changes in keloids treated with kenacort. J Trauma 1995; 38: 299–302.

185. Tang YW. Intra- and postoperative steroid injections for keloids and hypertrophic scars. Br J Plast Surg 1992; 45: 371–3.

186. Kiil J. Keloids treated with topical injections of triamcinolone acetonide (kenalog). Immediate and long-term results. Scand J Plast Reconstr Surg 1977; 11: 169–72.

187. Ardehali B, Nouraei SA, van Dam H, et al. Objective assessment of keloid scars with three-dimensional imaging: Quantifying response to intralesional steroid therapy. Plast Reconstr Surg 2007; 119: 556–61; LEVEL A.

188. Fitzpatrick RE. Treatment of inflamed hypertrophic scars using intralesional 5-FU. Dermatol Surg 1999; 25: 224–32.

189. Nanda S, Reddy BS. Intralesional 5-fluorouracil as a treatment modality of keloids. Dermatol Surg 2004; 30: 54–7.

190. Skuta GL, Parrish RK II. Wound healing in glaucoma filtering surgery. Surv Ophthalmol 1987; 32: 149–70.

191. Gressel MG, Parrish RK II, Folberg R. 5-Fluorouracil and glaucoma filtering surgery: I. an animal model. Ophthalmology 1984; 91: 384–93.

192. Heuer DK, Parrish RK II, Gressel MG, et al. 5-Flourouracil and glaucoma filtering surgery: II. A pilot study. Ophthalmology 1984; 91: 384–93.

193. Heuer DK, Parrish RK II, Gressel MG, et al. 5-Fluorouracil and glaucoma filtering surgery. III. intermediate follow-up of a pilot study. Ophthalmology 1986; 93: 1537–46.

194. The Fluorouracil Filtering Surgery Study Group. Three-year follow-up of the fluorouracil filtering surgery study. Am J Ophthalmol 1993; 115: 82–92.

195. Wendling J, Marchand A, Mauviel A, Verrecchia F. 5-Fluorouracil Blocks Transforming Growth Factor-beta-induced Alpha 2 Type I Collagen Gene (COL1A2) Expression in Human Fibroblasts Via c-Jun NH2-Terminal Kinase/Activator Protein-1 Activation. Mol Pharmacol 2003; 64: 707–13.

196. de Waard JW, de man BM, Wobbles T, van der Linden W, Hendriks T. Inhibition of fibroblast collagen synthesis and proliferation by levamisole and 5-fluorouracil. Eur J Cancer 1998; 34: 162–7.

197. Levinson H, Liu W, Peled Z. 5-Fluorouracil inhibits keloid fibroblast proliferation and keloid fibroblast populated collagen lattice contraction. J Burns 2002; 1: 1–9.

198. Al-Attar A, Mess S, Thomassen JM, Kauffman CL, Davison SP. Keloid pathogenesis and treatment. Plast Reconstr Surg 2006; 117: 286–300.

199. Davison SP, Dayan JH, Clemens MW, et al. Efficacy of intralesional 5-fluorouracil and trimcinolone in the treatment of keloids. Aesth Surg J 2009; 29: 40–6.

200. Wang X-Q, Liu Y-K, Wang Z-Y, et al. Antimitotic drug injections and radiotherapy: A review of the effectiveness of treatment for hypertrophic scars and keloids. Int J Low Extrem Wounds 2008; 7: 151–9.

201. Atiyeh BS, Costagliola M, Hayek SN. Keloid of hypertrophic scar: The controversy. Review of the literature. Ann Plast Surg 2005; 54: 676–80.

202. Bulstrode NW, Mudera V, McGrouther DA, Grobbelaar AO, Cambrey AD. 5-Fluorouracil selectively inhibits collagen synthesis. Plast Reconstr Surg 2005; 116: 209–21.

203. Occleston NL, Daniels JT, Tarnuzzer RW, et al. Single exposures to antiproliferatives: Long-term effects on ocular fibroblast wound-healing behavior. Invest Ophthalmol Vis Sci 1997; 38: 1998–2007.

204. Uppal RS, Khan U, Kakar S, et al. The effects of a single dose of 5-fluorouracil on keloid scars: A clinical trial of timed wound irrigation after extralesional excision. Plast Reconstr Surg 2001; 108: 1218–24.

205. Haurani MJ, Foreman K, Yang JJ, Siddiqui A. 5-Fluorouracil treatment of problematic scars. Plast Reconstr Surg 2009; 123: 139–48.

206. Khaw PT, Sherwood MB, MacKay SL, Rossi MJ, Schultz G. Five-minute treatments with fluorouracil, floxuridine and mitomycin have long-term effects on human tenon's capsule fibroblasts. Arch Ophthalmol 1992; 110: 1150.

207. Ghoshal K, Jacobs ST. An alternative molecular mechanism of action of 5-fluorouracil, a potent anti-cancer drug. Biochem Pharmacol 1997; 53: 1569.

208. Costa AM, Peyrol S, Porto LC, et al. Mechanical forces induce scar remodeling study in non-pressure-treated versus pressure-treated hypertrophic scars. Am J Pathol 1999; 155: 1671–9.

209. Berman B, Viera MH, Amini S, Huo R, Jones IS. Prevention and management of hypertrophic scars and keloids after burns in children. J Craniofac Surg 2008; 19: 989–1006.

210. Apikian M, Goodman G. Intralesional 5-fluorouracil in the treatment of keloid scars. Australas J Dermatol 2004; 45: 140.

211. Gupta S, Kalra A. Efficacy and safety of intralesional 5-fluorouracil in the treatment of keloids. Dermatology 2002; 204: 130–2.

212. Kontochristopoulos G, Stefanaki C, Panagiotopoulos A, et al. Intralesional 5-fluorouracil in the treatment of keloids: an open clinical and histopathologic study. J Am Acad Dermatol 2005; 52: 474–9.

213. Darougheh A, Asilian A, Shariati F. Intralesional trimacinolone alone or in combination with 5-fluorouracil for the treatment of keloid and hypertrophic scars. Clin Exp Dermatol 2007; 34: 219–23.

214. Goldan O, Weissman O, Regev E, Haik J, Winkler E. Treatment of postdermabrasion facial hypertrophic and keloid scars with intralesional 5-fluorouracil injections. case report. Aesth Plast Surg 2008; 32: 389–92.

215. Mutalik S, Patwardhan N. Use of injection Five Fluorouracil (FFU) with or without injection triamcinolone in the management of hypertrophic scars and keloids. J Cutan Aesthet Surg 2008; 1: 36.

216. Yang GP, Longaker MT. Invited discussion: 5-fluorouracil treatment of problematic scars. Plast Reconstr Surg 2009; 123:139–51.

217. Hatamipour E, Mehrabi S, Hatamipour M, Shirazi HRG. Effects of combined intralesional 5-fluorouracil and topical silicone in prevention of keloids: A double blind randomized clinical trial study. Acta Med Iran 2011; 49: 127–30.

218. Katz TM, Glaich AS, Goldberg LH, Friedman PM. 594-nm long pulsed dye laser and 1450-nm diode laser in combination with intralesional triamcinolone/5-fluorouracil for hypertrophic scarring following a phenol peel. J Am Acad Dermatol 2010; 62: 1045–9.

219. Gupta S, Sharma VK. Standard guidelines of care: keloids and hypertrophic scars. Indian J Dermatol Venereol Leprol 2011; 77: 94–100.

220. Wu XL, Liu W, Cao YL. Clinical study on keloid treatment with intralesional injection of low concentration 5-fluorouracil. Zhonghua Zheng Xing Wai Ke Za Zhi 2006; 22: 44–6.

221. Wu XL, Gao Z, Song N, Liu W. Clinical study of auricular keloid treatment with both surgical excision and intralesional injection of low-dose 5-fluorouracil and corticosteroids. Zhonghua Yi Xue Za Zhi 2009; 89: 1102–5.

222. Liu W, Wu X, Gao Z, Song N. Remodeling of Keloid tissue into normal-looking skin. Presented at Scar Meeting, Montpellier Franc, March 29-April 1 2006.

223. Huang L, Wong YP, , et al. Low-dose 5-fluorouracil induces cell cycle G2 arrest and apoptosis in keloid fibroblasts. Br J Dermatol 2010; 163: 1181–5.

10 Photodynamic therapy

Mitchel P. Goldman and Ane B.M. Niwa Massaki

INTRODUCTION

Aminolevulinic acid (ALA) was the first photosensitizer prodrug to be approved by the US Food and Drug Administration (FDA) for use in topical photodynamic therapy (PDT). Since its approval over a decade ago, many aspects of ALA-PDT have been examined. Studies investigating the treatment of nonhyperkeratotic actinic keratoses (AKs) with ALA-PDT have led to advances in treatment. Incubation times of ALA have decreased, multiple light sources have been used to elicit the reaction, and cosmetic benefits of treatment have been discovered. In the discussion that follows, background on topical 5-ALA and methyl aminolevulinic acid (MAL), the most commonly used agents in topical PDT, is provided. In addition, clinical studies regarding the treatment of AKs, nonmelanoma skin cancer (NMSC), acne, and photorejuvenation are summarized. There is now growing interest in the use of PDT for other skin tumors, such as lymphoma, as well as for nononcological indications, such as psoriasis, localized scleroderma, viral warts, onychomycosis, and many other dermatological conditions. Finally, a practical guide for treatment is provided for the reader to optimize treatment while avoiding common pitfalls of treatment.

HISTORY

In 1900, Raab (1) first noted that paramecia cells (*Paramecium caudatum*) were unaffected when exposed to acridine orange or light, but when exposed to both at the same time, they died within 2 hours. In 1904, Von Tappeiner and Jodblauer (2) were the first to use the term "photodynamic effect" to an oxygen-consuming reaction process in protozoa after aniline dyes were applied with fluorescence. In 1905, topical 5% eosin was successfully used as a photosensitizer with artificial light to treat NMSCs, lupus vulgaris, and condylomata lata in humans by Jesionek and Von Tappeiner (3). The authors theorized that the eosin was incorporated into cells and triggered a cytotoxic reaction when exposed to a light source and oxygen.

Most photosensitizers used in PDT are derivatives of hematoporphyrin, an endogenous porphyrin that was first synthesized from heme in the mid-19th century. In 1913, Meyer-Betz (4) was the first to demonstrate the "photodynamic effect" in vivo after he injected himself with hematoporphyrin and noticed that the areas exposed to light became swollen and painful. Unfortunately, the phototoxic reaction lasted for 2 months. In 1942, Auler and Banzer (5) demonstrated the ability of hematoporphyrin to concentrate more in certain dermatologic tumors than in their surrounding tissues. Histological analysis also showed that tumors were necrotic, confirming the photodynamic response of hematoporphyrin. However, large doses of hematoporphyrins were required for photosensitization, resulting in subsequent severe phototoxic reactions.

A new photosensitizer hematoporphyrin purified derivative (HPD) was presented in 1978 by Dougherty and colleagues (6) that successfully treated cutaneous malignancies using red light as the primary light source. HPD was a complex mixture of porphyrin subunits and byproducts. A complete or partial response in 111 of 113 malignant lesions, including carcinomas of the breast, colon, prostate, squamous cell, basal cell, and endometrium; malignant melanoma; mycosis fungoides; chondrosarcoma; and angiosarcoma, was observed with systemic HPD (dose of 2.5 or 5.0 mg/kg).

Subsequently, other studies (7,8) using a purified hematoporphyrin derivative, known as Photofrin (porfimer sodium), were conducted and Photofrin received approvals for PDT of selected stages of lung, esophageal, gastric, and cervical cancer in several European countries and Japan. Therefore systemic HPD became the standard for PDT research. However, practical use in dermatology was difficult due to the cutaneous accumulation of porphyrin-based photosensitizing drugs and their slow clearance leading to prolonged photosensitivity (4–6 weeks).

Second-generation photosensitizers were then developed, consisting of several synthetic purified compounds that have been proposed as potentially useful for anticancer PDT. Successful treatment of multiple NMSCs has been reported (6,9–11) using those synthetic purified systemic photosensitizers, including chlorine derivatives (benzoporphyrin derivative-monoacid ring A, *N*-aspartyl-chlorin e6, Tin etiopurpurin, lutetium texapyrin, porphines, and phthalocyanines (chloro-aluminum phthalocyanine tetrasulfonate and silicon phthalocyanine). Those compounds present strong light absorption at 660–850 nm range, allowing deeper penetration of tissue by the activating light as compared with porphyrins, which exhibit a maximum absorption in the Soret band (360–400 nm) followed by four smaller peaks between 500 and 635 nm (Q bands) (12). Furthermore, rapid drug accumulation in neoplastic tissue (1–8 hours after intravenous administration) enabled patients to be treated in the same day. In view of low accumulation levels in normal skin and rapid drug elimination, those synthetic compounds also presented mild photosensitivity for a few days after administration, although cutaneous reaction occurring one or more months after PDT was still possible (13). A randomized multicenter phase II study conducted at four North American university-based dermatology clinics evaluated 54 patients with 421 multiple NMSC treated with vertoporfin (benzoporphyrin derivative monoacid ring A)-PDT (intravenous dose 14–18 mg/m^2) using red light-emitting diode (LED) (688 ± 10 nm; 60, 120, or

180 J/cm^2; 200 ± 40 mW/cm^2) (14). After 6 months, the authors found higher histopathologic response with the higher light dose, ranging from 69% at 60 J/cm^2 to 93% at 180 J/cm^2. No significant systemic adverse events were observed and 65% of tumors were judged to have good-to-excellent cosmesis at 24 months.

In 1990, Kennedy and colleagues (15) introduced the first topical porphyrin derivative, known as 5-δ-ALA, which is a natural precursor of protoporphyrin IX (PpIX) in the heme pathway. Therefore, ALA is the prodrug photosensitizing agent with the ability to penetrate the stratum corneum of the skin and be absorbed by actinically damaged skin cells as well as pilosebaceous units, whereas PpIX is the photosensitizer. Exogenous ALA-forming PpIX is rapidly cleared from the body, reducing the potential for phototoxicity to days instead of several months.

Later, lipophilic ALA ester derivatives were developed, showing stronger porphyrin fluorescence and better tumor selectivity, most likely because of better penetration through cellular membranes compared with the hydrophilic ALA (16).

MECHANISM OF PDT
PDT Mechanism of Action

PDT involves the activation of a photosensitizer by light in the presence of an oxygen-rich environment. Topical PDT involves the application of ALA or its methylated derivative (MAL) to the skin for varying periods. This leads to the conversion of ALA to PpIX, an endogenous photoactivating agent. PpIX accumulates in rapidly proliferating cells of premalignant and malignant lesions (17), as well as in melanin, blood vessels, and sebaceous glands (18). Upon activation by a light source and in the presence of oxygen, the sensitizer (PpIX) is oxidized, a process called "photobleaching" (19). During this process, free radical oxygen singlets are generated, leading to selective destruction of tumor cells by apoptosis without collateral damage to surrounding tissues (20,21). Selective destruction of malignant cells is due in part to their reduced ferrochelatase activity, leading to excessive accumulation of intracellular PpIX (22). In vitro research suggests that any remaining malignant cells following PDT have reduced survival (23).

Although the precise mechanisms (at a cellular level) underlying the efficacy of topical PDT in the treatment of NMSC are not fully known, both apoptosis (24,25) and necrosis (26,27) have been described, with their respective importance being related to intracellular localization of the photosensitizer and illumination parameters. In addition to direct damage of neoplastic cells, vascular injury plays an important role for the tumor destruction (28–30), particularly with systemic photosensitizers. Oxygen radicals produced during the photodynamic process decrease the barrier function of endothelial cells, exposing the vascular basement membrane that leads to the activation of platelets and polymorphonuclear leukocytes (31,32), resulting in arteriolar vessel constriction, thrombus formation, and blood flow stasis causing indirect tumor cell kill (28,29). In addition, the impairment of vascular functions activates acute-phase proteins (proteinases, peroxidases, complement factors, and cytokines), resulting in massive accumulation of neutrophils and macrophages (32,33) that will contribute to the destruction of tumor tissue. The establishment of immune response against the treated malignancy by inflammatory processes leads to the generation of tumor-specific immune cells (34,35), which represents a unique feature of PDT and a major advantage over conventional anticancer therapy (34).

TOPICAL PHOTOSENSITIZERS
Aminolevulinic Acid /Methyl Aminolevulinate

5-δ-ALA is a hydrophilic, low-molecular weight molecule within the heme biosynthesis pathway (17,36). ALA is considered a prodrug (37). In vivo, it is converted to PpIX, a photosensitizer in the PDT reaction. In the USA, ALA is available as a 20% topical solution manufactured under the name Levulan® Kerastick (DUSA Pharmaceuticals, Inc., Wilmington, Massachusetts, USA). FDA-approved since 1999, Levulan is approved for the treatment of nonhyperkeratotic AKs in conjunction with a blue light source, such as the Blu-U (DUSA Pharmaceuticals, Inc.) (38). It is supplied as a cardboard tube housing two sealed glass ampules, one containing 354 mg of δ-ALA hydrochloride powder and the other 1.5 mL of solvent (22). The separate components are mixed within the cardboard sleeve just prior to use.

Esters of ALA [methyl ester methyl aminolevulinate (MAL)] are lipophilic derivatives of the parent molecule. Their chemical structure provides increased lipophilicity, allowing superior penetration through cellular lipid bilayers compared with ALA (18,39). MAL is available as a 16.8% cream in a 2 g tube and is produced under the name of Metvixia® (Galderma, SA, Switzerland; PhotoCure ASA, Norway). Since 2004, Metvixia® and the CureLight BroadBand (Model CureLight 01) were FDA-approved for the treatment of nonhyperkeratotic AKs of the face and scalp in immunocompetent patients. Metvixia® can be used in conjunction with the Aktilite CL128 lamp (Galderma, SA, Switzerland; PhotoCure ASA, Norway) as well. MAL may offer better tumor selectivity (39–42) and less pain (42,43) during PDT with less patient discomfort (43) compared with ALA.

Light Irradiation

A range of light sources can be used for topical PDT, including lasers, pulsed light sources, filtered xenon arc and metal halide lamps, fluorescent lamps and LEDs. However, certain laser and light sources are predictably chosen for PDT activation. Their wavelengths correspond closely with the four absorption peaks along the porphyrin curve. The Soret band (400–410 nm), with a maximal absorption at 405–409 nm, is the highest peak along this curve for photoactivating PpIX. Smaller peaks designated as the "Q bands" exist at approximately 505–510 nm, 540–545 nm, 580–584 nm, and 630–635 nm (Fig. 10.1) (17,18,36). There are advantages and disadvantages to exploiting the wavebands in either the Soret or Q bands for PDT. The Soret band peak is 10- to 20-fold larger than the Q bands, and blue light sources are often used to activate PpIX within this portion of the porphyrin curve, however, longer wavelengths found within the Q bands produce a red light that penetrates more deeply and can be used to treat NMSC up to a thickness of 2–3 mm (44), but necessitates higher energy requirements (17,36).

Light Sources

Light sources utilized in PDT can be categorized in a variety of ways, including incoherent versus coherent sources, or by color (and wavelengths) emitted. Incoherent light is emitted as noncollimated light and is provided through broadband

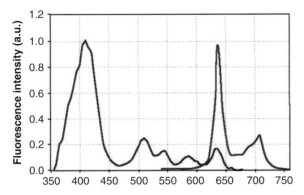

Figure 10.1 Porphyrin absorption curve displays maximum absorption in the Soret band (360–400 nm) followed by four smaller peaks between 500 and 635 nm (Q bands).

lamps, LEDs, and intense pulsed light (IPL) systems. Noncoherent light sources are easy to use, affordable, easily obtained, and portable due to their compact size (45). The earliest uses in PDT were filtered slide projectors that emitted white light (17). Metal halogen lamps such as the Curelight (Photocure, Oslo, Norway, 570–680 nm) are often employed in PDT as they provide an effective light source in a time, power, and cost-effective manner (17,46). In Europe, the PDT 1200 lamp (Waldmann Medizintechnik, VS-Schwennigen, Germany) gained in popularity, providing a unit with high power density emitting a circular field of light radiation from 600 to 800 nm (40,46). Short arc, tunable xenon lamps have also been used, emitting light radiation from 400 to 1200 nm (40). The only widely available fluorescent lamp used in conjunction with PDT is the Blu-U (DUSA Pharmaceuticals, Inc.) with a peak emittance at 417 ± 5 nm. LEDs provide a narrower spectrum of light irradiation, usually in a 20–50 nm bandwidth that matches the absorption spectrum of porphyrins via a compact, solid, but powerful semiconductor (17,47). LEDs are simple to operate, emitting light from the ultraviolet (UV) to infrared (IR) portion of the electromagnetic spectrum (47), and are relatively inexpensive compared with lasers. In addition, they can also provide wide area illumination fields. IPL is yet another source of incoherent light, emitting a radiation spectrum from approximately 500 to 1200 nm (47). Cutoff filters allow customization of the delivered wavelengths. This light source is particularly useful in photorejuvenation, targeting pigment, blood vessels, and even collagen.

Lasers provide precise doses of light radiation. As a collimated light source, lasers deliver energy to target tissues at specific wavelengths chosen to mimic absorption peaks along the porphyrin curve. Lasers used in PDT include the tunable argon dye laser (blue-green light, 450–530 nm) (40), the copper vapor laser-pumped dye laser (510–578 nm), pulsed dye laser (PDL, LPDL) (585–595 nm), the neodymium-doped yttrium aluminum garnet potassium-titanyl-phosphate dye laser (532 nm), the gold vapor laser (628 nm), and solid-state diode lasers (630 nm) (46). Although laser sources allow the physician to deliver light with exact specifications in terms of wavelength and fluence, the fluence rate should be kept in the range of 150–200 mW/cm² to avoid hyperthermic effects on the tissue (17,42). In fact, there is evidence to support that cumulative light doses of greater than 40 J/cm² can deplete all available oxygen sources during the oxidation reaction, making higher doses of energy during PDT unnecessary (19).

CLINICAL APPLICATIONS
Introduction: Actinic Keratoses
Background and Epidemiology

AKs are a premalignant skin condition, comprising the third most common reason and 14% of all dermatology office visits (48,49). Approximately 4 million Americans are diagnosed with AKs annually (50), with a prevalence of AKs within the US population ranging from 11% to 26% and the highest incidence in southern regions and older Caucasian patients (51).

The concern for untreated AKs is their rate of transformation to cutaneous squamous cell carcinoma (SCC). A small percentage of SCC metastasizes (52), and this is more likely in higher risk areas, such as mucous membranes (e.g., lips) (53). The reported conversion rate of AK to SCC varies widely, estimated as 0.025–16% per lesion per year (54–58). AKs may be considered an SCC-in situ (59,60), with AK resting on the precancerous end of a spectrum that leads toward invasive SCC. It has been suggested that the AK/SCC continuum be graded as "cutaneous intraepithelial neoplasia," in a manner analogous to cervical malignancy. Further histopathologic evidence supports the link between AKs and SCC. Both lesions express tumor markers, including the tumor suppressor gene p53 (61), and over 90% of biopsied SCCs have adjacent AKs within the examined histopathologic field (62).

Clinical Presentation and Diagnosis

AKs typically appear as 1–3 mm, slightly scaly plaques on an erythematous base, often on a background of solar damage. They are often detected more easily through palpation than visual detection (63), due to their hyperkeratotic nature. The surrounding skin often shows signs of moderate-to-severe photodamage, including dyspigmentation, telangiectasias, and sallow coloration due to solar elastosis (Fig. 10.2). Individual AK lesions may converge, creating larger contiguous lesions. Most AKs are subclincial and not readily apparent to visual or palpable examination. The evidence for subclinical AKs is their fluorescence when exposed to ALA + Wood's lamp or a specialized charge-coupled device (CCD) camera (64).

Although often asymptomatic, AKs may have accompanying burning, pruritus, tenderness, or bleeding (49). Several variants of AK exist, including nonhyperkeratotic (thin), hyperkeratotic, atrophic, lichenoid, verrucous, horn-like (cutaneous horn), and pigmented variants (51). AKs on the lip, most often occurring on the lower lip, are designated as actinic cheilitis (53). As AKs often result from a long history of UV exposure, the lesions usually arise in heavily sun-exposed areas, including the scalp, face, ears, lips, chest, dorsal hands, and extensor forearms (65). Risk factors for AKs include fair skin (Fitzpatrick skin type I–III), history of extensive, cumulative sun exposure, increasing age, elderly males (due to UV exposure), history of arsenic exposure, and immunosuppression (48,49).

Histopathology

Histopathologic examination of AKs is characterized by atypical keratinocytes and architectural disorder (49). Early lesions demonstrate focal keratinocyte atypia originating at the basal layer of the epidermis and extending variably upward within the epidermis (66). Hyperchromatic and pleomorphic nuclei and nuclear crowding characterize the cellular findings while architectural disorder is comprised of alternating ortho- and hyperkeratosis, hypogranulosis, and focal areas of downward budding in the basal layer of the epidermis (49,51). Solar elastosis is invariably present. Well-developed lesions may have apoptotic cells, mitotic figures, involvement of adnexal structures, lichenoid infiltrates, and a focal tendency toward

full-thickness involvement (Fig. 10.3). Full-thickness atypia indicates transformation into SCC-in situ (51).

Treatment Rationale

Treatment Options for AKs

Given the premalignant potential of AKs, and the metastatic potential of SCC, early treatment is paramount to preventing disease progression. Treatment options for AKs depend on a variety of factors, including severity of involvement, duration or persistence of lesions, patient tolerability or desire for cosmesis, affordability/insurance coverage, and physician comfort with available treatment modalities (49,58). Although AKs can reliably be diagnosed by clinical examination alone (67), a low threshold for biopsy should be exercised on atypical lesions, or lesions not responsive to prior treatment.

Although singular or few lesions may be approached with local surgical treatments, such as cryotherapy, curettage, excision, or dermabrasion, field treatment may be more appropriate when numerous lesions are identified. In addition, field therapy will treat subclinical AKs. Chemical peels, laser resurfacing, 5-fluorouracil (5-FU), topical diclofenac, topical retinoids, and topical immunomodulators (imiquimod) are all reasonable treatment options in addition to PDT.

A comparison of PDT to other field treatment options for AKs yields comparable clearance rates (68,69). In fact, a comparison of 100% clearance rates from phase III clinical trials reported complete AK clearance with ALA-PDT of 72%, comparable to 5-FU (72%), and superior to imiquimod (49%) and diclofenac (48%) (50). A direct comparison study by Kurwa and coworkers (70) found comparable lesion area reduction rates between ALA-PDT (73%) and 5-FU (70%).

Advantages/Disadvantages of ALA-PDT for AKs

Clearance rates of AKs following PDT has ranged from 68% to 98% (71,72). Assuming near equivalent or even superior clearance rates of PDT compared with other field treatment options, PDT has several advantages in the treatment of AKs. Improvement of photodamage, superior cosmesis, and better

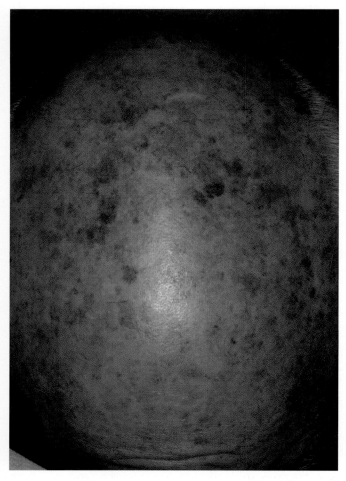

Figure 10.2 Frontal scalp of a 71-year-old white male demonstrating moderate-to-severe photodamage. Numerous actinic keratoses characterized by erythematous scaly slightly elevated plaques are visible on a background of extensive solar lentigines.

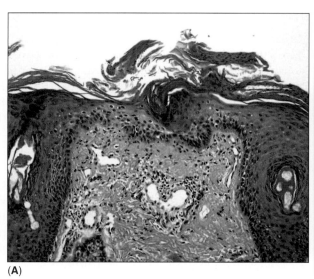

(A)

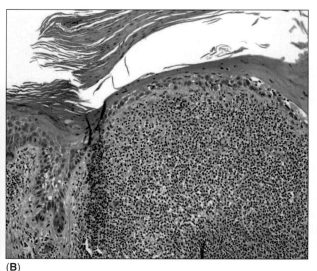

(B)

Figure 10.3 (**A**) Histopathologic section of actinic keratosis stained with hematoxylin and eosin at 20× magnification. Lesion is characterized by alternating ortho- and hyperkeratosis with nuclear atypia and architectural disorder. Keratinocyte atypia approaches full-thickness in middle area of lesion. Note the gray, fragmented nature of the papillary dermis representing expensive solar elastosis. (**B**) Actinic keratosis, lichenoid variant. A brisk lymphocytic infiltrate in the papillary dermis accompanies cytologic atypia of epidermal keratinocytes and marked architectural disorder. Numerous apoptotic cells are visible within the epidermis. *Source*: Courtesy of Wenhua Liu, MD, Consolidated Pathology Consultants, Inc., Libertyville, Illinois, USA.

patient satisfaction were documented in two studies by Szeimies et al. and Goldman and Atkin (69,72). Other procedures used for the clearance of AKs, such as cryotherapy or chemical peels, can result in hypopigmentation or even scarring (69,73). PDT, perhaps surprisingly to some, is a cost-effective means of treating AKs. Gold found ALA-PDT with a blue light source to be the least expensive treatment option for AKs compared with 5-FU, imiquimod, and diclofenac. In fact, ALA-PDT was approximately half the cost of a similar course of imiquimod for field AK treatment (50). Additionally, PDT accomplished field treatment of precancerous lesions, including subclinical ones (73).

Disadvantages of PDT are largely related to minor and expected adverse events following the procedure. Minor pain and erythema may occur during or following the procedure. Mild crusting and edema may occur, lasting up to 1 week. However, other treatment modalities for AKs have similar if not longer recovery periods. There are financial costs associated with the procedure. If PDT is performed for AK treatment and photorejuvenation, there is an associated out-of-pocket cost to the patient. The physician must also make an initial investment in the laser and light devices, although many of the light sources have multiple applications beyond PDT.

Treatment Results of ALA-PDT for AKs

Kennedy, in 1990, was the first to exploit the use of topical ALA in the treatment of NMSCs (74). Using a 20% ALA compound and a filtered slide projector for a light source, a complete response rate of 90% was achieved in patients with AKs. Since this initial study, a variety of light sources have been investigated for use in PDT for the treatment of AKs. As the PDT reaction is activated from an emission spectra ranging from 400 to 800 nm (75), we have organized clinical studies according to the light source utilized. Table 10.1 provides a summary of peer-reviewed articles on the use of ALA- and MAL-PDT in AK treatment.

Blue Light

Perhaps the most popular emission spectrum utilized in the USA, blue light was the first FDA-approved form of light for activating ALA (Fig. 10.4). As a result, numerous published studies exist on the use of blue light in ALA-PDT not only for the treatment of AKs, but also for other skin conditions responsive to this treatment modality. As the relatively shorter wavelength of blue light only penetrates 1–2 mm but is potent in its photochemical effect, blue light is often selected for the treatment of superficial lesions, such as nonhyperkeratotic AK lesions (76).

In 2001, Jeffes et al. (68) published the results of a multicenter, phase II study of ALA-PDT using blue light (417 nm). A 14- to 18-hour incubation was used on AK lesions of the face and scalp in 36 patients. A total of 70 lesions were treated. Light exposure duration was 16 minutes and 40 seconds, now considered standard of treatment. At 8 weeks following a single treatment, 88% of lesions cleared. Due to the extended time of incubation, an increased rate of phototoxicity-related side effects was observed. These adverse effects included erythema and edema. A second phase II study was conducted with the same protocol, this time in a total of 64 patients (77). All of the patients had 75% or more clearance of AK lesions

following one treatment. However, 14% of patients required reduced power density during blue light irradiation due to intolerable side effects, including stinging and burning. A final phase II study was a dose-ranging study of ALA solution from concentrations of 2.5% to 30% ALA. Clearance of AKs occurred in a dose-dependent manner, and a 20% concentration was selected as the most ideal concentration for use in ALA-PDT with blue light (77).

Piacquadio and coworkers (78) followed in 2004, publishing the results of a phase III clinical trial. The same long incubation and illumination times were used as in the phase II trial. A total of 243 patients with nonhyperkeratotic AKs were treated. Complete clearance at 12 weeks following one PDT session was 70%. A second treatment resulted in a complete clearance rate of 88%. Facial lesions responded more favorably than scalp lesions, with complete response rates of 78% and 50%, respectively, at week 12 following treatment. In terms of patient feedback, 94% of patients rated their cosmetic outcome following PDT as good or excellent. A recurrence rate analysis for this treatment cohort between 8 and 12 weeks posttreatment was 5% (77).

Work by Tschen and coworkers (67) confirmed earlier findings. This phase IV study of 101 patients with six to 12 AKs used a 14- to 18-hour ALA incubation time. After the first PDT, a complete clearance of 72–76% was observed, which increased to 86% with a second treatment.

Several other studies examined the use of blue light in ALA-PDT for the treatment of nonhyperkeratotic AKs and observed photorejunative effects on the treated area in addition to the reduction of AKs (72,79).

In 2004, Touma et al. (22) reported on the efficacy of short-contact ALA-PDT. Not only did this allow for PDT to be conducted in a single clinic visit rather than over 2 days, but side effects related to the longer 14- to 18-hour incubations were reduced. In this study, 17 patients with AKs of the face and scalp were treated with ALA using incubation times of 1, 2, or 3 hours. A clearance rate of 93%, 84%, and 90% were achieved in the 1-, 2-, and 3-hour incubation groups, respectively. Clearance rates were maintained through 5 months of follow-up. In addition, this study with blue light showed a modest but significant improvement in photoaging.

Green Light

One study by Fritsch and coworkers (80) used a green light source for the treatment of AKs with ALA-PDT. The focus of this study was on patient discomfort. Compared to a red light source, light irradiation with a green light source (543–548 nm) was less painful in the treatment of facial AKs during PDT.

Yellow-Orange Light

Pulsed Dye Laser

PDLs (585–595 nm) (Fig. 10.5) target the chromophore oxyhemoglobin, allowing selective destruction of blood vessels. As AKs often appear as erythematous scaly plaques, the inflammatory nature of these lesions can be targeted with this vascular laser. Alexiades-Armenakas and coworkers (73) were the first to report on its use in ALA-PDT. Thirty-six patients and a total of 3622 lesions were treated. Location of lesions included the face and scalp (2620 lesions), extremities (949), and trunk (79). ALA was applied with either a 3-hour unoccluded incubation or a 14- to 18-hour incubation. No difference in

Table 10.1 Published Clinical Studies on ALA- and MAL-PDT for AKs

Reference	ALA Preparation	Location of AKs	Incubation Period (hr)	# Lesions Treated (# Patients)	Light Source (Wavelength in nm)	Response Rate	Follow-up (mo)
Kennedy (74) (1990)	20% Emulsion	Not specified	3–6	10	Tungsten (>600)	90% CR	18
Wolf (21) (1993)	20% Emulsion	Face and scalp	4–8	9	Tungsten, unfiltered	100% CR	3–12
Calzavara-Pinton (17) (1995)	20% Cream	Face	6–8	50 (from pool of 85 patients with AKs, BCCs, SCCs, Bowen's disease)	Argon dye laser (630)	100% CR	24–36
Morton (263) (1995)	20% Emulsion	Face and scalp	4	4	Xenon (630)	100% CR	12
Fijan (264) (1995)	20% Emulsion	Not specified	20, Occluded	43 (9)	Halogen (570–690)	81% CR	3–20
Szeimies (265) (1996)	10% Emulsion	Head, hands, arms	6, Occluded	36 (10)	Waldmann red lamp (580–740)	71% CR head	1
Fink-Puches (89) (1997)	20% Emulsion	Head, neck, forearms, dorsal hands	4, Occluded	251 (28)	Halogen slide projector (300–800) with cutoff filters at 515, 530, 570, 610	71% CR	36
Fritsch (80) (1997)	10% Ointment	Face and scalp	6, Occluded	(6)	Green lamp (543–548) vs. red Waldmann lamp (570–750)	100% CR for both green and red light	15
Jeffes et al. (1997)	0–30% Emulsion	Face, scalp, trunk, extremities	3, Occluded	240 (40)	Argon dye laser (630)	91% CR face and scalp; 45% CR trunk and extremities	2
Karrer et al. (1999)	20% Emulsion	Scalp, face	6, Occluded	200 (24)	Red light lamp (580–740) or PDL (585)	84% CR (red light) 79% CR (PDL)	1
Kurwa et al. (1999)	20% Emulsion	Hands	4, Occluded	(14)	Metal halide lamp (580–740)	73% Lesion area reduction; comparable to 5–FU	6
Itoh (85) (2000)	20% Emulsion, 2 or more sessions	Face, neck, extremities	4, Occluded	53 (10)	Red lamp (peak 630, range 600–700), excimer dye laser (630)	82% CR face and neck; 56% CR extremities	12
Dijkstra (75) (2001)	20% Gel, 2 sessions	Unspecified	8, Occluded	4	Violet lamp (400–450)	50% CR	3–12
Jeffes (68) (2001)	20% Solution	Face, scalp	14–18	70 (36)	Blue light (417)	85% CR	4
Markam (48) (2001)	% Concentration unspecified, cream	Scalp	4, Occluded	(4)	Red light (580–740)	75% CR	6

(Continued)

Table 10.1 Published Clinical Studies on ALA- and MAL-PDT for AKs (*Continued*)

Reference	ALA Preparation	Location of AKs	Incubation Period (hr)	# Lesions Treated (# Patients)	Light Source (Wavelength in nm)	Response Rate	Follow-up (mo)
Varma (86) (2001)	20% Ointment	Not specified	4, Occluded	127 (88 Patients with mixed diagnoses)	Waldmann red lamp (580–740)	77% CR after 1st session, 99% after 2nd session, RR of 28%	6
Ruiz-Rodriguez (166) (2002)	20% Emulsion	Face, scalp	4, Occluded	38	IPL (590–1200)	76% CR 1 session; 91% CR 2 sessions	3
Alexiades-Armenakas (73) (2003)	20% Solution	Head, extremities, trunk	3 with Occlusion; 14–18 without occlusion	3622 (36)	PDL (595)	90–100% CR	8
Clark (46) (2003)	20% Ointment	Not specified	4	23	Metal halide (590–730); halogen lamp (570–680), diode laser (630)	91% CR	11
Goldman (72) (2003)	20% Solution	Face, long-incubation PDT	15–20	(32)	Blue light (417)	94% CR of AKs; improved skin texture, pigmentation	3–6
Smith (81) (2003)	20% Solution, 2 sessions	Face, scalp	1	(35)	Blue light (417) or PDL (595)	80% CR for blue light; 60% CR for PDL	1
Dragieva (101) (2004)	20% Emulsion; transplant patients	Face, scalp	5, Occluded	32 (20)	Red light (580–740)	94% CR at 4 wk; 72% at 48 wk	12
Piacquadio (78) (2004)	20% Solution, 1–2 sessions	Face, scalp	14–18	1402 (243)	Blue (417)	91% CR 1st session; 83% CR 2nd session	3
Touma (22) (2004)	20% Solution	Face	1–3	(17)	Blue lamp (417)	87–94% CR	5
Gilbert (107) (2005)	20% Solution, 5-FU daily × 5 days pre-PDT	Face	0.5–0.75	(15)	IPL (560–1200)	90% CR with combination therapy	12
Kim (87) (2005)	20% Emulsion	Face	4, Occluded	12 (7)	IPL (555–950)	50%	3
Tschen (67) (2006)	20% Solution, (1–2 treatment sessions)	Face, scalp	14–18	968 (110)	Blue (417)	72–76% CR 1st session; 86% CR 2nd session	12
Nakano (83) (2009)	20% Cream (3 treatment sessions)	Face	4, Occluded	(30)	Excimer dye laser (630 nm)	100% CR in lesions <10 mm; 70% CR in lesions >10 mm diameter	12

Table 10.1 Published Clinical Studies on ALA- and MAL-PDT for AKs (Continued)

Reference	MAL-PDT Study Design	Location	Incubation Period (hr)	# Lesions Treated (# Patients)	Light Source (Wavelength in nm)	Response Rate	Follow-up (mo)
Szeimies (90) (2002)	1× MAL-PDT vs. 2× freeze–thaw cryotherapy	Face, scalp, other	3, Occluded	699 AK (367 treated by MAL-PDT) in 193 patients	Noncoherent red light (570–670 nm), total light dose of 75 J/cm^2 and a light intensity of 70–200 mW/cm^2	MAL-PDT 69% and cryotherapy 75%	3
Freeman (91) (2003)	2× MAL-PDT vs. 2× placebo-PDT vs. 1 freeze cycle cryotherapy	Face and scalp	3, Occluded	763 AKs in 200 patients (295 treated by MAL-PDT)	Noncoherent Red light (570–670 nm) and a total light dose of 75 J/cm^2, light intensity of 50–250 mW/cm^2	MAL-PDT 91%, placebo-PDT 30%, and cryotherapy 68%	3
Pariser (92) (2003)	2× MAL-PDT vs. 2× placebo-PDT	Face and scalp	3, Occluded	502 AKs (260 treated with MAL-PDT) in 80 patients	Noncoherent red light (wavelength 570–670 nm, light dose of 75 J/cm^2, light intensity of 50–200 mW/cm^2	MAL-PDT 89%, placebo-PDT 38%	3
Dragieva (99) (2004)	MAL-PDT in transplant patients, 2× MAL-PDT vs. 2× placebo-PDT 1 wk apart	Face, scalp, neck, and extremities	3, Occluded	34 Lesional areas comprising 129 AKs (17 areas with 62 AKs treated with MAL-PDT) in 17 OTR patients	Noncoherent light source (600–730 nm), light dose of 75 J/cm^2, light intensity of 80 mW/cm^2	MAL-PDT 13 of 17 lesional areas with CR, placebo-PDT no response	4

(Continued)

Table 10.1 Published Clinical Studies on ALA- and MAL-PDT for AKs (Continued)

Reference	MAL-PDT Study Design	Location	# Lesions Treated (# Patients)	Incubation Period (hr)	Light Source (Wavelength in nm)	Response Rate	Follow-up (mo)
Tarstedt (97) (2005)	Comparison: 1× MAL-PDT repeated if necessary at 3 mo vs. 2× MAL-PDT	Face and scalp	400 AKs in 211 patients	3, Occluded	Red LED light source (634 ± 3 nm, 37 J/cm², 50 mW cm²)	1× MAL-PDT repeated if necessary-92% (81% after first treatment) vs. 2× MAL-PDT-87%	3 After last treatment
Morton (93) (2006)	1× MAL-PDT vs. cryotherapy (2 freeze cycle), repeat at 12 wk, if required	Face and scalp	1505 AK in 119 patients	3, Occluded	Red LED light source (634 ± 3 nm, 37 J/cm², 50 mW/cm²)	MAL-PDT-89% (84% after 1 treatment) vs. cryotherapy 86% (75% after 1 treatment)	3 After last treatment
Perrett (99) (2007)	MAL-PDT in transplant patients, 2× MAL-PDT vs. topical 5-FU twice daily for 3 wk	Head, trunk, and extremities	18 lesional areas were treated (10 Carcinoma in situ and 8 AK) in 8 OTR patients	3, Occluded	Noncoherent red light source (633 ± 15 nm light dose of 75 J cm, light intensity of 80 mW/cm²)	8 of 9 lesional areas (89%) cleared with MAL-PDT vs. 1 of 9 lesional areas (11%) cleared with 5-FU	6
Kauffman (94) (2008)	1× MAL-PDT vs. 2× freeze-thaw cryotherapy, repeat at 12 wk, if required	Extremities (98%), trunk, and neck	1343 AK in 121 patients (691 treated with MAL-PDT)	3, Occluded	Red LED light source (634 ± 3 nm, 37 J/cm², 50 mW/cm²)	MAL-PDT-78% vs. cryotherapy-88%	6
Palm (106) (2011)	MAL-PDT blue light vs. red light	Face, scalp, chest, and back	(18)	1	PDL (7 mm, 10–12 J/cm², 40 ms) +/– IPL, + blue light (407 nm, 10 J/cm², 16 min, 40 s) vs. Red LED light (630 nm, 37 J/cm², 8 min, 49 s)	No difference in improvement in AKs, wrinkles, pigmentation, or erythema between red and blue light	1

Abbreviations: AKs, actinic keratoses; ALA, aminolevulinic acid; BCC, basal cell carcinoma; MAL, methyl aminolevulinic acid; PDT, photodynamic therapy; SCC, squamous cell carcinoma; RR, relapse rate; CR, clearance rate; IPL, intense pulsed light; OTR, organ transplant recipients; 5-FU, 5-fluorouracil; LED, light-emitting diode; PDL, pulsed dye laser; mo, month.

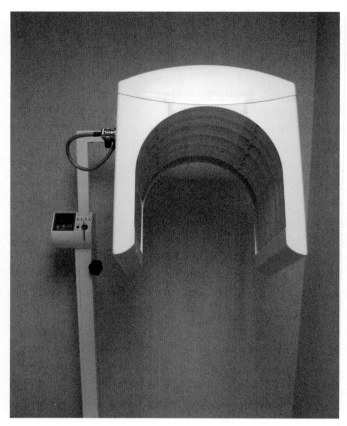

Figure 10.4 Noncoherent blue lamp is a common choice for photoactivating, aminolevulinic acid in the USA. The Blu-U (DUSA Pharmaceuticals, Inc., Wilmington, Massachusetts, USA) emits light at a bandwidth of approximately 417 ± 5 nm. *Source*: Courtesy of DUSA Pharmaceuticals, Inc.

clearance was observed between the two incubation time groups. Clearance rates were highest for head lesions at 100%. According to this large cohort study, it appeared that PDL at subpurpuric doses allows an efficient and less painful means of accomplishing PDT.

In 2003, Smith and coworkers (81) published a three-arm study on 36 patients with AKs. One arm received treatment with low concentration 5-FU, the other two arms received ALA-PDT—using either a PDL or blue light for photoactivation. A short, 1-hour unoccluded incubation was used. Clearance rates at 4 weeks follow-up were similar for 5-FU and ALA-PDL (79% vs. 80%). Clearance rates of PDT using a blue light source were lower (60%). Additionally, improvements in global photodamage, hyperpigmentation, and tactile roughness were observed (81).

Red Light Sources
The longer wavelength of red light allows deeper tissue penetration. Red light is used frequently during PDT with MAL. Red light may also be used for photoactivation of PpIX during ALA-PDT. Several laser and light sources emit wavelengths in the red light spectrum, usually targeted around 630 nm. These include the argon pumped dye laser, excimer laser, metal halide lamps, and red LED lamps.

Red Light from Laser Sources
One of the earliest studies reporting on ALA-PDT was completed by Calzavara-Pinton et al. (17) using an argon pumped dye laser (630 nm). In the treatment of 50 facial AK lesions, 20% ALA cream was applied topically for 6–8 hours. The study's patient population also included a mixed pool of 85 total patients

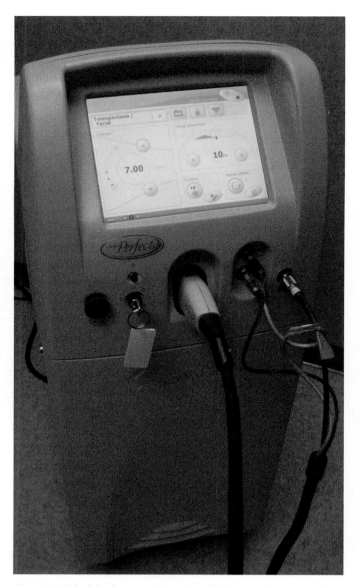

Figure 10.5 Pulsed dye lasers may be used as a light source for aminolevulinic acid-photodynamic therapy to target individual lesions, including actinic keratoses, sebaceous hyperplasia, and solar lentigines. *Source*: Vbeam Perfecta (595 nm) laser image, courtesy of Candela Corporation, Wayland, Massachusetts, USA.

with diagnoses of Bowen's disease (BD), SCCs, basal cell carcinomas (BCCs), and AKs. In terms of AK outcomes, a clearance rate of 100% was achieved at 24–36 months posttreatment.

The initial phase I clinical study for FDA-approval of ALA in PDT also utilized an argon-pumped dye laser. Thirty-nine of the 40 enrolled patients completed the dose-ranging study. Jeffes and coworkers (82) used 0–30% ALA topically with an extended incubation time of 14–18 hours. Ninety-one percent clearance was obtained in thin to well-developed AKs on the face and scalp that were treated with 30% ALA. Extremity treatment was not as successful with only 45% clearance of AKs on the limbs. Hyperkeratotic AKs did not respond well to therapy, and the small number of treated hyperkeratotic lesions precluded statistical analysis.

Nakano and coworkers (83) reported on the use of an excimer laser (630 nm) in patients of darker skin types. Thirty Japanese patients with AKs were divided into two groups based on lesion appearance. The first group included subjects with AK lesions 10 mm or less in diameter with the second group including larger lesions greater than 10 mm in diameter. Patients received three ALA-PDT sessions weekly for 3 weeks.

A clinical and histologic clearance of 100% was obtained in the small AK lesions group during the 1-year follow-up period. In the cohort with larger AK lesions, six of the 20 patients experienced residual lesions or recurrence. These findings are consistent with the poor penetration of ALA through thicker, hyperkeratotic lesions and resulting lower AK clearance rates.

Incoherent Red Light Sources

Metal halide lamps emitting a spectrum of light from 580 to 740 nm have been used in numerous ALA-PDT studies. Using the Waldmann/PDT 1200 lamp, 36 lesions in 10 patients were treated topically with ALA for 6 hours under occlusion followed by red light irradiation. At 28 days following treatment, the clearance of face and scalp lesions was 71%. Patients experienced pain and burning and mild postprocedure erythema.

Several studies followed shortly thereafter reporting clearance rates of facial AKs between 77% and 99%. Karrer et al. (84) treated 24 patients and 200 scalp and facial lesions with a clearance rate of 84% at 1 month following PDT. Kurwa et al. (70) used a metal halide lamp for ALA-PDT to treat the dorsal hands, resulting in a 79.5% decrease in AKs lesions. Itoh and coworkers (85) treated Japanese patients with AKs on the face, neck, and extremities. With two or more treatments, clearance rates at 12 months were higher for lesions on the head and neck (81.8%) compared with the extremities (55.6%). No serious adverse effects were reported in these patients with darker skin types. Markham and Collins (48) treated four patients with topical ALA under occlusion for 4 hours for scalp AKs. Three patients cleared following treatment, and the remaining patients had significant improvement at 6 months. Varma et al. (86) treated 88 patients with ALA-PDT using a red lamp for a variety of diagnoses, including AKs (127 lesions), BD (76), and

superficial BCC (87). Complete clearance rate for AKs after one and two treatments were 77% and 99%, respectively. However, the recurrence rate at 12 months was 28%. Mild stinging, tingling, or burning was reported by most patients. Another study also treated patients of mixed diagnoses. AKs, BCC, and SCC-in situ in 762 patients were treated by Moseley and coworkers (88). Ninety-two percent of AKs cleared after two treatments, with 100% clearance after three PDT sessions. Finally, Clark et al. (46), using a topical 20% ointment, treated 207 patients with 483 lesions. An impressive 91% clearance was observed clinically at a median of 48 weeks following treatment.

Broadband/Visible Light Sources

The earliest light sources used for the treatment of AKs during the modern PDT era produced unfiltered, noncollimated light for photoactivation. Following the work by Kennedy et al. (74), Wolf (21) in 1993 reported on the complete clearance of nine AKs after one round of treatment using a slide projector for a light source. Fink-Puches and coworkers (89) used a modified halogen slide projector with four filter cutoffs at 515, 530, 570, and 610 nm. AK lesions of the head, neck, forearms, and dorsal hand lesions were treated with 20% ALA for 4 hours under occlusion prior to light irradiation. Overall, complete response after one treatment was 64%, increasing to 85% with a second treatment. Head and neck lesions responded better than extremity lesions. Head and neck complete response rates varied from 93% to 100% depending on the spectrum of light used for treatment. Forearms and hands had a lower response rate ranging from 33% to 53%. Overall complete response rate at 36 months was 23% for filtered light and 71% for full spectrum light.

IPL devices (Fig. 10.6) are powerful tools for treating the signs of photoaging. Their use in photorejuvenation with

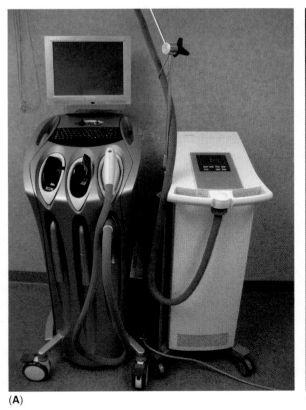
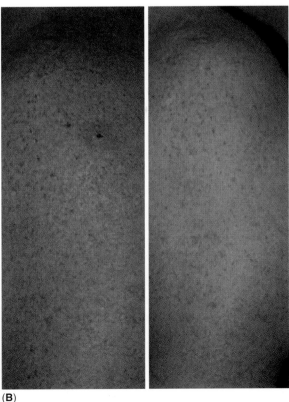

(A)   **(B)**

Figure 10.6 IPL devices are particularly effective in ALA-PDT for photorejuvenation. Cooled conductive gel and forced air cooling units minimize discomfort during treatment. (**A**) Patient with basosquamous carcinoma on the shoulder before and 8 months after two sessions of ALA-PDT (**B**). *Abbreviations:* ALA-PDT, aminolevulinic acid-photodynamic therapy; IPL, intense pulsed light. *Source:* Image of Lumenis One IPL device, courtesy of Lumenis, Inc., Santa Clara, California, USA.

ALA-PDT is discussed in a separate section of this chapter. However, a small study by Kim et al. (87) documented the use of ALA-IPL for the treatment of AKs exclusively. Twelve facial AK lesions in seven patients were treated with one session of ALA-PDT. At 12 weeks follow-up, 50% of lesions cleared. This clearance rate is markedly lower than reported averages, but it is difficult to formulate sound conclusions based on the small sample size.

TREATMENT RESULTS OF MAL-PDT FOR AKs

Three randomized comparison/control studies of MAL-PDT using the same protocol (MAL 3 hours, 570–670 nm, 75 J/cm^2, 50–250 mW/cm^2) cleared 69% of predominantly thin and moderately thick AKs of the face or scalp after a single treatment (90), increasing to 89–91% when two treatments 7 days apart were performed (13,91). In comparison, cryotherapy cleared 68% and 75% (90,91) in two of these studies, with placebo responses of 30–38% (92,91). Superior cosmetic response was observed in the MAL-PDT group in both studies that compared PDT with cryotherapy (90,91).

A large randomized intraindividual study of 1501 face/scalp AKs in 119 patients compared MAL-PDT (3-hour application) using routine initial double therapy 7 days apart with double freeze–thaw cryotherapy, repeating treatments at 3 months if required (93). In this study, Morton et al. used red LED light source (634 ± 3 nm, 37 J/cm^2, 50 mW/cm^2). PDT resulted in a significantly higher cure rate than cryotherapy (87% vs. 76%), after initial cycle of treatments; however, final outcome after all nonresponders were retreated was equivalent. PDT also exhibited significantly superior cosmesis and overall subject preference (efficacy and skin discomfort).

It should be noted that a multicenter intraindividual randomized trial comparing MAL-PDT versus cryotherapy for multiple AKs on the extremities demonstrated inferior efficacy with PDT, with clearance of 78% of lesions at 6 months compared with 88% for cryotherapy (94). The same red LED light source and settings described above were used in this study, but one single treatment was performed, to be repeated 3 months later if complete response was not achieved, which might help explain the different results found for facial/neck AKs. Besides, AK on the extremities may also be modestly more resistant to this treatment, according to results of previous smaller studies of topical ALA-PDT (95,96). One possible explanation for an increased resistance of AK of the extremities would be the lack of pilosebaceous units in these areas, which are important to a better absorption of prodrug and so to a better response. However, regarding cosmetic outcome in terms of both investigator assessment and patient preference, MAL-PDT was superior to cryotherapy. Patients also confirmed their general preference for MAL-PDT as a therapeutic option.

Using the same LED and MAL dosing parameters as above, Tarstedt et al. (97) found that for thin lesions a single treatment with MAL-PDT, repeated after 3 months in cases in which lesions remained, was equally as effective (93% with single MAL-PDT vs. 89% with double treatment) as using two treatments, 7 days apart. However, for thicker lesions, they found that clearance rates were greater after double treatment (84% vs. 70% with single treatment). After this study, most countries in Europe revised their MAL-PDT license in AK and started to recommend an initial single treatment for thin AK, with repeat after 3 months if necessary.

Solid organ transplant recipients (OTRs) suffer from a 10- to 250-fold increase in AKs due to their ongoing immunosuppressive therapy (98). In addition, the precancerous and cancerous lesions developing in the OTR population are often more aggressive (98), requiring frequent and ongoing cancer surveillance. PDT, a safe and effective treatment option for precancerous and malignant lesions, offered a new treatment modality for controlling AKs and NMSCs in the OTR population. Dragieva et al. assessed the response of AK in 17 transplant recipients, each with two suitable sites, in a randomized, placebo-controlled, double-blind study (99). Two MAL-PDT treatments 7 days apart were compared with placebo-PDT. At 4 months, there was lesion clearing in 13 of 17 sites with a partial response in three while there was no reduction in size or number of lesions in the sites treated by placebo-PDT. A randomized intrapatient comparative study of 5-FU cream, applied twice daily for 3 weeks, and topical MAL-PDT, two treatments 7 days apart, in eight OTRs demonstrated that at 3 and 6 months after completion of treatment, PDT was more effective than 5-FU in achieving complete resolution (100). Eight of nine lesional areas cleared with PDT (Clearance rate (CR) 89%, 95% CI: 0.52–0.99), compared with one of nine lesional areas treated with 5-FU (CR 11%, 95% CI: 0.003–0.48) ($P = 0.02$). In this study, a noncoherent red light source (633 ± 15 nm; Paterson PDT Omnilux, Phototherapeutics Ltd, Altrincham, UK) with an irradiance of 80 mW/cm^2, and a total dose of 75 J/cm^2 was applied to illuminate the treatment area after 3-hour MAL incubation. Although initial response rates of AKs following PDT were comparable in the OTR patient population and normal controls (101), longer-term follow-up demonstrated statistically significant decreases in clearance rates in the OTR population. In addition, SCC of the dorsal hands and forearms were not prevented in OTRs in a 2-year follow-up study, although there was a trend toward decreased keratotic regions in the areas treated (102). PDT may still be a viable treatment option in this population, but it may require adjustments to typical treatment protocols, including increased frequency of PDT sessions (101) and use of longer wavelengths (red light) for deeper skin penetration (102).

Finally, multiple AKs, particularly those that develop within the context of the field of cancerization (103) with (pre-) neoplastic processes at multiple sites, frequently challenge our clinical routine. In these patients, PDT appears to be very effective, with a patient complete response rates varying from 82% to 68% (92,91,104) and generally well tolerated. A recent randomized study by Serra-Guillen (105) compared tolerance and satisfaction in the treatment of AK of the face and scalp between 5% imiquimod cream and MAL-PDT. Among 58 patients included, there was a significantly greater percentage of patients very satisfied with the MAL-PDT treatment than in the imiquimod group (93% in MAL-PDT vs. 62% in imiquimod). Although the percentage of patients with good tolerance to the MAL-PDT was higher (38% for PDT vs. 21% for imiquimod), the differences were not statistically significant.

A randomized split-area study conducted by Palm and Goldman compared the use of red versus blue light sources in the treatment of AKs and photodamage in 18 patients with AKs using MAL-PDT with 60-minute incubation. All patients received illumination with PDLs and/or IPL, followed by split-area treatment of either blue or red light. No statistically significant differences in signs of photodamage and in improvement of AKs following MAL-PDT were observed between blue light– and red light–treated sides. Additionally, side effects were mild and did not differ between treatment sides (106).

Combination Therapy for AK Treatment

Several small case studies have demonstrated a possible synergistic effect of ALA-PDT with other treatment options for AKs. Combination 5-FU cream with PDT was tested in a study by Gilbert (107). Fifteen patients with multiple AKs completed a five-day course of nightly 5-FU cream to the face followed by short-contact PDT activated by an IPL light source. A clearance rate of 90% was observed at 1 year follow-up. Martin (108) performed a split-area study with three patients treated with ALA-PDT alone versus sequential therapy with 5-FU (7–10 days) and short-contact ALA-PDT (1 hour ALA incubation followed by blue light 417–432 nm illumination). At follow-up visit, 6 months after initial visit, the combined regimen showed enhanced efficacy in treating AK, suggesting synergistic effects of 5-FU and ALA-PDT. Shaffelburg (109) conducted a split-face study of 24 patients with multiple AKs, in which ALA-PDT was performed on the entire face. A half of the face was also randomized to receive additional subsequent treatment with a 12-week regimen of imiquimod. Clearance rates at 12 months were superior on the combination treatment side, with 89.9% complete lesion clearance compared with 74.5% on the ALA-PDT treatment side alone.

NONMELANOMA SKIN CANCER

BCC is the most common malignant skin tumor in the Caucasian population and is classified together with SCC as NMSC. It is estimated that NMSC affects at least 1–2% of the population annually (110,111), with 0.9–1.2 million new cases of NMSC diagnosed each year in the USA; of these 80% are BCC and 16% are SCC (110). Risk factors to NMSC include exposure to UV radiation, light complexion, male gender, increasing age, immunosuppression, precancerous skin lesion, and ionizing radiation (111,112).

Treatment of NMSC usually is based on clinical type, tumor size, and location; and also other important factors should be considered, such as maintaining close to normal skin appearance, downtime, treatment compliance, therapeutic risks related to comorbidities, and medications (anticoagulants, immunosuppressive therapy). Apart from surgical excision, which is the standard treatment for cutaneous SCC, other treatment options exist, including curettage and electrocautery, cryotherapy, radiotherapy, cytotoxic agents, and immunoresponse modifiers.

PDT with methylaminolevulinate is an innovative treatment modality that has been approved in Europe for the treatment of superficial BCC (sBCC), nodular BCC (nBCC), AKs, and BD (114). Herein, we revise the evidence for the efficacy and safety of PDT in the treatment of NMSC.

Figure 10.6A illustrates a case of basosquamous carcinoma on the shoulder treated with ALA-PDT.

BOWEN'S DISEASE

BD typically presents as an enlarging, erythematous plaque, well demarcated with a crusted or scaling surface (111). This epidermal dysplasia, histologically corresponding to SCC-in situ, is particularly common in elderly patients, frequently occurring on the lower part of the legs (92) and is associated with a small risk of progression (about 3%) to an invasive SCC (97).

This condition has been widely proposed as an indication for topical PDT with several studies confirming the efficacy of ALA-PDT. Topical ALA-PDT clears, on average, 86–93% of lesions of BD following one or two treatments (115). Three small randomized trials using nonlicensed ALA formulations and identical protocols demonstrated that PDT was equivalent in efficacy to cryotherapy (116), superior to 5-FU (117) and significantly more effective when delivered narrowband red instead of green light (118), possibly related to deeper tissue penetration. Table 10.2 provides a summary of peer-reviewed articles on the use of ALA-PDT and MAL-PDT in BD treatment.

A large multicenter study has been completed by Morton and colleagues comparing MAL-PDT with cryotherapy or topical 5-FU (119). In this randomized placebo-controlled study, 225 patients with 275 lesions had histologically confirmed intraepithelial SCC, with 111 lesions treated with two MAL-PDT treatments, 7 days apart, with a repeat cycle after 3 months if necessary. Cryotherapy was performed as a single freeze–thaw cycle to achieve an ice field that persisted for at least 20 seconds and 5-FU was topically applied once daily for 3 weeks. Both the treatment modalities were also repeated if required. After 3 months, MAL-PDT achieved clearance of 93% in comparison with 86% and 83% for cryotherapy and topical 5-FU, respectively. The remission rate after 12 months was 80% with MAL-PDT versus 67% with cryotherapy ($P = 0.047$) and 69% ($P = 0.19$) with 5-FU. At 24 months following final treatment lesion, clearance rates were 68% for MAL-PDT, 60% for cryotherapy, and 59% for 5-FU (120). Cosmetic outcome at 3 months was good or excellent for 94% of patients from the PDT group in comparison with 66% for the cryotherapy and 76% for 5-FU.

Data concerning long-term clearance are limited, but in one retrospective study of 617 patients, Thestrup-Pedersen and colleagues (121) found relapse rates (>5 years) of 34% for cryotherapy, 19% for curettage, 14% for 5-FU, 6% for radiotherapy, and 5% for surgery. With a 64-month recurrence rate of 17% in BD as noted by Leman et al. (122) following ALA-PDT, PDT, comparing with more established therapies, seems to have an acceptable long-term efficacy.

Topical PDT seems to be an especial option for the treatment of large and multiple patches of BD (123). Morton et al. found an initial clearance rate after ALA-PDT for 40 large, 20–55 mm diameter lesions after one to three treatments of 88% falling to 78% at 12 months.

Case reports and series have demonstrated a beneficial use of topical PDT to clear BD in unusual sites (nipple, subungueal) (124–126) and in cases of poor healing settings (epidermolysis bullosa and radiation dermatitis (127,128) as well.

Tolerability of MAL-PDT in BD was generally excellent and superior to standard treatments in the study by Morton et al. (129). Most patients experienced a certain degree of pain, but it was less severe than that caused by cryotherapy, whereas 5-FU was associated with poor local tolerability, eczematous reaction, ulceration, and erosion.

Topical PDT may represent a valuable treatment option for BD as a tissue-sparing, noninvasive therapy with high efficacy and good tolerability. MAL-PDT has been approved in most

Table 10.2 Published Clinical Studies on ALA- and MAL-PDT for Bowen's Disease

Reference	ALA Preparation	Location of BD	Incubation Period (hr)	# Lesions Treated (# Patients)	Light Source (Wavelength in nm)	Response Rate	Follow-up (mo)
Morton (116) (1996)	20% Emulsion vs. cryotherapy; repeated after 2 mo if required		4	40 (20 lesions were treated with ALA-PDT)	Desktop lamp 300 W xenon short arc (125 J/cm² at a fluence rate of 70 mW/cm²)	15/20 Lesions cleared after 1 ALA-PDT session, the remaining 5 after the 2nd session; 10/20 lesions cleared after 1 session of cryotherapy	12
Morton (118) (2000)	20% Emulsion using red vs. green light	Legs	4	61 (32 with red light) in 16 patients	Red (630 ± 15 nm, 125 J/cm²) or green (540 ± 15 nm, 62.5 J/cm²) light	88% CR red light; 48% green light	12
Morton (123) (2001)	20% Emulsion	Face, trunk, and limbs	4–6	40 Large lesions greater than 20 mm in diameter	Filtered red light (Xenon source, 630 ± 15 nm, 125 J/cm²)	78%	12
Leman (122) (2002)	20% Emulsion	Unspecified	4	107 (68)	Filtered red light (Xenon source, 630 ± 15 nm, 100–125 J/cm²)	83%	64 (range 34–84 mo)
Salim (117) (2003)	20% Emulsion vs. 5-FU for 4 wk, repeated after 6 wk if required	Legs	4	66 Lesions (33 treated with ALA-PDT) in 40 patients	Red light (630 +/- 15 nm, 100 J cm²)	ALA-PDT 88% CR vs. 5-FU 67% CR	12

(Continued)

Table 10.2 Published Clinical Studies on ALA- and MAL-PDT for Bowen's Disease (*Continued*)

Reference	MAL-PDT Study Design	Location of BD	Incubation Period (hr)	# Lesions Treated (# patients)	Light Source (wavelength in nm)	Response Rate	Follow-up (mo)
Morton (119) (2006)	MAL-PDT (2 sessions 1 wk apart) vs. placebo-PDT vs. cryotherapy vs. 5-FU for 4 wk; repeated at 3 mo if required	Face, scalp, trunk, and limbs	3	275 (124 treated with MAL-PDT) in 225 patients	Broadband red light (570–670 nm, 75 J/cm^2)	MAL-PDT-80% CR vs. placebo-PDT 10% CR vs. cryotherapy 67% CR vs. 5-FU 69% CR	12
Morton (120) (2005)	MAL-PDT (2 sessions 1 wk apart) vs. placebo-PDT vs. cryotherapy vs. 5-FU for 4 wk; repeated at 3 mo if required	Face, scalp, trunk, and limbs	3	275 (124 treated with MAL-PDT) in 225 patients	Broadband red light (570–670 nm, 75 J/cm^2)	MAL-PDT-68% CR vs. placebo-PDT 11% CR vs. cryotherapy 60% CR vs. 5-FU 59% CR	24

Abbreviations: ALA, aminolevulinic acid; BD, Bowen's disease; MAL, methyl aminolevulinic acid; PDT, photodynamic therapy; 5-FU, 5-fluorouracil; CR, clearance rate.

European countries for the treatment of BD, using a protocol with dosimetry as with MAL-PDT for AK (red LED light source 634 ± 3 nm, 37 J/cm^2, 50 mW/cm^2), but with two treatments 7 days apart, repeated at 3 months, if required (130).

Invasive SCC treated with ALA-PDT has been described in three open-label studies with initial complete response rates of 54–100% for superficial lesions, but with recurrence rates of up to 69% (mean 24%, 12 of 49, after 3–47 months) and a clearance rate of only 40% (4 of 10) of nodular SCCs after 12–36 months (131–133). In 2008, Calzavara-Pinton et al. treated 112 biopsy-proven lesions of BD and SCC in 55 patients with MAL-PDT using the red LED with the settings described above. After 3 months, the overall complete response was 73.2% and 53.6%, respectively, at 2 years (134). Cell atypia was a statistically significant independent predictor of the treatment outcome at 3 months. Therefore, the high efficacy of topical PDT for SCC-in situ suggests that depth of therapeutic effect is the limiting factor for PDT in invasive SCC. Although topical PDT has shown efficacy, in view of its metastatic potential, topical PDT cannot be currently recommended for the treatment of invasive SCC (135,136).

SUPERFICIAL BASAL CELL CARCINOMA

BCCs are locally aggressive tumors that very rarely metastasize and can be divided into three major groups: superficial, nodular, and infiltrating morpheaform lesions. sBCC usually differs from the other subtypes as it tends to appear at a younger age, frequently occurs on the trunk, limbs, and neck and often is multiple (137). A large number of treatment modalities exist, including surgical techniques [excisional surgery, curettage, and electrocautery, Mohs micrographic surgery (MMS), cryosurgery], immune response modifiers, cytotoxic agents, and PDT. Table 10.3 shows the main clinical studies of topical ALA- and MAL-PDT in sBCC.

In 1990, Kennedy et al. (138) were the first to report a 79% complete response rate at 3 months for 300 cases of sBCC treated with ALA-PDT (3–6 hours application of 20% ALA followed by filtered red light, 600+ nm). In 2001, Morton and colleagues (139) treated 98 large or multiple sBCCs with ALA-PDT and noted an 89% clearance rate after one or more treatments. In another study by Clark et al. (140), patients were treated up to four times with ALA applied for 6 hours followed by irradiation with red lamps (570–720 nm), or a 630 nm diode laser with a light dose of 125 J/cm^2 and found a 97% clearance for sBCC. The number of treatments increased with lesion diameter and the recurrence rate was 4.8% with a median follow-up of 55 weeks. A comparison study by Wang et al. (141) with ALA-PDT and cryotherapy (6-hour application of ALA followed by illumination with a 635-nm dye laser; 60 J/cm^2) for the treatment of sBCC and nodular BCC (nBCC) noted no significant difference in efficacy between the two groups. However, ALA-PDT was associated with fewer adverse events, faster healing times, and better cosmetic results. It should be noted that lesions were followed clinically and biopsied at 3 months; they were re-treated on clinical grounds or for histopathologic tumor and biopsied again at 12 months. They found that despite only 5% of the ALA-PDT–treated sBCC were clinical failures at 12 months, an additional 20% of the treatment sites that were clinically clear had residual BCCs on biopsy. Blume and colleagues used higher light doses

(200–300 J/cm^2 at 150 mW/cm^2) of a 633-nm laser irradiation combined with 20% ALA in a cream base applied under occlusion for either 4–6 hours or 18–24 hours (142). After 6 months of a single treatment, they found complete clearance in 94 of 95 (99%) sBCC with 4- to 6-hour ALA, and in 93 of 98 (94%) sBCCs with 18- to 24-hour ALA. There was no improvement going from 200 to 300 J/cm^2, which is consistent with the sigmoidal shape of the response versus light dose curve. At 3 years, recurrences were about 14% and the authors found that retreatment of recurrences had about the same efficacy as did initial treatments.

Several trials in Europe, USA, and Australia have been performed to investigate the efficacy and safety of MAL-PDT for the treatment of both sBCC and nBCC. Initial efficacy is consistently high, with clearance rates at 3 months after MAL-PDT ranging from 80% (in difficult-to-treat cases, recurrent or large lesions, or H-zone lesions) (143,144) to 97% in primary sBCC. In terms of long-term responses as nearly two-thirds of all recurrent BCC lesions appear in the first 3 years after treatment (145,146). A 5-year follow-up of a randomized trial (147) showed that recurrence with MAL-PDT (one PDT treatment session only, retreatment after 3 months with two sessions 7 days apart if required vs. double freeze–thaw cycle also repeated after 3 months if necessary) is comparable with cryotherapy (22% for MAL-PDT vs. 20% for cryotherapy at 60 months). However, more patients had an excellent outcome with MAL-PDT (60% vs. 16% with cryotherapy).

Another clinical study by Szeimies and colleagues (148) compared MAL-PDT (one cycle of two treatment sessions, 7 days apart, retreatment after 3 months with a second cycle if required) and surgery in sBCC. Three months after last treatment, the efficacy of MAL-PDT was similar to that of surgery: 92.2% showed complete clearance at 3 months with MAL-PDT versus 99.2% with surgery. However, at 12 months, 9.3% of lesions recurred with MAL-PDT compared with none with surgery. Cosmetic outcome was superior for MAL-PDT at all time points, with 94.1% lesions treated with MAL-PDT having an excellent or good cosmetic result compared with 59.8% with surgery.

In difficult-to-treat populations, that is, large lesions, in the H-zone, or in patients at a high risk for surgical complications, Vinciullo et al. (149) treated 95 patients having 148 BCC lesions (superficial, nodular or mixed superficial, and nodular) with MAL-PDT (3-hour occlusion, 570–670 nm, 75 J/cm^2, 50–200 mW/cm^2) and achieved an estimated lesion complete response rate of 90% at 3 months, 84% at 12 months, and 78% at 24 months. Overall cosmetic outcome was rated as excellent or good in 79% and 84% of the patients at 12 and 24 months, respectively. Therefore, MAL-PDT does show good efficacy and is an attractive option when surgery would be inappropriate or the patient wants to maintain normal skin appearance.

NODULAR BASAL CELL CARCINOMA

Clinical results for nBCC using ALA-PDT varied more markedly than those obtained for sBCC, with clearance rates ranging from 64% to 92% (150). This difference might be due to inadequate penetration of ALA into the deeper portions of the skin and the malignancy (142), therefore, several strategies have been studied to enhance effectiveness. One approach is to debulk the lesion before PDT. Thissen and colleagues (151)

Table 10.3 Published Clinical Studies on ALA- and MAL-PDT for Superficial Basal Cell Carcinoma

Reference	ALA Preparation	Location of sBCC	Incubation Period (hr)	# Lesions Treated (# Patients)	Light Source (Wavelength in nm)	Response Rate	Follow-up (mo)
Kennedy (138) (1990)	20% Emulsion	Not specified	3	80 Lesions	Slide projector with a cutoff filter at 600 nm	90% CR	2–3
Calzavara-Pinton (132) (1995)	20% emulsion ALA-PDT repeated EOD until clinical disappearance	Head, trunk, and limbs	6–8 occluded	23 lesions	Argon dye laser (630)	91% CR	24–36
Fijan (264) (1995)	1× ALA-PDT in combination with desferrioxamine (no lesion preparation specified), repeated after 3–6 mo if required	Face, scalp, trunk, and extremities	Not specified	34 (32)	Halogen lamp with a red filter	88% CR after 1 treatment, 97% after 2 treatments	20
Wennberg (265) (1996)	20% emulsion 1× ALA-PDT	Not specified	3 Occluded	190 (37)	Filtered xenon lamp (620–670 nm)	92% CR	6
Fink-Puches (131) (1998)	20% Emulsion 1× ALA-PDT	Face, scalp, neck, trunk (65 lesions), and lower extremity	4 Occluded	95 (47)	UV-A or full-spectrum visible light, >515, >570, or >610 nm)	Initial response (2–4 wk) : 86% CR, recurrence rate of 44% after median of 19 mo	Median of 19 mo
Haller (266) (2000)	20% cream Routine 2× ALA-PDT, 7 days apart	Face, trunk, and limbs	3–4 occluded	26 (6)	Red light (630 ± 15 nm)	1–2 mo lesion CR: 100%; 1 lesion recurred at 16 mo	Median of 27 mo

Reference	MAL-PDT Study Design	Location	Incubation Period (hr)	# Lesions Treated (# Patients)	Light Source (wavelength in nm)	Response Rate	Follow-up (mo)
Soler (267) (2000)	ALA-PDT 15 min of pretreatment with 99% DMSO before topical 20% ALA with DMSO (2%) and ethylene-diaminetetraacetic acid (2%)	Face, scalp, trunk, and extremities	3 occluded	245 (83)	Broadband lamp with continuous spectrum (570–740 nm) or a red-light laser (630 nm)	Red light : 86% CR vs. Broadband lamp : 82% CR	6
Wang (141) (2001)	20% cream 1× ALA PDT × Cryotherapy 2× freeze–thaw cryotherapy; repeat at 12 wk, if required	Head and neck, trunk, and limbs	6 occluded	39 sBCC (22 treated with ALA-PDT) 49 nodular BCC (25 treated with ALA-PDT)	Frequency doubled Nd:YAG laser pumping a dye laser (635 nm, 60 J/cm², 80 ± 20 mW cm²)	12 mo histologically recurrences: 38% for ALA-PDT vs. 7% for cryotherapy; Excellent or good cosmetic outcome (sBCC + nBCC) in 93% treated with ALA-PDT vs. 54% with cryotherapy	12
Soler (162) (2001)	1× MAL-PDT (lesion preparation)	Face, scalp, trunk, and extremities	Mean 4 occluded	131 sBCC	Broadband halogen light (570–670 nm) mean light dose of 50–200 J/cm², light intensity of 100–180 mW/cm²	91% CR after 3 mo, 9% relapse at 35 mo	24–48
Horn (143) (2003)	MAL-PDT "difficult to treat" BCC (European trial) 2× MAL-PDT retreated after 3 mo if necessary (lesion preparation)	Face, scalp, neck, trunk, and extremities	3, Occluded	49 sBCC	Red light (570–670 nm), dose of 75 J/cm², light intensity of 50–200 mW/cm²	85% CR after 3 mo (histological control);22% recurrence at 24 mo	24

(Continued)

Table 10.3 Published Clinical Studies on ALA- and MAL-PDT for Superficial Basal Cell Carcinoma (Continued)

Reference	MAL-PDT Study Design	Location	Incubation Period (hr)	# Lesions Treated (# Patients)	Light Source (wavelength in nm)	Response Rate	Follow-up (mo)
Vinciullo (149) (2005)	MAL-PDT "difficult to treat" BCC (Australian trial) 2× MAL-PDT retreated after 3 mo if necessary (lesion preparation)	Face, scalp, neck, trunk, and extremities	3, Occluded	92 sBCC	Red light (570–670 nm), dose of 75 J/cm², light intensity of 50–200 mW/cm²	93% CR at 3 mo, 82% at 24 mo	24
Surrenti (268) (2007)	2× MAL-PDT (7 days apart) with additional monthly MAL-PDT sessions up to a maximum 8 where necessary (lesion preparation)	Face, neck, trunk, and extremities	3, Occluded	94 (69)	Red LED light source (634 ± 3 nm, 37 J/cm², 50 mW/cm²)	89%CR 1 mo after 2 sessions, 2.4% recurrence at 12 mo; no additional clinical benefit beyond 2 MAL-PDT sessions	12
Basset-Seguin (147) (2008)	1× MAL-PDT vs. double freeze-thaw cryotherapy retreated with 2× MAL-PDT (7 days apart) or double freeze-thaw cryotherapy after 3 mo if necessary (lesion preparation)	Face, scalp, neck, trunk, and extremities	3, Occluded	219 (114 treated with MAL-PDT)	Red light (570–670 nm), dose of 75 J/cm², mean light intensity of 150 mW/cm²	MAL-PDT 97% at 3 mo vs. cryotherapy 95%	60
Szeimies (148) (2008)	2× MAL-PDT (7 days apart), retreated after 3 mo if necessary vs. surgery	Face, scalp, neck, trunk, and extremities	3, Occluded	246 (128 treated with MAL-PDT)	Red LED light source (634 ± 3 nm, 37 J/cm², 50 mW/cm²)	MAL-PDT 92% at 3 mo vs. cryo-therapy 99%; 9.3% recurrence with MAL-PDT vs. none with surgery at 12 mo	12
Fantini (269) (2010)	1 or 2× MAL-PDT (7 days apart), a third PDT session after 3 mo if required (lesion preparation)	Head, neck, trunk, and limbs	3, Occluded	116	Red LED light source (634 ± 3 nm, 37 J/cm², 50 mW/cm²)	CR: 82%	Mean of 23.5

Abbreviations: ALA, aminolevulinic acid; DMSO, dimethyl sulfoxide; EOD, every other day; LED, light-emitting diode; MAL, methyl aminolevulinic acid; Nd: YAG, neodymium-doped yttrium aluminum garnet; PDT, photodynamic therapy; nBCC, nodular basal cell carcinoma; sBCC, superficial basal cell carcinoma; UV-A, ultraviolet-A.

reported a clearance rate of 92% (22 of 24 tumors) after a single cycle of ALA-PDT (noncoherent red light, 100 mW/cm^2, 120 J/cm^2) with debulking curettage performed three weeks earlier. Another approach used to increase ALA within the lesion was iontophoresis and the addition of dimethylsulfoxide (DMSO) or ethylenediaminetetraacetic acid (152,153). Christensen and colleagues (154) demonstrated clearance of 91% BCC lesions (24 sBCC and 36 nBCC) at 3 months and 81% remained disease-free at 72 months with one or two sessions of DMSO-supported ALA-PDT following curettage.

Topical MAL has shown superior tissue penetration over ALA due to its decreased charge and increased lipophilicity (155). Whether these properties make MAL more efficacious than ALA is unknown with only one small randomized study by Kuijpers and colleagues (156) showing similar effectiveness of MAL and ALA-PDT for nBCC.

Five phase III studies in which a total of 220 nBCCs were treated (143,149,157–159) with MAL-PDT have demonstrated significant efficacy with 3-month complete response rates of 73–94%. It should be noted that histologically controlled studies have confirmed the reliability of efficacy data (73% and 79%). Two studies by Horn et al. (117) and Vinciullo et al. (149) examined the use of MAL-PDT in "difficult-to-treat" and high-risk cases and still found 3-month response rates of 87% and 82% for nBCC, respectively. However, at 24 months after treatment, Vinciullo found a lower sustained lesion clearance rate of 67% for nodular lesions.

A comparison study of MAL-PDT versus surgery for nBCC (159,160) has provided a 3-month response rate noninferior to surgery (91% compared with 98% for surgery) and a 60-month recurrence rate of 14% compared with 4% with surgery. However, estimated sustained lesion complete response rates were 76% for MAL-PDT compared with 96% for surgery. The authors concluded that a favorable cosmetic outcome, with 82% rating as excellent or good versus 33% in the surgery group, combined with moderately low 5-year lesion recurrence with MAL-PDT supports a clinical role for this modality of treatment for nBCC.

In 2009, Foley et al. (161) published favorable results for nBCC (≤5 mm in depth) from two randomized studies, showing histologically verified lesion complete response rates of 73% with MAL-PDT (two sessions, 7 days apart repeated after 3 months if necessary) versus 27% with placebo at 6 months after last treatment. Although curettage was used to debulk rather than remove the tumor, repeat curettage and inflammation associated with the debridement procedure could have contributed to high response rate with the placebo-PDT. Although thickness of nBCC has not specifically been assessed in other trials, a retrospective study of MAL-PDT for nBCC found recurrence rates of 7% and 14% for thin (<2 mm) and thick (>2 mm) nBCC, respectively, at a median 35-month of follow-up, suggesting that thin nBCC might be particularly responsive to MAL-PDT (162).

In terms of cosmetic outcome, PDT in nBCC usually achieves superior results compared with other modalities, such as cryotherapy (141) and surgery (159), with 82–95% (141,143,151,157,159,162) of patients rating as "excellent" or "good."

Since the penetration of MAL is higher than that of ALA and a standardized protocol involving lesion preparation, light source (red light), and dose has been developed for nBCC in the countries where MAL-PDT is approved for this particular condition, current evidence supports the use of MAL rather than ALA for PDT of nBCC (163). Table 10.4 shows the main clinical trials of topical ALA- and MAL-PDT in nBCC.

More recently, photodynamic diagnosis using MAL in conjunction with a Wood's lamp examination has been reported as an adjunctive to accentuate tumor margins before MMS (164), showing a high degree of consistency between post-MMS defect and fluorescent examination size. Therefore, this technique has the potential for increasing the efficiency of MMS, by decreasing the number of stages. It should be noted that Tierney and colleagues (164) used a 13-hour preincubation time in order to maximize the signal-to-noise ratio of tumor fluorescence relative to background fluorescence of non–tumor-laden skin. Another study by Lee and colleagues (165), using 20% ALA ointment 6 hours before MMS for NMSC, failed to find any efficacy of photodynamic diagnosis though; the authors concluded that many variables such as tumor thickness, type of photosensitizer, incubation time might affect the fluorescence, therefore future large-scale studies are still needed.

Photorejuvenation
Definition of Photoaging
Photodamage is a marker of cumulative UV exposure and senescent changes to the skin. Not only can the appearance be concerning to the patient, but it can also lead to precancerous conditions with the development of AKs (166). The characteristic appearance of photodamaged skin includes sallow discoloration, inelasticity, rhytid formation, pigmentary alteration, ecstatic vessels/telangiectasias, and textural alterations (45). Global photodamage scales have been developed for scoring the severity of skin involvement. Dover used a 5-point scale in evaluating several categories of photodamage, including fine surface lines, mottled pigmentation, sallowness, tactile roughness, coarse wrinkling, and global photodamage (167). Working from this initial scale, others have added facial erythema, telangiectasias, sebaceous gland hyperplasia, and facial AKs as separate categories in the evaluation of photodamage (168,169).

Light Sources in ALA- and MAL-PDT Photorejuvenation
Many of the same lasers and light sources effective in ALA- and MAL-PDT for the treatment of AKs have the added benefit of inducing photorejunative effects on the skin. Chromophores targeted during PDT treatment may include vessels, melanin, and even collagen (168). Blue light only allows for a photochemical effect in PDT with less tissue penetration than other light sources, such as IPL and PDL. The latter sources penetrate deeply enough to target vessels, pigment, and collagen (170). The choice of which light source to use ultimately depends on such factors as the condition being treated, efficacy, cost of use, and availability of equipment.

Treatment Results of ALA- and MAL-PDT in Photorejuvenation
Studies relating to the treatment of photodamage with ALA- and MAL-PDT are organized in the section below according to the light source employed. A summary of these studies is provided in Table 10.5.

Table 10.4 Published Clinical Studies on ALA- and MAL-PDT for Nodular Basal Cell Carcinoma

Reference	ALA Preparation	Location of nBCC	Incubation Period (hr)	# Lesions Treated (# Patients)	Light Source (Wavelength in nm)	Response Rate	Follow-up (mo)
Fijan (264) (1995)	1× ALA-PDT in combination with desferrioxamine (no lesion preparation specified), repeated after 3–6 mo if required	Face, scalp, trunk, and extremities	Not specified	22 (32)	Halogen lamp with a red filter	32% CR after 1 treatment, 59% after 2 treatments	3–20
Calzavara-Pinton (132) (1995)	Various cutaneous malignancies. ALA20% emulsion ALA-PDT repeated EOD until clinical disappearance	Head, trunk, and limbs	6–8	30	Argon dye laser (630)	1-mo lesion CR (histologically controlled) : 61% 33% Recurrence after median of 29 mo	24–36
Thissen (151) (2000)	1× ALA-PDT using 20% ALA cream and DMSO (lesion preparation)	Not specified	6 Occluded	24 (23)	Red light (630–635 nm, 120 J/cm², 100 mW/cm²)	3–6 mo lesion CR: 92% 5% recurrence after median of 17 mo	17
Wang (141) (2001)	20% ALA cream 1× ALA-PDT × Cryotherapy 2× freeze-thaw cryotherapy, repeat at 12 wk, if required	Head and neck, trunk, and limbs	6 Occluded	49 nBCC (25 treated with ALA-PDT) 39 sBCCs (22 treated with ALA-PDT)	Frequency doubled Nd:YAG laser pumping a dye laser (635 nm, 60 J/cm², 80 ± 20 mW cm²)	12 mo histologically recurrences: 13% for ALA-PDT vs. 21% for cryotherapy	12
Christensen (154) (2009)	1 or 2× ALA-PDT (7 days apart) using 20% ALA cream and DMSO (lesion preparation)	Face, scalp, trunk, and extremities	3 Occluded	36 nBCC 24 superficial BCC	Broadband halogen light source (550–700 nm, 150–230 mW/cm²)	3 mo CR (sBCC + nBCC): 91%, 17% of nBCC recurred after 72 mo	72

Reference	MAL-PDT Study Design	Location	Incubation Period (hr)	# Lesions Treated (# Patients)	Light Source (Wavelength in nm)	Response Rate	Follow-up (mo)
Soler (162) (2001)	1× MAL-PDT (lesion preparation)	Face, scalp, trunk, and extremities	Mean 4 occluded	82 Thin nBCC (<2 mm thickness), 86 thick nBCC (>2 mm)	Broadband halogen light (570–670 nm) light dose of 50–200 J/cm², light intensity of 100–180 mW/cm²	Thin nBCC: 93% CR and thick nBCC: 86% CR after 3 mo, 7% of thin nBCC and 14% of thick nBCC relapsed at 35 mo	24–48
Horn (143) (2003)	MAL-PDT "difficult-to-treat" BCC (European trial) 2× MAL-PDT retreated after 3 mo if necessary (lesion preparation)	Face, scalp, neck, trunk, and extremities	3, Occluded	52 nBCC	Red light (570–670 nm), dose of 75 J/cm², light intensity of 50–200 mW/cm²	75% CR after 3 mo (histologic control); 14% recurrence at 24 mo	24
Rhodes (159) (2004)	2× MAL-PDT (7 days apart) vs. surgery (lesion preparation), retreatment after 3 mo if required	Face, scalp, neck, trunk, and extremities	3, Occluded	105 nBCC (53 treated with MAL-PDT)	Red light (570–670 nm), dose of 75 J/cm², light intensity of 50–200 mW/cm²	MAL-PDT: 91% CR vs. Surgery: 98% 3 mo after last treatment, NR, or recurrence after 24 mo: 19% in the MAL-PDT vs. 4% in the surgery group	24
Vinciullo (149) (2005)	MAL-PDT "difficult to treat" BCC (Australian trial) 2× MAL-PDT retreated after 3 mo if necessary (lesion preparation)	Face, scalp, neck, trunk, and extremities	3, Occluded	36 nBCC	Red light (570–670 nm), dose of 75 J/cm², light intensity of 50–200 mW/cm²	82% CR at 3 mo, 67% at 24 mo	24

(Continued)

Table 10.4 Published Clinical Studies on ALA- and MAL-PDT for Nodular Basal Cell Carcinoma (*Continued*)

Reference	MAL-PDT Study Design	Location	Incubation Period (hr)	# Lesions Treated (# Patients)	Light Source (Wavelength in nm)	Response Rate	Follow-up (mo)
Kuijpers (156) (2006)	2×MAL-PDT × 2× ALA-PDT (20% cream) 7 days apart (lesion preparation)	Face, neck, trunk, and extremities	3, Occluded	43 (22 Treated with ALA-PDT and 21 with MAL-PDT)	Broadband halogen light (600–730 nm), dose of 75 J/cm², light intensity of 100 mW/cm²	CR at 2 mo (histologically controlled): 72.7% with ALA-PDT vs. 71.4% with MAL-PDT	8
Rhodes (160) (2007)	2×MAL-PDT 7 days apart (repeated if necessary, lesion preparation) × surgery	Face, scalp, neck, trunk, and extremities	3, Occluded	105 (53 treated with MAL-PDT)	Red light (570–670 nm), dose of 75 J/cm², light intensity of 50–200 mW/cm²	Sustained CR at 5 years: MAL-PDT 76% vs. surgery 96%; recurrence at 5 yr: 14% in the MAL-PDT vs. 4% in the surgery group	60
Surrenti (268) (2007)	2× MAL-PDT (7 days apart) with additional monthly MAL-PDT sessions up to a maximum 8 where necessary (lesion preparation)	Face, neck, trunk, and extremities	3, Occluded	24	Red LED light source (634 ± 3 nm, 37 J/cm², 50 mW/cm²)	52.2% CR 1 mo after 2 sessions, no additional clinical benefit beyond 2 MAL-PDT sessions	12
Foley (161) (2009)	2× MAL-PDT (7 days apart) retreated after 3 mo if required (lesion preparation) × placebo-PDT for nBCC <5 mm in depth	Face, scalp, neck, trunk, and extremities	3, Occluded	150 (75 lesions treated with MAL-PDT)	Red light (570–670 nm), dose of 75 J/cm², light intensity of 50–200 mW/cm²	Histologically verified CR: 73% with MAL-PDT vs. 27% with the Placebo-PDT	6
Fantini (269) (2010)	1 or 2× MAL-PDT (7 days apart), a third PDT session after 3 mo if required (lesion preparation)	Head, neck, trunk, and limbs	3, Occluded	78	Red LED light source (634 ± 3 nm, 37 J/cm², 50 mW/cm²)	CR:33%(tumor thickness superior o 0.5 mm and the presence of ulceration were predictors of negative outcome)	Mean of 23.5

Abbreviations. ALA, aminolevulinic acid; CR, clearance rate; DMSO, dimethyl sulfoxide; EOD, every other day; LED, light-emitting diode; MAL, methyl aminolevulinic acid; nBCC, nodular basal cell carcinoma; NR, nonresponse; sBCC, superficial basal cell carcinoma; PDT, photodynamic therapy.

Table 10.5 Published Clinical Studies on ALA- and MAL-PDT for Photorejuvenation

Reference	ALA Preparation	Location of Photodamage/ Study Design	Incubation Period (hr)	# Patients	Light Source (Emission λ, nm)	Response	Follow-up (mo)
Ruiz-Rodriguez (166) (2002)	20% Emulsion	Face and scalp, ≥1 AK and chronic photodamage; 2 PDT sessions	4, Occluded	17 (38 AKs)	IPL (590–1200)	87% CR of AKs; excellent cosmesis	3
Goldman (72) (2003)	20% Solution	Face, long-incubation PDT	15–20	32	Blue light (417)	94% CR of AKs; improved skin texture, pigmentation	3–6
Smith (81) (2003)	20% Solution, 2 sessions	Face, scalp	1	35	Blue light (417) or PDL (595)	80% CR for AKs with blue light; 60% CR for PDL; both demonstrated improvement in global photodamage, tactile roughness, and hyperpigmentation	1
Touma (22) (2004)	20% Solution	Facial AK and mild-to-moderate photodamage	1–3	17	Blue light (417)	Improvement in photodamage markers, including skin quality, fine rhytides, and sallowness	1–5
Avram (178) (2004)	20% Solution	Facial photodamage (with AKs) treated with 1 ALA-IPL session	1	17	IPL	69% CR of AKs; improvement in telangiectasias, dyspigmentation, skin texture	3

(Continued)

Table 10.5 Published Clinical Studies on ALA- and MAL-PDT for Photorejuvenation (*Continued*)

Reference	ALA Preparation	Location of Photodamage/ Study Design	Incubation Period (hr)	# Patients	Light Source (Emission λ, nm)	Response	Follow-up (mo)
Alster (179) (2005)	20% Solution	Split-face comparison, IPL vs. ALA-IPL	1–3	10	IPL (500–1200)	ALA-IPL-treated side showed greater improvement	6
Dover (167) (2005)	20% Solution	Split-face comparison, IPL vs. ALA-IPL (5 treatment sessions)	0.5–1	20	IPL (515–1200)	Greater improvement in ALA-IPL over IPL only for global photoaging, pigmentation, and fine lines only	1
Key (183) (2005)	20% Solution	Face, subpurpuric doses of PDL	1	12	PDL (585)	Improvement in majority of photodamage parameters with ALA-PDL; no improvement with PDL alone	1
Lowe (175) (2005)	5–20% Cream	Forearm, periorbital	0.5–2	6	Red light (633)	Mild improvement noted in photoaging	0.25
Marmur (180) (2005)	20% Solution	Split-face comparison, IPL vs. ALA-IPL (1 treatment)	1	7	IPL	Microscopic changes demonstrated greater type I collagen on ALA-IPL side	N/A
Gold (169) (2006)	20% Solution	Split-face comparison, IPL vs. ALA-IPL (3 treatment sessions)	0.5–1	16	IPL (550/570 cutoff filters-1200)	ALA-IPL results superior to IPL alone	1–3

Serrano (181) (2009)	1–2% Gel	Multiple application, low concentration ALA-PDT to face, neck, hands (3 treatment sessions)	0.5–1	8/26 Patients with photoaging; 18/26 treated for acne, vitiligo	IPL (530–1200) or yellow-red lamp (550–630)	90% of cases with hyperpigmentation improvement; erythema (85%), skin texture (100%)	6
Park (176) (2010)	20% cream	2 ALA-PDT at 1-mo interval, repeated (2 sessions) after 1 mo if required	4	14 with 1–3 AKs on the face and photodamage	Red light (580–740 nm), dose of 100 J/cm^2, 100 mW/cm^2	82.6% CR of Aks 1 mo after last treatment, microscopic analysis showed increased expression of type I and III procollagen, reduced elastotic material, decreased levels of matrix metalloproteinases-1,-3, and -12	1 mo after last treatment
Clementoni (184) (2010)	20% Solution	Face, pretreatment with a microneedle roller followed by ALA-PDT	1	21	IPL (560 cutoff filter-1200) and red LED light (630 nm)	Improvement in photodamage markers, including fine lines, mottled pigmentation, sallowness, tactile roughness, and telangiectasias	6
Xi et al. (182) (2011)	5% and 10% Cream	Face, split-face comparison, IPL vs. ALA-IPL (3 treatment sessions) in Chinese patients	1	26	IPL (560 and 590 cutoff filter-1200 nm)	Greater improvement in global score for photoaging, fine lines, and coarse wrinkles. PIH was higher on the ALA-IPL PDT side (22% vs. 15% on the IPL-only side)	2

(Continued)

Table 10.5 Published Clinical Studies on ALA- and MAL-PDT for Photorejuvenation (*Continued*)

Reference	MAL-PDT Study Design	Location of Photodamage	Incubation Period (hr)	# Patients	Light Source (Emission λ, nm)	Response	Follow-up (mo)
Zane (173) (2007)	2 Sessions, 1-mo interval	Facial AK and severe photodamage	3, Occluded (2–3 tubes for each session)	20 (137 AKs)	Red LED (634 ± 3 nm, 37 J/cm²)	88.3% CR of AKs, improvement of hyperpigmented spots, sallowness, skin texture, and fine lines, erythema, telangiectasia, sebaceous gland hypertrophy, and deep wrinkles, showed no change	2 mo after last treatment
Ruiz-Rodriguez (185) (2007)	2 Sessions, 3 wk apart	Perioral, pretreatment with fractional resurfacing (1550 nm), a half followed by MAL-PDT	3, Occluded	4	Red LED (634 ± 3 nm, 37 J/cm²)	Increased improvement in superficial wrinkles in 3 out of 4 patients on the combined treatment side	12 wk after last treatment
Issa (174) (2010)	2 sessions, 1-mo interval	Facial AK and photodamage (Glogau classification types II and III)	2, Occluded (1/2 tube for each session)	14	Red LED (634 ± 3 nm, 37 J/cm²)	89.1% CR of AKs after 6 mo; 10/14 patients: improvement of skin texture, wrinkles and firmness and pigmentation; increase in collagen fibers density and decrease in elastotic material assessed through morphometric exam 6 mo after treatment	6

Abbreviations. AKs, actinic keratoses; ALA, aminolevulinic acid; CR, clearance rate; DMSO, dimethyl sulfoxide; IPL, intense pulsed light; LED, light-emitting diode; MAL, methyl aminolevulinic acid; nBCC, nodular basal cell carcinoma; PDL, pulsed dye laser; PDT, photodynamic therapy; PIH, postinflammatory hyperpigmentation.

PDT with Blue Light

Despite the shallow penetration of blue light, it still appears to improve the signs of photoaging following ALA-PDT. The first indication that blue light had photorejuvenative effects in PDT was with the phase II/III clinical trials for FDA-approval of Levulan for nonhyperkeratotic AKs. In these studies, significant improvement in the signs of photoaging were noted after treatment (68,78,171).

Photorejuvenation studies using the blue light source have also been conducted by Goldman and Atkin (72), where a blue light source was used to illuminate the face after the topical application of ALA. Thirty-two patients with photodamage and AKs were treated with one session of ALA-PDT using a 1-hour ALA incubation followed by Blu-U activation. AKs showed a 90% improvement in terms of photorejuvenation parameters, a 72% improvement in skin texture, and a 59% improvement in skin pigmentation. Gold (79) reported on the dual use of blue light ALA-PDT for AKs and photoaging. The treatment of nonhyperkeratotic facial AKs also resulted in an improvement of skin elasticity and texture in patients with photodamaged skin.

Touma et al. (22) studied the effectiveness of ALA and blue light illumination in the treatment of AKs and diffuse photodamage. Eighteen patients with facial nonhypertrophic AKs and mild-to-moderate facial photodamage were evaluated. Short-contact ALA was applied from 1 to 3 hours with subsequent exposure to blue light. At 1 and 5 month follow-up intervals, there was a significant reduction in AKs. In addition, marked improvement in photodamage parameters, such as skin quality, fine wrinkling, and sallowness, were observed. Other markers of photodamage, such as pigmentary changes and coarse wrinkling, showed little to no improvement. Patients were also satisfied with the procedure, with 80% of patients rating their results as good to excellent. Other findings make this an intriguing study. This clinical study was pivotal in shifting treatment of AKs from long, 14- to 18-hour incubation times to shorter contact times. In addition, study patients were pretreated with microdermabrasion prior to topical ALA application, leading to more uniform and rapid penetration of ALA.

A final study by Smith and coworkers (81) examined the use of blue light ALA-PDT in diffuse photodamage. As discussed in the AK section of this chapter, this study was a three-arm study comparing topical, low concentration 5-FU to two forms of short-contact ALA-PDT—one arm with activation from a blue light source, the other with a PDL. While one patient in the 5-FU group discontinued due to a confluent erythematous reaction, all patients in the ALA-PDT group completed the study. In both ALA-PDT groups, patients experienced improvement in global photodamage, hyperpigmentation, and tactile roughness. The ALA-PDL was more successful in treating pigmentation, while blue light had lower response rates to global photoaging. Interestingly, the blue light ALA-PDT was the only treatment arm to have photoaging completely resolved in one patient.

PDT with Red Light

Many of the studies regarding red light PDT for the treatment of photoaging utilized MAL rather than ALA. These studies by Szeimies et al. (69) and Pariser (172) demonstrated excellent cosmetic results. Zane and colleagues (173) evaluated the efficacy and tolerability of MAL-PDT in 20 patients with multiple AKs and photoaging of the face. Two treatments (MAL under occlusion for 3 hours before red LED 37 J/cm^2) were performed at 1-month interval. The clearance rate of AKs found was 88.3%, and global improvement was observed in mottled hyperpigmentation, fine lines, and roughness of the skin. A recent randomized, clinical, histopathologic, and morphometric study by Issa and colleagues (174) using MAL-PDT and red light (LED 635 nm, 37 J/cm^2) evaluated 14 patients treated with two sessions, 4 weeks apart. Clinical improvement with regard to texture, firmness, wrinkle depth, skin coloration, and AK was observed. Histopathologic and morphometric studies were consistent, showing increased collagen fibers, and decrease in the fragmented elastic fibers 6 months after treatment.

One small pilot study conducted by Lowe and Lowe (175) investigated the use of ALA-PDT for the treatment of photoaging on the forearm and periorbital region. Escalating concentrations of ALA (5–20%) and increasing incubation times (30–120 minutes) were used prior to light irradiation with a red light source (633 nm). Mild improvement in signs of photoaging was noted at 7 days following treatment.

A histologic and immunohistochemical analysis conducted by Park and colleagues (176) in 14 patients with AKs and photodamage treated with ALA-PDT (twice at 1-month interval, using red light 580–740 nm, dose of 100 J/cm^2, 100 mW/cm^2) showed significant increase in type I and III procollagen expression. Elastotic material with fibrillin-1 and tropoelastin expression in the dermis decreased after treatment as well as the expression of matrix metalloproteinases-1, -3, and -12. Although the study was limited by the small sample size, those histologic changes indicated restoration of photoaged skin with ALA-PDT.

Photodynamic Therapy with Intense Pulsed Light

IPL is a light source that emits noncollimated, noncoherent light with wavelengths in the range of 515–1200 nm, which corresponds to the visible light and near-IR spectrum (47). Various filters can be used to block certain wavelengths below the cutoff point of the desired filter. IPL treatments improve many of the signs of photoaging, including pigmentation in the form of solar lentigines, erythema, and telangiectasias due to vascular ectasia/damage, as well as fine wrinkling (47). Like the PDL, IPL treatments also promote neocollagenesis (177). Although IPL alone has been proven effective in the treatment of photodamage, the addition of ALA to IPL treatment (ALA-IPL) appears to be more effective in treating photodamaged skin. Clinical examples of ALA-IPL treatment for photorejuvenation are illustrated in Figures 10.7–10.10.

In 2002, Ruiz-Rodriguez et al. (166) investigated the treatment of photodamage and AKs using ALA-PDT with IPL as the light source for photorejuvenation. Seventeen patients with various degrees of photodamage and AKs (38 AKs total) underwent therapy with ALA-IPL. A total of two treatments were performed 1 month apart. Treatments were well tolerated. At 3 months follow-up, 87% of AKs disappeared and marked cosmetic improvement was noted in wrinkling, coarse skin texture, pigmentary changes, and telangiectasias.

Multiple studies followed the initial results of Ruiz-Rodriguez and coworkers. Avram and Goldman (178) evaluated the

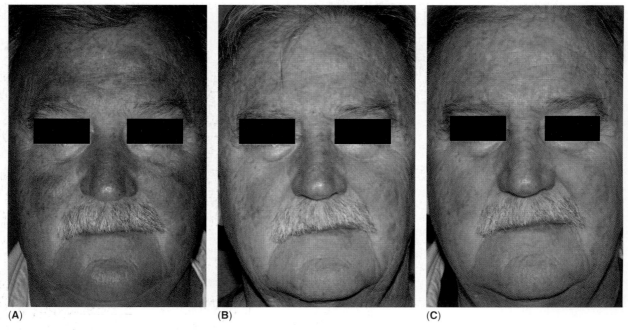

Figure 10.7 Here we can see greatest improvement with the first two aminolevulinic acid-photodynamic therapy sessions (**A,B**) as the patient presented more photodamage, but further improvement is achieved in vascularity, pigmentation, and skin sallowness after one additional session (**C**).

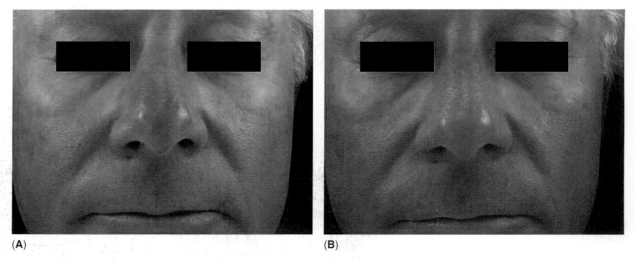

Figure 10.8 (**A**) White male with moderate erythema and telangiectasias concentrated over the nose on a background of mild-to-moderate photodamage. The patient had received a single treatment of intense pulsed light without significant clearance. (**B**). Significant improvement after one treatment of aminolevulinic acid-photodynamic therapy.

combined use of ALA-IPL for the treatment of photorejuvenation with one treatment session. Sixty-nine percent of the AKs responded to the use of ALA-IPL. Additionally, a 55% improvement in telangiectasias, 48% improvement in pigment irregularities, and 25% improvement in skin texture were observed.

Alster and colleagues (179) also examined the use of IPL in ALA-PDT. Ten patients with mild-to-moderate photodamage underwent two sessions of split-face treatment. Patients received treatment with ALA-IPL on one side and IPL alone on the contralateral side at 4-week intervals. Clinical improvement scores were noted to be higher on the side of the face treated with the combination of ALA-IPL. They concluded that the combination of topical-ALA + IPL is safe and more effective than IPL alone for the treatment of facial rejuvenation.

Another split-face study on ALA-IPL versus IPL alone was performed by Dover et al. (167). In this study, 20 subjects had three split-face treatments 3 weeks apart. Half of the face was treated with ALA followed by IPL treatment and the other half was treated with IPL alone. A blinded investigator was used to evaluate global photodamage, fine lines, mottled pigmentation, tactile roughness, and sallowness during the study. They concluded that pretreatment with ALA followed by IPL resulted in greater improvement in global photoaging (80% vs. 50%) and mottled pigmentation (95% vs. 65%). Successful results were also noted for fine lines for the ALA-IPL side compared with the IPL side alone (55% vs. 20%). Although tactile roughness and sallowness were noticeably better, pretreatment with ALA did not enhance the results of using IPL alone. It was important to note that both modes of treatment were well

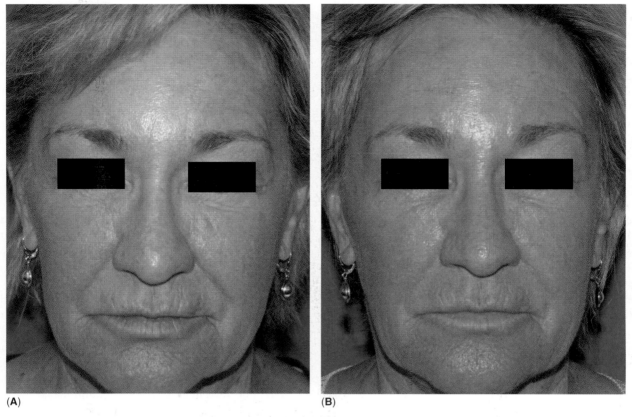

Figure 10.9 (**A**) Before and (**B**) 1 month following multilaser aminolevulinic acid-photodynamic therapy with a significant improvement in fine lines, sallowness, and skin texture.

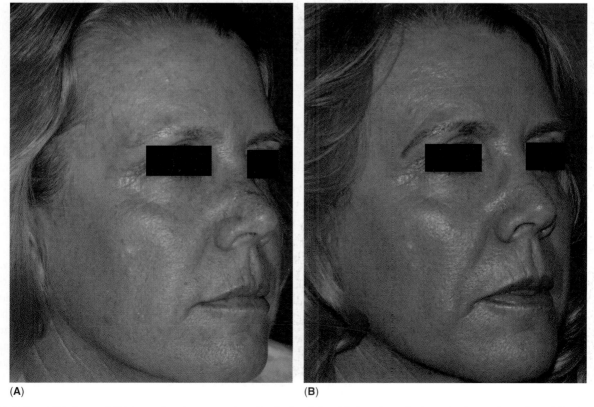

Figure 10.10 Patient (**A**) before and (**B**) 3 months after one session of aminolevulinic acid-photodynamic therapy. Of note, the quality of the skin texture has improved with a reduction in the sebaceous hyperplasia lesions.

tolerated and that no significant differences in the side effect profiles were observed. This study was important not only for its demonstration and safety of IPL in the use of ALA-PDT, but for the development of a photodamage rating scale.

Another split-face comparative study for photorejuvenation using ALA-IPL versus IPL alone was performed by Gold and coworkers (169). Thirteen patients received short-contact ALA-IPL on one side of the face and IPL alone on the contralateral side. Photoaging categories, including fine wrinkling (crow's feet), tactile skin roughness, mottled pigmentation, telangiectasias, and AKs, were evaluated. All demonstrated a better response on the side of the face treated with ALA-PDT. This study also confirmed the enhancing effects of ALA-PDT in IPL photorejuvenation.

Marmur et al. (180) conducted a pilot study to assess the ultrastructural changes seen after ALA-IPL photorejuvenation. Seven adult subjects were treated with a full-face IPL treatment. Half of the face in the study subjects received pretreatment with topical ALA before the IPL treatment. Pre- and posttreatment biopsies were reviewed by electron microscope for changes in collagen. A greater increase in type I collagen was noted in the subjects that were pretreated with ALA-IPL as opposed to the group treated with IPL alone. They concluded that the addition of ALA-PDT using IPL could be superior to IPL alone.

A study by Serrano et al. (181) in 2009 examined the use of ALA-IPL for the treatment of acne, vitiligo, and photoaging. Twenty-six patients in total completed the study, eight of which were in the photoaging treatment arm. Low-concentration ALA (1–2%) was used for incubation prior to light exposure. Improvement in several photoaging parameters were noted in the majority of patients. One hundred percent of cases had skin texture improvement; erythema/telangiectasia and hyperpigmentation were improved in 85% and 90% of cases, respectively. Eighty-eight percent of patients were satisfied with the results after three sessions of ALA-PDT.

Regarding treating patients with Fitzpatrick skin types III and IV, particularly Asians, a double-blind split-face controlled study examined the safety and efficacy of ALA-IPL PDT (182) using lower concentrations of ALA. Twenty-six patients were pretreated with 5% and 10% (regions with severe photodamage) ALA cream applied to half of the face for 1 hour followed by full-face IPL (520–1200 nm) treatment. Three treatments at 1-month intervals were done followed at 1 and 2 months after the final treatment. Higher success rates for fine lines and coarse wrinkles were seen on ALA-IPL PDT side at the final visit. However, postinflammatory hyperpigmentation was higher on the ALA-IPL PDT side (22%) than on the IPL-only side (15%), although this was transient (2 months) and reversible. The authors concluded that by using ALA in low concentration (5%), incubation time as short as 1 hour and relatively low energy of IPL irradiation (on average 15 J/cm^2 for double-pulse mode and 19 J/cm^2 for triple-pulse mode) satisfactory results could be achieved in patients with Fitzpatrick skin types III and IV.

PDT with PDL

PDLs have also been studied as a light source for photorejuvenation in ALA-PDT. PDL targets oxyhemoglobin as a chromophore according to the theory of selective photothermolysis. But thermal energy generated in the surrounding areas adjacent to targeted blood vessels may also result in photorejuvenative effects. Subpurpuric doses from the PDL alter dermal collagen and may improve skin texture (47).

Alexiades-Armenakas et al. (73) found ALA-PDT with the 595 nm PDL was successful in treating face and scalp AKs. Additionally, in this large study of 2561 lesions, areas treated showed signs of photorejuvenation.

Key (183) treated 14 patients with long-incubation ALA (12 hours) followed by photoactivation using a PDL. Improvement was noted following ALA-PDL in terms of skin texture, tactile quality, and brown spots, although the degree of vascularity and seborrheic keratoses were unaffected by treatment. The lack of improvement in blood vessel lesions is curious given that PDL targets the vasculature.

Combination Therapy for Photorejuvenation

A combination of microneedling roller (108 µm in width and 300 µm in depth) prior to ALA incubation (1 hour) to maximize epidermal penetration and irradiation of both red light (630 nm) and broadband pulsed light in a single treatment has been studied in 21 patients by Clementoni and colleagues (184). At 6 months posttreatment, 76.2% scored themselves an overall improvement greater than 75% and statistically significant improvement was observed in the global photoaging scores, fine lines, mottled pigmentation, sallowness, tactile roughness, and telangiectasias at 3 months posttreatment.

Enhanced efficacy of PDT after fractional resurfacing was observed by Ruiz-Rodriguez (185) in four patients treated in the perioral area. Two sessions of a 1550 nm fractional laser were immediately followed by MAL-PDT (3 hours occlusion, illumination with red LED 634 nm, 37 J/cm^2) on half of the perioral area. Twelve weeks after last treatment, a blinded investigator found increased improvement in superficial wrinkles in three out of four patients on the combined treatment side.

A study by Hædersdal and colleagues has demonstrated enhanced delivery of topical MAL deeply into in vivo porcine skin with ablative fractional CO$_2$ laser (186). They found significantly higher PpIX fluorescence throughout the entire skin depth where pretreatment with CO$_2$ ablative fractional laser was performed before MAL-application, compared with conventional topical MAL application, suggesting that ablative fractional resurfacing could be a clinically practical means for enhancing uptake of MAL and even many other topical skin medications.

Summary of Findings for ALA- and MAL-PDT in AK Treatment and Photorejuvenation

These results show the potential usefulness of a variety of lasers and light sources in the treatment of AKs and in the improvement of photodamage and photorejuvenation utilizing ALA- and MAL-based PDT treatments. Current studies have been focused on novel photosensitizer drugs and reformulations of ALA, such as nanoemulsions or patch-based applicators, with ALA patch PDT appearing to be superior to cryosurgery in the treatment of mild-to-moderate AK (187). Beyond the treatment of AKs, ALA- and MAL-PDT offer beneficial cosmetic outcomes in photorejuvenation.

Pain Experienced During PDT

During illumination, a sensation of stinging or burning sensations is frequently observed, which can range from mild to severe and varies from patient to patient. The precise mechanism of pain is not fully elucidated but likely involves nerve stimulation and/or tissue damage (188).

A review study by Warren and colleagues (188) of 43 articles consisting of clinical PDT trials (2000–2008) that used ALA or MAL was performed to summarize the effectiveness of interventions to reduce ALA-PDT–related pain and to explore contributing factors to pain induction. Their consensus opinion is that, in general, topical anesthetics do not work and cooling the skin with either ice water or with a high-airflow cooling device (such as Zimmer MedizinSystems, Irvine, California, USA) represents the best topical intervention to control the pain during PDT. They also found that pain intensity is associated with lesion size and location; certain diagnoses, particularly plaque-type psoriasis, appear to generate the highest PDT-related pain scores. Inconsistent results were encountered for the correlation of pain with light source, wavelength of light, fluence rate, and total light dose.

Although the use of forced airflow cooling device (ACD) appears to be effective in reducing pain during PDT, a recent nonrandomized retrospective observational controlled study conducted by Tyrrell and colleagues (189) demonstrated that patients using ACD throughout treatment presented significantly less PpIX photobleaching than the control group. The 100 lesions (in 100 patients) investigated in this study included: 39 AK, 29 sBCCs, and 32 BD. After comparing the data from 50 patients who utilized the ACD throughout irradiation with the other 50 patients not requiring any pain relief, the authors found 82% complete response in the non-ACD group versus only 68% complete response in the ACD group (including all three lesion types). As demonstrated by previous studies (190,191), the level of PpIX photobleaching correlates to cell death and therefore tumor clearance rates and might be the reason that utilization of the ACD during light irradiation lowers the potential efficacy of the treatment. Furthermore, AK lesions using the ACD were more susceptible to reduced PpIX photobleaching when compared with PpIX accumulation indicating a potential reduction in treatment efficacy. It is proposed that the low temperature of air used may cause local vasoconstriction, reducing reactive oxygen species (ROS) production and thus limiting clinical effectiveness.

The efficacy of subcutaneous infiltration anesthesia (SIA) on pain in PDT was demonstrated in a study conducted by Borelli and colleagues (192). They compared the pain related to ALA-PDT in 16 patients who received oral analgesics (1 g paracetamol, 20 mg codeine) and SIA on one side of the face, containing a mixture of ropivacaine, prilocaine, and epinephrine. Significantly less pain was reported by 94% of the patients with SIA. However, subcutaneous infiltration anesthesia should not contain vasoconstrictors, such as epinephrine, as their use could reduce the oxygen supply in the skin and thus compromise the effectiveness of PDT.

It should be noted that the influence of irradiation on the pain experienced during topical PDT is still a matter of debate. Preliminary studies of prototype devices consisting of portable LED sources (2 cm diameter, 45–60 J/cm², red light,

550–750 nm, irradiance 5 mW/cm²) showed that low-irradiance PDT could be effectively used and was significantly less painful (193). Twelve patients (eight with BD and four with sBCC <2 cm in diameter) received two treatments, 1 month apart following ALA 20% cream incubation of 4 hours. At 12-month follow-up, seven of the 12 patients had a complete response while the pain scores using a numerical rating scale were referred as <2 by all 12 patients.

Another study conducted by Wiegell and colleagues (194) evaluated continuous activation of PpIX by daylight and found to be as effective as and less painful than conventional PDT for AK. Twenty-nine patients with AK of the face and scalp had two symmetrical areas treated with MAL-PDT: one was illuminated by red LED light using standard parameters (632 nm, 37 J/cm²) after 3 hours of incubation and the other was treated with daylight for 2.5 hours after half hour incubation. At the 3-month follow-up, no significant difference in the treatment effect between the two was observed, with a reduction in AK of 71% in the LED-treated area versus 79% in the daylight-treated area. Treatment with daylight was significantly less painful than with LED light with a mean maximal score (numerical scale from 0 to 10) during daylight exposure of 2 compared with 6.7 during LED exposure. Therefore the authors concluded that daylight PDT could be an effective, nearly pain-free alternative to conventional PDT for patients with thin AK. However, it is unlikely that ambient light exposure can offer a practical, safe, and consistent method to the delivery of PDT.

PRACTICAL CONSIDERATIONS

Patient Selection for ALA-PDT

Thoughtful selection of eligible patients for ALA-PDT benefits both physician and patient. Patients should be carefully screened at an initial clinical consultation for inclusion and exclusion criteria for PDT. Physicians should gauge whether a patient has an accurate understanding and realistic expectations of the procedure. This will maximize patient results, reduce patient anxiety, and ensure the PDT is conducted smoothly on the day of the procedure. A comprehensive consent that explains the risks, benefits, and complications of therapy as well as treatment alternatives should be reviewed with patients carefully prior to treatment.

Exclusion Criteria

Patients should be screened for important exclusion criteria prior to undergoing PDT. A history of photosensitivity, including porphyria, photodermatoses, and photosensitizing medication use should preclude treatment (72,82,168). Many studies have excluded patients from treatment if they have undergone treatment with systemic retinoids, chemotherapeutic agents, or immunotherapy in the past 6 months (68,82,175). Pregnant or nursing women and individuals with an active infection should not undergo treatment (67,68). Patients should refrain from topical retinoids, alpha hydroxy acids, and chemical peels approximately 1 month prior to treatment (82).

Treatment Protocol

Skin Preparation

Optimal results following ALA-PDT can be achieved with proper preparation prior to the procedure itself. The stratum corneum is a major barrier to the penetration of ALA (49,77). Hyperkeratotic lesions must be treated with light curettage prior to ALA application. Otherwise, ALA is preferentially absorbed by the hyperkeratotic scale rather than the lesion intended for treatment (48). Some physicians use occlusion to improve delivery of ALA through thicker lesions. Tegaderm™, opaque Mepore®, or Glad Press-N-Seal® may be used for these purposes.

Methods of proper skin preparation to reduce stratum corneum thickness also include light chemical peels, tape stripping, microdermabrasion, and degreasing of the skin with acetone (170,195–197). All of the above measures can improve the absorption of ALA by the skin (49). We routinely use a vibrating microdermabrasion system (Vibraderm, Great Plains, Texas, USA) (Fig. 10.11) with subsequent acetone degreasing to prepare the skin for ALA application (Fig. 10.12).

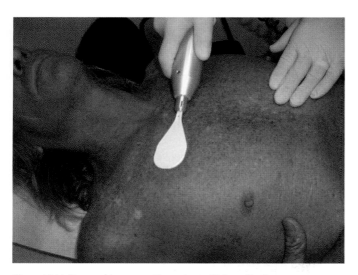

Figure 10.11 Proper skin preparation prior to ALA application removes excess layers of the stratum corneum and improves ALA penetration. We use a vibrating microdermabrasion device for 5 minutes prior to acetone degreasing. *Abbreviation*: ALA, aminolevulinic acid.

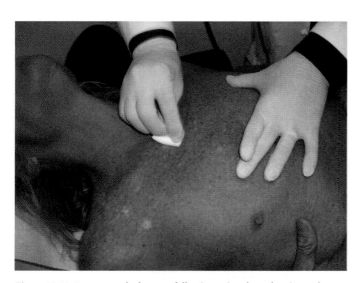

Figure 10.12 Acetone-soaked gauze following microdermabrasion enhances aminolevulinic acid delivery. Firm pressure should be used during scrubbing to remove excess skin lipids and keratinocytes.

Incubation Time

ALA is FDA-approved for use with a 14- to 18-hour incubation and subsequent photoactivation with blue light (38). However, longer incubation times often result in an increased severity of adverse effects following ALA-PDT (Fig. 10.13) (68), and furthermore, shorter incubation times (1–3 hours) have demonstrated similar efficacy in AK clearance (22,81).

We routinely use a 60-minute incubation time in the treatment of AKs or for photorejuvenation. When treating thicker, larger, or more invasive lesions, we extend the incubation time to 3 hours and occlude the treated area with Glad Press'N Seal®. Current FDA approval for MAL-PDT involves applying a 16.8% cream under occlusive dressing for 3 hours followed by illumination with a narrow spectrum red light lamp.

Light Sources

Blue, red, green, and broadband light sources may be used to activate PpIX during ALA-PDT for AKs or photorejuvenation. There is some evidence that blue light may be more effective for superficial AKs due to the shorter wavelength and increased potency during PDT of blue light (170). However, other authors found no difference in efficacy between blue and red light for the treatment of AKs and photorejuvenation (106). Green light was found to cause less pain than red light in the treatment of AKs (80). Red light has a deeper depth of penetration, but is often used with MAL rather than ALA. Broadband light sources, including IPL, have the advantage of improving signs of photodamage. It is our practice, both in the treatment of AKs and photorejuvenation, to use multiple light sources

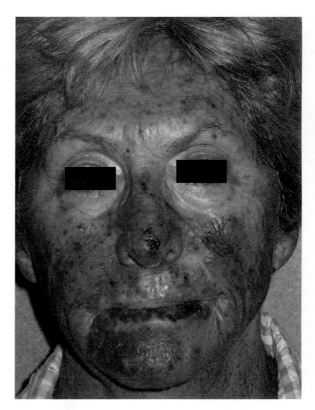

Figure 10.13 Moderate-to-severe phototoxic reaction due to extended ALA incubation period. This woman had ALA-PDT with a 3-hour, unoccluded incubation. The patient denied UV exposure for the 36 hours following PDT. *Abbreviations*: ALA, aminolevulinic acid; PDT, photodynamic therapy; UV, ultraviolet.

during ALA-PDT. With a typical treatment, we treat individual lesions first with subpurpuric doses of a PDL, followed by full-face treatment by an IPL, and lastly illumination with a blue and/or red light source. It should be noted that the IPL also results in hair reduction, so judicious use should be exercised in hair-bearing areas, such as the scalp and beard area.

Patient Comfort and Photoprotection and Follow-Up

We do not routinely use topical or intralesional anesthesia prior to ALA-PDT. With a 1-hour incubation time, our clinical experience is that the procedure is well tolerated by the overwhelming majority of patients. We use forced air cooling (Fig. 10.6) and refrigerated conductive gel during the IPL portion of photoactivation, and the forced air cooling during blue light and red light exposure. For longer incubation periods, the use of oral analgesics, topical lidocaine preparations, and ice packs in conjunction with PDT may increase patient comfort (72).

Immediately following treatment, we apply an aloe vera-based gel to the treated skin to calm erythema and irritation. A sunblock (physical blocker) containing zinc oxide and titanium dioxide is applied to the treated skin. To avoid phototoxicity during daylight hours, our patients are scheduled for treatment in the late afternoon, so they may depart the clinic during twilight hours. Patients are given a protective visor if the face was treated, and patients are asked to wear sunglasses and protective clothing during their ride home.

We instruct patients to avoid sunlight and bright indoor light sources for 36 hours following treatment. We request patients return to clinic at 1 week and 2 months following PDT for routine follow-up. We perform subsequent rounds of ALA-PDT at 1–2 month intervals. We counsel patients to anticipate two ALA-PDT sessions for the treatment of AKs, while photorejuvenation, especially when sebaceous hyperplasia is present, usually requires 3–4 sessions. These recommendations are consistent with consensus guidelines from the American Society of Photodynamic Therapy (37).

CLINICAL TECHNIQUE

Summarized below is our treatment protocol for ALA-PDT (18). This is supplied as an example, but is by no means the only way to successfully perform PDT. This may be used as a general guideline and practitioners must decide for themselves the most effective and efficient use of ALA-PDT in their office.

AMINOLEVULINIC ACID-PHOTODYNAMIC THERAPY FOR ACTINIC KERATOSES AND PHOTOREJUVENATION

1. Cleanse the patient's skin with mild soap and water (Cetaphil cleanser or Neutrogena Foaming Facial Wash).
2. Perform microdermabrasion with the Vibraderm over the treated area (Fig. 10.11).
3. Scrub the skin vigorously using a 4 × 4 inch acetone-soaked gauze (Fig. 10.12).
4. Break the two glass ampules in the Levulan Kerastick as per the package insert (38). Shake the stick for about 2 minutes.
5. Apply the ALA solution to the treatment area. This is best accomplished by painting the Levulan on using the application stick. At least two coats of the solution are recommended, and the entire contents of the Kerastick should be used. It is important to get close to the eyes, otherwise it will be apparent that the periorbital skin was not treated.
6. Allow the Levulan to incubate for 60 minutes on the skin. The patient should remain indoors during the incubation period.
7. Remove the Levulan prior to any light treatment by requesting the patient to wash his/her face with a gentle soap and water.
8. Activate the Levulan with the appropriate light source(s):

- AKs: PDL is used to target individual lesions at subpurpuric settings, followed by treatment with blue light and red LED simultaneously. The blue light (Blu-U, DUSA Pharmaceuticals, Inc.) should be positioned approximately 25–50 mm from the treatment area (Fig. 10.14) and the red light source (Aktilite CL 128, Galderma, Fort Worth, Texas, USA) should be positioned 50–80 mm from the skin.
- Photorejuvenation +/− AKs: PDL is used to target individual lesions at subpurpuric settings, including AKs, sebaceous hyperplasia, solar lentigines, and telangiectasias. IPL treatment follows using a double-pulse and 560 nm cutoff filter for Fitzpatrick skin types I–III and the 590 nm filter for skin types IV. Fluence, pulse duration, and pulse delay settings are determined according to skin type and type of photodamage. Lastly, the patient is treated with the Blu-U and the red LED (Aktilite) simultaneously in a similar manner to the AK protocol.

1. Wash the patient's face again to remove any residual Levulan on the skin's surface.
2. Apply soothing gel or lotion (we recommend an aloe vera-based gel) to the treated area after the illumination period.
3. Apply a physical sunblock containing zinc oxide and titanium dioxide to the treated area. Instruct the patient on strict photoprotection for the following

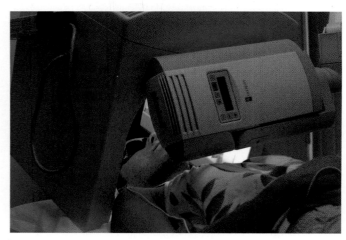

Figure 10.14 Simultaneously illumination with blue (Blu-U®) and red light (Aktilite®).

36 hours. The patient is to remain indoors, out of direct sunlight.

4. Patients are given Avene Thermal Spring Water spray to apply to their skin 4–6 times a day.
5. Repeat the treatment in 4–8 weeks. If there was little reaction, increase the incubation time or reevaluate your skin preparation technique.

Clinical examples of AKs treated with a multilaser PDT approach are presented in Figures 10.15 and 10.16.

Safety, Adverse Effects, and Complications

Expected side effects following PDT are related to the phototoxic nature of treatment and are usually mild in nature. Pain and burning may be experienced during light irradiation. Shorter incubation times decrease the severity of side effects. Expected phototoxic side effects include erythema, edema, stinging/burning, pruritus, and crusting. Pigmentary changes, whealing, and vesiculation may also occur (40,67,69). Erythema and mild crusting occur in most patients following treatment (Fig. 10.17), usually resolving in 1–2 weeks (88). Hypopigmentation is rare, and hyperpigmentation, with an incidence as high as 27% following ALA-PDT (67), is usually mild in nature. More pronounced reactions are correlated with disease burden. Typically, repeat treatments are less painful than previous ones.

In patients with extensive phototoxic reactions (Fig. 10.18), especially in cases when patients are exposed to UV radiation in the 24–36 hours following treatment, topical therapy may be necessary to address erythema, edema, and crusting. Topical steroid creams and ice packs may be used on the treated area until the symptoms subside. All patients should be screened for

a history of cold sores and appropriate HSV prophylaxis begun prior to treatment in such cases (18).

Pain management, especially with shorter incubation times (e.g., 1 hour), is usually a nonissue. Reassurance to the patient and "talk-esthesia" by a caring member of the clinical staff is usually more than adequate to comfort any patient anxiety and pain. However, the use of cooling fans, Avene Thermal Water Spray, forced air cooling systems, Xylocaine spray, and even oral non-narcotic pain medication have been used successfully to mitigate pain during ALA-PDT (22,67,88).

Patients should be counseled to practice strict photoprotection for 24–36 hours following treatment. Titanium dioxide- and zinc oxide-containing sunblocks are preferred, in addition to protective clothing and sunglasses. Excessive UV radiation from sunlight, as well as intense spotlights, photocopy machines, photographic flashlights, and medical examining lights/lamps should be avoided during the period of photosensitivity. Indoor light is usually not a concern, but patients should avoid bright sources of light, even while indoors (40).

Not unexpectedly, if patients require a second treatment, the adverse effects as well as treatment pain are usually much less than those experienced with the initial treatment. We believe that the decrease is due to the resolution of most of the clinical and subclinical photodamage which occurs during the initial treatment.

Expected Benefits

Many of the benefits of ALA- and MAL-PDT treatment have been addressed in the discussion of clinical studies regarding the treatment of AKs and photorejuvenation. Both ALA- and MAL-PDT are safe, efficacious, and well-tolerated treatment

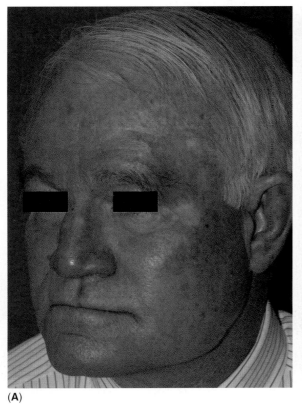
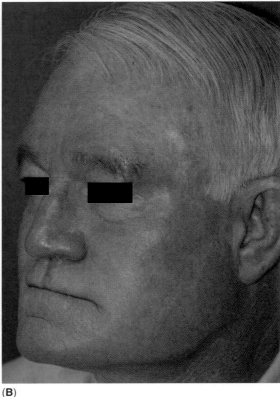

(A)   **(B)**

Figure 10.15 (**A**) Before and (**B**) 1 month after a single multilaser aminolevulinic acid-photodynamic therapy to the face of a middle-aged male with reduction in actinic keratosis along with improvement in signs of photoaging, including solar lentigines and erythema.

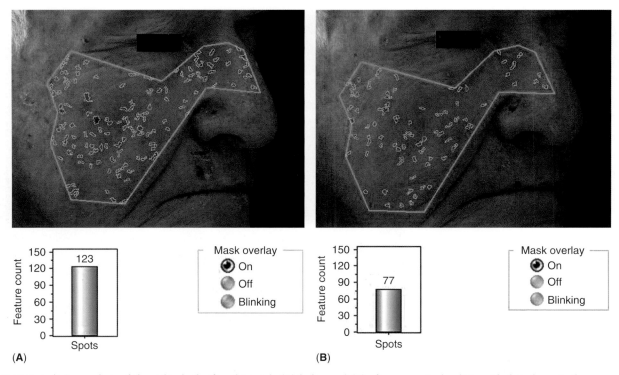

Figure 10.16 Complexion analysis of the right cheek of a white male (**A**) before and (**B**) after one aminolevulinic acid-photodynamic therapy session for photorejuvenation. A 47% decrease in brown spots (solar lentigines) was quantified using the computer software system.

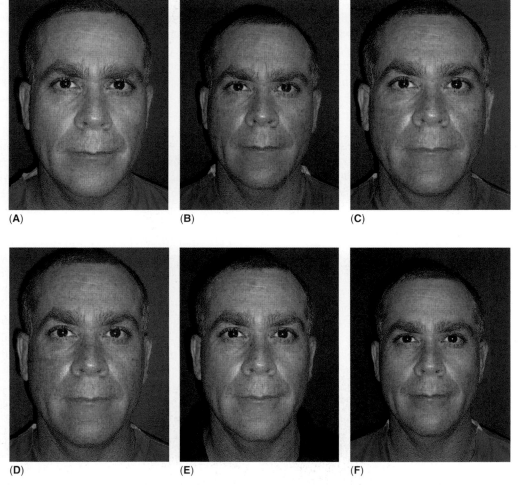

Figure 10.17 (**A**) Frontal view of a 51-year-old male with photodamage consisting of numerous solar lentigines. (**B**) One day after ALA-PDT treatment. Levulan ALA was applied to the entire treatment area for 1 hour, unoccluded. IPL treatment with Lumenis One using a 560 nm cutoff filter, double pulse of 4 and 4 ms with a 10 ms delay at a fluence of 18 J/cm² followed by a 10-minute exposure with the Blu-U. Note the erythema and crusting of all actinically damaged skin. (**C**) Two days after PDT, treatment, further increase in erythema is seen in areas of actinically damaged skin. (**D**) Three days after PDT treatment, resolution of erythema begins. (**E**) Four days after PDT treatment, further resolution of erythema. (**F**) Seven days after PDT treatment, complete resolution of erythema. *Abbreviations*: ALA, aminolevulinic acid; IPL, intense pulsed light; PDT, photodynamic therapy. *Source*: From Ref. 64.

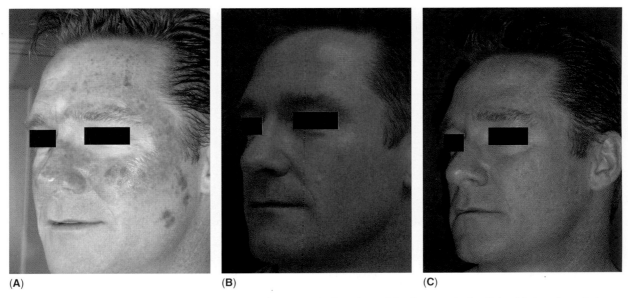

(A)   **(B)**   **(C)**

Figure 10.18 (**A**) Mild-to-moderate phototoxic reaction due to sunlight exposure in the 24 hours following an aminolevulinic acid-photodynamic therapy session. (**B**) Six months postprocedure, the patient demonstrated marked improvement in photodamage without postinflammatory hyperpigmentation. (**C**) Four-year follow-up with durable photorejuvenative effects.

for AKs, with the added benefit of addressing photoaging. Clearance of AK lesions with PDT is superior from a cosmetic standpoint compared with conventional treatments such as liquid nitrogen (72). In terms of patient satisfaction with PDT, a study by Tierney and colleagues followed 39 patients treated with ALA-PDT (71). In this study, patients reported statistically significant better recovery compared with other treatments, including cryotherapy or surgical excision. A borderline statistically significant improvement was achieved with PDT for overall cosmetic outcome and patient satisfaction compared with other therapies. Morton (198) also found that patients preferred the overall treatment procedure and cosmetic outcome of ALA-PDT compared with cryotherapy. Patient satisfaction was high in the stage III clinical trial by Piacquadio et al. (78) Ninety-four percent of patients thought the cosmetic results following PDT were good to excellent.

TOPICAL PHOTODYNAMIC THERAPY FOR INFLAMMATORY AND INFECTIOUS DERMATOSES

Acne Vulgaris

Acne results from the obstruction and inflammation of the sebaceous glands, and it affects 80% of the human population. The pathogenic mechanisms of acne are complex and include epithelial hyperproliferation, follicular plugging with formation of comedones, increased sebum production by sebaceous glands, inflammation, and the presence and proliferation of *Propionibacterium acnes* within the follicle (199). Acne typically begins in adolescence with hormonal changes and more often affects males, but in 30% of women can persist during the entire fertile period (200). There are several different presentations of acne ranging from comedonal (blackheads and whiteheads), papular, pustular, and cystic acne. In many cases, many of these presentations of acne can be present on an individual simultaneously.

The firstline treatments for acne vulgaris are conventional topical and/or oral medications. However, many patients have

contraindications, partial response, or significant adverse effects. Oral isotretinoin is the current most effective treatment that is known to reduce 80–90% of the acne lesions after 4 months of treatment (201,202); however, despite its undeniable effectiveness isotretinoin is not a curative drug. Relapse within 2 years may be seen in up to half of the patients that will require two or more courses of treatment (203,204). Besides, its use is associated with many side effects, some of which can be very serious. The most important issue is its teratogenicity, but common adverse events include dry skin/lips, ophthalmologic and gastrointestinal symptoms, and headaches. Laboratory abnormalities have been described, warranting adequate monitoring of liver functions and serum lipids (205). In addition, bone mineralization abnormalities (206) and depression (207) have been reported. PDT and light-based treatments can offer alternative treatments for acne with their own advantages and disadvantages.

PDT may promote acne improvement via antibacterial activity against *P. acnes*, selective damage to sebaceous glands, reduction of follicular obstruction and hyperkeratosis, and via immunologic host responses (208,209). Visible light is able to activate natural endogenous porphyrins produced by *P. acnes*, generating ROS that destroy the bacteria (209). Therefore, it is expected that topical application of ALA, producing additional porphyrins, makes the combination more effective than light alone (210).

A variety of light sources for the treatment of acne with PDT have been studied, including noncoherent red and blue light, PDL, IPL, and a combination of these.

Hongcharu and colleagues (211) first described the efficacy of topical ALA followed by light exposure (20% ALA 3 hours, 550–700 nm, 150 J/cm^2) for acne on the back of 22 subjects in a randomized controlled study. Porphyrin fluorescence, sebum output, and acne severity were measured at baseline and at intervals after treatment. Histologic examinations have demonstrated vacuolization of sebocytes and keratinocytes followed by sustained atrophic glands, granulomatous reaction, and perifollicular fibrosis up to 3 weeks after irradiation. Significant improvement in inflammatory acne was observed for 10 weeks after a single treatment and for at least 20 weeks after four treatments. Both sebum excretion and bacterial porphyrin fluorescence were decreased with sustained reduction of sebum output for at least 20 weeks of follow-up.

Another study conducted by Itoh and colleagues (212) using lower fluence red light (600–700 nm, 17 mW/cm^2, total dose of 13 J/cm^2) and 20% topical ALA under occlusion for 4 hours reported improvement of acne lesions in 13/13 patients treated with one session. Recurrence of lesions started after 3–6 months, suggesting that one session might not be enough for sustained results.

Since then, several open studies report a clinical benefit of ALA-PDT in facial acne with application times varying from 0.25 to 4 hours and a variety of light sources, including blue light, IPL, and PDL. Unfortunately, reports of these studies are difficult to compare because of protocol variations with small number of patients, short follow-up periods, and variable light dosimetry. Table 10.6 provides a summary of peer-reviewed articles on the use of ALA- and MAL-PDT in acne treatment.

PDT with Blue Light

The blue light-PDT studies for acne treatment demonstrated a range of 25–75% decrease in inflammatory lesions (213–215) compared with the lower response (25% reduction) in patients treated with blue light alone (214). A pilot study conducted by Taub (213) treated 18 patients with two to four treatments using short-contact ALA 20% (15–30 minutes) followed by illumination with blue light or electro-optical synergy or both. Eleven of these patients had at least 50% improvement and acne lesions have not recurred in five patients for at least 6 months of follow-up.

Goldman and Boyce (214) compared blue light with and without 20% ALA in 22 patients with mild-to-moderate acne. Patients were treated twice with short-contact ALA-PDT/blue light (15 minutes incubation) at 2 week intervals, whereas patients in the blue light alone treatment group received two treatments at 1-week interval. Reductions in papule count from baseline were 68% in patients treated with ALA-PDT/blue light versus 40% in the blue light alone group.

A split-face study by Akaraphanth et al. (215) compared 1-hour incubation with 10% ALA blue light PDT versus blue light treatment alone. Twenty patients received four sessions at 1-week intervals. At 16 weeks after first treatment, the mean percent reduction of inflammatory lesions tended to be higher in the ALA-PDT group: 71.1% versus 56.7% in the blue light treatment alone; however, it did not reach statistical significance. It is possible that the lower concentration of ALA used in the study and the short incubation time contributed to those results.

Photodynamic Therapy with Intense Pulsed Light

In 2004, Gold and colleagues (216) treated 15 patients with moderate to severe inflammatory acne with 1 hour of 20% ALA incubation followed by IPL (430–1100 nm at 39 J/cm^2) for four treatments per week. The authors reported clinical improvement in 12/15 patients, with a 71.8% reduction in inflammatory lesions after 12 weeks. Subsequently, Gold and colleagues (217) evaluated 15 patients treated with four

sessions of ALA-PDT, 2 weeks apart, using a pulsed light source (420–950 nm) and a short incubation of 15–30 minutes with 20% ALA. The total reductions of inflammatory and noninflammatory lesion counts were 54.5% and 37.5%, respectively, after 11 weeks.

Rojanamatin and Choawawanich (218) performed a split-face study in Thai patients, using IPL (550–700 nm) and 20% ALA. Fourteen patients received three sessions of IPL on one side and a combination of short contact (30 minutes incubation) ALA and IPL on the other side. There were very few adverse events and they observed a statistically significant improvement (87.7% vs. 66.8%) in lesion counts 3 months after the last treatment for ALA-PDT and IPL only, respectively. In another split-face study conducted by Santos and colleagues (219), 20% ALA was incubated for 3 hours on half of the face, followed by IPL (560–1200 nm) irradiation to the whole face. Thirteen patients were treated with two sessions at 2-week interval. At 8 weeks after initial treatment, 10/13 patients presented greater improvement in the ALA-PDT side compared with the side treated with IPL alone, however, results were evaluated by a subjective grading system and lesion counts were not reported.

Taub (220) compared the efficacies of IPL (680–850 nm), combination radiofrequency and IPL (580–980 nm), and blue light (417 nm) for activating ALA-induced PpIX for the treatment of acne vulgaris. All three groups used 30-minute incubation with 20% ALA and received three treatments at 2-week intervals. They found that IPL-PDT group was superior to blue light group, although the differences did not reach a statistical significance. The author attributed these results to IPL's deeper penetration in the dermis compared with blue light.

Surprisingly, Yeung and colleagues (221) found that MAL-PDT using IPL and MAL in Asians did not lead to significant improvement of moderate inflammatory acne compared with the control group. It should be noted that a short incubation time (30 minutes) of 16% MAL cream was used and a relatively small sample size (23 Chinese patients) was evaluated. They received four treatment sessions at 3 week intervals in a randomized half-facial treatment study with IPL (530–750 nm) alone, IPL with PDT or as controls. The mean reduction of the inflammatory lesion count was 65% in the PDT group, 23% in the IPL group, and 88% in control group at 12 weeks after last treatment. Significant reductions of noninflammatory lesions were observed in the MAL-PDT group (38%) and IPL group (43%) compared with 15% increase in the control group though.

In 2009, a randomized half-facial treatment study by Oh and colleagues (222) compared two different incubation times (30 minutes and 3 hours) in 20 Korean patients with moderate-to-severe acne. Three sessions at 1-month intervals were performed, with short incubation of 20% ALA plus IPL (590 nm cutoff filter) or long incubation with ALA plus IPL on one side of the face and IPL alone on the other side. At 12 weeks after the third session, the reduction of inflammatory acne lesions was greater in the long incubation time group than the short incubation time group or the IPL-alone group, but this difference was statistically significant only between the long incubation group and the IPL-only group. The authors believe that those results could be due to the small subject size or different number of inflammatory lesions in each group before treatment. Moreover, the mean reduction of inflammatory acne lesions in the short incubation time was not statistically

Table 10.6 Published Clinical Studies on ALA- and MAL-PDT for Acne Vulgaris

Reference	Photosensitizer/ Duration/ Study Design	Location/ Pretreatment	Number of Sessions	# Patients	Light Source (Emission λ, nm)	Response	Follow-up (wk)
Hongcharu (212) (2000)	20% ALA, 3 hr occlusion/3 test sites and 1 control site on back per patient (ALA-PDT, red light only, control); 2 randomized groups: 1 vs. 4 sessions (1 wk apart)	Back/70% isopropyl alcohol	1 vs. 4	22	Broad-spectrum (550–700 nm, 150 J/cm²)	Only ALA-PDT showed significant reduction in inflammatory lesions, 4 sessions better than 1	20
Itoh (213) (2001)	20% ALA, 4 hr occlusion	Face/not mentioned	1	13	Broad-spectrum (600–700 nm, 17 mW/cm², 13 J/cm²)	100% with some improvement, new lesions after 3–6 mo	24
Goldman (215) (2003)	20% ALA, 15 min/ blue light only vs. ALA-PDT	Face/2% salicylic acid cleanser	2 Sessions of blue light alone weekly, 2 sessions of ALA-PDT at 2 wk-intervals	22 (12 blue light vs. 10 ALA-PDT)	Blue light (417 nm)	68% Decrease of papules in the ALA-PDT vs. 40% decrease in the blue light alone	2 wk after last treatment
Pollock (210) (2004)	20% ALA, 3 hr occlusion/3 test sites and 1 control site on back per patient (ALA-PDT, red light only, control)	Back/not mentioned	3, 1 wk apart	10	Diode laser (635 nm, 25 mW cm², 15 J cm²)	Significant reduction of mean acne lesions count (69%) in the ALA-PDT site only	3 wk after last treatment
Gold (217) (2004)	20% ALA, 1 hr	Face/Cetaphil cleanser	4 (1 wk apart)	15	IPL (430–1100 nm, 3–9 J/cm²)	3 Patients did not respond, 12 patients had 71.8% reduction in acne lesions	12
Taub (214) (2004)	20% ALA, 15–30 min	Face, back and chest/acetone scrub and alcohol scrub	2–4 (4–8 wk apart)	18	Blue light (417 nm) or IPL (400–980 nm, 18–25 J/cm² + radiofrequency)	5 Patients did not improve, 11 had at least 50% improvement	Average follow-up time of 4 mo
Hong (226) (2005)	20% ALA, 4 hr under occlusion/ split-face ALA-PDT vs. controls	Face/not mentioned	1	8	Halogen lamp red light (630 ± 63 nm, 30 mW/cm², 18 J/cm²)	41.9% (treated) vs. 15.4% (control) reduction of inflamed lesions at 6 mo	6 mo

Santos (220) (2005)	20% ALA, 3 hr/ split-face: IPL alone vs. IPL+ALA	Face/not mentioned	2 (2 wk apart)	13	IPL cutoff filter, 560 nm, 26–34 J/cm²	Improvement significantly higher in ALA-PDT side: 10/13 had good or excellent results vs. IPL only: 3/13 had good results at 8 wk	8 wk
Rojanamatin (219) (2006)	20% ALA, 30 min under occlusion/ split-face IPL + placebo vs. IPL + ALA	Face/soap and water	3 (3–4 wk apart)	14	IPL cutoff filter 560–590 nm, 25–30 J/cm²	IPL + ALA: 87.7% vs. IPL + placebo: 66.8% reduction of inflammatory lesions	12 wk
Alexiades-Armenakas (224) (2006)	20% ALA, 45 min/ ALA topical + LPDL or blue light vs. LPDL only vs. conventional therapy. Superficial chemical peels in 6 patients (2 control and 4 ALA-LPDL)	Face/Cetaphil cleanser	1–6 (monthly)	19: 1 ALA + blue, 14 ALA+LPDL, 4 control (2 LPDL only and 2 conventional therapy)	LPDL (595 nm, 7–7.5 J/cm², 6–10 msec, 10 mm spot size, blue light	ALA+LPDL: 77% clearance rate per treatment vs. LPDL only: 32% vs. conventional therapy: 20%	13 mo
Wiegell (229) (2006)	16.8% MAL, 3 hr under occlusion/ treatment × control group	Face/curettage	2 (2 wk apart)	31 (19 treatment vs. 12 control)	Noncoherent red (630 nm), 37 J/cm²	MAL-PDT: 68% reduction of inflammatory lesions vs. 0% in control	12 wk
Wiegell (228) (2006)	Split-face 20% ALA vs. 16.8% MAL, 3 hr under occlusion	Face/not mentioned	1	15	Noncoherent red (630 nm), 37 J/cm², 34 mW/cm²	59% reduction of inflammatory lesions for both MAL and ALA	12 wk
Hörfelt (227) (2006)	16.8% MAL, 3 hr under occlusion/ split-face treatment × control group	Face/nodular lesions were prepared using a cannula (1–2 mm)	2 (2 wk apart)	30	Noncoherent red (630 nm), 37 J/cm²	MAL-PDT-side: 54% clearance of inflammatory vs. control-side: 20%	10 wk after last treatment
Gold (218) (2007)	20% ALA, 15–30 min	Face/cleanser	4 (2 wk apart)	15	IPL (420–950 nm), 5–7 J/cm², 30–50 msec	54.5% reduction of inflammatory lesions	11 wk

(Continued)

Table 10.6 Published Clinical Studies on ALA- and MAL-PDT for Acne Vulgaris (Continued)

Reference	Photosensitizer/ Duration/ Study Design	Location/ Pretreatment	Number of Sessions	# Patients	Light Source (Emission λ, nm)	Response	Follow-up (wk)
Akaraphanth (216) (2007)	10% ALA in acne spots, 1 hr/ split-face blue light + ALA vs. blue light alone	Face/not mentioned	4 (1 wk apart)	20	Blue LED (409–410 nm), 48 J/cm², 40 mW/cm²	Blue + ALA: 71.1% reduction of inflammatory lesions vs. blue light alone: 56.7%; (no statistical difference)	16
Yeung (222) (2007)	16.8% MAL, 30 min/split-face MAL + IPL, IPL alone or control (ratio of 1:2:1); all patients used 0.1% adapalene during the study	Face/soap followed by alcohol scrub	4 (3 wk apart)	23 (11 with MAL-PDT)	IPL (530–750 nm), 7–9 J/cm²	MAL-PDT: 65% reduction of inflammatory lesions vs. IPL: 23% vs. control: 88% (no statistical difference)	3 mo after last treatment
Hörfelt (230) (2007)	20% ALA, 3 hr/ split-area with different light doses	Face and back/not mentioned	1	14 (9 Cheek, 5 Back)	Noncoherent red (600–730 nm), 50 mW/cm², 50 or 30 J/cm² (cheek); 50 or 70 J/cm² (back)	No difference in clinical results between the 2 doses for face and back, 8/9 patients with face acne had some improvement	10 (cheek) and 20 wk (back)
Oh (222) (2009)	20% ALA/split-face 30 min or 3 hr incubation ALA-IPL vs. IPL only	Face/soap and 70% alcohol	3 (4 wk apart)	20	IPL cutoff filter 590 nm, 12–15 J/cm²	Clearance of 89.5% (3 hr), 83% (30 min), and 74% (IPL only). Long incubation group and IPL-only group were statistically different	12 wk after last treatment
Yin (230) (2010)	5%, 10%, 15%, and 20% ALA, 1.5 hr occlusion/ split-face ALA-PDT vs. placebo- red light cm²	Face/70% isopropyl alcohol	4 (10 days apart)	180	Red light (633 ± 3 nm), 126 J/cm²	Statistically significantly more patient treated with 20% ALA achieved complete clearance, no statistical difference between 15 and 20% at 12 wk or more.	24 wk

Abbreviations. ALA, aminolevulinic acid; IPL, intense pulsed light; LED, light-emitting diode; LPDL, long-pulsed dye laser; MAL, methyl aminolevulinic acid; PDT, photodynamic therapy.

different from the IPL-alone group, suggesting that 30 minutes is not sufficient incubation time before PDT in acne patients. It should be noted that prolonged incubation time did not result in more adverse effects than in the short incubation time group.

Photodynamic Therapy with Pulsed Dye Lasers

A randomized controlled trial conducted by Hædersdal and colleagues (223) compared MAL-Long-pulsed dye laser (LPDL) to LPDL alone in 15 patients treated with three sessions at 2 week intervals. Twelve patients completed the study and were found to present significantly greater reduction in inflammatory lesions on the MAL-LPDL side versus the LPDL-alone side (80% vs. 67%, respectively) at 12 weeks after the final treatment.

Alexiades-Armenakas (224) treated 14 patients with 20% ALA with 45 minutes incubation time followed by activation with LPDL (595 nm, 7–7.5 J/cm^2, 10 ms, 10 mm spot size). Patients received 1–6 monthly treatments and were maintained on topical regimen. Complete clearance was achieved in 100% (14/14 patients) with a mean of 2.9 treatments required to achieve complete clearance for a mean follow-up time of 6.4 months. Moreover, a reduction in the erythema in erythematous acne scars was observed.

PDT with Red Light Sources

The studies (78,211,225) investigating red light have demonstrated an overall range of 20–69% reduction of acne lesions. Hong and Lee (225) performed a split-face study in eight patients comparing the use of red light (630 ± 63 nm, 30 mW/cm^2, and 18 J/cm^2) plus 20% ALA incubated for 4 hours to red light alone. Six months after one treatment, the authors reported a 41.9% reduction in inflammatory lesions on the red light plus ALA side and a 15.4% reduction on the red light side alone. Hörtfelt and colleagues (226) compared MAL-pretreated red light (3 hours occlusion, 635 nm, and 37 J/cm^2) therapy to red light treatment alone in 27 patients. After two treatment sessions, the authors found 54% and 20% reductions in inflammatory lesion on the red light plus MAL side and red light alone side, respectively. The improvement observed in the placebo/red light side was attributed to activation of endogenous porphyrins leading to photoinactivation of *P. acnes*.

Wiegell and Wulf (227) conducted a randomized controlled investigator-blinded study with 15 patients to compare the efficacy and tolerability of ALA-PDT versus MAL-PDT. MAL and ALA were applied to each half of the face for 3 hours, followed by illumination with red light (635 nm, 34 mW/cm^2, 37 J/cm^2). Thirteen patients completed the study and presented at 12 weeks follow-up similar response rates for the two treatment regimens (59% reductions in inflammatory lesions). The two treatments were equally painful during illumination but ALA-PDT resulted in more prolonged and severe adverse effects after treatment. A previous study by Wiegell and Wulf (228) had treated 21 patients with two MAL-PDT sessions at 2-week intervals. Approximately 2 g of MAL cream was applied to the face and occluded for 3 hours followed by illumination with red light (635 nm, 37 J/cm^2). After 12 weeks, there was a reduction of inflammatory lesions of 68% in the PDT group versus 0% in the control group (who received no treatment). It should be noted that seven patients were unable to undergo the second treatment due to side effects.

Another study by Hörtfel and colleagues (229) aimed to determine the optimal light dose for effective PDT treatment of acne and mechanism of action. Fifteen patients with mild-to-severe acne were treated with 20% ALA cream occluded for 3 hours followed by illumination with red light (635 nm). A light dose of 30 J/cm^2 was used on the left cheek and 50 J/cm^2 on the right cheek. At 10 weeks of clinical follow-up, the authors found that the improvement of lesions was the same for the two light doses and no significant reduction in *P. acnes* or sebum excretion was found at any time after PDT. Therefore, the authors theorize that other mechanisms of actions should be considered such as effect on infiltrating inflammatory cells around the acne lesion or decrease of follicular obstruction by affecting keratinocyte shedding and hyperkeratosis as suggested by Hongcharu and colleagues (211).

A recent study conducted by Yin and colleagues (230) compared the efficacy and safety of different ALA concentrations in 180 Chinese patients. Patients received four sessions (10 days apart) using different concentrations (5%, 10%, 15%, and 20%) of ALA (1.5 hour occlusion) on one side and placebo on the other side as control followed by irradiation with red light (633 ± 3 nm, 126 J/cm^2). The authors found a significant statistical difference among the four groups with different ALA concentrations, with a clear positive correlation between global improvement scores and ALA concentration. However, there was no statistical difference in clinical outcomes between 15% and 20% ALA at 12 weeks of follow-up or more. Regarding side effects, particularly hyperpigmentation was positively correlated to the ALA concentration. Therefore, the authors suggest that 10% and 15% ALA for 1.5 hours and red light source should provide ideal treatment for moderate-to-severe acne in patients with Fitzpatrick skin type III and IV.

Adverse Reactions and Summary of Findings for ALA- and MAL-PDT for Acne Vulgaris

Both ALA and MAL have shown effective with PDT for the treatment of acne. The most prevalent side effects reported in the studies were erythema, edema, and pain at the time of the treatment. Other adverse reactions reported include crusting (214,215), photosensitivity following posttreatment sun exposure (214,224), pustular eruptions (223,228), and postinflammatory hyperpigmentation (219,221).

In conclusion, PDT has shown safety and efficacy in the treatment of inflammatory acne vulgaris with many effective light sources and photosensitizers. Unfortunately, PDT has been limited by the fact that both the cost of the medicine and the cost of the laser or light procedure must be borne by the patient. Clinicians should use topical PDT in the treatment of acne particularly for those patients who are refractory to standard therapy, who have been on numerous medical therapies in the past and who are looking for clinical results to occur at a faster time interval. Further studies are warranted to establish consensus for optimal photosensitizer, ideal concentration, incubation time, activating light source, and frequency of treatment.

CLINICAL TECHNIQUE

Our treatment protocol using ALA-PDT for acne vulgaris involves the same steps described above for AKs and photorejuvenation except that we use longer incubation times

(120–180 minutes). We also use red LED (633 ± 5 nm) in addition to the blue light because sebaceous glands are deeply located, approximately 0.5–1.0 mm from the cutaneous surface (231). Therefore, PDL is used to target individual lesions at subpurpuric settings, followed by blue and red light irradiation.

Figure 10.19 illustrates a case of acne vulgaris after one session of ALA-PDT.

Vulgar Warts and Genital Warts

Although many therapeutic modalities for viral warts exist, sometimes the human papillomavirus causes highly refractory skin disorders. Original guidelines reported clearance rates of 56–100% (232). Fabbrocini and colleagues conducted a controlled study with 64 plantar warts treated with 20% ALA under occlusion for 5 hours (400–700 nm, peaking at 630 nm, 50 J/cm²), while 57 lesions (controls) received only the vehicle (233). Pretreatment with an ointment containing 10% urea and 10% salicylic acid was applied for 7 days to remove the superficial hyperkeratotic layer of the warts. All lesions were treated once and repeated weekly if required for a maximum of three sessions. After two months, the authors found 75% clearance rate in the ALA-PDT group compared with 22% reduction in the untreated warts. A comparison study with ALA-PDT using either PDL or LED versus PDL alone (ALA 3 hours, PDL at 595 nm and 20 J/cm², LED at 635 nm and 50 J/cm²) found that a combination of PDT and PDL is the most effective, with clearance rates of 100% (mean 1.96 treatments), 96% (mean 2.54 treatments), and 81% (mean 3.34 treatments), respectively (234). It should be noted that the verruca was curetted until visible bleeding occurred before ALA gel was applied.

Successful treatment of periungueal warts was reported by Schroeter and colleagues with complete clearance in 90% of warts after a mean of 4.5 treatments (235). Forty periungueal and subungueal warts were pretreated with scalpel curettage 48 hours before the application of 20% ALA, with a mean incubation time of 4.6 hours. Irradiation with light at 580–720 nm with 100 mW/cm² for 5–30 minutes was used in the study. During the follow-up of 5.9 months, only two recurrences were observed.

PDT results for the treatment of genital warts in case series and comparison trials reported clearance rates varying from 66% to 73% (236,237). A large study with 164 patients with urethral condylomata reported 95% clearance rate after one to four sessions with ALA-PDT (10% ALA, 3 hours incubation, 630 nm, 100 J/cm², 100 mW/cm²) (238). High remission rates were also reported by Chen and colleagues (239) in the treatment of condylomatas of the urethra and external genitalia. They compared ALA-PDT (20% ALA, 3 hours incubation, 633 nm, 100 J/cm², 100 mW/cm²) with conventional carbon dioxide (CO_2) laser in 86 patients and found 100% clearance after two PDT treatments and one CO_2 laser treatment, respectively. Moreover, during follow-up of 12 weeks, they found a recurrence rate of 6.3% and 19.1% for the ALA-PDT and CO_2 laser, respectively, which was significantly different between these two groups ($P < 0.05$). However, disappointing results of PDT were seen in 175 patients with condylomata acuminate treated with CO_2 laser vaporization plus adjuvant ALA-PDT or adjuvant placebo-PDT (240). This prospective, randomized, double-blind study compared 20% ALA or placebo ointment applied to the lesion, 4–6 hours before CO_2 laser vaporization, followed by red light (600–740 nm, 100 mW/cm², 100 J/cm²).

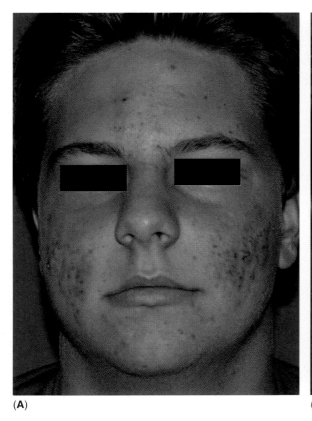
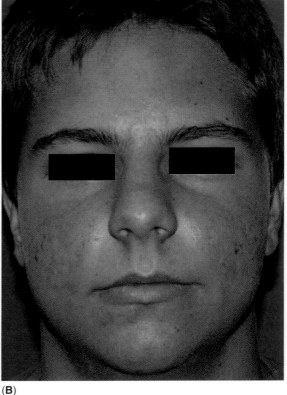

(A)   **(B)**

Figure 10.19 Patient with acne vulgaris (**A**) at baseline and (**B**) 3 months after one session of aminolevulinic acid-photodynamic therapy showing significant improvement of inflammatory papules and pustules.

They found no significant difference (50% in the ALA-PDT group vs. 52.7% in the placebo-PDT group) between groups with regard to recurrence rates up to 12 months after treatment. Interestingly, use of an ablative CO_2 fractional laser for removing the upper parts of hyperkeratotic wart lesions followed by MAL application showed 100% clearance in 90% of lesions after a mean of 2.2 treatments (241). Thus, perhaps use of MAL or ALA ointment applied after CO_2 laser ablation of the lesion should allow better penetration of the drug and allow enhanced efficacy of PDT in the treatment of warts.

Therefore, topical PDT appears to be a potential resource against viral warts. It is a safe and wart-selective therapy, leaving excellent esthetic results. The treatment, however, is time-consuming for patients, requires the use of a keratolytic agent pre-PDT and it can be very painful as well.

Psoriasis Vulgaris

Limited evidence indicates PDT to be of benefit for psoriasis (242). A small study of four patients comparing topical PDT (20% ALA, 4 hours under occlusion, 630 nm, 10 J/cm², 120 mW/cm²) with narrowband UV-B therapy showed that topical PDT was inferior in inducing clinical response and remission and was poorly tolerated by patients because of pain (243).

Schleyer and colleagues (244) conducted a randomized, double-blind intrapatient comparison study in 12 patients with psoriasis treated with 0.1%, 1%, and 5% ALA (4–6 hours under occlusion, 600–740 nm, 20 J/cm², 60 mW/cm²) and found limited mean improvement of 37.5%, 45.6%, and 51.2%, respectively. Furthermore, irradiation had to be interrupted several times because of severe burning and pain sensation.

Apparently, good results were achieved in a dose-ranging PDT study with a single oral dose of 5–15 mg/kg ALA and irradiation with blue light, 1–6 hours after ALA administration (245). Improvement was noted in the 15 mg/kg group only, with a 42% reduction in plaque severity compared with baseline. In contrast to topical ALA-PDT, tolerability was excellent, with no patient complaining about pain during systemic PDT.

Overall, topical PDT does not appear to be a practical therapy for psoriasis, due to the disappointing clinical response, very slow improvement and unpredictable occurrence of pain related to irradiation.

OTHER INDICATIONS

Topical PDT has been studied in many other dermatologic conditions that are beyond the scope of this chapter. Other oncologic cutaneous conditions studied include cutaneous lymphoma T-cell lymphoma (CTCL) with case reports and case series (246,247) showing successful topical ALA- and MAL-PDT for early-stage localized CTCL after multiple treatment sessions and extramammary Paget's disease (EMPD). Although there are limited cases reported with high recurrence rates (248,249), PDT, particularly using systemic photosensitizers, might be a useful, surgery-sparing therapeutic option for management of noninvasive EMPD in selected patients.

In inflammatory skin diseases, modulation of cellular functions, rather than cell death, is the main mechanism of action. It appears that PDT is involved in a minor immunosuppression due to temporary suppression of Langerhans cells in the epidermis (250). In addition, transcription factors, especially AP-1, NfκB, and subsequently different cytokines are induced, which influence inflammatory cells within the epidermis and the dermis as well as fibroblasts (251,252). Case series and individual reports describe the potential of topical PDT in a variety of other indications that include localized scleroderma (253), lichen sclerosus (254), hidradenitis suppurativa (255), sarcoidosis (256), necrobiosis lipoidica (257), inflammatory linear verrucous epidermal nevus (258), among others.

Finally, there is evidence that topical PDT can be effective in cutaneous infectious disorders that include cutaneous leishmaniasis (259,260), recalcitrant molluscum contagiosum (261), and onychomycosis (262).

FUTURE DIRECTIONS

PDT, with a variety of lasers and light sources, is changing how many dermatologists and laser surgeons look at a variety of diseases/entities for which they are using the devices in their clinical practices. ALA- and MAL-PDT has found its niche in the treatment of photorejuvenation and associated AKs, if present. It has also found its niche in the treatment of moderate to severe inflammatory acne vulgaris. Other entities, including sebaceous gland hyperplasia and recalcitrant hidradenitis suppurativa are also being treated successfully and routinely with ALA-PDT. Superficial skin cancers and BD are also regularly treated with ALA- and MAL-PDT. More and more entities will continue to be studied with PDT and its use expanded in the next several years. The future for this type of therapy looks very bright.

CONCLUSION

PDT is a safe and effective treatment for nonhyperkeratotic lesions. Although FDA-approved for use with a blue and red light source, other laser and light sources have demonstrated promise in the treatment of AKs during PDT. Shorter incubation times maintain AK clearance rates but decrease the occurrence of phototoxic adverse events. With careful patient selection, PDT allows selective field treatment of precancerous skin lesions with improvement in overall photodamage. Patient satisfaction is high and cosmetic results can be excellent. Strong evidence confirms the high efficacy of topical PDT in BD, superficial BCC, and also in thin nBCC, following lesion preparation, as demonstrated by comparison studies.

REFERENCES

1. Raab O. Ueber die wirkung fluoreszierenden stoffe auf infusorien. Z Biol 1900; 39: 524–6.
2. Von Tappeiner H, Jodblauer A. Uber die wirkung der photodynamischen (fluorescierenden) staffe auf protozoan und enzyme. Dtsch Arch Klin Med 1904; 80: 427–87.
3. Jesionek A, Von Tappeiner H. Behandlung der hautcarcinome nut fluorescierenden stoffen. Dtsch Arch Klin Med 1905; 85: 223–7.
4. Meyer-Betz F. Untersuchungen uber die bioloische (photodynamische) wirkung des hamatoporphyrins und anderer derivative des blut-und gallenfarbstoffs. Dtsch Arch Klin Med 1913; 112: 476–503.
5. Auler H, Banzer G. Untersuchungen ueber die rolle der porphyrine bei geschwulstkranken menschen und tieren. Z Krebsforsch 1942; 53: 65–8.
6. Dougherty TJ, Kaufman JE, Goldfarb A, et al. Photoradiation therapy for the treatment of malignant tumors. Cancer Res 1978; 38: 2628–35.
7. Van Hillegersberg R, Kort WJ, Wilson JH. Current status of photodynamic therapy in oncology. Drugs 1994; 48: 510–27.

8. Evensen JF. The use of porphyrins and non-ionizing radiation for treatment of cancer. Acta Oncol 1995; 8: 1103–10.

9. Keller GS, Razum NJ, Doiron DR. Photodynamic therapy for non-melanoma skin cancer. Facial Plast Surg 1989; 6: 180–4.

10. Wilson BD, Mang TS, Stoll H, et al. Photodynamic therapy for the treatment of basal cell carcinoma. Arch Dermatol 1992; 128: 1597–601.

11. Sommer CA, Van Leengoed H, Conti CM, et al. Photodynamic therapy for cutaneous carcinomas using the second generation photosensitizer tin ethyl etiopurpurin (SnET2). Lasers Surg Med 1995; 7: 45.

12. Soret JL. Recherches sur l'absorption des rayons ultra violets par diverses substances. Arch Sci Phys Nat 1883; 10: 430–85.

13. Garbo GM. Purpurins and benzochlorins as sensitizers for photodynamic therapy. J Photochem Photobiol B 1996; 34: 109–16.

14. Lui H, Hobbs L, Tope WD, et al. Photodynamic therapy of multiple nonmelanoma skin cancers with verteporfin and red light-emitting diodes. Two-year results evaluating tumor response and cosmetic outcomes. Arch Dermatol 2004; 140: 26–32.

15. Kennedy JC, Pottier RH, Pross DC, et al. Photodynamic therapy with endogenous protoporphyrin IX: basic principles and present clinical experiences. J Photochem Photobiol B 1990; 6: 143–8.

16. Peng Q, Warloe T, Berg C, et al. 5-Aminolevulinic acid-based photodynamic therapy:clinical research and future challenges. Cancer 1997; 79: 2282–308.

17. Calzavara-Pinton PG, Venturini M, Sala R. Photodynamic therapy: update 2006. Part 1: Photochemistry and photobiology. JEADV 2007; 21: 293–302.

18. Nootheti PK, Goldman MP. Aminolevulinic acid-photodynamic therapy for photorejuvenation. Dermatol Clin 2007; 25: 35–45.

19. Ericson MB, Sandberg C, Stenquist B, et al. Photodynamic therapy of actinic keratosis at varying fluence rates: assessment of photobleaching, pain and primary clinical outcome. Br J Dermatol 2004; 151: 1204–12.

20. Nakaseko H, Kobayashi M, Akita Y, et al. Histological changes and involvement of apoptosis after photodynamic therapy for actinic keratoses. Br J Dermatol 2003; 148: 122–7.

21. Wolf P, Rieger E, Kerl H. Topical photodynamic therapy with endogenous porphyrins after application of 5-aminolevulinic acid. J Am Acad Dermatol 1993; 28: 17–21.

22. Touma D, Yaar M, Whitehead S, et al. A trial of short incubation, broad-area photodynamic therapy for facial actinic keratoses and diffuse photodamage. Arch Dermatol 2004; 140: 33–40.

23. Tsai T, Ji HT, Chiang PC, et al. ALA-PDT results in phenotypic changes and decreased cellular invasion in surviving cancer cells. Lasers Surg Med 2009; 41: 305–15.

24. Gad F, Viau G, Boushira M, Bertrand R, Bissonnette R. Photodynamic therapy with 5-aminolevulinic acid induces apoptosis and caspase activation in malignant T cells. J Cutan Med Surg 2001; 5: 8–13.

25. Kuzelova K, Grebenova D, Pluskalova M, Marinov I, Hrkal Z. Early apoptotic features of K562 cell death induced by 5-aminolaevulinic acid-based photodynamic therapy. J Photochem Photobiol B 2004; 73: 67–78.

26. Noodt BB, Berg K, Stokke T, Peng Q, Nesland JM. Apoptosis and necrosis induced with light and 5-aminolaevulinic acidderived protoporphyrin IX. Br J Cancer 1996; 74: 22–9.

27. Webber J, Luo Y, Crilly R, Fromm D, Kessel D. An apoptotic response to photodynamic therapy with endogenous protoporphyrin in vivo. J Photochem Photobiol B 1996; 35: 209–11.

28. Dougherty TJ, Gomer CJ, Henderson BW, et al. Photodynamic therapy. J Natl Cancer Inst 1998; 90: 889–905.

29. Henderson BW, Dougherty TJ. How does photodynamic therapy work? Photochem Photobiol 1992; 55: 145–57.

30. Wieman TJ, Fingar VH. Photodynamic therapy. Surg Clin North Am 1992; 72: 609–22.

31. Klausner JM, Paterson IS, Kobzik L, et al. Oxygen free radicals mediate ischemia-induced lung injury. Surgery 1989; 105: 192–9.

32. Doukas J, Hechtman HB, Shepro D. Vasoactive amines and eicosanoids interactively regulate both polymorphonuclear leukocyte diapedesis and albumin permeability in vitro. Microvasc Res 1989; 37: 125–37.

33. Gollnick SO, Liu X, Owczarczak B, Musser DA, Henderson BW. Altered expression of interleukin 6 and interleukin 10 as a result of photodynamic therapy in vivo. Cancer Res 1997; 57: 3904–9.

34. Korbelik M. Induction of tumor immunity by photodynamic therapy. J Clin Laser Med Surg 1996; 14: 329–34.

35. Canti G, Lattuada D, Nicolin A, et al. Antitumor immunity induced by photodynamic therapy with aluminium phthalocyanine and laser light. Anticancer Drugs 1994; 5: 443–7.

36. MacCormack MA. Photodynamic therapy in dermatology: An update on applications and outcomes. Semin Cutan Med Surg 2008; 27: 52–62.

37. Nestor MS, Gold MH, Kauvar ANB, et al. The use of photodynamic therapy in dermatology: Results of a consensus conference. J Drugs Dermatol 2006; 5: 140–54.

38. Product information (package insert): Levulan R Kerastick TM (aminolevulinic acid HCl) for topical solution, 20%. Wilmington, MA, USA: DUSA Pharmaceuticals, Inc, 2009.

39. Fotinos N, Campo MA, Popowycz F, et al. 5-aminolevulinic acid derivatives in photomedicine: characteristics, application and perspectives. Photochem Photobiol 2006; 82: 994–1015.

40. Kalka K, Merk H, Mukhtar H. Photodynamic therapy in dermatology. J Am Acad Dermatol 2000; 42: 389–413.

41. Gaullier JM, Berg K, Peng Q, et al. Use of 5-aminolevulinic acid esters to improve photodynamic therapy on cells in culture. Cancer Res 1997; 57: 1481–6.

42. Peng Q, Warloe T, Berg K, et al. 5-aminolevulinic acid-basedd photodynamic therapy. Cancer 1997; 79: 2282–308.

43. Kasche A, Luderschmidt S, Ring J, Hein R. Photodynamic therapy induces less pain in patients treated with methyl aminolevulinate compared to aminolevulinic acid. J Drugs Dermatol 2006; 5: 353–6.

44. Babilas P, Schreml S, Landthaler M, Szeimies RM. Photodynamic therapy in dermatology: state-of-the-art. Photodermatol Photoimmunol Photomed 2010; 26: 118–32; Review.

45. Zakhary K, Ellis DAF. Applications of aminolevulinic acid-based photodynamic therapy in cosmetic facial plastic practices. Facial Plast Surg 2005; 21: 110–16.

46. Clark C, Bryden A, Dawe R, et al. Topical 5-aminolevulinic acid photodynamic therapy for cutaneous lesions: outcome and comparison of light sources. Photodermatol Photoimmunol Photomed 2003; 19: 134–41.

47. DeHoratius DM, Dover JS. Nonablative tissue remodeling and photorejuvenation. Clin Dermatol 2007; 25: 474–9.

48. Markham T, Collins P. Topical 5-aminolaevulinic acid photodynamic therapy for extensive scalp actinic keratoses. Br J Dermatol 2001; 145: 502–4.

49. Kalisiak MS, Rao J. Photodynamic therapy for actinic keratoses. Dermatol Clin 2007; 25: 15–23.

50. Gold MH. Pharmacoeconomic analysis of the treatment of multiple actinic keratoses. J Drugs Dermatol 2008; 7: 23–5.

51. Stockfleth E, Kerl H. Guidelines for the management of actinic keratoses. Eur J Dermatol 2006; 16: 599–606.

52. Lehmann P. Methyl aminolaevulinate-photodynamic therapy: A review of clinical trials in the treatment of actinic keratoses and nonmelanoma skin cancer. Br J Dermatol 2007; 156: 793–801.

53. Berking C, Herzinger T, Flaig MJ, et al. The efficacy of photodynamic therapy in actinic cheilitis of the lower lip: a prospective study of 15 patients. Dermatol Surg 2007; 33: 825–30.

54. Marks R. Epidemiology of nonmelanoma skin cancer and solar keratoses in Australia: a tale of self-immolation in Elysian fields. Australas J Dermatol 1997; 38: S26–9.

55. Diepgen TL, Mahler V. The epidemiology of skin cancer. Br J Dermatol 2002; 146: 1–6.

56. Osborne JE. Skin cancer screening and surveillance. Br J Dermatol 2002; 146: 745–54.

57. Marks R, Rennie G, Selwood TS. Malignant transformation of solar keratoses to squamous cell carcinoma. Lancet 1988; 1: 795–7.

58. Glogau RG. The risk of progression to invasive disease. J Am Acad Dermatol 2000; 42: 23–4.

59. Czarnecki D, Meehan CJ, Bruce F, Culjak G. The majority of cutaneous squamous cell carcinomas arise in actinic keratoses. J Cutan Med Surg 2002; 6: 207–9.

60. Cockerell CJ, Wharton JR. New histopathological classification of actinic keratosis (incipient intraepithelial squamous cell carcinoma). J Drugs Dermatol 2005; 4: 462–7.

61. Ortonne JP. From actinic keratoses to squamous cell carcinoma. Br J Dermatol 2002; 146: S20–3.

62. Hurwitz RM, Monger LE. Solar keratosis: an evolving squamous cell carcinoma. Benign or malignant? Dermatol Surg 1995; 21: 184.

63. Moy RL. Clinical presentation of actinic keratoses and squamous cell carcinoma. J Am Acad Dermatol 2000; 42: 8–10.

64. Bäumler W, Wetzig T. Clinical application of fluorescence diagnosis. In: Goldman MP, Dover JS, Alam M, eds. Procedures in Cosmetic Dermatology: Photodynamic Therapy, 2nd edn. Philadelphia, PA: Elsevier, 2008: 149–60.

65. Salasche SJ. Epidemiology of actinic keratoses and squamous cell carcinoma. J Am Acad Dermatol 2000; 42: 4–7.

66. Cockerell CJ. Histopathology of incipient intraepidermal squamous cell carcinoma ("actinic keratosis"). J Am Acad Dermatol 2000; 42: 11–17.

67. Tschen EH, Wong DS, Pariser DM, et al. Photodynamic therapy using aminolaevulinic acid for patients with nonhyperkeratotic actinic keratoses of the face and scalp: phase IV mulicentre clinical trial with 12-month follow up. Br J Dermatol 2006; 155: 1262–9.

68. Jeffes EW, McCullough JL, Weinstein GD, et al. Photodynamic therapy of actinic keratoses with topical aminolevulinic acid hydrochloride and fluorescent blue light. J Am Acad Dermatol 2001; 45: 96–104.

69. Szeimies RM, Karrer S, Radakovic-Fijan S, et al. Photodynamic therapy using topical methyl 5-aminolevulinate compared with cryotherapy for actinic keratosis: a prospective, randomized study. J Am Acad Dermatol 2002; 47: 258–62.

70. Kurwa HA, Yong-Gee SA, Seed PT, et al. A randomized paired comparison of photodynamic therapy and topical 5-fluorouracil in the treatment of actinic keratoses. J Am Acad Dermatol 1999; 41: 414–18.

71. Tierney EP, Eide MJ, Jacobsen G, Ozog D. Photodynamic therapy for actinic keratoses: survey of patient perceptions of treatment satisfaction and outcomes. J Cosmet Laser Ther 2008; 10: 81–6.

72. Goldman MP, Atkin DH. ALA/PDT in the treatment of actinic keratosis: spot versus confluent therapy. J Cosmet Laser Ther 2003; 5: 107–10.

73. Alexiades-Amenakas MR, Geronemus RG. Laser-mediated photodynamic therapy of actinic keratoses. Arch Dermatol 2003; 139: 1313–20.

74. Kennedy JC, Pottier RH, Pross DC. Photodynamic thereapy with endogenous protoporphyrin IX: basic priniciples and present clnical experience. J Photochem Photobiol Biol B 1990; 6: 143–8.

75. Dijkstra AT, Majoie IML, van Dongen JWF, van Weelden H et al. Photodynamic therapy with violet light and topical δ-aminolaevulinic acid in the treatment of actinic keratosis, Bowen's disease and basal cell carcinoma. J Eur Acad Dermatol Venereol 2001; 15: 550–554.

76. Ross EV, Anderson RR. Laser-tissue interactions. In: Goldman MP, ed. Cutaneous and Cosmetic Laser Surgery. Philadelphia, PA: Elsevier, 2006: 1–26.

77. Ormrod D, Jarvis B. Topical aminolevulinic acid HCl photodynamic therapy. Am J Clin Dermatol 2000; 2: 133–9.

78. Piacquadio DJ, Chen DM, Farber HF, et al. Photodynamic therapy with aminolevulinic acid topical solution and visible blue light ini the treatment of multiple actinic keratoses of the face and scalp: investigator-blinded, phase 3, multicenter trials. Arch Dermatol 2004; 140: 41–6.

79. Gold MH. The evolving role of aminolevulinic acid hydrochloride with photodynamic therapy in photoaging. Cutis 2002; 69: 8–13.

80. Fritsch C, Stege H, Saalmann G, et al. Green light is effective and less painful than red light in photodynamic therapy of facial solar keratoses. Photodermatol Photoimmunol Photomed 1997; 13: 181–5.

81. Smith S, Piacquadio D, Morhenn V, Atkin D. Short incubation PDT versus 5-FU in treating actinic keratoses. J Drugs Dermatol 2003; 2: 629–35.

82. Jeffes WJ, McCullagh JL, Weinstein GD, et al. Photodynamic therapy of actinic keratosis with topical 5-aminolaevulinic acid. Arch Dermatol 1997; 133: 727–32.

83. Nakano A, Tamada Y, Watanabe D, Ishida N et al. A pilot study to assess teh efficacy of photodynamic therapy for Japanese patients with actinic keratosis in relation to lesion size and histological severity. Photodermatol Photoimmunol Photomed 2009; 25: 37–40.

84. Karrer S, Bäumler W, Abels C, et al. Long-pulse dye laser for photodynamic therapy: investigations in vitro and in vivo. Lasers Surg Med 1999; 25: 51–9.

85. Itoh Y, Nineomiya Y, Henta T, et al. Topcal delta-aminolevulinic acid-based photodynamic therapy for Japanese actinic keratoses. J Dermatol 2000; 27: 513–18.

86. Varma S, Wilson H, Kurwa HA, et al. Bowen's disease, solar keratoses and superficial basal cell carcinomas treated by photodynamic therapy using a large-field incoherent light source. Br J Dermatol 2001; 144: 56–574.

87. Kim HS, Yoo JY, Cho KH, et al. Topical photodynamic therapy using intense pulsed light for treatment of actinic keratosis: clinical and histopathologic evaluation. Dermatol Surg 2005; 31: 33–7.

88. Moseley H, Ibbotson S, Woods J, et al. Clinical and research applications of photodynamic therapy in dermatology: experience of the Scottish PDT centre. Lasers Surg Med 2006; 38: 403–16.

89. Fink-Puches R, Hofer A, Smolle J, et al. Primary clinical response and long-term follow-up of solar keratoses treated with topically applied 5-aminolevulinic acid and irradiation by different wave bands of light. J Photochem Photobiol 1997; 41: 145–51.

90. Szeimies RM, Karrer S, Radakovic-Fijan S, et al. Photodynamic therapy using topical methyl 5-aminolevulinate compared with cryotherapy for actinic keratosis: a prospective, randomized study. J Am Acad Dermatol 2002; 47: 258–62.

91. Freeman M, Vinciullo C, Francis D, et al. A comparison of photodynamic therapy using topical methyl aminolevulinate (Metvix) with single cycle cryotherapy in patients with actinic keratosis: a prospective, randomized study. J Dermatolog Treat 2003; 14: 99–106.

92. Pariser DM, Lowe NJ, Stewart DM, et al. Photodynamic therapy with topical methyl aminolevulinate for actinic keratosis: results of a prospective randomized multicenter trial. J Am Acad Dermatol 2003; 48: 227–32.

93. Morton CA, Campbell S, Gupta G, et al. Intraindividual, right-left comparison of topical methyl aminolaevulinate-photodynamic therapy and cryotherapy in subjects with actinic keratoses: a multicentre, randomized controlled study. Br J Dermatol 2006; 155: 1029–36.

94. Kaufmann R, Spelman L, Weightman W, et al. Multicentre intraindividual randomized trial of topical methyl aminolaevulinate photodynamic therapy vs. cryotherapy for multiple actinic keratoses on the extremities. Br J Dermatol 2008; 158: 994–9.

95. Kurwa HA, Yong-Gee SA, Seed PT, et al. A randomized paired comparison of photodynamic therapy and topical 5-fluorouracil in the treatment of actinic keratoses. J Am Acad Dermatol 1999; 41: 414–18.

96. Szeimies RM, Karrer S, Sauerwald A, Landthaler M. Photodynamic therapy with topical application of 5-aminolevulinic acid in the treatment of actinic keratoses: an initial clinical study. Dermatology 1996; 192: 246–51.

97. Tarstedt M, Rosdahl I, Berne B, Svanberg K, Wennberg AM. A randomized multicenter study to compare two treatment regimens of topical methyl aminolevulinate (Metvix)-PDT in actinic keratosis of the face and scalp. Acta Derm Venereol 2005; 85: 424–8.

98. Oseroff A. PDT as a cytotoxic agent and biological response modifier: implications for cancer prevention and treatment in immunosuppressed and immunocompetent patients. J Invest Dermatol 2006; 126: 542–4.

99. Dragieva G, Prinz BM, Hafner J, et al. A randomized controlled clinical trial of topical photodynamic therapy with methyl aminolaevulinate in the treatment of actinic keratosis in transplant patients. Br J Dermatol 2004; 151: 196–200.

100. Perrett CM, McGregor JM, Warwick J, et al. Treatment of post-transplant premalignant skin disease: a randomized intrapatient comparative study of 5-fluorouracil cream and topical photodynamic therapy. Br J Dermatol 2007; 156: 320–8.

101. Dragieva G, Hafner J, Dummer R, et al. Topical photodynamic therapy in the treatment of actinic keratoses and Bowen's disease in transplant recipients. Transplantation 2004; 17: 115–21.

102. de Graaf YGL, Kennedy C, Wolterbeek R, et al. Photodynamic therapy does not prevent cutaneous squamous-cell carcinoma in organ-transplant recipients: results of a randomized-controlled trial. J Invest Dermatol 2006; 126: 569–74.

103. Vatve M, Ortonne JP, Birch-Machin MA, et al. Management of field change in actinic keratosis. Br J Dermatol 2007; 157: 21–4.

104. Szeimies RM, Matheson RT, Davis SA, et al. Topical Methyl aminolevulinate photodynamic therapy using red light-emitting diode light for multiple actinic keratoses: a randomized study. Dermatol Surg 2009; 35: 586–92.

105. Serra-Guillen C, Nagore E, Hueso L, et al. A randomized comparative study of tolerance and satisfaction in the treatment of actinic keratosis of the face and scalp between 5% imiquimod cream and photodynamic therapy with methylaminolaevulinate. Br J Dermatol 2011; 164: 429–33.

106. Palm MD, Goldman MP. Safety and efficacy comparison of blue versus red light sources for photodynamic therapy using methyl aminolevulinate in photodamaged skin. J Drugs Dermatol 2011; 10: 53–60.

107. Gilbert D. Treatment of actinic keratoses with sequential combination of 5-fluorouracil and photodynamic therapy. J Drugs Dermatol 2005; 4: 161–3.

108. Martin G. Prospective, case-based assessment of sequential therapy with topical fluorouracil cream 0.5% and ALA-PDT for the treatment of actinic keratosis. J Drugs Dermatol 2011; 10: 372–8.

109. Shaffelburg M. Treatment of actinic keratoses with sequential use of photodynamic therapy and imiquimod 5% cream. J Drugs Dermatol 2009; 8: 35–9.

110. Diepgen TL, Mahler V. The epidemiology of skin cancer. Br J Dermatol 2002; 146: 1–6.

111. Lehmann P. Methyl aminolaevulinate-photodynamic therapy: a review of clinical trials in the treatment of actinic keratoses and nonmelanoma skin cancer. Br J Dermatol 2007; 156: 793–801.

112. Albert MR, Weinstock MA. Keratinocyte carcinoma. CA Cancer J Clin 2003; 53: 292–302.

113. Krosl G, Korbelik M, Dougherty GJ. Induction of immune cell infiltration into murine SCCVII tumor by photofrin-based photodynamic therapy. Br J Cancer 1995; 71: 549–55.

114. Szeimies RM, Morton CA, Sidoroff A, Braathen LR. Photodynamic therapy for nonmelanoma skin cancer. Acta Derm Venereol (Stockh) 2005; 85: 483–90.

115. Morton CA, Brown SB, Collins S, et al. Guidelines for topical photodynamic therapy: report of a workshop of the British Photodermatology Group. Br J Dermatol 2002; 146: 552–67.

116. Morton CA, Whitehurst C, Moseley H, et al. Comparison of photodynamic therapy with cryotherapy in the treatment of Bowen's disease. Br J Dermatol 1996; 135: 766–71.

117. Salim A, Leman JA, McColl JH, et al. Randomized comparison of photodynamic therapy with topical 5-fluorouracil in Bowen's disease. Br J Dermatol 2003; 148: 539–43.

118. Morton CA, Whitehurst C, Moore JV, MacKie RM. Comparison of red and green light in the treatment of Bowen's disease by photodynamic therapy. Br J Dermatol 2000; 143: 767–72.

119. Morton C, Horn M, Leman J, et al. Comparison of topical methyl aminolevulinate photodynamic therapy with cryotherapy or fluoracil for treatment of squamous cell carcinoma in situ. Arch Dermatol 2006; 142: 729–35.

120. Morton CA, Horn M, Leman J, et al. A randomised, placebo-controlled, European study comparing MAL-PDT with cryotherapy and 5-fluorouracil in subjects with Bowen's disease: results from a 24 months follow-up. Poster presented at the 10th World Congress on Cancers of the Skin, Vienna, 2005. P129.

121. Thestrup-Pedersen K, Ravnborg L, Reymann F. Morbus Bowen. A description of the disease in 617 patients. Acta Derm Venereol 1988; 68: 236–9.

122. Leman JA, Mackie RM, Morton CA. Recurrence rates following aminolaevulinic acid photodynamic therapy for intraepidermal squamous cell carcinoma compare favourably with outcome following conventional modalities. Br J Dermatol 2002; 147: 35.

123. Morton CA, Whitehurst C, McColl JH, et al. Photodynamic therapy for large or multiple patches of Bowen's disease and basal cell carcinoma. Arch Dermatol 2001; 137: 319–24.

124. Brookes PT, Jhawar S, Hinton CP, et al. Bowen's disease of the nipple – a new method of treatment. Breast 2005; 14: 65–7.

125. Tan B, Sinclair R, Foley P. Photodynamic therapy for subungual Bowen's disease. Australas J Dermatol 2004; 45: 172–4.

126. Usmani N, Stables GI, Telfer NR, Stringer MR. Subungual Bowen's disease treated by topical aminolevulinic acid-photodynamic therapy. J Am Acad Dermatol 2005; 53: S273–6.

127. Souza CS, Felicio LB, Bentley MV, et al. Topical photodynamic therapy for Bowen's disease of the digit in epidermolysis bullosa. Br J Dermatol 2005; 153: 672–4.

128. Guillen C, Sanmartin O, Escudero A, et al. Photodynamic therapy for in situ squamous cell carcinoma on chronic radiation dermatitis after photosensitization with 5-aminolaevulinic acid. J Eur Acad Dermatol Venereol 2000; 14: 298–300.

129. Morton CA, Horn M, Leman J, et al. A randomized, placebo-controlled, European study comparing MAL-PDT with cryotherapy and 5-fluoracil in subjects with Bowen's disease. J Eur Acad Dermatol Venereol 2004; 18: 415.

130. Morton CA. Methyl aminolevulinate: actinic keratosis and Bowen's disease. Dermatol Clin 2007; 25: 81–7.

131. Fink-Puches R, Soyer HP, Hofer A, et al. Long-term follow-up and histological changes of superficial nonmelanoma skin cancers treated with topical delta-aminolevulinic acid photodynamic therapy. Arch Dermatol 1998; 134: 821–6.

132. Calzavara-Pinton PG. Repetitive photodynamic therapy with topical delta-aminolaevulinic acid as an appropriate approach to the routine treatment of superficial non-melanoma skin tumours. J Photochem Photobiol B 1995; 29: 53–7.

133. Fritsch C, Goerz G, Ruzicka T. Photodynamic therapy in dermatology. Arch Dermatol 1998; 134: 207–14.

134. Calzavara-Pinton PG, Venturini M, Sala R, et al. Methylaminolaevlinate-based photodynamic therapy of Bowen's disease and squamous cell carcinoma. Br J Dermatol 2008; 159: 137–44.

135. Morton CA, McKenna KE, Rhodes LE; British Association of Dermatologists Therapy Guidelines and Audit Subcommittee and the British Photodermatology Group. Guidelines for topical photodynamic therapy: update. Br J Dermatol 2008; 159: 1245–66.

136. Braathen LR, Szeimies RM, Basset-Seguin N, et al. International Society for Photodynamic Therapy in Dermatology. Guidelines on the use of photodynamic therapy for nonmelanoma skin cancer: an international consensus. International Society for Photodynamic Therapy in Dermatology, 2005. J Am Acad Dermatol 2007; 56: 125–43.

137. McCormack CJ, Kelly JW, Dorevitch AP. Differences in age and body site distribution of the histological subtypes of basal cell carcinoma. A possible indicator of differing causes. Arch Dermatol 1997; 133: 593–6.

138. Kennedy JC, Pottier RH, Pross DC. Photodynamic therapy with endogenous protoporphyrin IX: basic principles and present clinical experience. J Photochem Photobiol B 1990; 6: 143–8.

139. Morton CA, Whitehurst C, McColl JH, et al. Photodynamic therapy for large or multiple patches of Bowen disease and basal cell carcinoma. Arch Dermatol 2001; 137: 319–24.

140. Clark C, Bryden A, Dawe R, et al. Topical 5-aminolaevulinic acid photodynamic therapy for cutaneous lesions: outcome and comparison of light sources. Photodermatol Photoimmunol Photomed 2003; 19: 134–41.

141. Wang I, Bendsoe N, Klinteberg CA, et al. Photodynamic therapy vs. cryosurgery of basal cell carcinomas: results of a phase III clinical trial. Br J Dermatol 2001; 144: 832–40.

142. Blume JE, Oseroff AR. Aminolevulinic acid photodynamic therapy for skin cancers. Dermatol Clin 2007; 25: 5–14.

143. Horn M, Wolf P, Wulf HC, et al. Topical methyl aminolevulinate photodynamic therapy in patients with basal cell carcinoma prone to complications and poor cosmetic outcome with conventional therapy. Br J Dermatol 2003; 149: 1242–9.

144. Vinciullo C, Elliott T, Gebauer K, Spelman L, Ngyen R. MAL-PDT in patients with basal cell carcinoma: results of an Australian multicenter study. Poster presented to the International Skin Cancer Conference 2004, Zurich, Switzerland, July 22-24, 2004.

145. Thissen MR, Neumann MH, Schouten LJ. A systematic review of treatment modalities for primary basal cell carcinomas. Arch Dermatol 1999; 135: 1177–83.

146. Rowe DE, Carroll RJ, Day CI Jr. Long term recurrence rates in previously untreated (primary basal cell carcinoma): implications for subject follow-up. J Dermatol Surg Oncol 1989; 15: 315–28.

147. Basset-Seguin N, Ibbotson SH, Emtestam L, et al. Topical methyl aminolaevulinate photodynamic therapy versus cryotherapy for superficial basal cell carcinoma: a 5 year randomized trial. Eur J Dermatol 2008; 18: 547–53.

148. Szeimies RM, Ibbotson S, Murrell DF, Rubel D, Frambach Y. A clinical study comparing methyl aminolevulinate photodynamic therapy and surgery in small superficial basal cell carcinoma (8-20 mm), with a 12-month follow-up. J Eur Acad Dermatol Venereol 2008; 22: 1302–11.

149. Vinciullo C, Elliott T, Francis D, et al. Photodynamic therapy with topical methyl aminolaevulinate for 'difficult-to-treat' basal cell carcinoma. Br J Dermatol 2005; 152: 765–72.

150. Tierney E, Barker A, Ahdout J, et al. Photodynamic therapy for the treatment of cutaneous neoplasia, inflammatory disorders and photoaging. Dermatol Surg 2009; 35: 725–46.

151. Thissen MR, Schroeter CA, Neumann HA. Photodynamic therapy with delta-aminolaevulinic acid for nodular basal cell carcinoma using a prior debulking technique. Br J Dermatol 2000; 142: 338–9.

152. Rhodes LE, Tsoukas MM, Anderson RR, et al. Iontophoretic delivery of ALA provides a quantitative model for ALA pharmacokinetics and PpIX phototoxicity in human skin. J Invest Dermatol 1997; 108: 87–91.

153. Choudry K, Brooke RC, Farrar W, et al. The effect of an iron chelating agent on protoporphyrin IX levels and phototoxicity in topical 5-aminolaevulinic acid photodynamic therapy. Br J Dermatol 2003; 149: 124–30.

154. Christensen E, Skogvoll E, Viset T, Warloe T, Sundstrm S. Photodynamic therapy with 5-aminolaevulinic acid, dimethylsulfoxide and curettage in basal cell carcinoma: a 6-year clinical and histological follow-up. J Eur Acad Dermatol Venereol 2009; 23: 58–66.

155. Peng Q, Soler AM, Warloe T, et al. Selective distribution of porphyrins in skin thick basal cell carcinoma after topical application of methyl 5-aminolevulinate. J Photochem Photobiol B 2001; 62: 140–5.

156. Kuijpers DI, Thissen MR, Thissen CA, et al. Similar effectiveness of methyl aminolevulinate and 5-aminolevulinate in topical photodynamic therapy for nodular basal cell carcinoma. J Drugs Dermatol 2006; 5: 642–5.

157. Tope WD, Menter A, El-Azhary RA, et al. Comparison of topical methyl aminolevulinate photodynamic therapy versus placebo photodynamic therapy in nodular BCC. J Eur Acad Dermatol Venereol 2004; 18: 413–14.

158. Foley P, Freeman M, Siller G, et al. MAL-PDT or placebo cream in nodular basal cell carcinoma: results of an Australian double-blind randomized multicenter study. Poster presented at the International Skin Cancer Conference 2004, Zurich, July 22-24, 2004.

159. Rhodes LE, de Rie M, Enstrom Y, et al. Photodynamic therapy using topical methyl aminolevulinate vs surgery for nodular basal cell carcinoma: results of a multicenter randomized prospective trial. Arch Dermatol 2004; 140: 17–23.

160. Rhodes LE, de Rie M, Leifsdottir R, et al. Five-year follow-up of a randomized, prospective trial of topical methyl aminolevulinate photodynamic therapy vs surgery for nodular basal cell carcinoma. Arch Dermatol 2007; 143: 1131–6.

161. Foley P, Freeman M, Menter A, Siller G, El-Azhary RA. Photodynamic therapy with methyl aminolevulinate for primary nodular basal cell carcinoma: results for two randomized studies. Int J Dermatol 2009; 48: 1236–45.

162. Soler AM, Warloe T, Berner A, Giercksky KE. A follow-up study of recurrence and cosmesis in completely responding superficial and nodular basal cell carcinomas treated with methyl 5-aminolaevulinate-based photodynamic therapy alone and with prior curettage. Br J Dermatol 2001; 145: 467–71.

163. Szeimies RF. Methyl aminolevulinate-photodynamic therapy for basal cell carcinoma. Dermatol Clin 2007; 25: 89–94.

164. Tierney E, Petersen J, Hanke CW. Photodynamic diagnosis of tumor margins using methyl aminolevulinate before Mohs micrographic surgery. J Am Acad Dermatol 2011; 64: 911–18.

165. Lee CY, Kim KH, Kim YH. The efficacy of photodynamic diagnosis in defining the lateral border between a tumor and a tumor-free area during mohs micrographic surgery. Dermatol Surg 2010; 36: 1704–10.

166. Ruiz-Rodriguez R, Sanz-Sánchez T, Córdoba S. Photodynamic photorejuvenation. Dermatol Surg 2002; 28: 742–4.

167. Dover JS, Bhatia AC, Stewart B, Arndt KA. Topical 5-aminolevulinic acid combined with intense pulsed light in the treatment of photoaging. Arch Dermatol 2005; 141: 1247–52.

168. Zane C, Capezzera R, Sala R, Venturini M, Calzavara-Pinton P. Clinical and echographic analysis of photodynamic therapy using methylaminolevulinate as sensitizer in the treatment of photodamaged facial skin. Lasers Surg Med 2007; 39: 203–9.

169. Gold MH, Bradshaw VL, Boring MM, et al. Split-face comparison of photodynamic therapy with 5-aminolevulinic acid and intense pulsed light versus intense pulsed light alone for photodamage. Dermatol Surg 2006; 32: 795–803.

170. Uebelhoer NS, Dover J. Photodynamic therapy for cosmetic applications. Dermatol Ther 2005; 18: 242–52.

171. Jeffes EWB. Levulan: the first approved topical photosensitizer for the treatment of actinic keratosis. J Dermatol Treat 2002; 13: S19–23.

172. Pariser DM, Lowe NJ, Stewart DM, et al. Photodynamic therapy with topical methyl aminolevulinate for actinic keratosis: Results of a prospective randomized multicenter trial. J Am Acad Dermatol 2003; 48: 227–32.

173. Zane C, Capezzera R, Sala R, et al. Clinical and echographic analysis of photodynamic therapy using methylaminolevulinate as sensitizer in the treatment of photodamaged facial skin. Lasers Surg Med 2007; 39: 203–9.

174. Issa MCL, Pineiro-Maceira J, Vieira MTC, et al. Photorejuvenation with topical methyl aminolevulinate and red light: a randomized, prospective, clinical, histopathologic, and morphometric study. Dermatol Surg 2010; 36: 39–48.

175. Lowe NJ, Lowe P. Pilot study to determine the efficacy of ALA-PDT photorejuvenation for the treatment of facial ageing. J Cosmet Laser Ther 2005; 7: 159–62.

176. Park MY, Sohn S, Lee E, Kim YC. Photorejuvenation induced by 5-aminolevulinic acid photodynamic therapy in patients with actinic keratosis: a histologic analysis. J Am Acad Dermatol 2010; 62: 85–95.

177. Goldberg DJ. New collagen formation after dermal remodeling with intense pulsed light sources. J Cutan Laser Ther 2000; 2: 59–61.

178. Avram DK, Goldman MP. Effectiveness and safety of ALA-IPL in treating actinic keratoses and photodamage. J Drugs Dermatol 2004; 3: S36–9.

179. Alster TS, Tanzi EL, Welch EC. Photorejuvenation of facial skin with topical 20% 5-aminolevulinic acid and intense pulsed light treatment: a split-face comparison study. J Drugs Dermatol 2005; 4: 35–8.

180. Marmur ES, Phelps R, Goldberg DJ. Ultrastructural changes seen after ALA-IPL photorejuvenation: a pilot study. J Cosmet Laser Ther 2005; 7: 21–4.

181. Serrano G, Lorente M, Reyes M, et al. Photodynamic therapy with low-strength ALA, repeated applications and short contact periods (40-60 minutes) in acne, photoaging, and vitiligo. J Drugs Dermatol 2009; 8: 562–8.

182. Xi Z, Shuxian Y, Zhong L, et al. Topical 5-aminolevulinic acid with intense pulsed light versus intense pulsed light for photodamage in chinese patients. Dermatol Surg 2011; 37: 31–40.

183. Key DJ. Aminolevulinic acid-pulsed dye laser photodynamic therapy for the treatment of photoaging. Cosmet Dermatol 2005; 18: 31–6.

184. Clementoni MT, B-Roscher M, Munavalli GS. Photodynamic photorejuvenation of the face with a combination of microneedling, red light, and broadband pulsed light. Lasers Surg Med 2010; 42: 150–9.

185. Ruiz-Rodriguez R, López L, Candelas D, Zelickson B. Enhanced efficacy of photodynamic therapy after fractional resurfacing: fractional photodynamic rejuvenation. J Drugs Dermatol 2007; 6: 818–20.

186. Hædersdal M, Sakamoto FH, Farinelli WA, et al. Fractional CO_2 laser-assisted drug delivery. Lasers Surg Med 2010; 42: 113–22.

187. Szeimies RM, Stockfleth E, Popp G, et al. Long-term follow-up of photodynamic therapy with self-adhesive 5-aminolaevulinic acid patch: 12 months data. Br J Dermatol 2010; 162: 410–14.

188. Warren CB, Karai LJ, Vidimos A, Maytin EV. Pain associated with aminolevulinic acid-photodynamic therapy of skin disease. J Am Acad Dermatol 2009; 61: 1033–43.

189. Tyrrell J, Campbell SM, Curnow A. The effect of air cooling pain relief on protoporphyrin IX photobleaching and clinical efficacy during dermatological photodynamic therapy. J Photochem Photobiol B 2011; 103: 1–7.

190. Tyrrell J, Campbell SM, Curnow A. The relationship between protoporphyrin IX photobleaching during real-time dermatological methyl-aminoluvinate photodynamic therapy (MAL-PDT) and subsequent clinical outcome. Lasers Surg Med 2010; 42: 613–19.

191. Ascencio M, Collinet P, Farine MO, Mordon S. Protoporphyrin IX fluorescence photobleaching is a useful tool to predict the response of rat ovarian cancer following hexaminolevulinate photodynamic therapy. Lasers Surg Med 2008; 40: 332–41.

192. Borreli C, Herzinger T, Merk K, et al. Effect of subcutaneous infiltration anesthesia on pain in photodynamic therapy: a controlled open pilot trial. Dermatol Surg 2007; 33: 314–18.

193. Attili SK, Lesar A, McNeill A, et al. An open pilot study of ambulatory photodynamic therapy using a werable low-irradiance organic light-emitting diode light source in the treatment of nonmelanoma skin cancer. Br J Dermatol 2009; 161: 170–3.

194. Wiegell SR, Hædersdal M, Philipsen PA, et al. Continuous activation of PpIX by daylight is as effective as and less painful than conventional photodynamic therapy for actinic keratosis: a randomized, controlled, single-blinded study. Br J Dermatol 2008; 158: 740–6.

195. Goldberg DJ. Photodynamic therapy in skin rejuvenation. Clin Dermatol 2008; 26: 608–613.

196. Lee WR, Tsai RY, Fang CL, et al. Microdermabrasion as a novel tool to enhance drug delivery via the skin: an animal study. Dermatol Surg 2006; 32: 1013–22.

197. Katz BE, Truong S, Maiwald DC, Frew KE, George BA. Efficacy of microdermabrasion preceding ALA application in reducing the incubation time of ALA in laser PDT. J Drugs Dermatol 2007; 6: 140–2.

198. Morton S, Campbell S, Gupta G, et al. Intraindividual, right-left comparison of topical methyl aminolaevulinate photodynamic therapy and cryotherapy in subjects with actinic keratosis: a multicentre, randomized controlled study. Br J Dermatol 2006; 155: 1029–36.

199. Harper JC. An update on the pathogenesis and management of acne vulgaris. J Am Acad Dermatol 2004; 51:s36–8.

200. Herane MI, Ando I. Acne in infancy and acne genetics. Dermatology 2003; 206: 24–8.

201. Strauss JS, Leyden JJ, Lucky AW, et al. A randomized trial of the efficacy of a new micronized formulation versus a standard formulation of isotretinoin in patients with severe recalcitrant nodular acne. J Am Acad Dermatol 2001; 45: 187–95.

202. Layton AM, Knaggs H, Taylor J, Cunliffe WJ. Isotretinoin for acne vulgaris—10 years later: a safe and successful treatment. Br J Dermatol 1993; 129: 292–6.

203. Quereux G, Volteau C, N'Guyen JM, Dreno B. Prospective study of risk factors of relapse after treatment of acne with oral isotretinoin. Dermatology 2006; 212: 168–76.

204. Zouboulis CC. The truth behind this undeniable efficacy—recurrence rates and relapse risk factors of acne treatment with oral isotretinoin. Dermatology 2006; 212: 99–100.

205. Zane LT, Leyden WA, Marqueling AL, Manos MM. A population-based analysis of laboratory abnormalities during isotretinoin therapy for acne vulgaris. Arch Dermatol 2006; 142: 1016–22.

206. DiGiovanna JJ, Langman CB, Tschen EH, et al. Effect of a single course of isotretinoin therapy on bone mineral density in adolescent patients with severe, recalcitrant, nodular acne. J Am Acad Dermatol 2004; 51: 709–17.

207. Wysowski DK, Pitts M, Beitz J. An analysis of reports of depression and suicide in patients treated with isotretinoin. J Am Acad Dermatol 2001; 45: 515–19.

208. Hongcharu W, Taylor CR, Chang Y, et al. Topical ALA-photodynamic therapy for the treatment of acne vulgaris. J Invest Dermatol 2000; 115: 183–92.

209. Pollock B, Turner D, Stringer MR, et al. Topical aminolaevulinic acid-photodynamic therapy for the treatment of acne vulgaris: a study of clinical efficacy and mechanism of action. Br J Dermatol 2004; 151: 616–22.

210. Ashkenazi H, Malik Z, Harth Y, Nitzan Y. Eradication of Propionibacterium acnes by its endogenic porphyrins after illumination with high intensity blue light. FEMS Immunol Med Microbiol 2003; 35: 17–24.

211. Hongcharu W, Taylor CR, Chang Y, et al. Topical ALA–photodynamic therapy for the treatment of acne vulgaris. J Invest Dermatol 2000; 115: 183–92.

212. Itoh Y, Ninomiya Y, Tajima S, Ishibashi A. Photodynamic therapy of acne vulgaris with topical delta-aminolevulinic acid and incoherent light in Japanese patients. Br J Dermatol 2001; 144: 575–9.

213. Taub AF. Photodynamic therapy for the treatment of acne: a pilot study. J Drugs Dermatol 2004; 3: S10–14.

214. Goldman MP, Boyce SM. A single-center study of aminolevulinic acid and 417 nm photodynamic therapy in the treatment of moderate to severe acne vulgaris. J Drugs Dermatol 2003; 2: 393–4.

215. Akaraphanth R, Kanjanawanitchkul W, Gritiyarangsan P. Efficacy of ALA–PDT vs blue light in the treatment of acne. Photodermatol Photoimmunol Photomed 2007; 23: 186–90.

216. Gold MH, Bradshaw VL, Boring M, et al. The use of a novel intense pulsed light and heat source and ALA-PDT in the treatment of moderate to severe inflammatory acne vulgaris. J Drugs Dermatol 2004; 3: S15–16.

217. Gold MH, Biron JA, Boring M, Bridges TM, Bradshaw VL. Treatment of moderate to severe inflammatory acne vulgaris: photodynamic therapy with 5-aminolevulinic acid and a novel advanced fluorescence technology pulsed light source (Clinical report). J Drugs Dermatol 2007; 6: 319–22.

218. Rojanamatin J, Choawawanich P. Treatment of inflammatory facial acne vulgaris with intense pulsed light and short contact of topical 5-aminolevulinic acid: a pilot study. Dermatol Surg 2006; 32: 991–7.

219. Santos MAV, Belo VG, Santos G. Effectiveness of photodynamic therapy with topical 5-aminolevulinic acid and intense pulsed light versus intense pulsed light alone in the treatment of acne vulgaris: comparative study. Dermatol Surg 2005; 31: 910–15.

220. Taub AF. A comparison of intense pulsed light, combination radiofrequency and intense pulsed light, and blue light in photodynamic therapy for acne vulgaris. J Drugs Dermatol 2007; 6: 1010–16.

221. Yeung CK, Shek SY, Bjerring P, et al. A comparative study of intense pulsed light alone and its combination with photodynamic therapy for the treatment of facial acne in Asian skin. Lasers Surg Med 2007; 39: 1–6.

222. Oh SH, Ryu DJ, Han EC, Lee KH, Lee JH. A comparative study of topical 5-aminolevulinic acid incubation times in photodynamic therapy with intense pulsed light for the treatment of inflammatory acne. Dermatol Surg 2009; 35: 1918–26.

223. Haedersdal M, Togsverd-Bo K, Wiegell SR, et al. Long-pulsed dye laser versus long-pulsed dye laser-assisted photodynamic therapy for acne vulgaris: a randomized controlled trial. J Am Acad Dermatol 2008; 58: 387–94.

224. Alexiades-Armenakas M. Long-pulsed dye laser-mediated photodynamic therapy combined with topical therapy for mild to severe comedonal, inflammatory, or cystic acne. J Drugs Dermatol 2006; 5: 45–56.

225. Hong S-B, Lee M-H. Topical aminolevulinic acid–photodynamic therapy for the treatment of acne vulgaris. Photodermatol Photoimmunol Photomed 2005; 21: 322–5.

226. Hörfelt C, Funk J, Frohm-Nilsson M, et al. Topical methyl aminolaevulinate photodynamic therapy for treatment of facial acne vulgaris: results of a randomized, controlled study. Br J Dermatol 2006; 155: 608–13.

227. Wiegell SR, Wulf HC. Photodynamic therapy using 5-aminolevulinic acid versus methyl aminolevulinate. J Am Acad Dermatol 2006; 54: 647–51.

228. Wiegell SR, Wulf HC. Photodynamic therapy of acne vulgaris using methyl aminolaevulinate: a blinded, randomized, controlled trial. Br J Dermatol 2006; 154: 969–76.

229. Hörfelt C, Stenquist B, Larko O, et al. Photodynamic therapy for acne vulgaris: a pilot study of the dose-response and mechanism of action. Acta Derm Venereol 2007; 87: 325–9.

230. Yin R, Hao F, Deng J, Yang XC, Yan H. Investigation of optimal aminolaevulinic acid concentration applied in topical aminolaevulinic acid-photodynamic therapy for treatment of moderate to severe acne: a pilot study in Chinese subjects. Br J Dermatol 2010; 163: 1064–71.

231. Sakamoto FH, Tannous Z, Doukas AG, et al. Porphyrin distribution after topical aminolevulinic acid in a novel porcine model of sebaceous skin. Lasers Surg Med 2009; 41: 154–60.

232. Morton CA, Brown SB, Collins S, et al. Guidelines for topical photodynamic therapy: report of a workshop of the British Photodermatology Group. Br J Dermatol 2002; 146: 552–67.

233. Fabbrocini G, Di Costanzo MP, Riccardo AM, et al. Photodynamic therapy with topical delta-aminolaevulinic acid for the treatment of plantar warts. J Photochem Photobiol B 2001; 61: 30–4.

234. Smucler R, Jatsova E. Comparative study of aminolevulinic acid photodynamic therapy plus pulsed dye laser versus pulsed dye laser alone in treatment of viral warts. Photomed Laser Surg 2005; 31: 51–3.

235. Schroeter CA, Kaas L, Waterval JJ, et al. Successful treatment of periungual warts using photodynamic therapy: a pilot study. J Eur Acad Dermatol Venereol 2007; 21: 1170–4.

236. Fehr MK, Hornung R, Degen A, et al. Photodynamic therapy of vulvar and vaginal condyloma and intraepithelial neoplasia using topically applied 5-aminolevulinic acid. Lasers Surg Med 2002; 30: 273–9.

237. Stefanaki IM, Georgiou S, Themelis GC, et al. In vivo fluorescence kinetics and photodynamic therapy in condylomata acuminata. Br J Dermatol 2003; 149: 972–6.

238. Wang XL, Wang HW, Wang HS, et al. Topical 5-aminolaevulinic acid-photodynamic therapy for the treatment of urethral condylomata acuminata. Br J Dermatol 2004; 151: 880–5.

239. Chen K, Chang BZ, Ju M, et al. Comparative study of photodynamic therapy vs. CO2 laser vaporization in treatment of condylomata acuminata: a randomized clinical trial. Br J Dermatol 2007; 156: 516–20.

240. Szeimies RM, Schleyer V, Moll I, et al. Adjuvant photodynamic therapy does not prevent recurrence of condylomata acuminata after carbon

dioxide laser ablation- a phase III, prospective, randomized, bicentric, double-blind study. Dermatol Surg 2009; 35: 757–64.

241. Yoo KH, Kim BJ, Kim MN. Enhanced efficacy of photodynamic therapy with methyl-5-aminolevulinic acid in recalcitrant periungual warts after ablative carbon dioxide fractional laser: a pilot study. Dermatol Surg 2009; 35: 1927–32.

242. Stringer MR, Collins P, Robinson DJ, et al. The accumulation of protoporphyrin IX in plaque psoriasis after topical application of 5-aminolaevulinic acid indicates a potential for superficial photodynamic therapy. J Invest Dermatol 1996; 107: 76–81.

243. Beattie PE, Dawe RS, Ferguson J, Ibbotson SH. Lack of efficacy and tolerability of topical PDT for psoriasis in comparison with narrowband UVB phototherapy. Clin Exp Dermatol 2004; 29: 560–2.

244. Schleyer V, Radakovic-Fijan S, Kerrer S, et al. Disappointing results and low tolerability of photodynamic therapy with topical 5-aminolaevulinic acid in psoriasis. A randomized, double-blind phase I/II study. J Eur Acad Dermatol Venereol 2006; 20: 823–8.

245. Bissonnette R, Zeng H, McLean DI, et al. Oral aminolevulinic acid induced protoporphyrin IX fluorescence in psoriatic plaques and peripheral blood cells. Photochem Photobiol 2001; 74: 339–45.

246. Edström DW, Porwit A, Ros AM. Photodynamic therapy with topical 5-aminolevulinic acid for mycosis fungoides: clinical and histological response. Acta Derm Venereol (Stockh) 2001; 81: 184–8.

247. Zane C, Venturini M, Sala R, Calzavara-Pinton P. Photodynamic therapy with methyl aminolevulinate as a valuable treatment option for unilesional cutaneous T-cell lymphoma. Photodermatol Photoimmunol Photomed 2006; 22: 254–8.

248. Shieh S, Dee AS, Cheney RT, et al. Photodynamic therapy for the treatment of extramammary Paget's disease. Br J Dermatol 2002; 146: 1000–5.

249. Housel JP, Izikson L, Zeitouni NC. Noninvasive extramammary Paget's disease treated with photodynamic therapy: case series from the Roswell Park Cancer Institute. Dermatol Surg 2010; 36: 1718–24.

250. Hayami J, Okamoto H, Sugihara A, Horio T. Immunosuppressive effects of photodynamic therapy by topical aminolevulinic acid. J Dermatol 2007; 34: 320–7.

251. Karrer S, Bosserhoff AK, Weiderer P, Landthaler M, Szeimies RM. Keratinocyte-derived cytokines after photodynamic therapy and their paracrine induction of matrix metalloproteinases in fibroblasts. Br J Dermatol 2004; 151: 776–83.

252. Karrer S, Szeimies RM. Photodynamic therapy: non-oncologic indications. Hautarzt 2007; 58: 585–96.

253. Karrer S, Abels C, Landthaler M, Szeimies RM. Topical photodynamic therapy for localized scleroderma. Acta Derm Venereol 2000; 80: 26–7.

254. Hillemanns P, Untch M, Prove F, et al. Photodynamic therapy of vulvar lichen sclerosus with 5-aminolevulinic acid. Obstet Gynecol 1999; 93: 71–4.

255. Schweiger ES, Riddle CC, Aires DJ. Treatment of hidradenitis suppurativa by photodynamic therapy with aminolevulinic acid: preliminary results. J Drugs Dermatol 2011; 10: 381–6.

256. Karrer S, Abels C, Wimmershoff MB, et al. Successful treatment of cutaneous sarcoidosis using topical photodynamic therapy. Arch Dermatol 2002; 138: 581–4.

257. Heidenheim M, Jemec GBE. Successful treatment of necrobiosis lipoidica diabeticorum with photodynamic therapy. Arch Dermatol 2006; 142: 1548–50.

258. Parera E, Gallardo F, Toll A, et al. Inflammatory linear verrucous epidermal nevus successfully treated with methyl-aminolevulinate photodynamic therapy. Dermatol Surg 2010; 36: 253–6.

259. Enk CD, Fritsch C, Jonas F, et al. Treatment of cutaneous leishmaniasis with photodynamic therapy. Arch Dermatol 2003; 139: 432–4.

260. Asilian A, Davami M. Comparison between the efficacy of photodynamic therapy and topical paromomycin in the treatment of Old World cutaneous leishmaniasis: a placebo-controlled, randomized clinical trial. Clin Exp Dermatol 2006; 31: 634–7.

261. Gold MH, Boring MM, Bridges TM, Bradshaw VL. The successful use of ALA-PDT in the treatment of recalcitrant molluscum contagiosum. J Drugs Dermatol 2004; 3: 187–90.

262. Watanabe D, Kawamura C, Masuda Y, et al. Successful treatment of toenail onychomycosis with photodynamic therapy. Arch Dermatol 2008; 144: 19–21.

263. Morton CA, Whitehurst C, Moseley H, et al. Development of an alternative light source to lasers for photodynamic therapy: clinical evaluation in the treatment of pre-malignant non-melanoma skin cancer. Lasers Med Sci 1995; 10: 165–71.

264. Fijan S, Honigsmann H, Ortel B. Photodynamic therapy of epithelial skin tumors with delta-aminolaevulinic acid and desferrioxamine. Br J Dermatol 1995; 133: 282–8.

265. Wennberg AM, Lindholm LE, Alpsten M, Larkö O. Treatment of superficial basal cell carcinomas using topically applied delta-aminolaevulinic acid and a filtered xenon lamp. Arch Dermatol Res 1996; 288: 561–4.

266. Haller JC, Cairnduff F, Slack G, et al. Routine double treatments of superficial basal cell carcinomas using aminolaevulinic acid-based photodynamic therapy. Br J Dermatol 2000; 143: 1270–5.

267. Soler AM, Angell-Petersen E, Warloe T, et al. Photodynamic therapy of superficial basal cell carcinoma with 5-aminolevulinic acid with dimethylsulfoxide and ethylediaminetetraacetic acid: a comparison of two light sources. J Photochen Photobiol 2000; 71: 724–9.

268. Surrenti T, De Angelis L, Di Cesare A, Fargnoli MC, Peris K. Efficacy of photodynamic therapy with methylaminolevulinate in the treatment of superficial and nodular basal cell carcinoma: an open-label trial. Eur J Dermatol 2007; 17: 412–15.

269. Fantini F, Greco A, Del Giovane D, et al. Photodynamic therapy for basal cell carcinoma: clinical and pathological determinants of response. J Eur Acad Dermatol Venereol 2011; 25: 896–901.

11 Treatment of leg telangiectasias with laser and high-intensity pulsed light

Mitchel P. Goldman

Lasers have been used to treat leg telangiectasias for various reasons (1). First, lasers have a futuristic appeal. By virtue of their advanced technology, lasers are perceived as "state of the art". The general public often equates "high tech" with treatment safety and superiority. Unfortunately, as described later, this perception by both the general public and the physician has often resulted in unanticipated adverse sequelae (scarring and pain) and higher costs; lasers cost considerably more in terms of purchase and maintenance than a needle, syringe, or sclerosing solution. In addition, lasers have theoretical advantages compared with sclerotherapy for treating leg telangiectasias. Sclerotherapy-induced pigmentation is caused by hemosiderin deposition through extravasated red blood cells (RBCs). Laser coagulation of vessels should not have this effect. In the rabbit ear model, approximately 50% of vessels treated with an effective concentration of sclerosing solution demonstrated extravasated erythrocytes, compared with a 30% incidence when treated with the flashlamp-pumped pulsed dye laser (PDL) (Goldman, unpublished observations). Furthermore, telangiectatic matting (TM), which occurs in a significant percentage of sclerotherapy-treated patients, has also not been seen after laser treatment of vascular lesions. Finally, specific allergenic effects of sclerosing solutions are not a concern when treating telangiectasias with a laser.

Both lasers and intense pulsed light (IPL) have been used to treat leg telangiectasias. Each acts in a different manner to induce vessel destruction. Effective lasers and IPL are pulsed so that their effects act within the thermal relaxation times of blood vessels to produce specific destruction of vessels of various diameters based on the pulse duration. Lasers of various wavelengths and the broad-spectrum IPL are used to selectively treat blood vessels by taking advantage of the difference between the absorption of the components in a blood vessel (oxygenated and deoxygenated hemoglobin) and the overlying epidermis and surrounding dermis (as described below) to selectively thermocoagulate blood vessels (Fig. 11.1). Each wavelength requires a specific fluence to cause vessel destruction. In addition, leg veins are not composed mostly of oxygenated hemoglobin, as are port-wine stains (PWSs) and hemangiomas. They are filled with predominantly deoxygenated hemoglobin, hence their blue color. Selective wavelengths for deoxyhemoglobin as opposed to oxyhemoglobin include approximately 545 and 580 nm and a broad peak between 650 and 800 nm.

Optical properties of blood are mainly determined by the absorption and scattering coefficients of its various oxyhemoglobin components. Oxyhemoglobin has three major absorption peaks at 418, 542, and 577 nm. A less selective and broader absorption peak spans from approximately 750 to 1100 nm. There is a strong absorption at wavelengths below 600 nm with less absorption at longer wavelengths. However, a vessel of 1 mm in diameter absorbs more than 67% of light even at wavelengths longer than 600 nm. This absorption is even more significant for blood vessels of 2 mm in diameter. Therefore, use of a light source above 600 nm would result in deeper penetration of thermal energy without negating absorption by oxyhemoglobin in vessels greater than 1 mm in diameter. This is because the absorption coefficient in blood is higher than that of surrounding tissue for wavelengths between 600 and 1000 nm. Shorter wavelengths heat only the portion of the vessel wall closest to the skin surface, which can result in incomplete thrombosis (2). The only caveat is that wavelengths greater than 900 nm are less specific and also target water, making higher fluences required to produce the desired effects on oxyhemoglobin, the desired chromophore (3). However, these higher fluences can cause unnecessary damage to surrounding tissue unless adequate cooling measures are employed.

Patients seek treatment for a leg vein largely for cosmetic reasons (4). Bernstein (5) has evaluated the clinical characteristics of 500 consecutive patients presenting for laser removal of lower extremity spider veins. Patients ranged in age from 20 to 70 years and had had noticeable spider veins for an average of 14 years. Twenty-eight percent of patients had leg veins less than 0.5 mm in diameter; 39% of patients had veins less than 1.5 mm in diameter. Fifty-six percent of patients who had had sclerotherapy (not stated how this was performed) developed TM. Therefore, any treatment that is effective should be relatively free of adverse sequelae. With recent advances, lasers or IPL systems have become methods for treating telangiectatic vessels with a minimum of adverse effects. However, for these advanced treatments to be effective and safe, they must be used appropriately.

Sclerotherapy has a number of potential adverse effects. Up to 30% of patients treated with sclerotherapy develop post-sclerosis pigmentation (6) and/or TM (7). As discussed earlier, at least one study determined that TM developed in 56% of patients who presented for laser treatment of leg veins (5). These adverse effects can occur even with optimal treatment but are more common when an excessive inflammatory reaction occurs. To minimize risks of an inflammatory response, lasers and IPL act by producing thermal damage with the ultimate goal being vaporization of the targeted vessel. When used

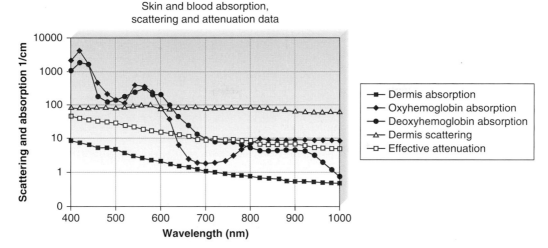

Figure 11.1 Coefficient of blood relative to dermis. *Source*: Courtesy of ESC Medical, Inc.; redrawn from Ref. 28.

with appropriate fluences, pulse durations, and epidermal cooling, the thermal effects of lasers and IPL present minimal inflammatory response compared with chemical irritation of the vessel wall through sclerotherapy. An understanding of the appropriate target vessel for each laser and/or IPL is important so that treatment is tailored to the appropriate target. Telangiectasia arises mostly from reticular veins. Therefore, the single most important concept for the treating physician is that feeding reticular veins must be treated completely before treating telangiectasia. This minimizes adverse sequelae and enhances therapeutic results. When no apparent connection exists between deep collecting and reticular vessels, telangiectasia may arise from a terminal arteriole or arteriovenous anastomosis (8). In this latter scenario, the telangiectasia may be treated without consideration of underlying forces of hydrostatic pressure. Failure to treat "feeding" reticular veins and short follow-up periods after the use of lasers may give inflated values to the success of laser treatment (9). This chapter reviews and evaluates the use of these nonspecific and specific laser and light systems in the treatment of leg venules and telangiectasias.

LASER TREATMENT OF LEG TELANGIECTASIA

Various lasers have been used in an effort to enhance clinical efficacy and to minimize the adverse sequelae of telangiectasia treatment. (Table 11.1) Unfortunately, most have also been associated with adverse responses far in excess of those associated with sclerotherapy. This is related to both the nonspecificity of the laser used and the lack of treatment of hydrostatic pressure from the "feeding" venous system. The optimal light source would have a wavelength specific for the vessel treated and would be able to penetrate to the depth of the vessel through its entire diameter. This wavelength has been proposed to be between 600 and 900 nm. Ideally, a light source should have a pulse duration that would allow the light energy to build up in the target vessel so that its entire diameter is thermocoagulated. Optimal pulse durations have been calculated for various diameter blood vessels (Table 11.2). During the process of delivering a sufficient packet of energy to thermocoagulate the target vessel, the overlying epidermis and perivascular tissue should be unharmed. This requires some

form of epidermal cooling. A number of different laser and IPL systems have been developed toward this end, as discussed in subsequent sections. In addition to the information presented in the following sections, the reader is encouraged to refer to an excellent summary of various laser treatments for leg veins by Kunishige et al. (3).

KRYPTON TRIPHOSPHATE
AND FREQUENCY-DOUBLED Nd:YAG (532 nm)

Modulated krypton triphosphate (KTP) lasers have been reported to be effective in removing leg telangiectasia, using pulse durations between 1 and 50 ms. The 532-nm wavelength is one of the hemoglobin absorption peaks. Although this wavelength does not penetrate deeply into the dermis (about 0.75 mm), relatively specific damage can occur in the vascular target by selection of an optimal pulse duration, enlargement of the spot size, and addition of epidermal cooling. Effective results have been achieved by tracing vessels with a 1-mm projected spot. Typically, the laser is moved between adjacent 1-mm spots with vessels traced at 5–10 mm/second. Immediately after the laser exposure, the epidermis is blanched. Lengthening of the pulse duration to match the diameter of the vessel is attempted to optimize treatment. Usually, more than one treatment is necessary for maximum vessel improvement, with only rare reports of 100% resolution of the leg vein. Efficacy is technique dependent, with excellent results achievable. Patients need to be informed of the possibility of prolonged pigmentation at an incidence similar to that with sclerotherapy, as well as temporary blistering and hypopigmentation that is predominantly caused by epidermal damage in pigmented skin (type III or above, especially when tanned) (Fig. 11.2).

FLASHLAMP-PULSED DYE LASER (585 OR 595 nm)

The PDL has been demonstrated to be highly effective in treating cutaneous vascular lesions consisting of very small vessels, including PWSs, hemangiomas, and facial telangiectasia. The depth of vascular damage is estimated to be 1.5 mm at 585 nm and 15–20 μm deeper at 595 nm. Therefore, penetration to the typical depth of superficial leg telangiectasia may be achieved. However, telangiectasia over the lower extremities has not

Table 11.1 Lasers and Light Sources for Leg Veins

Supplier	Product Name	Device Type	Wavelength (nm)	Energy (J)	Pulse Duration (ms)	Spot Diameter (mm)	Cooling
American BioCare	OmniLight FPL	Fluorescent pulsed light	480, 515, 535, 550, 580–1200	Up to 90	Up to 500		External continuous
Adept Medical	Ultrawave II/III	Alexandrite	755	5–55	5–50	8, 10, 12	None
	Ultrawave	Nd:YAG	1064	5–500	5–100	2, 4, 6, 8, 10, 12	None
Aerolase	LightPod Neo XT	Nd:YAG	1064	Up to 1274	0.65 or 1.5		
Alderm	Prolite	IPL	550–900	10–50		10 × 20, 20 × 25	
Alma (formerly Orion)	Harmony	Fluorescent pulsed light	515–950	5–30	10, 12, 15	40 × 16	None
		Nd:YAG	1064	30–450	10, 15, 45, 60	2, 6	
Asclepion-Meditech	Pro Yellow	CuBr	578	55	300	1.5	None
Candela	Vbeam Perfecta	Pulsed dye	595	Up to 40	0.45–40	Multiple, up to 12	DCD
	Vbeam Platinum	Pulsed dye	595	Up to 40	0.45–40	Multiple	DCD
	Vbeam Aesthetica	Pulsed dye	595	Up to 20	0.45–40	Multiple, up to 10	DCD
	Cbeam	Pulsed dye	585	8–16	0.45	5, 7, 10	DCD
	Gentle YAG VR	Nd:YAG	1064	Up to 600	Up to 300	1.5–3	DCD
	GentleLASE	Alexandrite	755	Up to 100	3	6, 8, 10, 12, 15, 18	DCD
	GentleMax	Alexandrite/Nd:YAG	755/1064	Up to 600	0.25–300	1.5–18	DCD and Cold air
CoolTouch	Varia	Nd:YAG	1064	Up to 500	300 continuous	2–10	DCD
Cutera	CoolGlide Excel	Nd:YAG	1064	5–300	1–300	3, 5, 7, 10	
	CoolGlide Vantage	Nd:YAG	1064	Up to 300	0.1–300	3, 5, 7, 10	Copper contact
	XEO	Nd:YAG and pulsed light	1064 and 600–850 (pulsed light)	Up to 300 and 6–40 (pulsed light)	0.1–300 and Automatic (pulsed light)	10 × 30	None
	Solera Opus	Pulsed light	500–635	3–24	Variable	6.35	

Company	Device	Type	Wavelength (nm)	Pulse duration (ms)	Fluence (J/cm²)	Spot size (mm)	Cooling
Cynosure/Deka	PhotoGenica V	Pulsed dye	585	20	0.45	3, 5, 7, 10	Cold air
	PhotoGenica V-Star	Pulsed dye	585–595	40	0.5–40	5, 7, 10, 12	Cold air
	SmartEpil II	Nd:YAG	1064	1–200	Up to 100	2, 5, 7, 10	Cold air
	Acclaim	Nd:YAG	1064	10–600	0.4–300	3, 5, 7, 10, 12	Cold air
	Cynergy	Pulsed dye/Nd:YAG	595/1064	2–40/10–600	0.5–40/0.3–300	1.5, 12, 15	Cold air
	Cynergy with XPL	Pulsed dye/ Nd:YAG/ Pulsed light	595/1064/560–950	0.5–40/0.3–300/ 5–50			Cold air
	Cynosure PL	Pulsed light	560–950	3–10	5–50	46 × 18, 46 × 10	None
	PhotoLight	Pulsed light	400–1200	3–30	5–50	46 × 18; 46 × 10	Cold air
	Elite	Alexandrite/ Nd:YAG	755/1064	25–50/10–600	0.5–300/0.4–300	1.5, 12, 15	
DDD	Elipse	IPL	400–950	Up to 21	0.2–50	10 × 48	
DermaMed USA	Quadra Q4 (Platinum and Gold Series)	Pulsed light	510–1200	10–20	48	33 × 15	None
Fotana	DermaYAG	Nd:YAG	1064	15–300	150	1, 2, 3, 4, 6, 8, 10, 12	None
	Dualis	Nd:YAG	1064	Up to 600	5–200	2–10	
Iridex	Apex-800	Diode	800	5–60	5–100	7, 9, 11	Cooling handpiece
	DioLite^XP	KTP	532	250	5–100	0.5, 0.7, 1.0	Cooling handpiece
	VariLite	KTP/Diode	532/940	250/850	5–100	0.7, 1, 2	Cooling handpiece
	Lyra i	Nd:YAG	1064	5–900	20–100	1–5 Cont. Adjustable	Cooling handpiece
	Aura i	KTP	532	1–240	1–50	1–5 Cont. Adjustable	Cooling handpiece
	Gemini	KTP	532	Up to 100	1–100	1–5 Cont. Adjustable	Cooling handpiece
		Nd:YAG	1064	Up to 990	10–100	1–5 Cont. Adjustable and 10	Cooling handpiece

(Continued)

Table 11.1 Lasers and Light Sources for Leg Veins (*Continued*)

Supplier	Product Name	Device Type	Wavelength (nm)	Energy (J)	Pulse Duration (ms)	Spot Diameter (mm)	Cooling
LightAge	Epicare	Alexandrite	755	25–40	3–300	7, 9, 12, 15	None
Lumenis	Quantum DL	Nd:YAG	1064	90–150	5–38	6	
	Quantum SR	Pulsed light	560–1200	15–45	6–26	34 × 8	Cooled sapphire crystal
	Vasculite Elite	Pulsed light	515–1200	3–90	1–75	35 × 8	Cooled sapphire crystal
		Nd:YAG	1064	70–150	2–48	6	Cooled sapphire crystal
	LightSheer	Diode	800	10–100	5–400	9 × 9	Cooled sapphire crystal
	Lumenis One	Pulsed light	515–1200	10–40	3–100	15 × 35, 8 × 15	Cooled sapphire crystal
		Nd:YAG	1064	10–225	2–20	2 × 4, 6, 9	Cooled sapphire crystal
		Diode	800	10–100	5–400	9 × 9	Cooled sapphire crystal
Med-Surge	Quantel Viridis	Diode	532	Up to 110	15–150	10 × 20, 20 × 25	None
OpusMed	ProliteII	Pulsed light	550–900	10–50	N/A	5,7	None
	F1	Diode	800	10–40	15–40		None
Palomar	MediLux	Pulsed light	470–1400	Up to 45	10–100	12 × 12+	None
	EsteLux	Pulsed light	470–1400	Up to 40	10–100	12 × 12	
	SLP1000	Diode	810	Up to 575	50–1000		DCD
	StarLux	Pulsed light/Nd:YAG	500–670, 870–1400/1064	Up to 60/700	0.5–500	1.5, 3, 6, 9	
Quantel	Athos	Nd:YAG	1064	Up to 80	3.5	4	None
Sciton	Profile	Nd:YAG	1064	4–400	0.1–200	30 × 30	Contact sapphire
	BBL	Pulsed light	400–1400	Up to 30	Up to 200	15 × 45, 15 × 15	Contact sapphire
	BBL/s	N/A	410–1400	Up to 30	Up to 500	15 × 45, 15 × 15	Contact sapphire
	Profile HMV	Nd:YAG/Pulsed light	1064/410–1400	Up to 400	0.1–200/1–15	30 × 30, 15 ×45	Contact sapphire
Syneron	eLight SR	Optical energy/RF	580–980	Up to 45/25	N/A	12 × 25	
	eLight SRA	Optical energy/RF	470–980	Up to 45/5	N/A	12 × 25	
	eLaser LV	Diode/RF	900	Up to 140/100	N/A	8 × 5	
	eLaser LVA	Diode/RF	900	Up to 350/10–100	N/A	8 × 2	
	Polaris Vascular	Diode/RF	900	Up to 50/100 RF			
WaveLight	Galaxy	Diode	580–980	Up to 140/100 RF	Up to 200	1.5, 3, 5, 7, 10	Contact or cold air
	Mydon	Nd:YAG	1064	10–450	0.5–90	1.5, 3, 3, 5	Contact or cold air
	Arion	Alexandrite	755	5–40	1–50	6, 8, 10, 12, 14	Cold air

Abbreviations: DCD, dynamic cooling device; ITP, intense pulsed light; Nd:YAG, neodymium-doped:yttrium-aluminum-garnet; KTP, krypton triphosphate; RF, radiofrequency.
Source: From Ref. 26.

responded as well, with less lightening and more post-therapy hyperpigmentation (10). This may be due to the larger diameter of leg telangiectasia as compared with dermal vessels in PWS and larger diameter feeding reticular veins as described previously. Vessels that should respond optimally to PDL treatment are predicted to be red telangiectasia less than 0.2 mm in diameter, particularly those vessels arising as post-sclerotherapy TM. This is based on the time of thermocoagulation produced by this relatively short-pulsed laser system. The PDL produces vascular injury in a histologic pattern that is different from that produced by sclerotherapy. In the rabbit ear vein, approximately 50% of vessels treated with an effective concentration of sclerosant demonstrated extravasated RBCs, whereas with PDL treatment, extravasated RBCs were apparent in only 30% of the vessels treated (unpublished observations). Thus, the PDL may produce less post-therapy pigmentation because of a decreased incidence of extravasated RBCs.

Similar to TM vessels, essential telangiectasia represents a network of fine red telangiectasia usually less than 0.2 mm in diameter. This condition responds well to the PDL at fluences of 7–7.25 J/cm^2 (11). Treatment, however, is tedious, with more than 2000, 5-mm diameter pulses are sometimes necessary to cover the entire affected area.

The reason for greater efficacy of treatment in Goldman and Fitzpatrick's report in comparison with others (10,12) may be due to the rigid criteria by which patients were selected for treatment. Patients who responded well to treatment had red telangiectasia less than 0.2 mm in diameter without associated "feeding" reticular veins. Many physicians have found that vessel location may affect treatment outcome, with vessels on the medial thigh being the most difficult to completely eradicate.

However, with the PDL, vessel location appears to be unrelated to treatment outcome if telangiectatic patches with untreated associated reticular veins are excluded. In addition, there appears to be no obvious difference in efficacy between telangiectatic patches that are treated with compression and those that are not (Fig. 11.3). Sadick et al. (13) conducted a study that further supported the notion that graduated compression stocking use for 7 days starting immediately after treatment of class I–II venulectasia with PDL yielded no additional therapeutic efficacy.

LONG PULSED ALEXANDRITE (755 nm)

A long-pulsed alexandrite laser was developed to treat hair. It soon became apparent that the wavelength, fluence, and pulse duration could also be used for telangiectasia. The 755-nm wavelength should penetrate 2–3 mm beneath the epidermis. This laser has been reported to be effective in thermocoagulating blood vessels in clinical and histological studies (14–16). One study of leg telangiectasia in 28 patients treated three times every 4 weeks at fluences ranging from 15 to 30 J/cm^2 found that a single-pulse technique with 20 J/cm^2, 5-ms pulse duration yielded the best resolution when combined with sclerotherapy using 23.4% hypertonic saline (HS) (15). When this technique was used without epidermal cooling with a chill tip at 4°C, focal crusting and scabbing were noted. With laser treatment alone, telangiectasia smaller than 0.2 mm in diameter improved by 23%, vessels between 0.4 and 1 mm improved by 48%, and telangiectasia 1–3 mm improved 32%. The bottom line is that the alexandrite laser is more painful, no more effective, and probably produces more adverse effects than other lasers at the parameters stated by the above-mentioned studies.

DIODE LASERS

Diode lasers generate coherent monochromatic light through excitation of small diodes. These devices are therefore lightweight and portable, with a relatively small desktop footprint. Dierickx et al. (17) evaluated an 800-nm diode laser system (LightSheer, Lumenis, Santa Clara, California, USA) on eight areas of leg veins. The laser was used at 15–40 J/cm^2 given in 5- to 30-ms pulses as double or triple pulses separated by a delay of 2 seconds. Veins were treated every 4 weeks for three sessions and evaluated 2 months after the last treatment. Optimal

Table 11.2 Thermal Relaxation Times of Blood Vessels

Diameter of Vessel (mm)	Thermal Relaxation Time (seconds)
0.1	0.01
0.2	0.04
0.4	0.16
0.8	0.6
2.0	4.0

Source: From Ref. 27.

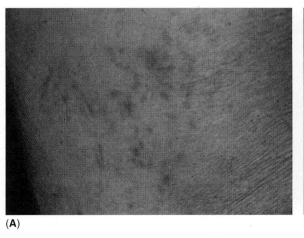 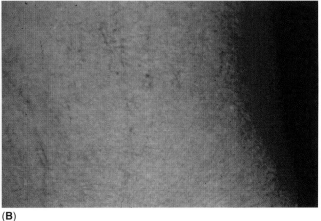

(A) **(B)**

Figure 11.2 (**A**) Before treatment. (**B**) 3 months after treatment, there is hyperpigmentation in the telangiectasia treated with the flashlamp-pumped pulsed dye laser at 15 J/cm^2. Of note, the side treated with the KTP (532-nm) laser at 15 J/cm^2 and a 10-ms pulse showed no change. *Source*: From Ref. 29.

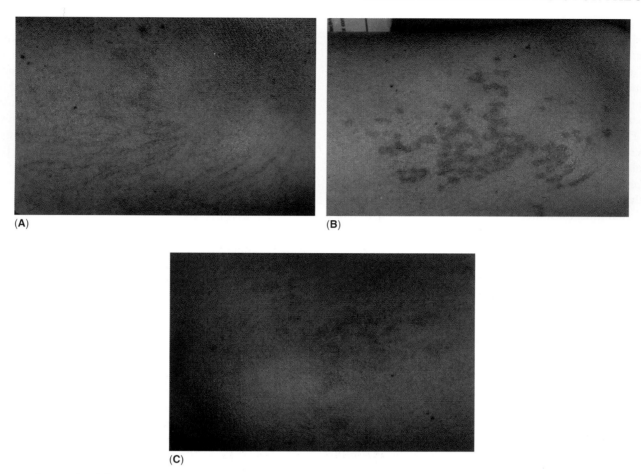

Figure 11.3 Photographic follow-up of telangiectatic flare on the lateral thigh treated with flashlamp-pumped pulsed dye laser at 7 J/cm², 125 pulses. (**A**) Immediately before treatment. (**B**) Immediately after treatment; note the characteristic, localized urticarial response. (**C**) 6 weeks after treatment; note slight hyperpigmentation and total resolution of telangiectasia. Pigmentation completely cleared over the subsequent 2–4 weeks. *Source*: From Ref. 30.

parameters were 30-ms pulses at 40 J/cm². At these parameters, vessels 0.4–1 mm in diameter showed 100% clearing in 22%, 75% clearing in 42%, and 50% clearing in 32%. Trelles et al. (18) evaluated both the subjective and the objective efficacy of an 800-nm diode laser for leg vein clearance in 10 women of various ages and skin types. Investigators used a sequence of five to eight stacked pulses with a pulse duration of 50 ms, a delay of 50 ms, and a 3-mm spot size. Treatments were administered at 2-month intervals until complete clearance occurred, and final efficacy was assessed 6 months following each patient's final treatment. To reach complete clearance, 50% of patients needed three treatment sessions and the remaining 50% needed less than three. Although treated leg veins varied from 1 to 4 mm in diameter, the best results were ultimately seen in those vessels that had initially measured 3–4 mm. Treatment of vessels located on the thigh as well as those in patients with Fitzpatrick skin type III also yielded superior efficacy. Of note, no correlation was found between patient age and efficacy of treatment. A subsequent study evaluated the dermal histologic and immunohistochemical changes induced by exposure of leg telangiectasias to either a combination 915-nm diode laser and radiofrequency device or a 1064-nm Nd:YAG laser (19). Among three patients having 0.1–2.0 mm telangiectasias, each had one leg treated with the combination diode and radiofrequency device and the opposite leg treated with the Nd:YAG laser. Punch biopsies from treated areas were taken 7 days after laser or radiofrequency exposure. Tissue

from each treatment type showed intermediate-sized vessels with complete thrombosis and hemorrhage within the dermis as well as the subcutis; focal full-thickness necrosis was seen in the overlying epidermis. A single-treatment session of both the combination diode and radiofrequency device and the Nd:YAG, each yielded an average of 50–75% clinical clearing. Thus, when comparing results from both treatment modalities, a similar degree of improvement in the clinical appearance of the telangiectasias was supported by histologic examination of tissue specimens.

In summary, diode laser use is limited by treatment pain and adverse effects. Of note, when feeding reticular veins are not treated, distal treated telangiectasias tend to recur at 6–12 months after treatment. Some authors appear to be able to achieve better results than others using similar parameters. Although most apparent in target vessels larger than 1–2 mm in diameter, the addition of radiofrequency to the diode appears to yield vessel clearance at lower diode fluences than would be necessary to achieve the same results if the diode was used alone.

HIGH-INTENSITY PULSED LIGHT
The high-IPL source was developed as an alternative to lasers to maximize efficacy in treating leg veins (Lumenis). This device permits sequential rapid pulsing, longer duration pulses, and penetrating longer wavelengths compared with other laser systems. Theoretically, a phototherapy device that

produces a noncoherent light as a continuous spectrum longer than 550 nm should have multiple advantages over a single-wavelength laser system. First, both oxygenated and deoxygenated hemoglobins absorb at these wavelengths. Second, blood vessels located deeper in the dermis are affected. Third, thermal absorption by the exposed blood vessels should occur with less overlying epidermal absorption, since the longer wavelengths penetrate deeper and are absorbed less by the epidermis, including melanin.

Treatment of essential telangiectasia, especially on the legs, is efficiently accomplished with the IPL (Fig. 11.4). A variety of parameters have been shown to be effective. We recommend testing a few different parameters during the first treatment session and using the most efficient and least painful parameter on subsequent treatments.

The use of IPL to treat leg veins requires significant experience and surgical ability to produce good results. Various parameters must be matched both to the patient's skin type and to the diameter, color, and depth of leg vein. With older machines that do not have integrated cooling through sapphire crystals, a cold gel must be placed between the IPL crystal and the skin surface to provide optimal elimination of epidermal heat. Many have compared using the IPL to playing a violin. A 2- to 3-year-old child playing a violin will make a squeaky noise, but, with practice, by the time the child is 7 or 8, he or she will make beautiful music. Regarding the IPL, it is the art of medicine that assumes an equal importance to its science. Fortunately, for those who do not play musical instruments, there are now dozens of IPLs available from many different manufacturers.

Nd:YAG LASER (1064 nm)

The 1064-nm Nd:YAG laser is probably the most effective laser available to treat leg telangiectasia. The average depth of penetration in human skin is 0.75 mm, and reduction to 10% of the incident power occurs at a depth of 3.7 mm (20). A narrow therapeutic fluence range, which reduces both its efficacy and safety, is associated with the 1064-nm Nd:YAG laser (16). This narrow range may be largely attributed to the formation of methemoglobin (metHb), an oxidized form of hemoglobin that appears during laser-induced blood vessel heating (21). At 1064 nm, metHb shows a significantly stronger absorption than either deoxyhemoglobin or oxyhemoglobin. Theoretically, this metHb formation effect is less pronounced at 755 nm.

Three mechanisms are available to minimize epidermal damage through heat absorption. First, the longer the wavelength, the less energy will be absorbed by melanocytes or melanosomes. This will allow darker skin types to be treated with minimum risks to the epidermis caused by a decrease in melanin interaction. Second, delivering the energy with a delay in pulses greater than the thermal relaxation time for the epidermis (1 to 2 ms) allows the epidermis to cool conductively between pulses. This cooling effect is enhanced by the application of cold gel on the skin surface that conducts away epidermal heat more efficiently than air. Finally, the epidermis can be cooled directly to allow the photons to pass through without generating sufficient heat to cause damaging effects.

Epidermal cooling can be given in many different ways. The simplest method is continuous contact cooling with chilled water, which can be circulated in glass, sapphire, or plastic housings. The laser impulse is given through the transparent housing, which should be constructed to ensure that the laser's

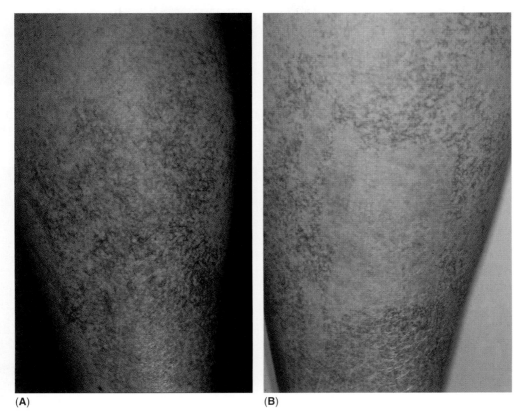

(A) **(B)**

Figure 11.4 A 63-year-old female with tanned, skin type III having isolated telangiectasias without associated varicosities. Previous attempt with sclerotherapy yielded no improvement. (**A**) Before treatment. (**B**) 10 minutes after treatment with intense pulsed light. Parameters were a double pulse of 2.4 and 7 ms with a 10-ms delay using a 570-nm filter, at 44 J/cm². *Source*: From Ref. 30.

effective fluence is not diminished. The benefit of continuous contact cooling is its simplicity. The disadvantage is that the cooling effect continues throughout the time that the device–crystal is in contact with the skin. This results in a variable degree and depth of cooling determined by the length of time the cold housing is in contact with the skin. This nonselective and variable depth and temperature of cooling may necessitate additional treatment energy so that the cooled vessel will heat up sufficiently for thermocoagulation.

Another method of cooling is contact precooling. In this approach, the cooling device contacts the epidermis adjacent to the laser aperture. The epidermis is precooled and then treated as the handpiece glides along the treatment area. Because the cooling surface is not in the beam path, no optical window is required and better thermal contact can be made between the cooling device and the epidermis. The drawback is the nonreproducibility of cooling levels and degrees that are based on the speed and pressure at which the surgeon uses the contact cooling device.

Yet another method for cooling the skin is to deliver a cold spray of refrigerant to the skin that is timed to precool the skin before laser penetration and also to postcool the skin to minimize thermal backscattering from the laser-generated

heat in the target vessel. The authors have termed this latter effect "thermal quenching" (Fig. 11.5). This method reproducibly protects the epidermis and superficial nerve endings. In addition, it acts to decrease the perception of thermal laser epidermal pain by providing another sensation (cold) to the sensory nerves. Finally, it allows an efficient use of laser energy because of the relative selectivity of the cooling spray that can be limited to the epidermis. The millisecond control of the cryogen spray prevents cooling of the deeper vascular targets and is given in varying amounts so that epidermal absorption of heat is counteracted by exposure to cryogen.

Since the target vessel poorly absorbs 1064-nm wavelength, a much higher fluence is necessary to cause thermocoagulation. Although a fluence of 10–20 J/cm^2 is sufficient to thermocoagulate blood vessels when delivered at 532 or 585 nm, a fluence of 70–150 J/cm^2 is required to generate sufficient heat absorption at 1064 nm. Various 1064-nm lasers are currently available that meet the criteria for selectively thermocoagulating blood vessels. Variabilities include the spot size, laser output (both in fluence and in how the extended time of the laser pulse is generated), pulse duration, and epidermal cooling (Fig. 11.6). In addition, although many claims are made by the laser

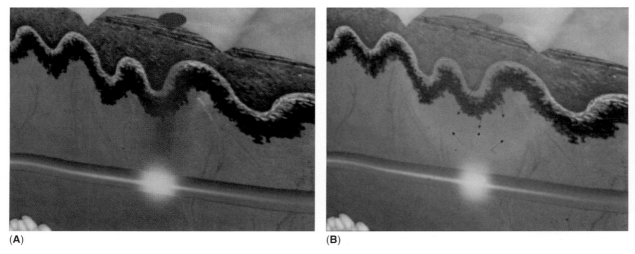

(A)   **(B)**

Figure 11.5 Thermal quenching through the application of dynamic cooling. (**A**) Laser pulse penetrates through the epidermis and dermis to be absorbed by the vascular target. (**B**) After absorption by the blood vessel, a pulse of cooling selectively protects the epidermis and quenches the heat rising from the thermocoagulated vessel. *Source*: From Ref. 28.

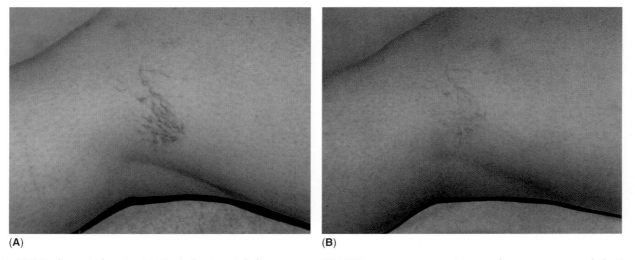

(A)   **(B)**

Figure 11.6 (**A**) Feeding reticular vein with distal telangiectasia before treatment. (**B**) 80% improvement, 3 months apart after one treatment with the Vasculight 6-mm spot, 120 J/cm^2 at 16-ms pulse duration. In comparison with sclero, would also require a second treatment to get to 95% clearance, concerning that there is some matting but no pigmentation.

manufacturers, few well-controlled peer-reviewed medical studies are available. A study on 30 women with leg telangiectasia compared treatment with 75% glucose solution sclerotherapy without the use of compression to long-pulsed 1064-nm Nd:YAG treatment using 100–120 J/cm², 15–30 ms, and 3-mm cooled spot (Xero, Cutera Inc., Brisbane, California, USA) and found that sclerotherapy was less painful and led to faster clinical improvement. This was significant since the sclerotherapy treatment utilized was suboptimal using no compression and a very low potency sclerosing solution (22).

To summarize, we have found the 1064-nm, long-pulsed Nd:YAG lasers to be beneficial in the treatment of leg telangiectasia not responsive to sclerotherapy or other lasers (Fig. 11.6). The benefit of using a 1064-nm laser is that its longer wavelength can penetrate more deeply, allowing effective thermosclerosis of vessels up to 3–4 mm in diameter. In addition, the 1064-nm wavelength permits treatment of patients of skin types I–VI with or without a tan, since melanin absorption is minimal. The 1064-nm, long-pulsed laser systems are not entirely without side effects. Cutaneous burns with resulting ulceration, pigmentation, and TM have been observed with each of these systems as parameters are being tested. The dynamically cooled 1064-nm Nd:YAG laser appears to produce the best clinical resolution with the least pain and adverse effects compared with other long-pulsed 1064-nm lasers. However, sclerotherapy still provides better results in fewer treatments, is associated with less pain, and has comparable adverse effects with lasers. Thus, the reader should evaluate the latest studies to ensure ideal results.

CONCLUSIONS

As sclerotherapy treatment is relatively cost-effective compared with laser or IPL treatment, when is it appropriate to use this advanced therapy? Obviously, needle-phobic patients will tolerate this technology even though the pain from lasers and IPL is more intense than that of sclerotherapy with all but hypertonic solutions. Patients who are prone to TM are also appropriate candidates. Finally, patients who have vessels that are resistant to sclerotherapy are excellent candidates. Efficacy of 75% clearance with two to three IPL treatments occurred in sclerotherapy-resistant vessels (23).

In a similar "vein," enhanced efficacy of treatment may occur when combining sclerotherapy with lasers or IPL. This technique is not new and was even reported approximately 30 years ago by the Italian vascular surgeon Leonardo Corcos, who used the argon laser to spot-weld telangiectasia so the sclerosing solution could have a prolonged contact with the vessel wall (24). This combination technique also gives the patient the opportunity to experience "laser" treatment, which is perceived as more advanced than merely injecting a solution into a vein. The optimal efficacy in treating common leg telangiectasia uses sclerotherapy to treat the feeding venous system and a laser or IPL to seal off superficial vessels, thus preventing extravasation with resulting pigmentation, recanalization, and TM.

So, is there a single laser that can adequately treat leg veins? The answer is yes and no. Yes, lasers are now available with pulse durations optimized to treat blood vessels of various sizes. One can select virtually any wavelength from 532 to 1064 nm, as well as a broad spectrum of IPL. It has been demonstrated that any wavelength can be used effectively as long as the pulse duration matches the diameter of the vessel and an appropriate fluence is utilized. This also assumes that the epidermis will be protected from nonspecific thermal effects by a variety of cooling and pulsing scenarios. One can cool the skin directly with a contact probe before and after the laser pulse or through a sapphire window before, during, and after the laser pulse. Cooling can also be given dynamically with a cryogen spray before, during, or after the laser pulse. Most patients prefer dynamic cooling as providing the highest degree of pain control. Contact cooling is unpredictable in adequately cooling the epidermis; unless optimal techniques are used, epidermal burns will occur.

However, the answer is also no, as presently available lasers still require skillful use for safe and effective treatment (Figs. 11.7 and 11.8). The ideal laser of the future (25) will have a built-in thermal sensor to detect both epidermal and vascular heating. This will automatically regulate the fluence so that the vessel is completely thermocoagulated while cooling the epidermis to maintain its temperature at that of one below a damaging threshold. Even better would be an infrared sensor that would determine the location of feeding dermal vessels so that they

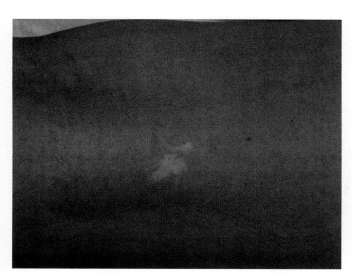

Figure 11.7 Hypopigmented scar 1 year after treatment of leg telangiectasia by a nurse in a plastic surgeon's office with an 800-nm diode laser.

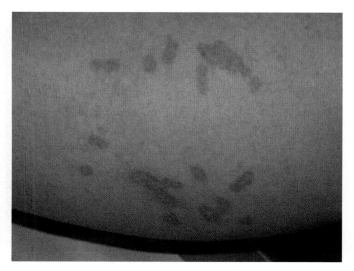

Figure 11.8 Hyperpigmentation 9 months after treatment of leg telangiectasia by a nurse at a medical spa with a long-pulsed alexandrite laser.

too can be treated along with the visible telangiectasia. One could imagine in the future the patient placing the leg into a laser machine that would map the visible veins to be thermocoagulated and automatically treat the entire superficial venous network. At this time, the only barrier preventing the development of such a laser is money and the willingness of a company to produce a machine of this type.

REFERENCES

1. Dover JS, Sadick NS, Goldman MP. The role of lasers and light sources in the treatment of leg veins. Dermatol Surg 1999; 25: 328.
2. Ross EV, Domankevitz Y. Laser treatment of leg veins: physical mechanisms and theoretical considerations. Lasers Surg Med 2005; 36: 105.
3. Kunishige JH, Goldberg LH, Friedman PM. Laser therapy for leg veins. Clin Dermatol 2007; 25: 454.
4. Weiss RA, Weiss MA. Resolution of pain associated with varicose and telangiectatic leg veins after compression sclerotherapy. J Dermatol Surg Oncol 1990; 16: 333.
5. Bernstein EF. Clinical characteristics of 500 consecutive patients presenting for removal of lower extremity spider veins. Dermatol Surg 2001; 27: 31.
6. Goldman MP, Kaplan RP, Duffy DM. Postsclerotherapy hyperpigmentation: a histologic evaluation. J Dermatol Surg Oncol 1987; 13: 547.
7. Duffy DM. Small vessel sclerotherapy: an overview. In: Callen JP, et al. eds. Advances in Dermatology. Chicago: Year Book Medical Publishers, 1988.
8. De Faria JL, Moraes IN. Histopathology of the telangiectasias associated with varicose veins. Dermatologia 1963; 127: 321.
9. Goldman MP. Laser and sclerotherapy treatment of leg veins: my perspective on treatment outcomes. Dermatol Surg 2002; 28: 969.
10. Polla LL, Tan OT, Garden JM, Parrish JA. Tunable pulsed dye laser for the treatment of benign cutaneous vascular ectasia. Dermatologica 1987; 174: 11.
11. Perez B, Nunez M, Boixeda P, et al. Progressive ascending telangiectasia treated with the 585nm flashlamp-pumped pulsed dye laser. Lasers Surg Med 1997; 21: 413.
12. Fajardo LF, Prionas SD, Kowalski J, Kwan HH. Hyperthermia inhibits angiogenesis. Radiat Res 1988; 114: 297.
13. Sadick NS, Sorhaindo L. An evaluation of post-sclerotherapy laser compression and its efficacy in the treatment of leg telangiectasias. Phlebology 2006; 21: 191.
14. Adrian RM. Long pulse normal mode alexandrite laser treatment of leg veins. Presented at the 18th Annual Meeting of the American Society of Laser Medicine and Surgery. San Diego, CA, April 5–7, 1998.
15. McDaniel DH, Ash K, Lord J, et al. Laser therapy of spider leg veins: clinical evaluation of a new long pulsed alexandrite laser. Dermatol Surg 1999; 25: 52.
16. Izikson L, Nelson JS, Anderson RR. Treatment of hypertrophic and resistant port wine stains with a 755-nm laser: A case series of 20 patients. Lasers Surg Med 2009; 41: 427.
17. Dierickx CC, Dugue V, Anderson RR. Treatment of leg telangiectasia by a pulsed 800nm diode laser. Presented at the 18th Annual Meeting of the American Society of Laser Medicine and Surgery. San Diego, Calif, April 5–7, 1998.
18. Trelles MA, Allones I, Álvarez J, et al. The 800-nm diode laser in the treatment of leg veins: Assessment at 6 months. J Am Acad Dermatol 2006; 54: 282.
19. Prieto V, Zhang P, Sadick NS. Comparison of a combination diode laser and radiofrequency device (Polaris®) and a long-pulsed 1064-nm Nd:YAG laser (Lyra®) on leg telangiectases. Histologic and immunohistochemical analysis. J Cosmet Laser Ther 2006; 8: 191.
20. Glassberg E, Lask GP, Tan EM, et al. The flashlamp-pumped 577-nm pulsed tunable dye laser: clinical efficacy and in vitro studies. J Dermatol Surg Oncol 1988; 14: 1200.
21. Black JF, Wade N, Barton JK. Mechanistic comparison of blood undergoing laser photocoagulation at 532 and 1,064 nm. Lasers Surg Med 2005; 36: 155.
22. Munia MA, Wolosker N, Munia CG, Puech-Leao P. Comparison of laser versus sclerotherapy in the treatment of lower extremity telangiectases: a prospective study. Dermatol Surg 2012; 38: 635.
23. Weiss RA, Weiss MA. Photothermal sclerosis of resistant telangiectatic leg and facial veins using the PhotoDerm VL. Presented at the Annual Meeting of the Mexican Academy of Dermatology. Monterey, Mexico, April 24, 1996.
24. Corcos L, Longo L. Classification and treatment of telangiectases of the lower limbs. Laser 1988; 1: 22.
25. Goldman MP. Are lasers or non-coherent light sources the treatment of choice for leg veins? A look into the future. Cosmet Dermatol 2001; 14: 58.
26. Goldman MP. Cosmetic and Cutaneous Laser Surgery. Elsevier: Philadelphia and THE Aesthetic Guide Primary Care Edition Autumn 2008, 2006: [Available from: www.miinews.com]
27. Anderson RA. Annual Meeting of the North American Society of Phlebology. Washington, DC, November, 1996.
28. Goldman MP, Weiss RA, Bergan JJ, eds. Varicose Veins and Telangiectasia: Diagnosis and Treatment. St Louis: Quality Medical Publishers, 1999.
29. West TB, Alster TS. Comparison of the long-pulsed dye and KTP lasers in the treatment of facial and leg telangiectasia. Dermatol Surg 1998; 24: 221.
30. Goldman MP, Guex JJ, Weiss RA, eds. Sclerotherapy Treatment of Varicose and Telangiectatic Leg Veins, 5th edn. London: Elsevier, Inc, 2011.

12 Body contouring: Noninvasive fat reduction

Lilit Garibyan, H. Ray Jalian, Mathew M. Avram, and Robert A. Weiss

INTRODUCTION

The rise in the rate of obesity and the increase in public, medical, and scientific awareness of the disadvantages of excess adipose tissue have made body-sculpting procedures more and more popular. Although diet, exercise, and bariatric surgeries may effectively control obesity and lead to dramatic weight loss, oftentimes cosmetic procedures are still necessary to remove excess fat deposition in selected, more focal areas. The improvement in shape and smoothness of the human physique is referred to as "body contouring." The traditional method of improving body contour is removal of fat via liposuction and it remains the gold standard in this field. Liposuction is the most commonly performed procedure worldwide for excess fat removal and currently is among the top five cosmetic surgical procedures performed in the USA (1). However, as liposuction is an invasive procedure there are inherent risks including postprocedural pain, infection, prolonged recovery, impaired social downtime, and anesthesia-related complications (2). All these factors have contributed to patients seeking less invasive methods for body contouring. Less invasive surgical techniques such as tumescent liposuction and laser-assisted lipoplasty are still invasive surgical procedures and therefore have higher risk compared with noninvasive fat removal. Of late, multiple different modalities using different methods to induce adipocyte apoptosis resulting in noninvasive fat reduction have become available. These modalities primarily aim at targeting the physical properties of fat that differentiate it from the overlying epidermis and dermis, thus resulting in selective removal of fat or lipolysis. Currently available noninvasive fat removal methods include heating, cryolipolysis, laser, radiofrequency, and ultrasound sources to more selectively target adipocytes. This chapter reviews currently available and novel approaches for noninvasive and intended selective destruction of fat. Devices utilizing cryolipolysis, lipid-selective wavelengths of laser light, thermal focused ultrasound (TFU) and nonthermal focused ultrasound (NTFU), and radiofrequency will be reviewed.

CRYOLIPOLYSIS

The selective destruction and noninvasive removal of fat with cooling is termed "cryolipolysis" (CoolSculpting®, Zeltiq, Pleasanton, CA). This novel approach for fat removal was introduced in 2007 and was cleared in 2010 by the U.S. Food and Drug Administration (FDA) for the treatment of localized fat of the flanks and later in 2012 for the abdomen. The concept behind the development of selective cold injury stems from the clinical observation of "popsicle panniculitis" reported in infants at the site of prolonged contact with an ice popsicle. Histologic analysis of these sites demonstrated panniculitis, which subsequently resolved with a temporary focal lipoatrophy (3). This report, along with other reports of cold-induced fat injury, suggests that fat cells are more susceptible to cold at certain temperatures compared with the surrounding tissue, particularly dermis (4). This concept of selective susceptibility to cold led to the development of cryolipolysis for the noninvasive removal of fat and body sculpting.

The initial preclinical animal studies aimed at determining the feasibility of selective destruction of fat in pigs with local, noninvasive controlled cooling. In these studies, a Yucatan pig was exposed to a prototype device with a copper plate cooled with antifreeze solution at a target temperature of −7°C, pressed firmly against the skin surface. After single treatment at ten different sites, lasting between 5 and 21 minutes, the animal was followed for 3.5 months for appearance and persistence of local fat loss. The amount of fat loss was estimated relative to the adjacent unexposed fat layer thickness. The results demonstrated that in all 10 sites tested, there was visible indentation noted, with a maximal relative loss of the superficial fat layer of nearly 80% (5). In addition, there was lack of apparent skin injury in the test sites and only one case of transient hyperpigmentation following the procedure. This selective loss of fat was not associated with elevated cholesterol or triglyceride levels when monitored up to 3 months posttreatment (5). This study demonstrated a significant reduction in fat layer thickness with no damage to skin or associated structures and no systemic elevation of cholesterol or triglyceride levels. A subsequent porcine study confirmed that cryolipolysis led to decreased thickness of the fat layer as measured by ultrasound and by histology. Histologic analysis showed approximately 50% reduction in the thickness of superficial fat layer (6). A lobular panniculitis and inflammatory infiltrate was present within the subcutaneous adipose tissue. The inflammatory infiltrate was seen approximately 2 days following treatment and was thought to be related to cold-induced adipocyte apoptosis. This response peaked approximately 1 month after treatment and then declined. The inflammatory infiltrate is predominantly composed of macrophages that are hypothesized to ingest and clear the apoptotic fat cells. This process occurs slowly over a period of 90 days posttreatment, with an end result of gradual reduction of fat that is observed clinically (6). Other hypothesized mechanisms of action include reperfusion injury following cooling of temperature-sensitive adipocytes, resulting in free radical damage, oxidative stress, and subsequent cell death (7).

Human clinical studies were conducted utilizing a cup-shaped treatment applicator with cooling panels on both sides.

Vacuum suction within the applicator was used to ensure tight contact and optimal positioning of the skin and area to be treated, between the two cooling plates (Fig. 12.1). This design also decreases blood flow within the skin fold, which allows for more rapid and efficient cooling of the skin. The clinician then selected a cooling intensity factor (CIF), a value representing the rate of heat flux in or out of the tissue. After 60 minutes of cooling at a set CIF, the treatment was complete and the device was removed, leaving a firm area of fat that becomes soft over several minutes after removing the applicator.

The latest generation of device requires no input from the treating physician. Early clinical studies demonstrated that compared with 30 minutes, 60 minutes of cooling fat led to far better results. To date, multiple clinical studies have demonstrated the efficacy and safety of cryolipolysis for fat layer reduction in humans. In a pivotal study, 32 patients with localized fat accumulation of the flanks ("love handles") demonstrated clinical improvement as measured by digital photography, physician assessment, and subject satisfaction. In this study, 10 patients underwent ultrasonography of their treated area, which showed an average reduction of 22.4% in fat layer thickness (Fig. 12.2) (8). In a subsequent study, 50 patients underwent treatment of one flank followed by photography of the treated and untreated sides. Based on these photographs, three blinded physicians were able to differentiate between pre- and posttreatment sites in 82% of patients (9). These studies resulted in FDA clearance in the summer of 2010.

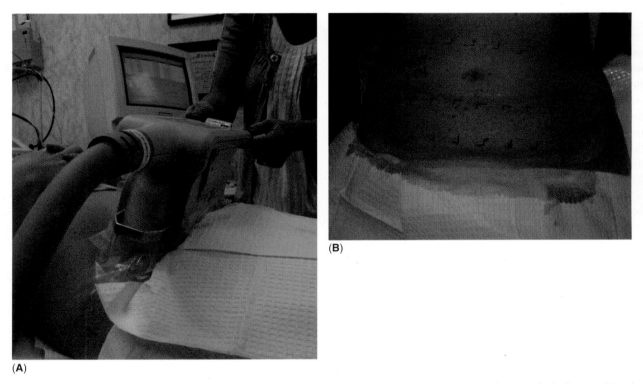

(A)

(B)

Figure 12.1 (**A**) The treatment applicator for cryolipolysis applied to the abdomen; notice the suction of fat into the applicator. (**B**) The fat is a solid wedge after removing the applicator after a 60-minute cycle; this clears within 10 minutes.

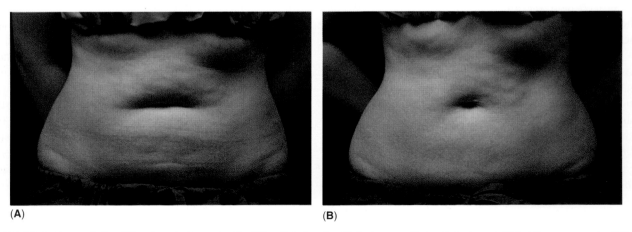

(A)   **(B)**

Figure 12.2 Clinical images before (**A**) and results 3 months after (**B**) a clinical study with the large applicator. Patients are told that they may expect a 25% reduction in fat from a single cycle. *Source*: Courtesy of Zeltiq Aesthetics, Inc.

Since FDA clearance in 2010, there have been more than hundreds of thousands of treatments completed. Data from all the clinical trials and studies thus far indicate that this device has a good safety profile without any systemic health effects. The most common reported and observed immediate adverse effect is localized erythema that can last for several hours after treatment. Localized ecchymosis at the site of device application has also been observed, especially in patients using aspirin or anticoagulants, and it is thought to be related to the vacuum suction of the applicator. Clinical studies have also reported reversible altered cutaneous sensation in the treated area, which is apparent immediately after treatment and can last up to 2 months. Typically soreness in the treated area is experienced for several days. Coleman et al. did a study to assess the effects of cryolipolysis on sensory function in humans and reported reduction in sensitivity to stimuli noted 1 week after treatment in all nine treated subjects that lasted 1–6 weeks (10). Six out of 9 subjects reported reduced pain or pinprick sensation. Some patients also reported reduction in light touch, 2-point discrimination, and temperature sensitivity on neurological examination of the treated area. A nerve biopsy taken from one patient 3 months following the procedure revealed no pathologic changes when compared with baseline biopsy specimens. In all cases, the neurologic side effects were transient and completely reversible by 2 months posttreatment.

The induction of adipocyte apoptosis did not significantly affect serum triglyceride or cholesterol levels or liver function tests, including aspartate aminotransferase, alanine aminotransferase, alkaline phosphatase, total bilirubin, and albumin (11). There have been rare reports of severe pain in approximately 0.05% of patients treated with cryolipolysis. This pain is characterized as a severe "shooting" and "jabbing" pain and the onset is usually within 4–7 days of treatment. The mechanism of action remains unclear, but it is more commonly seen with the treatment of a large surface area with the larger applicator. It is believed to be related to lax muscle with muscle being subject to prolonged cooling or may be related to a more robust panniculitis, nerve inflammation, or ischemia reperfusion injury resulting in allodynia and hyperneuralgia. In the 23 reported cases, rare severe pain was adequately controlled with topical and oral analgesics and resolved spontaneously within 1–4 weeks (12). The effect of cryolipolysis on patients with cold-induced dermatologic syndromes, such as cryoglobulinemia, cold-induced urticaria, Raynaud's syndrome, or paroxysmal cold-induced hemoglobinuria, is not yet known as most studies have excluded them from treatment (13).

When patients are seen for body contouring and they are deemed an appropriate candidate by a physician, the patients are informed that they may expect about 20–30% improvement with a single treatment and that multiple treatments may be required. We recommend waiting for 4–5 months to observe the maximal result from a single treatment. Cryolipolysis leads to induction of apoptosis, or programed cell death, for adipocytes. These slowly drop out, so the patient needs to understand that this will be a slow and steady process. The trade-off is minimal to no social downtime for a procedure that can reduce fat in selected areas on the flanks, abdomen, and even off-label uses such as inner thighs, male gynecomastia, and fat accumulations below the bra line in women.

ULTRASOUND

Ultrasound has been used to selectively target adipocytes through noninvasive mechanical and thermal mechanisms. Ultrasound is a cyclic sound pressure wave with frequency above the range of human hearing (>20 kHz). Ultrasound waves are capable of traveling through tissues and in the process they lose energy and become attenuated as they are reflected, scattered, or absorbed by the tissue they pass through. However, if sufficient quantities of ultrasound wave-generated energy reach the target tissue, they can induce molecular vibrations in the tissue, thus generating thermal heat (thermal-based ultrasound lipolysis). Ultrasound waves are also capable of creating holes (cavities) when they have sufficient negative pressure to overcome the adhesion of the medium molecules to each other (nonthermal or cavitation-based ultrasound lipolysis). In the latter case, mechanical energy of ultrasound is used to induce damage to targeted adipocytes. Ultrasound used for body sculpting is divided into two broad categories: cavitation-based lower-frequency nonthermal ultrasound that uses mechanical energy to disrupt adipocyte cells and high-intensity, thermal focused ultrasound (HIFU) that uses thermal energy to ablate adipose tissue (14).

NONTHERMAL FOCUSED ULTRASOUND

Cavitation-based NTFU (UltraShape™, Syneron/Candela Inc, Irvine, CA) uses focused ultrasound waves to deliver concentrated energy into a precise depth in the subcutaneous tissue resulting in cavitation. Focusing the ultrasound requires parabolic reflectors in the transducer. Target distances within the fat layer may be varied. Nonthermal, mechanical energy is used to disrupt fat cells without damaging the neighboring structures such as skin, blood vessels, and nerves. This technique takes advantage of the differential susceptibility of fat cells to mechanical stresses induced by the ultrasound. The device is composed of a parabolic transducer and an external visual guidance system to direct a focused beam of ultrasound energy (Fig. 12.3). Low-frequency ultrasound waves (~220 kHz) are delivered in pulse waves to the targeted tissue, where they generate cavitation causing cell death and apoptosis due to mechanical cell disruption (14,15).

One of the initial studies to demonstrate efficacy of NTFU was conducted in Spain on 30 healthy patients using Ultra-Shape *Contour I* (UltraShape Ltd., Syneron/Candela), a noninvasive, NTFU device. In this study, all patients underwent three treatments at 1-month interval and were evaluated 1 month after the last treatment. Outcomes were assessed on the basis of change in fat thickness, ultrasound measurements, and circumference measurements. Results showed that after three treatments, there was a mean reduction of fat thickness by 2.28 ± 0.80 cm and circumference reduction by a mean of 3.95 ± 1.99 cm, while weight was unchanged (15). A larger study with 137 patients reported a mean reduction of approximately 2 cm in treatment area circumference and approximately 2.9 mm in skin fat thickness after a single treatment. Most of the effect was notable within 2 weeks and lasted for 12 weeks (16). Overall, the treatments were well tolerated with patient experiencing only mild pain, but there were scattered reports of blister formation on the skin as a consequence of wave reflection of ultrasound waves over bony prominences. Studies for Asian patients using the same device were reported

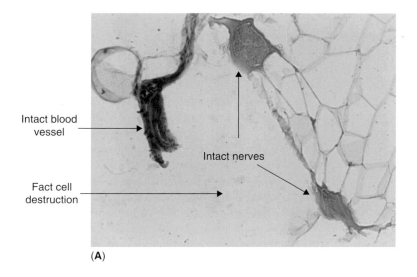

(A)

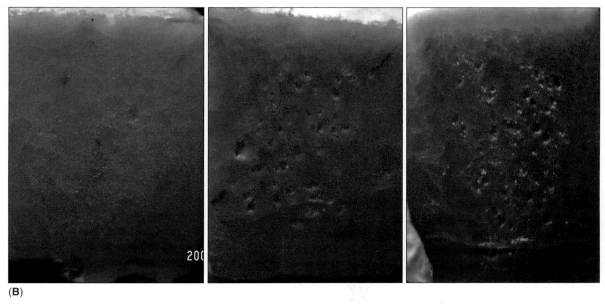

(B)

Figure 12.3 (**A**) Histology of porcine fat showing minimal impact for cavitation-based NTFU on nerves and blood vessels. (**B**) Porcine fat treated with NTFU shows cavitation without thermal effects; the third panel on the right shows a pass with a new variable depth focusing handpiece, which increases the vertical impact of cavitation. *Source*: Courtesy of UltraShape, Syneron/Candela. *Abbreviation*: NTFU, nonthermal focused ultrasound.

as well, but with less clinical result (17). Further studies are needed to determine the efficacy and the exact mechanism of fat loss. NTFU is pending clearance by the FDA for circumference reduction of the waist. Porcine studies have shown reduction in fat with a minimal impact on nerve tissue and blood vessels, so resultant risks of purpura are low (data on file, UltraShape, Syneron/Candela) (Fig. 12.3). The newest versions of this device allow multiple depth focal points. Clinical results have been documented after three treatments spaced 1 month apart (Fig. 12.4).

THERMAL FOCUSED ULTRASOUND

TFU (Liposonix®, Solta) has been used to thermally and selectively target adipose tissue leading to ablation. TFU delivers focused, high-intensity ultrasonic energy (~2 MHz) into subcutaneous tissue, which quickly raises the temperature above 56°C resulting in coagulative necrosis of the adipocytes and a subsequent reduction in fat layer. Passive heat diffusion to the overlying dermis is also hypothesized to possibly induce collagen remodeling in the skin. The prototype first-generation

device used a proprietary pattern generator that could be programed to move the ultrasound wave to predetermined focal points within the treatment area, thus allowing generation of a homogeneous matrix of lesions. The second-generation device that received FDA clearance in September 2011 for noninvasive fat removal is smaller in size. The ability of this device to focus into the appropriate plane allows individual lower-energy ultrasound beams to pass through the skin and intervening tissue layer above the focal zone providing less heating. When the target zone is reached, intensity is increased resulting in a high heating rate and ablation of subcutaneous fat.

Initial preclinical animal studies used to demonstrate the feasibility of selective fat destruction in porcine model showed localized damage within the fat with intact vasculature and nerve fibers within the treatment area (14). There was no evidence of fat accumulation or emboli on gross examination of tissue from various organs of these animals. Two case series were published to demonstrate the efficacy and safety in humans. The first reported a retrospective case series of 282 patients who underwent a single TFU treatment of their anterior abdomen

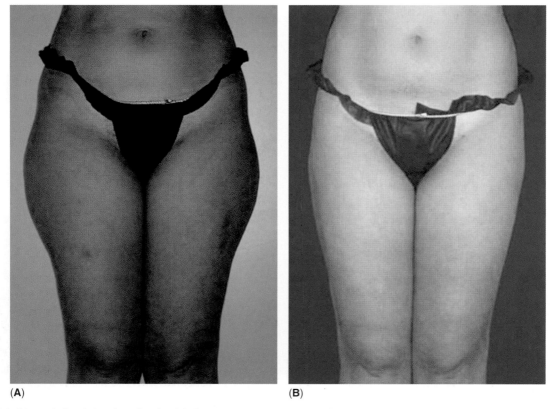

Figure 12.4 Clinical image before (**A**) and results after (**B**) three treatments spaced 1 month apart with nonthermal focused ultrasound (UltraShape). *Source*: Courtesy of UltraShape, Syneron/Candela.

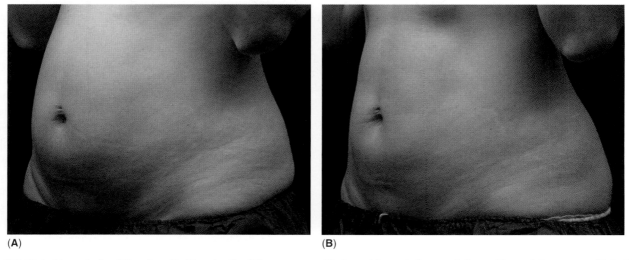

Figure 12.5 Clinical image before (**A**) and results 12 weeks after (**B**) a treatment with thermal focused ultrasound. *Source*: Liposonix®; courtesy of Solta Medical Aesthetic Center.

and flanks. Waist circumference measured before and 3 months after single treatment was one of the primary outcomes (Fig. 12.5) (18). The second study treated the abdomen and flank of 85 patients with a single session of HIFU (19). Both studies reported an average waist circumference reduction of 4.4 and 4.7 cm, respectively. In addition, greater than 70% subject satisfaction was reported in both studies at 3 months after treatment. Unfortunately, diet was not controlled in either study.

The seminal study that led to the approval of this device by FDA for body contouring, was a randomized controlled trial done by Jewell et al. (20). In this study, 180 patients were randomized to 1:1:1 to two treatment groups with variable

energy levels or sham-treated control group. Primary outcome measures included waist circumference measured at the iliac crest. Statistically significant decrease in waist circumference in treatment groups when compared with sham-treated control group was noted at 12 weeks following single treatment. During the study period, patients were instructed to continue their routine diet and exercise regimen in all treatment groups, and no significant change in body mass was noted in all treatment groups.

Histologic analysis of tissue from abdominal sites treated with TFU was obtained from patients who had subsequent abdominoplasty after TFU treatments. Evaluation of these tissues revealed clearly demarcated zones of necrosis visible on gross inspection of the treatment areas. The overlying dermis and epidermis were intact with no evidence of injury. Immediately after treatment, adipocyte necrosis was present in histologic specimens. Two weeks following treatment, a localized inflammatory infiltrate consisting primarily of scavenger macrophages is observed. It is presumed that these macrophages engulf cellular debris and extracellular lipids released from necrotic adipocytes, as lipid-laden macrophages were present within the treatment zone. The inflammatory and healing process is completed in about 14 weeks after treatment, which is the time that clinical reduction in fat is also observed (18).

From the limited clinical data available thus far, TFU has demonstrated a favorable safety profile when used for body contouring. Prolonged tenderness, edema, ecchymosis, and hard lumps were seen in less than 12% of patients. Importantly, all adverse events resolved within 1–3 months after treatment. Some treatments were terminated due to excessive pain during the treatment, but this pain resolved completely upon the termination of treatment (18,19). This illustrates the difference between thermal and NTFU, with nonthermal being much less painful during treatment application. Importantly, like all the devices used to affect adipocytes, TFU did not lead to elevation in serum lipid levels or liver function tests in multiple clinical studies. The first- and second-generation HIFU devices received FDA clearance in 2011 for body contouring.

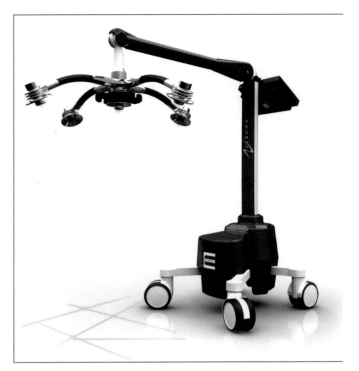

Figure 12.6 An FDA cleared multiple head, low-level laser therapy device for fat reduction. *Source*: Courtesy of Zerona.

LOW-LEVEL LASER THERAPY

The use of low-level light to affect cell biology and metabolic activity is termed photomodulation. The modulation of cell activity is believed to be the effect on mitochondria cell organelles. It is believed by some that low-level light may influence adipocytes making their membranes less stable. Low-level laser therapy (LLLT; Zerona™, Erchonia) claim for fat reduction was based on in vivo observation that a 635-nm laser caused a transitory pore within adipocytes, leading to deflation of the adipocyte through the release of lipids into the interstitial space. The theory was that this pore does not damage the cells but allows for the efflux of lipid contents from the cell into the interstitial space (21). The mechanism of action was thought to result from photoexcitation of cytochrome-*c* oxidase, an enzyme component of respiratory chain within the mitochondria as in other LLLT devices (22). LLLT received FDA clearance in 2010 for fat reduction (Fig. 12.6).

Several commercial devices are available and are various iterations of multiple low power laser diode modules operating at a wavelength of 635 nm. Current treatment recommendations are to undergo six to eight sessions, each lasting up to 30 minutes. In addition, some device manufacturers recommend concomitant proprietary nutritional supplements aimed at enhancing the lymphatic and circulatory systems. Although numerous studies exist on the role of laser-induced adipocyte modification as an adjunct to liposuction, there are limited data regarding the use of LLLT alone for fat reduction. The results from the limited number of studies are mixed. An initial, double-blind, placebo-controlled trial demonstrated an overall combined reduction of 3.51 inches when the results of all treatment sites (waist, hip, and thighs) were combined together, compared with 0.6 inches in the control group (23). This is based on subjective circumference measurements, not

on objective ultrasound or 3D imaging modalities. Critics have also noted the short follow-up time of these studies. A nonrandomized, uncontrolled retrospective study analyzed data from 689 patients who had the LLLT procedure to evaluate the circumferential reduction across the treatment site of the waist, hips, and thighs as well as untreated systemic regions (24). They reported a mean circumferential reduction in all treated sites 1 week after the treatment regimen of 3.27 inches. Most importantly, reduction was not attributed to fluid or fat relocation as all measurement points, including the untreated areas, demonstrated circumferential reduction. Study subjects were not asked to abstain from receiving any other treatment to promote body contouring and/or weight loss while receiving LLLT. Subsequent investigator-initiated trials using the same device with less number of patients failed to show statistically significant reduction in fat using waist circumference and more objective ultrasound measurements of fat layer thickness (22).

INFRARED LASERS

Infrared lasers use the concept of selective photothermolysis to specifically target fat. This involves the selection of a wavelength of light and pulse duration that can selectively heat up adipose tissue without damage to the surrounding tissue. Individual chromophores within the target tissue allow confinement of heat, specifically within target tissue. Infrared bands have been found to be useful for the selective targeting of lipid-rich tissues such as fat. The absorption spectrum of fat has two unique peaks at 1210 and 1720 nm, which were greater than that of water. It has been demonstrated that exposure of intact, full-thickness porcine tissue samples to infrared lasers with a wavelength of 1210 nm causes reproducible thermal damage to subcutaneous fat without injuring the overlying skin or surrounding tissues (25).

In a pilot human study, 24 subjects were treated noninvasively on the abdomen to a 1210 nm laser with variable fluences, a 10-mm spot size, and a 3-second exposure time. Six-millimeter punch biopsies were taken either at 1–3 days or at 4–6 weeks after treatment. Using nitroblue tetrazolium chloride (NTC) staining, which is a marker for viability, a dose-dependent damage to the subcutaneous fat and dermis was demonstrated. There was clear histologic evidence of laser-induced damage to fat, but no evidence was presented to support the clinical efficacy of this technique in fat removal due to the single pulse nature of this study (26). This treatment can be painful. Further studies and optimization of treatment parameters are still ongoing to one day allow this laser to be a useful tool for the noninvasive selective destruction of fat leading to fat removal.

RADIOFREQUENCY

Radiofrequency (RF) energy has been used for decades for a variety of medical applications such as tissue electrodessication, electrocoagulation, cardiac electroconduction ablation, and neoplasm eradication (27). In the past few years, researchers have attempted to harvest energy generated through RF for selective targeting of dermal and adipose tissues. RF energy is produced by an electric current that is able to pass through tissue. Heat is generated by RF through the transfer of energy from the electric field to the charges in target tissue. Because RF is not produced by a light source, the RF heating is not dependent on chromophores or skin type, and therefore patients of different skin phototypes and ethnicity can safely be treated with RF-based systems (Exilis™, BTL, Prague, The Czech Republic; Thermage™, Solta, Hayward, California, USA; Endymed™, Caesarea, Israel).

RF has different clinical and biological effects depending upon the depth of tissue targeted. The depth of penetration of RF energy is inversely proportional to the frequency. Therefore, at lower frequencies, energy is able to penetrate deeper. RF technology has the ability to noninvasively and selectively heat large volumes of subcutaneous adipose tissue. By selecting the appropriate electric field, one can obtain greater heating of fat. RF can be delivered using monopolar, bipolar, and unipolar devices. In monopolar devices, a delivery electrode is placed over a target area and a return electrode is applied at a distant site. This allows current to be generated, which passes through the target tissue and returns to the grounding pad somewhere else on the body inducing deeper thermal damage. In general, monopolar devices have more deeply penetrating effects than bipolar or unipolar devices. Pain is related to the duration of the pulse with some devices being painful and some being more like gentle thermal heating. Monopolar devices can be static where a short cycle is given while the handpiece is held in place or dynamic where the handpiece is continuously moved. Generally the dynamic devices (Exilis) tend to be more like a warm massage.

For bipolar RF devices, both electrodes are incorporated into a single handpiece. The distance between electrodes determines the depth of penetration and heating, which is typically confined to within 1–4 mm of the skin surface. Unipolar RF systems function with one electrode and no grounding pad. Some RF devices have controlled cooling built-in to allow protection of epidermis and dermis from thermal damage.

Most of the studies, including the initial animal and human studies, using radiofrequency devices have been aimed at skin tightening and cellulite. Although RF devices have been shown to produce tissue tightening, there are some data to suggest that they also can be effective in the removal of localized fat. Few studies have analyzed the use of RF devices on subcutaneous fat and circumferential reduction in size of treated areas. A study used ThermalCool TC (Solta Medical, Inc.) device with the Thermage Multiplex Tip to evaluate its effect on abdominal skin laxity and waist circumference. ThermalCool TC is a type of noninvasive monopolar RF device that provides precooling, parallel cooling, and postcooling for epidermal protection. Twelve subjects were treated in this study and results demonstrated an average decrease in waist circumference of 1.4 cm at 1-month follow-up visit. All patients tolerated the procedure with only mild-to-moderate tenderness but 10 out of 12 patients did have to take NSAIDs, oxycodone, and acetaminophen combination, and diazepam 1 hour before treatment (28). Although no histologic assessment of treated tissue was performed in this study, another study using a different monopolar RF device was able to demonstrate that adipocyte cell death from the thermal injury, which was evident starting at 9 days after treatment. Foamy histiocytic and granulomatous infiltrates were observed after cell death around the adipose tissue, but no increase in circulating lipid levels was seen (29). Another human study with a monopolar RF device, the Exilis (BTL) was used in a study to evaluate its effect on body contouring. The device is shown and body applicator is detailed in Figure 12.7. Exilis is a dynamic monopolar device as it has a handpiece that is in continuous motion allowing areas of skin with the most laxity to be specifically targeted. It has been utilized for reduction for body contouring around the abdomen, hips, thighs, and other areas of fat. Results are shown for the hips and abdomen for the body handpiece in Figure 12.8. In a study using this device, 20 subjects had four circumferential treatment sessions with the Exilis device for the upper arm. Treatment outcome was not measured by images or circumference but by ultrasound thickness of fat layer. Measurements were taken at very precise reproducible points on the arm. Authors reported average posterior fat reduction for the arm of 0.5 versus 0.02 cm for untreated control arms. (Weiss et al., in press, 2013). This was a statistically significant measurement of fat reduction by ultrasound fat layer thickness. So it has been demonstrated that RF can be utilized for fat reduction although ultimate clinical benefits of RF for fat reduction await further studies with larger numbers of patients.

CONCLUSION

In our current body-image conscious society, there is a growing demand for noninvasive body contouring. Few patients can devote the social downtime required of more invasive procedures. Patient demand and social media awareness over the past few years have led to the development of a number of ultrasound, laser, radiofrequency, light, and cold-based noninvasive systems. There is tremendous interest in methods of fat reduction and body contouring with more limited downtime and fewer serious side effects. These various modalities allow selective targeting of fat tissue taking advantage of the unique properties of adipocytes. Certain devices may provide the added benefit of tissue tightening. As shown in Table 12.1, these devices have different mechanisms of action, treatment times,

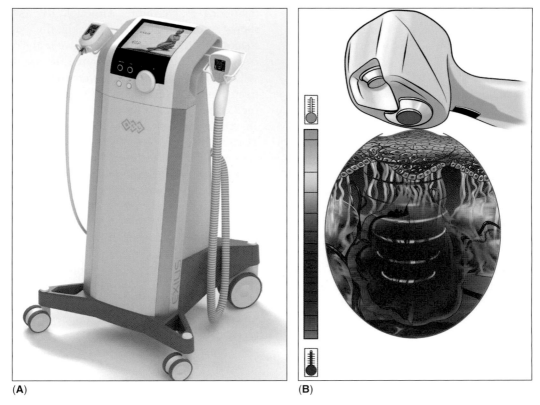

(A)   (B)

Figure 12.7 (**A**) Dynamic monopolar radiofrequency device with two heads. Face applicator and body applicator in a single unit. Temperature is monitored during treatment with body applicator seen on the right. (**B**) Schematic of body handpiece applicator with variable depth of heating cooling applied at the transducer protects the skin, allowing deeper penetration into fat without epidermal injury. *Source*: Exilis; courtesy of BTL, Prague, The Czech Republic.

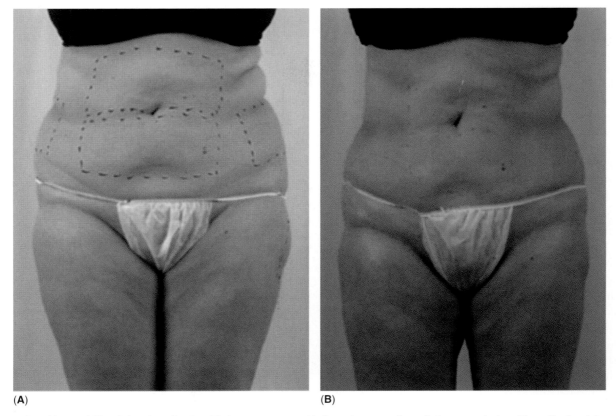

(A)   (B)

Figure 12.8 Clinical images before (**A**) and results after (**B**) three treatments with dynamic monopolar radiofrequency device with cooling handpiece shown in abdomen area.

Table 12.1 Devices and Treatments for the Selective Targeting of Fat Tissue

Treatment	Brand Names	Mechanism of Adipocyte Damage	Indications	Areas Treated	Anesthesia and Analgesia	Time per Treatment per Site	Time to Results (Reported)	Clearance Status
Cryolipolysis	Zeltiq	Cold-induced apoptosis	Focal adiposity	Flanks and abdomen	None	60 min	3 mo	FDA cleared
TFU	LipoSonix	Thermal destruction	Focal adiposity and skin tightening	Abdomen, flanks, and buttocks	Oral analgesics	90 min	90 d	FDA approved
NTFU	UltraShape	Cavitation reduction	Focal adiposity	Abdomen	None	30–90 min	3–4 wk	FDA clearance pending
Low-level laser therapy	Various	Nonthermal deflation (in vitro)	Focal adiposity and skin tightening	Abdomen, thighs, flanks, and neck	None	20–30 min	2–4 wk	FDA cleared
Infrared laser		Photothermolysis	Focal adiposity	Abdomen	Topical or injected anesthesia	~10 min	4–6 wk	Not FDA cleared
Radiofrequency	Thermage Exilis Endymed	Thermal reduction	Focal adiposity and skin tightening	Abdomen, thighs, buttocks, extremities, and face	None	~30 min to 2 hr	4–12 wk	FDA cleared

Abbreviations: d, day; mo, month; NTFU, nonthermal focused ultrasound; TFU, thermal focused ultrasound; wk, week.

level of pain associated with each treatment, and the time to final results. Based on patient's needs, the appropriate modality can be chosen. In choosing the device, the clinical efficacy should be reviewed with each patient to set the expectations correctly. Managing realistic expectations are key to ensuring satisfaction with results. Although many of the devices reviewed in this chapter have shown clinical efficacy in preliminary clinical trials, one should approach the results with healthy skepticism, especially when clinical outcome is measured only by images or circumferential measurements in small circumference areas of the body. Most of these clinical studies were based on limited number of patients, although once in regular daily use after FDA clearance, clinical experience accelerates incredibly quickly. Already hundreds of thousands of patients have been treated worldwide with cryolipolysis, NTFU and TFU, and rapidly proliferating RF devices. These devices achieve measurable clinically significant end points for patients without the downtime of invasive procedures, although the effects of individual treatments and individual devices may be quite variable and of course less dramatic than invasive fat reduction and body contouring procedures.

Regardless of the modality chosen for noninvasive fat removal, there are certain important points that each physician should discuss with patient before initiating noninvasive fat removal. First and foremost, patients should understand that these modalities are not a substitute for weight loss and healthy living. Second, patients should be thoroughly informed about the relatively modest nature of fat reduction with these techniques, which does not compare with the efficacy or results seen with liposuction. Maximal reduction for a single treatment is typically in the 20–30% range. Multiple treatments are typically necessary to obtain the desired results, which also can take up to 6 months after treatment to be appreciated. The devices reviewed in this chapter have demonstrated favorable safety results and when evaluated, they did not lead to liver function or lipid level abnormalities, with some modalities achieving better results than others.

REFERENCES

1. The American society of plastic surgeons: national clearinghouse of plastic surgery procedural statistics: the American society of plastic surgeons. [Available from: http://www.asps.org] [accessed November 8, 2011].
2. Matarasso A, Swift RW, Rankin M. Abdominoplasty and abdominal contour surgery: a national plastic surgery survey. Plastic Reconstruct Surg 2006; 117: 1797–808.
3. Epstein EH Jr, Oren ME. Popsicle panniculitis. N Engl J Med 1970; 282: 966–7.
4. Beacham BE, Cooper PH, Bushanan CS, et al. Equestrian cold panniculitis in women. Arch Dermatol 1980; 116: 1025–7.
5. Manstein D, Laubach H, Watanabe K, et al. Selective cryolysis: a novel method of non-invasive fat removal. Lasers Surg Med 2008; 40: 595–604.
6. Zelickson B, Egbert BM, Preciado J, et al. Cryolipolysis for noninvasive fat cell destruction: initial results from a pig model. Dermatol Surg 2009; 35:1462–70.
7. Preciado JA, Allison JW. The effect of cold exposure on adipocytes: Examining a novel method for the non-invasive removal of fat. Cryobiology 2008; 57: 327–7.
8. Dover J, Burns J, Coleman S, et al. A prospective clinical study of noninvasive cryopolysis for subcutaneous fat layer reduction—Interim report of available subject data. In Annual Meeting of the American Society for Laser Medicine and Surgery. National Harbor, Maryland, 2009.
9. Kaminer M, Weiss R, Newman J, et al. Visible cosmetic improvement with cryolipolysis: Photographic evidence. In Annual Meeting of the American Society for Dermatologic Surgery. Phoenix, AZ, 2009.
10. Coleman SR, Sachdeva K, Egbert BM, et al. Clinical efficacy of noninvasive cryolipolysis and its effects on peripheral nerves. Aesthetic Plast Surg 2009; 33: 482–8.
11. Klein KB, Zelickson B, Rieopelle JG, et al. Non-invasive cryolipolysis for subcutaneous fat reduction does not affect serum lipid levels or liver function tests. Lasers Surg Med 2009; 41: 785–90.
12. Dover J, Saedi N, Kaminer M, Zachary C. Side effects and risks associated with cryolipolysis. In Annual Meeting of the American Society for Laser Medicine and Surgery. Grapevine, Texas, 2011.
13. Avram MM, Harry RS. Cryolipolysis for subcutaneous fat layer reduction. Lasers Surg Med 2009; 41: 703–8.
14. Jewell ML, Solish NJ, Desilets CS. Noninvasive body sculpting technologies with an emphasis on high-intensity focused ultrasound. Aesthetic Plast Surg 2011; 35: 901–12.
15. Moreno-Moraga J, Valero-Altés T, Riquelme AM, et al. Body contouring by non-invasive transdermal focused ultrasound. Lasers Surg Med 2007; 39: 315–23.
16. Teitelbaum SA, Burns JL, Kubota J, et al. Noninvasive body contouring by focused ultrasound: safety and efficacy of the Contour I device in a multicenter, controlled, clinical study. Plast Reconstr Surg 2007; 120: 779–89; discussion 790.
17. Shek S, Yu C, Yeung CK, et al. The use of focused ultrasound for non-invasive body contouring in Asians. Lasers Surg Med 2009; 41: 751–9.
18. Fatemi A. High-intensity focused ultrasound effectively reduces adipose tissue. Semin Cutan Med Surg 2009; 28: 257–62.
19. Fatemi A, Kane MA. High-intensity focused ultrasound effectively reduces waist circumference by ablating adipose tissue from the abdomen and flanks: a retrospective case series. Aesthetic Plast Surg 2010; 34: 577–82.
20. Jewell ML, Baxter RA, Cox SE, et al. Randomized sham-controlled trial to evaluate the safety and effectiveness of a high-intensity focused ultrasound device for noninvasive body sculpting. Plast Reconstr Surg 2011; 128: 253–62.
21. Neira R, Arroyave J, Ramirez H, et al. Fat liquefaction: effect of low-level laser energy on adipose tissue. Plast Reconstr Surg 2002; 110: 912–22; discussion 923-5.
22. Elm CM, Wallander ID, Endrizzi B, et al. Efficacy of a multiple diode laser system for body contouring. Lasers Surg Med 2011; 43: 114–21.
23. Jackson RF, Dedo DD, Roche GC, et al. Low-level laser therapy as a non-invasive approach for body contouring: a randomized, controlled study. Lasers Surg Med 2009; 41: 799–809.
24. Jackson RF, Stern FA, Neira R, et al. Application of low-level laser therapy for noninvasive body contouring. Lasers Surg Med 2012; 44: 211–17.
25. Anderson RR, Farinelli W, Laubach H, et al. Selective photothermolysis of lipid-rich tissues: a free electron laser study. Lasers Surg Med 2006; 38: 913–19.
26. Wanner M, Avram M, Gagnon D, et al. Effects of non-invasive, 1,210 nm laser exposure on adipose tissue: results of a human pilot study. Lasers Surg Med 2009; 41: 401–7.
27. Alster TS, Lupton JR. Nonablative cutaneous remodeling using radiofrequency devices. Clin Dermatol 2007; 25: 487–91.
28. Anolik R, Chapas AM, Brightman LA, et al. Radiofrequency devices for body shaping: a review and study of 12 patients. Semin Cutan Med Surg 2009; 28: 236–43.
29. Franco W, Kothare A, Ronan SJ, et al. Hyperthermic injury to adipocyte cells by selective heating of subcutaneous fat with a novel radiofrequency device: feasibility studies. Lasers Surg Med 2010; 42: 361–70.

13 Use of lasers on Asian skin

Woraphong Manuskiatti

INTRODUCTION

The approximately 4.2 billion Asians in China, India, Japan, the Middle East, Southeast Asia, and elsewhere represent the majority of the world's population (1). Asian population is a diverse group with various skin phototypes ranging from Fitzpatrick types III to V. Racial differences in skin pathophysiology have been well documented (2–4). The high risk of pigmentary alterations and scarring following any procedure that produces inflammation of the skin continues to influence physicians to exercise caution with this group of patients. This caution also applies to laser therapy. Even with the highly selective characteristics of current laser and pulsed light therapy, when results are expected to be similar between the races, they are not. Both genetic background and environmental factors are involved in these differences.

Skin laser surgery for Asians is different from that for Caucasians in several important characteristics. Asian skin is often more pigmented than Caucasian skin, resulting in interference by epidermal melanin when using lasers to treat dermal lesions. Consequently, adverse pigmentary reactions, especially postinflammatory hyperpigmentation, are more likely to develop following laser surgery (5,6). Another important issue is the differences in the biological behavior of melanocytes among patients from different genetic backgrounds. A controversial deleterious effect of laser exposure is malignant transformation. Unlike the Caucasian population, melanoma is uncommon among Asians, and differences in skin types are uncertain to be the main explanation. Therefore, the risk of using laser for the removal of nevomelanocytic lesions in Asians differs from that in Caucasians.

Race is also a critical factor in the response of the skin to inflammation. Asians are far more likely than Caucasians to develop keloids. Some conditions such as nevus of Ota or acquired bilateral nevus of Ota-like macules (ABNOMs, Hori's nevus) are more commonly seen in Asians (5,6). Furthermore, photoaging in Asians tends to occur at a later age and have more pigmentary problems but less wrinkling than that in Caucasians (7).

DIFFERENCES BETWEEN PIGMENTED AND WHITE SKIN

The surgeon who considers performing laser surgical procedures in non-Caucasian patients should have an understanding of the morphological differences between white and nonwhite skin, especially in patients of Asian and black descent. The major determinant of differences in skin color between nonwhite and white skin is the amount of epidermal melanin. Although there is no difference in the quantity of melanocytes between the two groups, the larger and more melanized melanosomes in nonwhite skin compared with white skin have been well documented (8). In addition, the degradation rate of melanosomes within the keratinocytes of dark skin is slower than that of white skin. The larger and more melanized melanosomes of black skin absorb and scatter more energy, thus providing higher photoprotection. Conversely, the melanocytes and mesenchyma in darker skin seem to be more vulnerable to trauma and inflammatory conditions than those in white skin (9).

The majority of cutaneous laser wavelengths have significant overlap with the absorption spectrum of melanin (see chap. 1). Therefore, nonwhite skin presents a significant challenge because of greater absorption of laser energy and resulting damage to melanin-laden cells, increasing the risk of adverse complications, including hypopigmentation, hyperpigmentation, and depigmentation. Interestingly, alterations in pigmentation may not be apparent for several months after laser therapy. Thus, when treating nonwhite skin, test sites and long-term follow-up should be considered.

Asian and black skins have a thicker dermis than white skin, the thickness being proportional to the intensity of pigmentation. This increased dermal thickness, along with photoprotection from an increase in the size and number of melanosomes, may account for a lower incidence of facial rhytides in Asians and blacks. Increased mesenchymal reactivity may result in hypertrophic scars and keloids. Like black skin, Asian skin has a greater tendency toward hypertrophic scarring. Asians may also have a greater tendency toward prolonged redness during scar maturation than whites do (10,11).

Fitzpatrick developed the classification of skin phototypes based on response to ultraviolet (UV) irradiation of the Caucasian population (Box 13.1) (12). However, it has often been found that a patient with skin phototype I or II may have genetic origins of skin phototypes III–VI. Given the same clinical expertise in a specific cosmetically sensitive procedure, such as laser surgery, the result would be significantly different in clinically similar patients if one had considered more distant ancestry. Lancer proposed the so-called Lancer Ethnicity Scale (Table 13.1), factoring in this additional historical information to provide a method to presurgically determine skin type of the patients and more clearly predict the outcome (13,14). Goldman proposed a "universal classification of skin type" that considers genetic racial heritage in the response of melanocytes to both UV light and inflammation (Box 13.2) (15).

Box 13.1 Fitzpatrick Classification of Skin Type

   I. Always burns, never tans
  II. Burns easily, tans minimally with difficulty
 III. Burns moderately, tans moderately and uniformly
 IV. Burns minimally, tans moderately and easily
  V. Rarely burns, tans profusely
 VI. Never burns, tans profusely

Table 13.1 Lancer Ethnicity Scale

LES Skin Type	Fitzpatrick Skin Phenotype	Background Geography
		European
LES Type 3	Type II	Ashkenazy Jewish
LES Type 1	Type I	Celtic
LES Type 2	Type III	Central, Eastern European
LES Type 1	Type I–II	Nordic
LES Type 1–2	Type I	Northern European (general)
LES Type 3–4	Type III	Southern European, Mediterranean
		North American
LES Type 3	Type II	Native American (including Inuit)
		Asian
LES Type 4	Type IV	Chinese, Korean, Japanese, Thai, Vietnamese
LES Type 4	Type IV	Filipino, Polynesian
		Latin/Central/South American
LES Type 4	Type IV	Central, South American Indian
		African
LES Type 5	Type V	Central, East, West African
LES Type 5	Type V	Eritrean and Ethiopian
LES Type 5	Type V	North African, Middle East Arabic
LES Type 4	Type III	Sephardic Jewish

Risk Factors: LES Type 1, very low risk; LES Type 2, low risk; LES Type 3, moderate risk; LES Type 4, significant risk; LES Type 5, considerable risk.
ªThe LES is a system to calculate healing efficacy and times. To calculate individual's skin on the LES, find the LES skin type numbers for each of his or her four grandparents. Add the numbers together and divide this total by four. The lower LES skin type, the better skin healing should be after laser surgery and the less risk there is of scarring, keloids, erythema, discoloration, and uneven pigmentation.
Abbreviation: LES, Lancer Ethnicity Scale.
Source: Adapted From Ref. 13.

CLINICAL APPLICATIONS

Current laser or light-source systems can be classified according to the desired target of destruction (see chap. 1). Similar to the clinical applications on white complexions, the indications of laser therapy in Asian skin include vascular-specific lasers, laser treatment for hypertrophic scars, keloids and striae, pigment-specific lasers, laser hair removal, ablative laser resurfacing, and nonablative and ablative fractionated resurfacing (11,16,17).

In general, these applications are well established in Asia, with devices having been available for many years. Treatment

Box 13.2 World Classification of Skin Type

1. European/Caucasian: white:
   a. Pale, cannot tan, burns easily, no postinflammatory pigmentation
   b. Tan, rarely burns, rarely develops postinflammatory pigmentation
   c. Deep tan, never burns, develops postinflammatory pigmentation
2. Arabic/Mediterranean/Hispanic: light brown:
   a. Pale, cannot tan, burns easily, no postinflammatory pigmentation
   b. Tan, rarely burns, rarely develops postinflammatory pigmentation
   c. Deep tan, never burns, develops postinflammatory pigmentation
3. Asian: yellow:
   a. Pale, cannot tan, burns easily, no postinflammatory pigmentation
   b. Tan, rarely burns, rarely develops postinflammatory pigmentation
   c. Deep tan, never burns, develops postinflammatory pigmentation
4. Indian: brown:
   a. Pale, cannot tan, burns easily, no postinflammatory pigmentation
   b. Tan, rarely burns, rarely develops postinflammatory pigmentation
   c. Deep tan, never burns, develops postinflammatory pigmentation
5. African: black:
   a. Pale, cannot tan, burns easily, no postinflammatory pigmentation
   b. Tan, rarely burns, rarely develops postinflammatory pigmentation
   c. Deep tan, never burns, develops postinflammatory pigmentation

of pigmented condition, including melasma, lentigines, seborrheic keratoses, and ABNOMs (Hori's nevus) is particularly popular, due to the condition's more frequent occurrence in Asia and the associated social stigma. In skin rejuvenation, nonablative procedures are more popular than ablative treatment. Fractional laser resurfacing is well received in Asia with a growing number of patients seeking treatment. Additionally, since Asian skin pigments easily and postinflammatory hyperpigmentation (PIH) is a common problem, preferred devices tend to be those that offer a gentler treatment (5,6).

The increase in epidermal melanin in Asian skin compared with that of white skin has been claimed to be a limiting factor for obtaining beneficial results and to be a critical factor for developing adverse sequelae in dermatological laser treatment. Patients with nonwhite skin are generally less responsive to treatment because of competition from epidermal melanin for the laser energy.

VASCULAR-SPECIFIC LASERS

The indications for laser treatment of microvascular lesions are similar in Asians and Caucasians. Oxyhemoglobin, with its major absorption peaks at 418, 542, and 577 nm, is the major chromophore in cutaneous microvessels (12). Various lasers and intense pulsed light (IPL) systems are available, producing a spectrum of wavelengths that can be selectively absorbed by oxyhemoglobin. These include argon laser (AL) (488 and 514 nm), copper vapor laser (CVL) (511 and 578 nm), potassium titanyl phosphate (KTP) laser (532 nm), variable pulse width frequency-doubled neodymium-doped:yttrium-aluminum-garnet (Nd:YAG) 532 nm (VP 532) laser, tunable dye lasers (577, 585, 595, and 600 nm), long-pulsed (LP) Nd:YAG laser (1064 nm) and IPL system (>515 nm). In Asian skin, melanin competes strongly for laser light absorption. Melanin has strong absorption in the 350–1200 nm wavelength regions, being strongest in the UV range and decreasing exponentially through visible and into near-infrared wavelengths. In dark-skinned individuals the abundance of this chromophore in relation to oxyhemoglobin in cutaneous blood vessels acts as a total barrier to light from microvascular lasers and IPL system (18). Epidermal pigmentation is perhaps the most fundamental limitation, because it diminishes laser light reaching the dermis and causes unwanted thermal damage to the epidermis (19–21).

Port-Wine Stain

A study on the treatment of port-wine stains (PWS) using a 585-nm flashlamp-pumped pulsed dye laser (PDL; SPTL-1; Candela Laser Corp., Wayland, Massachusetts, USA) has shown that patients with skin types IV and V responded to treatment more slowly and required more treatment sessions to reach the same degree of clearing than patients with skin types I–III (22). In addition, patients with skin types IV–V had a higher overall percentage of none to poor, and slight responders than those of the skin types I–III group (30% vs. 16%). In contrast, when using the 585-nm PDL to treat facial telangiectasia, the same investigators found that skin type had no measurable influence on treatment response.

The influence of preoperative skin pigmentation on adverse effects following treatment with CVL, AL, and 585-nm flashlamp-pumped PDL has been well documented (23–25). Studies have shown that the risk of inducing clinically visible pigmentary alterations and textural changes increases with higher preoperative skin pigmentation, and with the application of increasing laser energy. However, pigmentary alteration (hyper- and hypopigmentation) was found to occur at a significantly lower intensity level than scarring (texture change, atrophy, hypertrophy, and skin shrinkage). Darkly pigmented individuals obtained more severe wounding than fair-skinned subjects from AL and CVL treatment (26). In addition, the immediate histological outcome after these laser treatments has been found to depend on the pretreatment pigmentation content (20,21).

Side effects after laser treatment of vascular malformations are theoretically due to three different mechanisms, all of which result in nonspecific energy deposition: (*i*) direct and competitive absorption by epidermal melanin; (*ii*) thermal diffusion away from the absorbing chromophores, primarily melanin and hemoglobin; and (*iii*) scattering effects that indirectly increase epidermal and dermal nonspecific injury (18,25).

Asian patients with PWS are less responsive to PDL and VP 532 laser treatment with higher risk for adverse effects, such as vesiculation and pigmentary alterations (Fig. 13.1). However, dark-skinned patients should not be excluded from laser

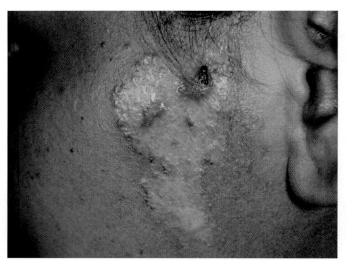

Figure 13.1 Atrophic scar and persistent hypopigmentation at 6 months after two, 585-nm pulsed dye laser treatments at average fluence of 7 J/cm^2 using a 7-mm spot size without epidermal cooling device.

(27–30) and IPL (31,32) therapies, provided that treatment expectation and risks are fully discussed. A retrospective study evaluating the results of a VP 532 laser, coupled with a cooling tip in the treatment of PWS in Chinese patients, found that this laser was only partially effective (27). Potential limitations of 532-nm light sources are that (although selective absorption of light by hemoglobin is equal to 585 nm) the shorter wavelength penetrates less deeply and is, therefore, less effective for deeper targets. Furthermore, melanin absorption is increased, making this wavelength suboptimal for Asian and darker skin types and also increasing the risk of hypopigmentation.

The development of a longer wavelength (595 nm), adjustable pulse width (0.45–40 ms) with a cooling device, is an alternative vascular-specific laser for dark-skinned patients. The laser operating at a longer wavelength of 595 nm is less absorbed by epidermal melanin. Therefore, it causes less nonspecific injury to the pigmented epidermis compared with that of the 585-nm PDL. The adjustable pulse width and longer wavelength also enables the pulsed light to target larger caliber and more deeply situated vessels in the skin. However, the conventional 585-nm PDL has demonstrated a significantly greater clearance rate than it did at the same setting of 595-nm PDL. In addition, the former also caused higher incidence of adverse effects, including pain, postoperative purpura, crusting, and transient hyperpigmentation (29,33,34). The higher incidence of complications is more likely due to the slightly higher absorption by epidermal melanin at the 585-nm wavelength.

The epidermal cooling device has been demonstrated to reduce adverse complications and improve the clinical efficacy of PDL for the treatment of PWS in Chinese patients (35,36). The use of cryogen spray cooling improves clinical efficacy, and a higher fluence can be used without an increase in complications such as permanent scarring or dyspigmentation. As a result, PDLs equipped with an epidermal cooling device of some types are considered to be the optimal lasers for treatment of PWS in Asians (Fig. 13.2). IPL treatment has been proved to be effective in PWS in Chinese patients (31,32). The clearing rate was reported to be better than that of PDL without cooling with fewer long-term complications. However, the authors emphasized that IPL can be effective and safe in the treatment of PWS only when used by an experienced operator.

LP 1064-nm Nd:YAG laser with epidermal cooling has also successfully treated vascular lesions in darkly pigmented skin. We have found that telangiectasias, both on the face and other body areas, can be successfully treated using a 1064-nm laser with a pulse duration of 25 ms, a 3.5-mm spot size, and fluencies between 200 and 250 J/cm². This is usually given in combination with dynamic cooling where a 30-ms cooling spray is given coincident with the laser pulse. Utilizing these parameters, we

have not found epidermal hypopigmentation to occur. These millisecond-domain 1064-nm lasers also offer a feasible treatment option for vascular birthmarks and deep cutaneous vascular lesions in patients with darker skin phototypes (30,31). As with the treatment of unwanted hair (as discussed later in this chapter), the long-pulsed, 1064-nm laser with epidermal cooling has become the laser of choice for the treatment of darkly pigmented skin.

The introduction of combined 595- and 1064-nm laser has also allowed for the treatment of recalcitrant and hypertrophic

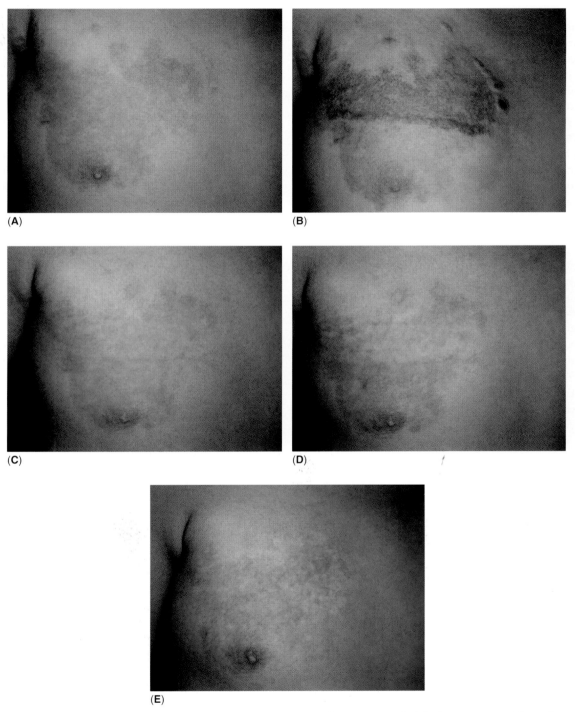

Figure 13.2 A 9-year-old Thai girl with port-wine stain (**A**) before and (**B**) immediately after a 595-nm pulsed dye laser treatment with a DCD, treatments were performed using a 7-mm spot size and a cryogen spurt duration of 80 ms, and a delay of 30 ms between spurt termination and onset of the laser pulse. The upper half was treated with a fluence of 8 J/cm² and a 0.45-ms pulse duration, whereas the lower half was treated with a fluence of 15 J/cm² and a 40-ms pulsed duration. (**C**) Two months after one treatment, the clearance rate corresponded to the extent of the postoperative purpura. (**D**) Two months after three treatments with the same parameter. (**E**) Two months after the 13th treatment. During the fourth to sixth treatments, the whole lesion was treated at a fluence of 8 J/cm² and a 0.45-ms pulse duration, whereas the seventh to the 13th treatments were performed at a fluence of 15 J/cm² and a 20-ms pulse duration. The DCD was set using the same parameters. *Abbreviation*: DCD, dynamic cooling device.

PWS. This laser system delivering sequential pulses of 595- and 1064-nm wavelengths provides another option that is likely to assist with removal of different vessels (37,38). The application of 595 nm light followed by the 1064-nm wavelength takes advantage of a chromic shift in blood when heated above 62°C; the oxyhemoglobin absorption coefficient peaks at 595 nm, whereas the methemoglobin absorption coefficient aligns with 1064 nm. The synergistic thermal effect of the dual wavelengths reduces the treatment fluence necessary for successful treatment. The combined 595- and 1064-nm laser has been used to successfully treat PWS and appears to have a more favorable side-effect profile than the 1064-nm laser used alone, but it is our experience that Asian patients have a greater risk of blistering, scabbing, and scarring associated with the combined 595- and 1064-nm device than with the PDL alone. Therefore, caution is warranted when treating any vascular lesion in Asian patients with the combined 595- and 1064-nm laser.

LASER TREATMENT OF HYPERTROPHIC SCARS, KELOIDS, AND STRIAE

The 585-nm PDL has also been used as a treatment of choice for hypertrophic scars and keloids in fair-skinned individuals (39,40). The efficacy of the PDL in treatment of scars in darker-skinned patients is not as good as that in white-skinned patients and the risk of pigmentary alterations is also higher. A study on the efficacy of the PDL performed in 20 patients with skin phototypes I–VI demonstrated no improvement of the hypertrophic scars on the laser-treated sites compared with untreated control. Eight of the 20 patients had skin phototype VI and two had type V. The effect of melanin was thought to be a factor of treatment failure (41). Similarly, our previous study (42) noted that clinical improvement of scars in patients with skin phototypes IV–VI after multiple treatment sessions with the PDL had a lower response rate, and the incidence of epidermal damage increased compared with that of the fair-skinned patients (Fig. 13.3). A previous study of PDL in the treatment and prevention of hypertrophic scars in Chinese patients also found that there was no significant objective improvement in terms of scar thickness and viscoelasticity compared with the controls (43). Our earlier study on the effect of pulse width of the PDL on the treatment response of hypertrophic scars also noted a lesser efficacy in Thai and Chinese patients with skin types III–V as well (44).

Treatment of stretch marks is another application of the 585-nm PDL that improves the appearance of these lesions (45,46). An increase in dermal elastin noted following PDL treatment was speculated to be the mechanism of improvement.

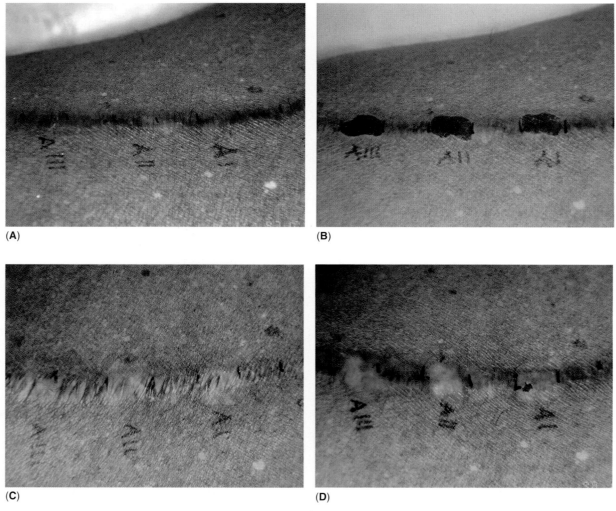

(A) (B) (C) (D)

Figure 13.3 (**A**) Linear hypertrophic scar on the thigh in an Indian patient with skin phototype V, before treatment. (**B**) One week following the first treatment with a 585-nm pulsed dye laser using a 5-mm spot size without epidermal cooling device; A I, treated with 3 J/cm²; A II, treated with 5 J/cm²; A III, treated with 7 J/cm²; E, untreated control. Epidermal necrosis is noted over all laser-irradiated segments. (**C**) Four weeks following the second treatment, erythema and hypopigmentation were seen on the laser-treated areas. (**D**) 12 Weeks after the sixth treatment, flattening of the scar without dyspigmentation was demonstrated.

In contrast, several studies by other investigators noted no clinical improvement of striae and no increase in dermal elastin content histologically (47,48). A study on the treatment of striae in skin types IV and VI patients has demonstrated no noticeable clinical improvement, with a higher risk of pigmentary alterations (48). In our experience, we also found that PDL provides a very minimal beneficial effect on the treatment of striae in Asian patients. Studies have demonstrated the ability of nonablative (49), ablative (50), and fractional lasers and radiofrequency device (51) to improve striae distensae in Asian skin with minimal side effects.

In summary, treatment technique and parameters for vascular-specific lasers in Asian skin are similar to those of white skin (see chap. 2), but more care should be taken in selecting an appropriate energy and in determining proper treatment intervals. Because melanin acts as a competing chromophore for vascular-specific lasers, to be effective the starting energy density has to be higher than that used on fair Caucasian skin. However, the improvement following this procedure seems to be less effective and with a higher incidence of epidermal damage than those seen in white-skinned patients. Laser-induced pigmentary alterations should be completely resolved before the delivery of additional laser treatment, and to effect the optimal result from each session, longer intervals may be necessary between laser treatments.

PIGMENT-SPECIFIC LASERS

Selective destruction of melanosomes has been well demonstrated by exposing skin to submicrosecond, Q-switched (QS), laser pulses (52,53). A wide range of these is available, including a PDL (510 nm), QS frequency-double Nd:YAG laser (532 and 1064 nm), QSRL (694 nm), and QS alexandrite laser (QSAL) (755 nm). All of these QS lasers are useful for treating superficial epidermal lesions, such as lentigines and ephelides, café-au-lait macules (CALMs), seborrheic keratosis, and dermal pigmented lesions, such as blue nevus, nevus of Ota/Ito, ABNOMs (Hori's nevus), infraorbital hyperpigmentation, drug-induced hyperpigmentaiton, and congenital melanocytic nevi.

Melanin absorption is stronger at shorter wavelengths, whereas longer wavelengths penetrate better into the skin (18). Several factors are involved in using QS lasers for treating benign pigmented lesions in Asian individuals. First, the greater amount of epidermal melanin results in greater damage to lesions and adjacent normal skin pigment during laser irradiation. This increased absorption may lead to posttreatment blistering (Fig. 13.4), hyperpigmentation (Fig. 13.5), hypopigmentation (Fig. 13.6), depigmentation, and even scarring. Second, larger amounts of epidermal melanin in persons with dark skin tones act as a competing chromophore for laser light while using these QS lasers for treating dermal pigmented lesions. Thus, a larger number of sequential treatments are required for complete clearing compared with those of white-complexioned persons. In addition, the adverse effects resulting from injury to epidermal melanin and the melanocytes responsible for producing normal skin color should be anticipated.

Benign Epidermal Pigmented Lesions

Benign epidermal pigmented lesions include lentigines, ephelides, CALMs, and seborrheic keratosis. In dark-skinned patients, these pigmented lesions have been successfully treated

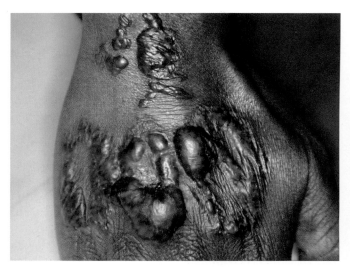

Figure 13.4 Blistering secondary to tattoo removal with the Q-switched ruby laser in a skin phototype IV Thai patient using a fluence of 6.5 J/cm² with a 5-mm spot size. *Source*: Courtesy of C. Vibhagool, Bangkok, Thailand.

with the argon [488 and 515 nm, continuous wave (CW)] laser (54), 510-nm short PDL (55), copper vapor (511 nm, CW) laser (56), QS frequency-doubled Nd:YAG (532 nm) laser (57,58), QSRL (54,59–61), QSAL (755 nm) (62,63), the low-fluence carbon dioxide (CO_2) (10,600 nm, CW) laser (64), and IPL (65,66). All of these lasers and light sources carry a small risk of depigmentation, hypopigmentation, and hyperpigmentation. However, when treating darkly pigmented skin, pulsed lasers with appropriate energy density provide a more selective destruction with a lower incidence of hyperpigmentation and scarring as compared with continuous wave lasers (5,67). The nonspecific injury to adjacent normal skin caused from CW lasers may result in "laser tanning," which has been hypothesized to result from feedback inhibition of melanogenesis, stimulation of tyrosinase activity, and/or release of intracellular or extracellular melanocyte-stimulating factors (68). This phenomenon is independent of PIH, which constitutes another effect of the nonspecific damage caused from CW laser energy.

Lentigines

Lentigines are a common sign of photoaging in Asians. This epidermal pigmented lesion has shown excellent response to QS (57) and LP Nd:YAG (532 nm) laser (69), QSRL (694 nm) (60,61), QSAL (755 nm) (51), and low-fluence CO_2 laser (52). Our experience in treating Asian patients shows that the pulsed dye (510 nm) laser, QS Nd:YAG laser (532 nm, 5–10 ns), QSRL, and QSAL provide excellent results, usually with a single treatment (Fig. 13.7).

The clinical endpoint is defined as the lowest fluence that can achieve immediate whitening (Fig. 13.8). This parameter is about 2.0–2.5 J/cm² for the 532-nm QS Nd:YAG laser (10 ns, 3-mm spot diameter) (46), and about 7.0 J/cm² for the QSAL (100-ns pulse width, 3-mm spot diameter) (62,66). For the LP 532-nm Nd:YAG laser the clinical endpoint, defined as a slate gray appearance, is usually about 3.2 J/cm² (2- to 50-ms pulse width, 2-mm spot diameter) (69).

QS (nanosecond domain) and LP (millisecond domain) laser systems have been found to be equally effective in

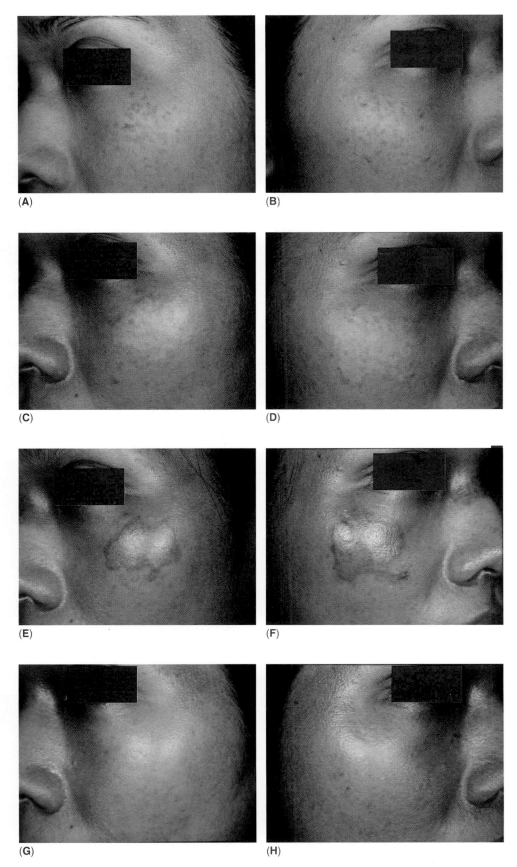

Figure 13.5 (**A**) A 23-year-old Thai woman with acquired bilateral nevus of Ota-like macules (Hori's nevus), before treatment (*left*) (**B**) before treatment (*right*). (**C**) One week after a 1064-nm Q-switched neodymium-doped:yttrium-aluminum-garnet laser treatment at a fluence of 6 J/cm² using a 3-mm spot size (*left*). (**D**) One week after treatment (*right*). (**E**) Development of postinflammatory hyperpigmentation at 4 weeks after treatment (*left*). (**F**) Postinflammatory hyperpigmentation (*right*) that cleared within 1–2 months after treatment with hydroquinone 4% cream. (**G**) Complete clearance of pigmented lesion after five laser treatments (*left*). (**H**) After five laser treatments (*right*).

treating freckles and lentigines in Oriental patients, with QS systems producing a higher incidence of PIH (69,70). It was explained that unlike LP lasers that cause tissue destruction purely by photothermolysis, QS lasers, with their short burst of high-energy nanosecond radiation, exhibit both photothermal and photomechanical effects. The undesirable photomechanical effect induces damage to surrounding oxyhemoglobin and melanin, resulting in inflammation

of superficial vessels, altered activity of melanocytes, and subsequent PIH (71).

Studies on the use of IPL sources for skin rejuvenation (57) and for the treatment of facial freckles in Asians (65,66) have demonstrated satisfactory outcome on facial pigmentation. Negishi et al. (72) addressed the use of the IPL device with integrated contact cooling for skin rejuvenation in Asian patients. A series of five or more treatments performed at 3- to 4-week intervals was given, using double-pulsing mode with a 560-nm cutoff filter and fluence of 23–27 J/cm². For patients with skin type III, the first and second pulse widths were set at 2.8 and 6.0 ms, respectively, at pulse intervals of 20 ms, whereas in patients with skin types IV–V, the first and second pulse widths were adjusted to 3.2 and 6.0, respectively, at the same pulse intervals. Greater than 60% improvement in pigmentation was noted in 81% of the 73 patients. Minor and transitory erythema with burning sensation was reported in 2.7% of those patients.

In our experience with Asian patients with skin types III–V, a longer-wavelength cutoff filter (590- or 640-nm) was used to minimize epidermal injury. A more conservative parameter using a longer pulse width, lower fluence, and proper epidermal cooling is recommended. The most common adverse complication was epidermal damage resulting in rectangular scale-crusts, matching the footprint of the IPL crystal, which came off in 1–2 weeks, followed by a rectangular hypopigmentation that spontaneously resolved in 4–16 weeks (Fig. 13.9).

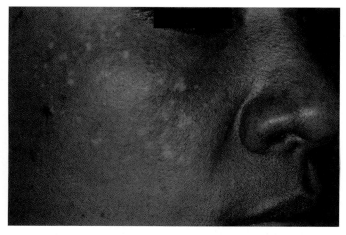

Figure 13.6 Hypopigmentation secondary to the Q-switched ruby laser treatment for Hori's nevus in a 40-year-old Thai woman using a fluence of 5 J/cm² with a 5-mm spot size.

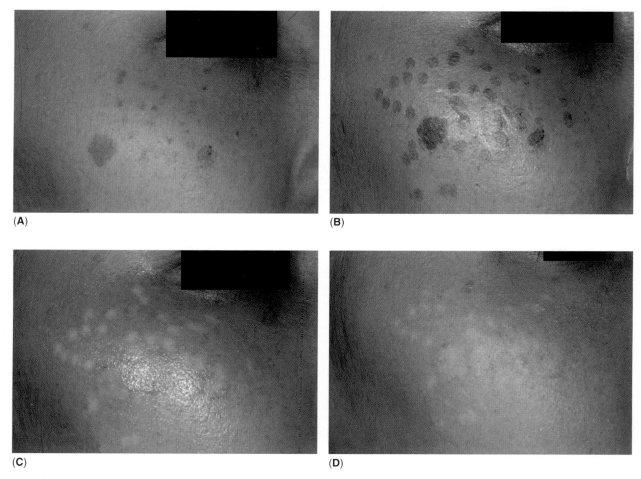

(A)

(B)

(C)

(D)

Figure 13.7 (**A**) Lentigines in a 20-year-old Thai woman, with skin phototype IV before treatment. (**B**) One day after one treatment with a 532-nm Q-switched neodymium-doped:yttrium-aluminum-garnet laser at a fluence of 1.8 J/cm² using a 3-mm spot size. Scabs developed on the laser-treated skin. (**C**) One week after treatment. The laser-treated are initially hypopigmented after the scabs resolve. (**D**) Two weeks after treatment. The hypopigmentation gradually improved. *Source*: From Ref. 283.

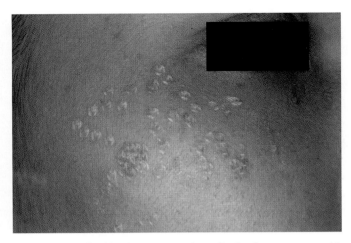

Figure 13.8 An ash-white tissue response immediately after a treatment with a 532-nm Q-switched neodymium-doped:yttrium-aluminum-garnet laser treatment of patient in Figure 13.7. *Source*: From Ref. 283.

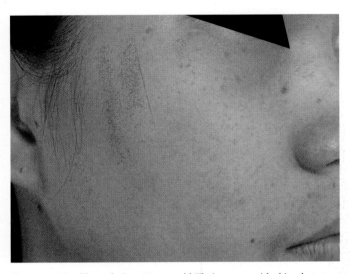

Figure 13.9 Bar-like scabs in a 28-year-old Thai woman with skin phototype III, one day after a full-face photorejuvenation with intense pulsed light equipped with an active skin cooling system delivered through a 560-nm cutoff filter using a fluence of 22 J/cm² by double pulsing (the first and second pulse widths were set at 3.2 and 6.0 ms, respectively, at a pulse interval of 20 ms). A chilled, colorless ultrasonic gel was applied directly to the filter surface prior to application to the skin.

Of interest is that we found much lower incidence of PIH compared with that of pigment-specific lasers. This observation is confirmed by a randomized, physician-blinded, split-face comparative trial showing that the improvement rates of lentigines after one QSAL treatment were comparable to those of after two IPL treatment sessions. However, the incidence of PIH caused by QSAL was significantly higher than hyperpigmentation associated with IPL (66).

When treating Asian patients, transient hyper- or hypopigmentation are the most common adverse effects of these pigment-specific lasers. However, the QSRL can cause long-term or permanent hypopigmentation, especially in dark-pigmented Asians (Fig. 13.6). The QS Nd:YAG laser is associated with purpura and more erythema, secondary to its increased absorption by oxyhemoglobin. A PIH incidence of 10–25% was reported in previous studies using QS Nd:YAG, QSRL, and QSAL for pigmented lesions in Asian patients (59,66,69). A low fluence CO_2 laser has been successfully used to remove lentigines in fair-skinned patients without posttreatment hyper- and hypopigmentation (64). In contrast, when treating lentigines in Chinese and Thai patients with dark complexion using the high-energy, pulsed CO_2 laser, transient posttreatment hyperpigmentation was the most common adverse sequelae noted in as much as 50% of the patients.

Café-Au-Lait Macules

Alster and Williams (55) successfully treated a boy with type V skin presented with a CALM, with six 510-nm short PDL treatment at an energy fluence of 2.5 J/cm², at 2-month intervals. Hypopigmentation or textural changes did not occur. No lesion recurrence was noted at a 2-year follow-up period. Treatment of CALMs with a copper vapor (511 nm) laser also provided favorable results in Thai patients (skin type V) (56). With a mean follow-up period of 22 months after one treatment, nine of 16 (60%) patients achieved 90–100% clearance, whereas the remainder of the 16 improved 40–80%. Repigmentation to normal skin color was complete within 1–2 months with slight hyperpigmentation at the periphery of the treated area, which responded favorably to topical hydroquinone. Transient hypopigmentation recovery after 2–3 months was observed in most cases. A hypertrophic scar developed in one of the 16 patients in the study. In essence, CALMs variably respond to laser treatments and may recur within a few weeks and up to years after complete clearance. Retreatment often results in rapid clearing (67). Studies on treatment of CALMs with lasers in white (73,74) and Asian (58,61,75) populations demonstrated a similar variable degree of repigmentation following a long-term follow-up period of up to 50%. This variable behavior of treated lesions implies a subset of lesions with unique biological behavior.

The 595-nm PDL delivered with compression has proved to be effective and safe for the treatment of epidermal pigmented lesions. The PDL has been the standard of care for many vascular lesions, and although it is well absorbed by blood, it is also well absorbed by melanin. By compressing a transparent flat optical element against the skin, the blood in the superficial vessels is squeezed out and displaced from the irradiated zone, thus minimizing absorption by blood in the superficial vessels and allowing the use of appropriate pulse width while reducing purpura and unwanted side effects.

For shorter pulse duration QS lasers, a study comparing the clinical efficacy and complications of QS and LP lasers indicated that although both were effective in the removal of lentigines, QS lasers were associated with a higher risk of PIH (59,69). LP lasers differ from QS lasers in the sense that they have a photothermal but not a photomechanical effect. It has been suggested that the photomechanical effect of QS lasers may not be desirable when used in the removal of lentigines in pigmented skin types (59,76,77). The pulse duration used for the aforementioned application was 1.5 ms, shorter than the predicted epidermal basal layer thermal relaxation time (1.6–2.8 ms for a basal layer thickness of 20 μm) (18,78). Following the principles of selective photothermolysis helps confine the zone of thermal damage to the epidermis and to minimize unnecessary adverse effects and pain (79).

Kono and coworkers used a compression technique with the 595-nm PDL, for the treatment of facial lentigines in Asian patients (80). The degree of clearing achieved after a single treatment was 70.3% and 83.3% for QSRL and PDL delivered

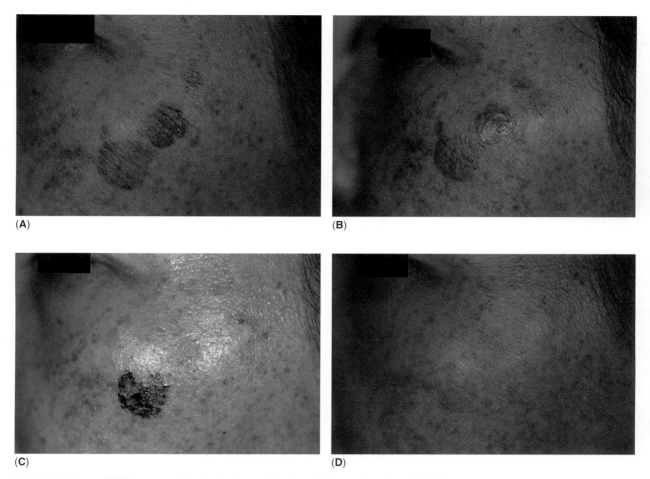

Figure 13.10 (**A**) A 60-year-old Thai woman with solar lentigo and flat seborrheic keratosis on her cheek, before treatment. (**B**) An ash-gray color change without purpura immediately after a treatment with a 595-nm PDL with compression at a fluence of 9.0 J/cm² using a 7-mm spot size. (**C**) One week after treatment. (**D**) Two weeks follow-up visit.

with compression, respectively. There was no significant difference in the efficacy between QSRL and PDL. However, complications after PDL treatment were substantially less frequent than after QSRL, presumably because of more optimal pulse duration for targeting the basal cell layer, with minimal photomechanical effect.

We achieved a similar degree of clearance when using this PDL with compression technique to treat facial lentigines in Thai and Chinese patients (Fig. 13.10). Lesions from various anatomical regions were successfully treated, including back, chest, upper/lower extremities, and face. We also treated a wide range of lesions, including dark and light lentigines and flat seborrheic keratoses. Seborrheic keratoses and lighter lentigines were more resistant to therapy. It is likely that the amount of delivered procedures and percentage of more resistant lesions in the patient group will dictate ultimate therapeutic outcome.

MIXED EPIDERMAL AND DERMAL PIGMENTED LESIONS

Postinflammatory Hyperpigmentation and Melasma

Mixed epidermal and dermal lesions, such as PIH or melasma, respond variably and unpredictably to QS lasers (81–83) and IPL (84–86). It is possible that not all pigment-producing structures are affected following a single irradiation. Therefore, residing melanocytes may cause additional pigmentation in patients tending to postlesional hyperpigmentation or melasma.

In addition, melasma tend to recur, often fairly soon, without ongoing topical bleaching medications. In our current practice, sunscreen use is mandatory.

"Laser toning" using low-fluence, large spot size, multi-passed QS 1064-nm Nd:YAG laser for skin rejuvenation and melasma has gained much popularity, especially in Asian countries; however, there are still very few evidence-based data supporting this approach in the treatment of PIH and melasma (87–90). In laser toning, multiple passes of low-fluence laser (e.g., 1.6–3.5 J/cm²) are delivered through a large spot size (e.g., 6–8 mm) to optimize energy delivery and to achieve mild erythema as the clinical endpoint. Some physicians have proposed the daily usage of laser toning for skin rejuvenation, whereas others offer treatments at weekly, 2-weekly, or monthly intervals with a wide variation in the total number of treatments.

Wattanakrai et al. (89) noted statistically significant improvement of melasma from baseline in colorimeter and modified Melasma Area and Severity Index (mMASI) score after five laser-toning treatments in 22 Thai patients. However, 18% of them developed rebound hyperpigmentation, and all had recurrence of melasma at 3 months after the last laser session. Although this treatment modality produced initial beneficial results to patients, it was not without adverse effects. During the course of five laser treatments, 14% of the patients experienced faint, spotty hypopigmentation.

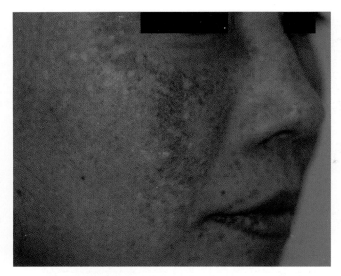

Figure 13.11 Confetti-like hypopigmented and recurrence of melasma at 6 months after low-fluence Q-switched 1064-nm neodymium-doped:yttrium-aluminum-garnet laser toning in Thai woman with skin phototype IV.

Confetti-like or spotty hypopigmented macules or punctate leukoderma is a common side effect associated with low-fluence QS 1064-nm Nd:YAG laser for skin rejuvenation and melasma (Fig. 13.11) (91,92). Chan et al. (91) assessed a case series of 14 Chinese patients with laser toning-associated facial depigmentation with cross-polarized and UV photographic images. Of all 14 patients, 9 received laser toning for nonablative skin rejuvenation and the other 5 for melasma. Treatment protocols received by these patients were highly variable. The total number of treatments received ranged from 6 to 50 (mean 22). In all cases, UV photographic images demonstrated facial mottled depigmentation. Laser toning failed to significantly improve melasma in all five patients.

The use of resurfacing lasers alone (93,94) or combined with a pigment-specific laser (95,96) have shown favorable results in the treatment of melasma. However, PIH commonly develops and can last for 3–6 months. This temporary worsening of the pigmentation may result from an inflammatory dermal reaction that stimulates the activity of melanocytes in the melasma-irradiated skin. Our own experience has found that PIH occurs in nearly 100% of the patients with skin types III and IV who underwent CO_2 laser resurfacing for treatment of melasma. Segmental hypopigmentation or pseudohypopigmentation is another common complication that develops when only the melasma area is resurfaced (Fig. 13.12). Pseudohypopigmentation, the situation in which the resurfaced area has a relatively light skin color, is similar in color to the pigmentation of non–sun-exposed skin but contrasts distinctively with the more darkly pigmented photodamaged adjacent skin.

The etiology of melasma remains unknown. The idea behind such an aggressive approach is that melasma may be caused by an abnormal epidermis, not abnormal melanocytes. This idea is supported by findings from previous studies showing that keratinocytes play a role in regulating distribution patterns of recipient melanosomes (97,98). Considering the expense and the risk of adverse effects, the use of laser resurfacing alone or combined techniques should be preserved for those refractory melasma that do not respond to conventional treatments.

A variable square pulse (VSP) erbium:yttrium-aluminum-garnet (Er:YAG) laser is an alternative of a minimally ablative laser resurfacing technique that has proved to be effective and safe for treatment of epidermal-type melasma (99). Significant improvement in visual analog scale (VAS) and MASI score from baseline were noted at 2 months following two treatment sessions (Fig. 13.13). Mild PIH developed in 18% of the patients and cleared spontaneously within 2 weeks. VSP Er:YAG pulses provide more-controlled heating of tissue and minimal epidermal vaporization. This minimally ablative laser resurfacing results in greater epidermal turnover and "washing out" of pigment. This results in a decrease in lesional hyperpigmentation but not elimination of the problem. When combined with a topical regimen of hydroquinone, retinoids, vitamin C, and sunscreens, a successful maintenance program can be crafted for melasma.

Nonablative fractional photothermolysis (FP) laser has increasingly been performed for treatment of recalcitrant melasma (49,100–103). The mechanism by which pigmented component is eliminated probably involves the extrusion and transepidermal vacuolar elimination of dermal and epidermal melanin content through a compromised dermoepidermal junction. This transport system is activated by FP whereby microscopic epidermal necrotic debris is shuttled through the epidermis to be eliminated by epidermal vacuoles (104). Pilot studies showed the effectiveness of FP in melasma, but most of them had a small sample size and/or a short follow-up period (102,105).

Lee et al. (101) treated Korean patients with melasma with four monthly FP sessions and followed up to 24 weeks after treatment completion. Clinical improvements of 60% were observed in 44% of the patients at 4 weeks after treatment, but the improvements decreased to 52% in 35% of the subjects at 24 weeks after treatment. Our experience in treating melasma with FP was similar to that of aforementioned study. We noted that FP led to some clinical improvements, but melasma tended to recur as early as 3 months after treatment was discontinued.

Wind and colleagues (106) compared efficacy and safety of nonablative 1550-nm fractional laser therapy (FLT) and triple topical therapy (TTT; hydroquinone 5%, tretinoin 0.05%, triamcinolone acetonide 0.1% cream) in 29 Chinese with melasma. Mean patient's global assessment and satisfaction were significantly lower at the FLT side. Physician's global assessment and melanin index showed a significant worsening of hyperpigmentation at the FLT side. At 6 months follow-up, most patients preferred TTT. Adverse effects of FLT were erythema, burning sensation, edema, and pain. Moreover, PIH developed in 31% of the patients after two or more laser sessions. Similarly, results from a recent prospective controlled single-blinded trial in 51 patients showed that four FP treatments at 3-week intervals did not provide a specific effect on melasma that is superior to an application of sunscreens alone (107).

A round table discussion among experienced physicians and a review of up-to-date literature findings also did not have complete consensus for the use of an erbium-doped 1550-nm fractionated laser for the treatment of melasma (103). Therefore, physicians should proceed with caution when treating melasma, especially in patients with dark-skin phototypes.

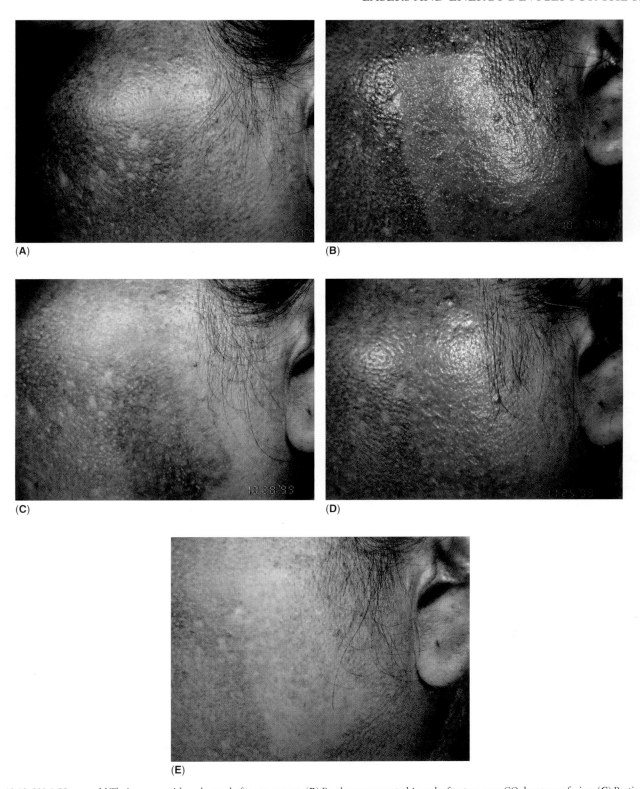

Figure 13.12 (**A**) A 55-year-old Thai woman with melasma, before treatment. (**B**) Erythema was noted 1 week after two-pass CO_2 laser resurfacing. (**C**) Postinflammatory hyperpigmentation developed 4 weeks after treatment. (**D**) Again 4 weeks after treated with hydroquinone 4% cream twice daily, hyperpigmentation had faded. (**E**) Pseudohypopigmentation without recurrence of melasma on the resurfaced area 4 years after treatment. She received no further topical bleaching agent but used only an SPF 30, broad spectrum sunscreen.

Dermal Pigmented Lesions

Nevus of Ota

Nevus of Ota, a dendritic melanocytosis of the papillary and upper reticular dermis involving the eye and surrounding skin innervated by the first and second branches of the trigeminal nerve, is a cosmetic problem commonly found in Asians but is also seen in blacks and whites. An incidence of 0.6% has been noted in the Japanese (108). Malignant degeneration has occasionally been reported (109,110). Studies in fair- and dark-skinned populations have demonstrated that red (QS ruby) (111–113), near infrared (QS alexandrite) (114–117), and QS Nd:YAG (76,118) lasers are very useful for treating nevus of Ota with fading over several months following each treatment session.

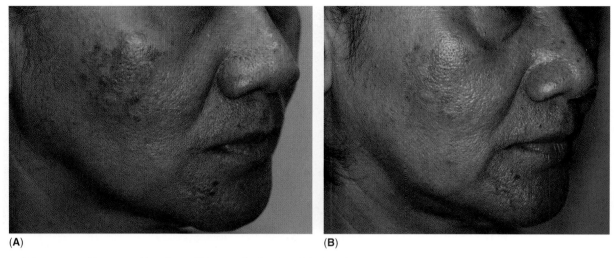

Figure 13.13 (**A**) A 50-year-old woman with melasma (skin type V) at baseline. (**B**) Clinical improvement 2 months after two variable square pulse erbium:yttrium-aluminum-garnet laser treatments. *Source*: From Ref. 99.

The "threshold" radiant exposure response defined as immediate whitening of pigmented lesions after short pulse laser exposure is a useful clinical endpoint with any QS laser because the whitening correlates directly with melanosome rupture and pigment cell injury. Geronemus (111) treated nevus of Ota in 15 patients of skin phototypes II–V with a QSRL and noted that this threshold response was based on the patients' skin phototype. Asian patients (skin types IV–V) required slightly lower energy fluence of 7.5–8.5 J/cm² to achieve immediate whitening compared with white and Hispanic patients (skin types II–IV) (8.5–10 J/cm²).

When treating nevus of Ota with QS lasers, lightening of the lesion is noted after the first session with additional clinical improvement noted after every session. Multiple, sequential treatments appear to increase the response rate and may be required for complete clearing of the lesion (Fig. 13.14). The response of nevus of Ota to QS laser treatment also appears to depend on the color of the lesion. The maximum response rate is found in the brown color, and gradually decreases in the brown-violet, violet-blue, and blue-green colors, respectively. On average, brown lesions can be cleared by three laser treatments, brown-violet lesions by four sessions, violet-blue lesions can be eliminated after five sessions, and blue-green lesions require at least six treatment sessions for complete clearance (119).

Studies comparing the use of QSAL and QS Nd:YAG laser showed that most patients more easily tolerated the former (118). However, the QS Nd:YAG laser was found to be more effective than the QSAL in the lightening of nevus of Ota after three or more laser treatment sessions (76). In terms of adverse effects, hypopigmentation is the most common adverse effect after treatment with QS lasers (82) and can be permanent, especially among those treated with QSRL (120). Transient hyperpigmentation can be found especially after the first treatment session. The incidence of textural changes and scarring are minimal.

Recurrence of original pigmentation could occur after complete laser-induced clearing. The rate of recurrence is estimated to be 0.6–1.2% (120). Laser treatment of nevus of Ota in children demonstrated a better response and a lower risk of adverse

effects than in adults (121). Early treatment, leading to complete clearance before school, may mean avoiding the childhood psychological trauma associated with the cosmetic disfigurement of the birthmark. This advantage must now be weighed against the risk of recurrence and the stress and cost associated with multiple sessions of laser treatment.

In our current practice, patients are treated with a 1064-nm QS Nd:YAG laser every 8–12 weeks. In a review of 125 patients 1–10 years postoperatively, we found that longer duration between treatments provides a decrease in the total number of treatments necessary over time (unpublished data, 2010). We encourage the parents and/or the patients to start the treatment as early as possible. Parents and patients are advised of the risks of complications, including hyperpigmentation and hypopigmentation, and are informed of the chance of recurrence after complete eradication. Ocular involvement including elevated intraocular pressure with or without glaucoma occurred in 10.3% of the patients; as a result, ophthalmologic assessment is necessary (122).

Acquired Bilateral Nevus of Ota-like Macules (Hori's Nevus)
ABNOMs (Hori's nevus) is a common condition that affects about 0.8% of the population with a marked female preponderance (a male:female ratio of 1:6) (123). Clinically, ABNOMs presents speckles or confluent blue-brown or slate gray pigmentation that usually affects the bilateral malar areas. Other involved sites include the temples, the root of the nose, the alae nasi, the eye lids, and the forehead. Unlike in nevus of Ota, the pigmentation in ABNOMs occurs in a symmetric bilateral distribution, has a late onset in adulthood, and does not involve mucosa. Histologically, lesions of ABNOMs demonstrate diffuse upper dermal melanocytosis and differ from nevus of Ota, in which dermal melanocytes occur not only in the upper dermis but also in the deep reticular dermis (124).

Pigment-specific lasers, including QSRL (125,126), QSAL (127), and QS Nd:YAG (124,128–130) lasers have proved to be effective in the treatment of ABNOMs. The treatment responses have been noted to be less effective than those of the nevus of Ota, and multiple sequential treatments are also required to achieve the desired improvement (Fig. 13.5).

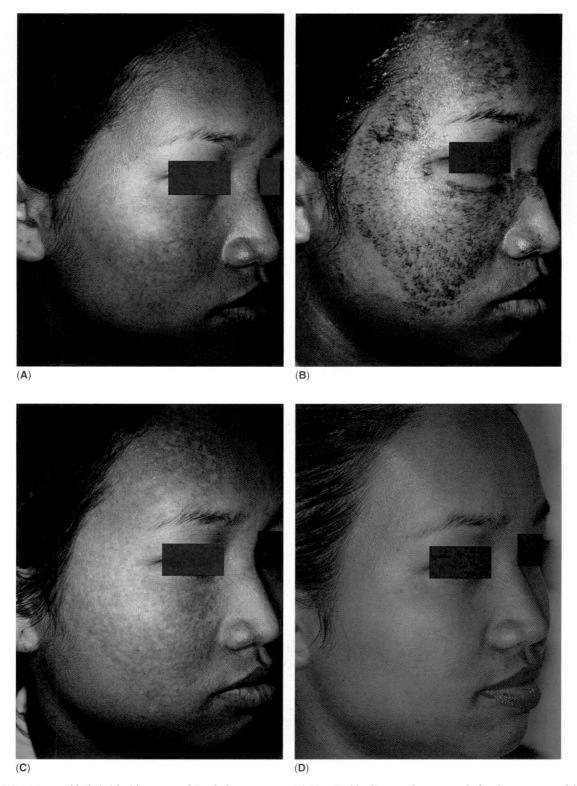

Figure 13.14 (**A**) A 22-year-old Thai girl with a nevus of Ota, before treatment. (**B**) Pinpoint bleeding was demonstrated after disappearance of the immediate whitening of the pigmented lesion following a 1064-nm Q-switched neodymium-doped:yttrium-aluminum-garnet laser treatment using a fluence of 7 J/cm^2 through a 4-mm spot size. (**C**) One month after the first treatment. (**D**) Two months after the seventh treatment. *Source*: From Ref. 283.

A total treatment of two to five sessions is usually required for complete clearance of the lesions. The treatment interval is controversial. Some groups (125,127) retreat the patients as soon as the wounds have healed, usually within 2–4 weeks. The rationale for early retreatment is to treat prior and prevent epithelial repigmentation so that more laser energy can reach the dermal target. However, a greater rate of complications,

especially persistent hypopigmentation, can occur. Polnikorn et al. (129) and our group (126) usually retreat the patients every 8–12 weeks, depending on the clearance of PIH. In fact, we noted the benefit of delayed treatment as significant lightening can sometimes be seen many months after the initial treatment session. Ee et al. (131) also noted continuous lightening of the residual pigmentation over a period of 6 months and suggested that resident macrophages continued scavenging of laser-damaged pigment cells.

PIH is more common than that of nevus of Ota, occurring in 50–73% of Asian patients (Fig. 13.5) (129). The benefit of using topical bleaching agents to prevent or to treat PIH in ABNOMs is also controversial. A previous study noted PIH in 73% of the 66 patients who underwent the treatment with a QS Nd:YAG laser despite the use of topical hydroquinone (129), whereas another series of 70 patients who developed PIH following the laser treatment responded readily to topical hydroquinone within a few days to weeks of application (128). In our experience, there is little beneficial effect in using topical bleaching agents preoperatively to decrease the rate of PIH. PIH usually persists for 2–3 months even with prompt postoperative treatment with hypopigmenting topical medications, sun-avoidance, and a broad-spectrum sunscreen with an SPF of at least 30.

As red (QS ruby) and near-infrared (QS alexandrite and QS Nd:YAG) wavelengths can be selectively absorbed by dermal pigment, the use of these lasers in the treatment of other melanocytic processes with dermal involvement, including nevus of Ito (67), Becker's nevus (132), nevus spilus (133), blue nevus (134), and congenital melanocytic nevus (135–138), may be effective. The café-au-lait background of nevus spilus and Becker's nevus frequently recurs after treatment (67). The short pulse width and low-energy fluence of these QS lasers are probably not able to damage clusters or nests of nevomelanocytic components. The development of dermal pigment-targeting lasers (139–141) and IPL systems (142) with long pulse widths shows encouraging results on the treatment of these pigmented lesions.

As described previously, multiple, sequential treatments are typically required for desired cosmetic results of the dermal pigmented lesions. Attempts to accelerate treatment response of dermal pigmentation have been employed including the use of multiple lasers on the same treatment session (126,131,143,144) and the application of bleaching agents prior to laser treatment (145).

Epidermal ablation with a resurfacing laser may enhance the effectiveness of laser for removing dermal pigmentation by eliminating competing epidermal melanin and melanocytes, and removing the epidermis itself, thereby reducing a scattering of the beam and physically placing it closer to the dermal target. Thus, a higher delivered energy fluence will have an impact on the target-dermal melanin.

To improve the response rate of treating dermal pigmented lesions, we developed a technique using a combination of scanned CO_2 and QSRL to treat ABNOMs in a series of 13 Thai women. A significantly higher percentage of clearing was noted on the sides treated with a combination of CO_2 and QSRL, compared with those with QSRL alone (Fig. 13.15) (126). By combining laser resurfacing and QSRL, a retrospective study in

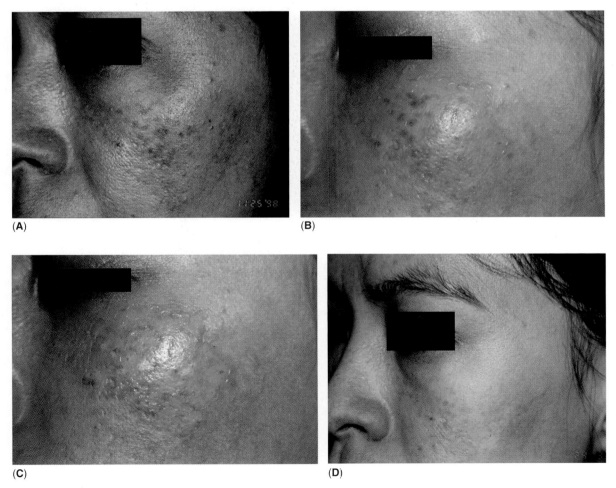

(A) (B)

(C) (D)

Figure 13.15 (**A**) Acquired bilateral nevus of Ota-like macules in a 40-year-old Thai woman, before treatment. (**B**) Just after epidermal ablation with carbon dioxide laser. (**C**) Immediately after Q-switched ruby laser irradiation on dermal pigmented lesions. (**D**) Four months after a combined laser treatment. *Source*: From Ref. 126.

Korean patients with nevus of Ota and congenital nevus showed that the treatment period had been reduced by 2–3 months, and the number of treatments had been reduced two- to threefolds (144). However, the use of this combined laser technique to nonfacial areas is yet to be fully evaluated. The risk of delayed healing time and adverse effects may be higher because of the decreased vascularity and the sparse adnexal structures relative to the face.

Concurrent use of the QS 532-nm Nd:YAG laser in combination with the 1064-nm laser has proven more effective in pigment lightening than the QS 1064-nm Nd:YAG laser alone for early lesion of Hori's nevi. Removal of the epidermal component of Hori's nevi as such, results in a lighter color. In addition, elimination of competing epidermal melanin may also assist in the penetration of longer wavelengths and result in more efficient removal of the dermal component with the 1064-nm laser (131).

Elimination of epidermal melanin by using topical bleaching agents has also been used to pretreat the skin 6–8 weeks prior to QSRL for acquired dermal melanosis (ADM) in Japanese patients. This combined therapy appeared to treat ADM consistently with a low occurrence rate of PIH and lessen the number of laser treatment sessions (144).

Nevomelanocytic Nevi
The treatment of congenital and acquired melanocytic nevi with laser irradiation is a very controversial issue. This concern has already been discussed in detail (see chap. 3). In Asian populations, melanocytic nevi are common and are often removed for cosmetic and superstitious concerns. The normal mode ruby laser (NMRL) alone (54,139,141), or together with QSRL or QSAL, has been employed to remove melanocytic nevi in Asians with good cosmetic results following multiple treatment sessions (146–148).

In spite of clinical improvement, complete histological clearance cannot be achieved. Long-term histological follow-up of congenital melanocytic nevi after NMRL treatment demonstrated that the subtle microscopic scar about 1 mm thick is required to mask the underlying residual pigmentation for good cosmetic results. The long-term follow-up for at least 8 years showed no histological or clinical evidence of the development of malignant change in the laser-irradiated areas (139). An NMRL appears to provide a more effective clearing on the basis that a longer pulse duration induces more melanocytic destruction to the clusters of nevus cells, and hence better clears pigmentation (136,141).

In our current practice, a CO_2 laser is commonly used to vaporize benign melanocytic nevi with promising outcomes and low risk of side effects (see also section "Ablative laser systems"). Importantly for Asians, laser treatment to remove melanocytic nevi is avoided if there is any risk of melanoma, including previous history or family history of melanoma, and clinical evidence of atypia. Although melanoma is uncommon in Asians, laser for the removal of nevomelanocytic nevus should be avoided if the lesion is located in the acral area, which is a common region of melanoma in Asian populations.

Tattoo Removal
In fair-skinned individuals, QS lasers have been proved to be effective in removing pigmented lesions and tattoos with minimal risk of adverse sequelae (149–152). Laser tattoo removal in darkly pigmented patients has often been presumed to have a greater risk of complications, such as hypertrophic scar (Fig. 13.16) and keloid formation, and pigmentary alterations (Fig. 13.17), as compared with fair-skinned patients.

The efficacy of the QS lasers on tattoo removal in dark-skinned patients is comparable to that of light-skinned patients. Studies on tattoo removal in dark-complexioned patients (skin phototypes III–VI) with QS lasers have shown favorable results without scarring or significant permanent pigment changes (153–160).

Grevelink et al. (154) determined the efficacy and side effects of QS lasers on a small series of skin phototypes V and VI patients. A QSRL at 694 nm, with a pulse duration of 20 ns using a 5-mm spot size at an energy fluence ranging from 4.5 to 6.0 J/cm², and a QS Nd:YAG laser at 1064 nm, with a pulse duration of 10 ns using a 3-mm spot size at an energy fluence ranging from 4.5 to 7.3 J/cm², were used to treat four of five patients presented with charcoal-injected tattoos on the face or neck, and one of five patients with a multicolored tattoo on the mid-chest region. Two of five patients (40%) cleared by more than 90% after six treatments. Lesions of the other three patients were 50% and 60% cleared after four to eight treatments, respectively.

A similar study on laser treatment of tattoos in skin phototype VI patients using a QS Nd:YAG laser demonstrated that after three to four treatments at 8-week intervals, 8 of 15 (53%) tattoos were 75–95% cleared, 5 of 15 (33%) were 50% cleared, and 2 of 15 (13%) were only 25% cleared (155). Compared to a study on light-skinned patients using a QS Nd:YAG laser for tattoo removal (156), 77% of patients' lesions cleared by more than 75% in four treatments, and in 28% of patients lesions cleared by more than 95% in four treatments. The QSAL (755 nm, 100 ns) has also been proved to be effective in the removal of various traumatic tattoos in Asian (skin phototypes III–V) (153,157) and Spanish (skin phototypes III–IV) (161) skin.

Multiple treatments are necessary. On average, 8–12 sessions may be required, with a minimum of 6–8 weeks between treatments with longer durations acceptable. Amateur tattoos require a fewer number of treatments than professional tattoos. There is rarely 100% clearing. Most tattoos clear to a point of being cosmetically acceptable.

When treating patients with dark skin types, pigmentary changes are the most commonly encountered side effect. Scarring can occur but is very rare when appropriate laser energy (the energy that produces nonexplosive effects on the skin) is selected (153–155,157,158). However, transient textural alterations associated with the healing response can occur during multiple treatments. The lack of clinical scarring noted with QS lasers, even when epidermal damage is noted, is most likely due to the lack of thermal injury to collagen, as evidenced by the absence of histological fibrosis in areas treated multiple times with both the QSRL (159) and QS Nd:YAG laser (156).

Transient pigmentary changes including hypopigmentation and hyperpigmentation, have been noted in the early healing phase but are commonly resolved in 6–8 weeks. Pre- and post-treatment epidermal cooling can minimize the nonspecific injury to the epidermis, and reduce postoperative pain and

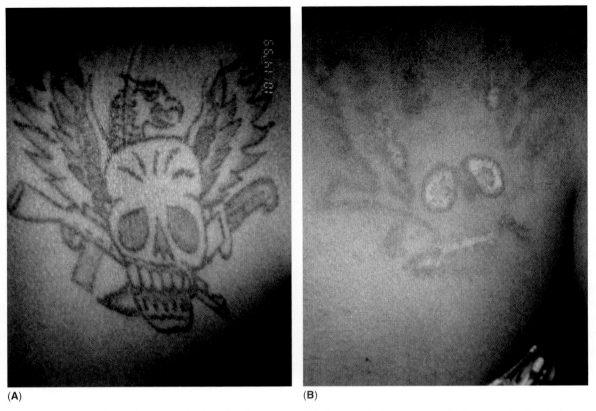

(A)   **(B)**

Figure 13.16 (**A**) Multicolored professional tattoo on the shoulder of a 20-year-old Thai woman, before treatment. (**B**) Four months after the last treatment with the Q-switched neodymium-doped:yttrium-aluminum-garnet laser. The dark blue and green inks received eight 1064-nm laser treatments, whereas the red ink got two 532-nm laser treatments. The green ink was incompletely eliminated. Hypertrophic scars developed on the previous red-ink portion.

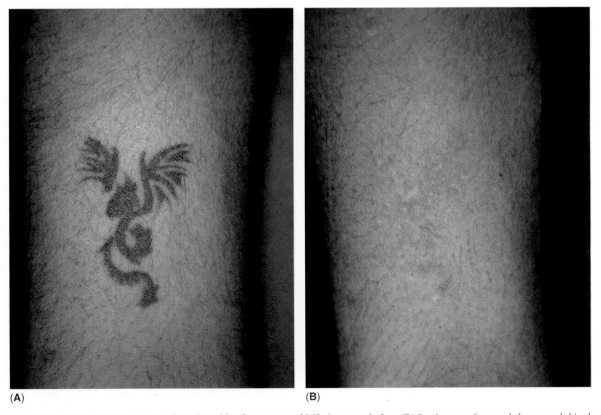

(A)   **(B)**

Figure 13.17 (**A**) A professional tattoo with blue ink on the ankle of an 18-year-old Thai woman, before. (**B**) Persistence of textural change and skin dyspigmentation, 3 months after five 1064-nm Q-switched neodymium-doped:yttrium-aluminum-garnet laser treatments. *Source*: From Ref. 284.

swelling. Laser tattoo removal on scar-prone areas, including presternal, deltoid areas, and back should be performed with the lowest fluence possible.

As with treatment of all other pigmented lesions in pigmented races, the incidence of hypopigmentation appears to be a wavelength-dependent phenomenon; the shorter the wavelength, the greater the incidence of hypopigmentation. The incidence of hyperpigmentation is comparable between QSRL and QS Nd:YAG laser, which is mostly transient, and has been reported only in darker-skinned patients (skin phototypes II–V) (156,159). A dose–response study on the treatment of tattoos by QSRL noted hypopigmentation at all doses greater than 1.5 J/cm². This persistent hypopigmentation was apparent in four of 10 tattoos followed-up 1 year after treatment (114). In contrast, hyperpigmentation was seen in only one of 13 skin phototype V patients. The QSRL treatment typically results in blistering at the dermoepidermal junction (Fig. 13.4) (68), transient hypopigmentation and, less frequently, hyperpigmentation (162).

As previously noted by others (154–156,159), we found that when treating tattoos in Asian patients, the QSRL commonly causes hypopigmentation, whereas the QS Nd:YAG laser at appropriate fluences has a very low incidence of hypopigmentation. At the wavelength of 1064 nm, the QS Nd:YAG laser light penetrates deeper and therefore might provide less injury to the unintentionally targeted melanosomes (163). We therefore agree with the recommendation of others (151,154) that the longer wavelength (1064 nm) QS Nd:YAG laser is preferable to the QSRL and QSAL in the treatment of deeper dermal and blue/black tattoo pigments in dark-skinned patients.

ABLATIVE LASER SYSTEMS

The use of pulsed or scanned CO_2 lasers for ablative skin resurfacing (ASR) is a popular procedure for similar indications as dermabrasion and chemical peels. The same principles of thermal confinement used in selective photothermolysis also apply to minimizing the thermal injury from CO_2 laser vaporization. In fair-skinned patients, the most common indication for skin resurfacing is to treat chronic sun damage, wrinkles, traumatic scars, surgical scars, and acne scars. In contrast, in non–white-skinned patients, acne scarring is the most common indication for this procedure. Unfortunately, the risk of prolonged or permanent dyspigmentation, especially PIH, parallels the degree of the patient's constitutive skin color or natural pigmentation: the darker the color, the greater the potential (164–166).

PIH, the most common complication seen following cutaneous CO_2 laser resurfacing in nonwhite patients, usually develops around the first month after treatment and becomes most significant within 4 months (Fig. 13.18). Various studies reported an incidence of 25% and 68% on laser resurfacing in Hispanic (skin phototypes II–V) (167) and other races with skin type IV patients (168), respectively. This is compared with a 3–7% incidence of PIH that occurs after CO_2 laser resurfacing in Caucasian patients with skin phototypes I–IV. In fact, in these studies, PIH occurred only in patients with skin phototypes III and IV (164,165).

In contrast to PIH, which typically resolves with time, the incidence of postlaser hypopigmentation is higher with a longer follow-up period. Incidence of PIH of 16–19% was noted in an 8-month follow-up (164) and our 2-year follow-up

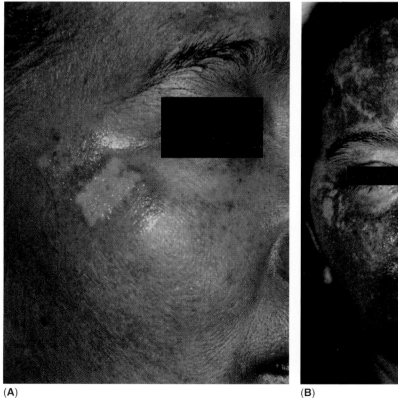
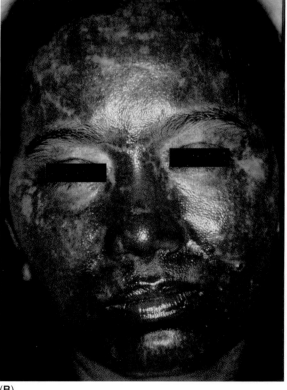

(A)   **(B)**

Figure 13.18 (**A**) Melasma in a 40-year-old Thai woman with skin phototype IV, 2 weeks after test area resurfacing using an ultrapulsed CO_2 laser. No PIH was seen. (**B**) Marked PIH developed 2 weeks after two passes of full-face CO_2 laser resurfacing. *Abbreviations*: CO_2, carbon dioxide; PIH, postinflammatory hyperpigmentation. *Source*: From Ref. 168.

studies (165), respectively. This may sometimes be a near permanent complication. The incidence of hypertrophic scars and keloids is comparable to that of fair-skinned patients. These later complications are usually the results of poor technique, postoperative infection, or other intrinsic patient factors.

We believe that the advantage of preoperative treatment is not so much in the prevention of PIH but in determining what medications a patient is sensitive to so they can be avoided in the postoperative period. A study by West and Alster (169) noted no significant difference in the incidence of post-CO_2 laser resurfacing hyperpigmentation between subjects who received pretreatment with either topical glycolic acid cream or combination tretinoin/hydroquinone creams and those who received no pretreatment regimen.

In our experience, PIH may occur in spite of careful preoperative treatment. Similarly, a retrospective study on facial resurfacing in patients with skin type IV indicated no correlation of pretreatment or types of laser used to incidence of PIH (168). However, PIH appears to respond to appropriate treatment once it has developed.

The application of broad-spectrum sunscreen and sun avoidance postoperatively is also beneficial in minimizing hyperpigmentation. The advantage of sun avoidance has been demonstrated in a study showing that preoperative and postoperative UV exposure on laser-treated skin resulted in a poor cosmetic appearance, including textural change and hyperpigmentation (170).

In 1996, the introduction of the Er:YAG laser represented an alternative to the pulsed and scanned CO_2 resurfacing lasers. Er:YAG laser resurfacing requires a shorter, less painful recovery time, and causes fewer long-term adverse effects. In general, the recovery time and the incidence of adverse sequelae are proportional to the extent of tissue injury, including the total anatomical depth of necrosis, ablation, and residual thermal damage (171–173). A layer of residual thermal damage observed after a typical Er:YAG laser resurfacing procedure is less than 50 μm versus the 80–200 μm typically observed after multiple passes of pulsed CO_2 laser resurfacing (174). Therefore, one advantage of the Er:YAG laser over the CO_2 laser is that it appears to offer a higher margin of safety when treating patients with darker complexions (skin phototypes III and higher), because the resultant inflammatory reaction caused by less extensive thermal trauma stimulates less melanocytic activity (93).

The incidence of transient PIH following CO_2 laser resurfacing ranges from 3% to 7% for all patients and nearly 68% among those with skin type IV and higher. Although postoperative hyperpigmentation and prolonged erythema seem to occur at roughly the same rate among patients with darker skin after Er:YAG laser resurfacing, it is often less severe and resolves more quickly compared with the CO_2 laser treatment (94). The Er:YAG laser, therefore, appears to be better suited for resurfacing of Asian skin.

With equal energy fluence and number of passes, the Er:YAG laser produces less total depth of tissue necrosis and hence less effective treatment of deeper wrinkles. The greater immediate collagen contraction effect and the hemostasis property provided by the CO_2 laser are the advantages of this laser resurfacing system over the Er:YAG laser. To combine the beneficial

properties of these two systems, Goldman and Manuskiatti (175) successfully developed a resurfacing technique using the combined CO_2 and Er:YAG lasers in the same treatment session. By using the Er:YAG laser to vaporize a portion of the layer of residual thermal damage created by the CO_2 laser, one can achieve a better cosmetic response with faster healing time and shorter duration of postlaser erythema, and hence a decreased incidence of adverse sequelae. The favorable result of this combined treatment method has also been confirmed by a study on the treatment of atrophic scars in Korean patients with skin phototypes IV–V (176).

The single-pass CO_2 or Er:YAG laser has been performed to help lessen the risks associated with multipass CO_2, Er:YAG, or combination techniques of laser skin resurfacing (177–179). Ruiz-Esparza and Gomez (179) evaluated 15 Hispanic patients after single-pass CO_2 laser resurfacing for a follow-up period of 18 months. All the patients were re-epithelialized by 7 days, and continued clinical improvement of rhytides was observed throughout the length of the study. However, the near universal incidence of transient postoperative hyperpigmentation has still been observed in patients with dark skin tones after CO_2 single-pass resurfacing. Although superficial resurfacing is definitely safer than deep resurfacing, it is no guarantee that PIH will not develop.

A less-aggressive technique in ablative facial resurfacing has emerged that offers modest clinical improvements in rhytides and atrophic facial scars with reduced postoperative morbidity and shorter recovery times, that is, the variable-pulsed, dual- or thermal-mode Er:YAG lasers emit light with extended pulse durations (up to 250 ms) producing larger zones of dermal heating compared with traditional short-pulsed Er:YAG laser systems (180–183). These larger zones of dermal collagen coagulation result in beneficial tissue effects that approximate those of the CO_2 laser. In addition, increased thermal coagulation of dermal vessels is effected, permitting deeper tissue penetration and improved intraoperative field visualization. The use of these newer methods are associated with a shorter and less severe postoperative course compared with traditional multipass CO_2 and short-pulsed Er:YAG laser skin resurfacing. The intensity and duration of such adverse sequelae as erythema and PIH are also reduced, making the variable-pulsed Er:YAG a potentially better choice when treating patients with darker skin tones (Fig. 13.19).

Studies on CO_2 (184–186), Er:YAG (94,181,187,188), and combined CO_2 and Er (176,189) lasers resurfacing on Asian skin (skin phototypes III–V) have shown that these procedures can be performed effectively and safely when proper pre- and postoperative management is implemented. Pre- and postoperative treatment regimens are necessary to achieve optimum results and reduce the incidence of PIH (190,191). In addition to topical retinoic acid applied each night, patients with skin phototypes III–VI are given topical preparations of hydroquinone, kojic acid, azelaic acid, or vitamin C to be used for 1–2 months preoperatively. Although an arbitrary minimum preoperative treatment time of 2 weeks is often recommended, achieving maximum benefit requires months of use. These agents are restarted as soon as possible postoperatively (2–4 weeks). Reinstitution of these topical preparations too early may induce inflammation on the newly regenerated treated skin and should be avoided (173,190).

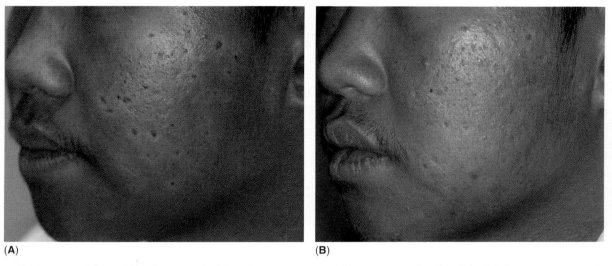

(A)   **(B)**

Figure 13.19 (**A**) A 19-year-old man (skin phototype V) with moderate to severe atrophic acne scars at baseline. (**B**) Clinical appearance 4 months after two variable square pulse erbium:yttrium-aluminum-garnet laser treatments. *Source*: From Ref. 183.

Inflammation in the postoperative period is a normal cascade of the healing process, but prolonged inflammation is not. Clinically, persistent postoperative erythema is a strong predictor of delayed-onset hyperpigmentation. Consequently, inflammation in darker-skinned individuals leads to hyperpigmentation and, if long-standing, may cause permanent depigmentation. All factors producing tissue inflammation during the healing process should be minimized or eliminated in these patients to reduce the risk of pigmentary alterations. Mechanical trauma (excessive rubbing of the tissue between laser passes), irritants, chemical causing an allergic contact dermatitis, and prolonging inflammation from an opportunistic infection should be prevented. Use of topical corticosteroid ointment from days 3–7 at night will help decrease inflammation. We recommend using an ointment that does not contain any stabilizing agents. We use fluocinolone ointment in petrolatum.

In brief, ASR is effective in treating photodamaged skin and acne scars in Asian patients with skin phototypes III–V. However, it must be performed with great caution, together with proper preoperative and postoperative treatment regimens, and sun avoidance. A test patch may be used when considering skin resurfacing for this group of patients. However, this is not always a reliable predictor of postoperative complications. Another application which the CO_2 laser offers definite advantage is in vaporization of selected epidermal and dermal lesions.

In the current practice, we successfully use the CO_2 laser to remove epidermal growth, such as seborrheic keratosis or verruca vulgaris, and benign nevomelanocytic nevi with low risk of adverse complications. The definite advantages of the CO_2 laser for removal of these lesions are the extreme precision in depth of ablation, leaving minimal damage to adjacent normal tissue, the speed of the treatment of multiple lesions, and near-bloodless field.

Clinical use of the CO_2 laser for this application must be guided by close attention to laser–tissue interaction during the procedure. The lesion is vaporized layer by layer by moving a defocused beam of the CW CO_2 laser with a spot size of 3 mm at 3–5 W across the surface of the lesion at a speed of approximately 1 cm/s. With thick lesion, several passes over the same area are necessary. A cotton-tipped applicator soaked in saline solution is used to remove vaporized debris after each pass. The endpoint of treatment is when the lesion is removed or a chamois yellow appearance is seen (Fig. 13.20). Treatment can be repeated at 4- to 6-week intervals if the lesion recurs.

When laser is used to remove nevomelanocytic nevi, several concerns should be judged. First, for Asians, the use of this technique should be avoided if there is any other risk of melanoma, including previous history or family history of melanoma, and clinical evidence of atypia. Second, for Caucasians, such use should be considered as the last resort of treatment. Third, recurrence of the treated nevus may show histologically atypical cells, termed pseudomelanoma (192).

NONABLATIVE LASER SYSTEMS

Despite the favorable results seen with CO_2 and Er:YAG laser resurfacing, the enthusiasm for these systems has been limited by the prolonged recovery time, long-lasting erythema, and dyspigmentation (hypo- and hyperpigmentation). To overcome the problems associated with ASR procedures, so-called nonablative dermal remodeling (NDR) techniques have been developed (193–196). The NDR technique involves the use of a cooling device to protect the epidermis, and in doing so allows high-energy laser light in the infrared spectrum to be delivered to the dermis. NDR induces the formation of new dermal collagen by creating a dermal wound without disruption to the epidermis and repair of tissue defects related to photoaging.

Although NDR lasers are not yet capable of results comparable with those of ablative laser systems, they have been shown to improve mild to moderate atrophic scars, rhytides, pigmentation, and telangiectasia. These NDR devices may be particularly suited to Asian patients because photoaging in Asians tends to have fewer wrinkles but higher pigmentary disorders (7). Furthermore, the adverse effects that are associated with ablative laser resurfacing systems, such as erythema and PIH, are particularly common and problematic in Asian skin.

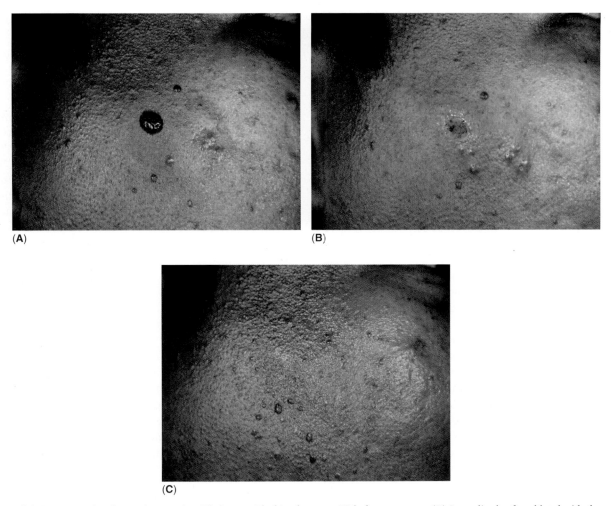

Figure 13.20 (**A**) A compound melanocytic nevus in a Thai man with skin phototype IV, before treatment. (**B**) Immediately after ablated with three passes of continuous wave CO_2 laser with a 3-mm spot size at 3 W. (**C**) Two years after one treatment with CO_2 laser vaporization. *Abbreviation*: CO_2, carbon dioxide.

Studies on the use of these nonablative laser devices in Asian patients have confirmed the effectiveness and safety of this technique (197–199). One important concern is the occurrence of prolonged or permanent skin dyspigmentation that might result from an improper parameter selection of a cryogen cooling device coupled to some nonablative laser systems or from an improper positioning of the laser handpiece, not from the thermal injury of laser light (Fig. 13.21) (200,201). Unfortunately, Asians with a higher epidermal melanin content are known to have an associated higher risk of PIH after skin injury which, although transient, is associated with a significant degree of patient dissatisfaction. Another more important concern is laser-induced hypopigmentation that can be prolonged or even permanent, particularly in pigmented Asian skin.

Nonablative laser skin remodeling remains a popular treatment choice for patients seeking noninvasive treatment modality and, although several systems have been shown to effect improvement in rhytides and atrophic scars, they still do not approximate the improvement typically seen after ablative laser treatment. In addition, none of these light systems has yet emerged as being clearly superior. While the absence of epidermal damage in NDR techniques significantly decreases the severity and duration of the treatment-related adverse effects, the major drawback of these techniques is their limited efficacy.

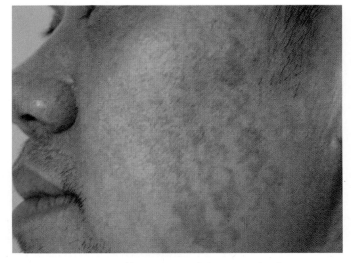

Figure 13.21 Persistence of hyperpigmented rings 3 months after a treatment with the 1450-nm diode laser equipped with a tetrafluoroethane spray cooling for nonablative dermal remodeling in a 36-year-old Thai man with skin phototype IV.

FRACTIONAL RESURFACING SYSTEMS

The latest concept of cutaneous remodeling called FP has been introduced in 2004 (202). Skin restoration by FP is achieved by applying an array of microscopic treatment zones (MTZs) of thermal injury to the skin. The concept behind this approach is to thermally alter a fraction of the skin, leaving intervening areas of normal skin untouched, which rapidly repopulate the ablated columns of tissue.

Clinical efficacy of FP for skin resurfacing depends in part on the dermal remodeling phase of MTZ repair. MTZs are intentionally designed to be small so that they can hardly be seen, if at all, without magnification. The macroscopic treatment effect of FP is characterized both by the arrangement and shape of these MTZs within the skin. Although there was visible necrosis of the epidermis and dermis in the MTZ, the stratum corneum remained histologically intact; thus, resurfacing with the prototype FP device was termed "nonablative" fractional resurfacing (NAFR) (203,204).

As compared with the full-ablative resurfacing, NAFR results in faster recovery and fewer side effects. Although erythema and edema resolve within a few days in most patients, the improvement in rhytides and photodamage is not as impressive as with full-ablative resurfacing. Mild-to-moderate improvement is observed, requiring multiple treatment sessions, ranging from 5 to 6 and spaced at 4- to 8-week intervals.

NAFR has been used for a wide range of skin conditions, beyond the initial studies demonstrating improvement in periorbital rhytides and forearm skin. NAFR has been useful in treating conditions such as mild-to-moderate rhytides (205,206), photodamaged skin (207), acne scarring (208,209), hypopigmented scars (210), melasma (101,102), and nonfacial skin rejuvenation (211).

Despite these safety advantages, the clinical efficacy profile of NAFR does not match that of the full-ablative process, especially with respect to moderate-to-severe rhytides. Hantash and colleagues (212,213) examined an application of a novel ablative CO_2 fractional resurfacing device that similarly produces an array of MTZs of a customizable density and depth but results in a confluent array of ablation and coagulation that extends through the stratum corneum, epidermis, and dermis. With the greater degree of injury with fractionated CO_2, a greater and prolonged effect on the induction of new collagen and remodeling of dermal collagen are anticipated. Immunohistochemistry studies demonstrating the histological and clinical effects of this prototype ablative fractionated CO_2 device confirmed that persistent collagen remodeling occurred for at least 3–6 months after treatment (214,215). The findings of these immunohistological studies are concordant with our previous study demonstrating clinical improvement of atrophic acne scars constantly increased up to 6 months postoperatively (216).

Previous studies have evaluated the clinical efficacy of ablative fractional resurfacing lasers, including CO_2 (10,600 nm) (216–218), Er:YAG (2940 nm) (219,220), and erbium yttrium scandium gallium garnet (Er:YSGG) (2790 nm) (221,222) fractional lasers and have confirmed the initial hypothesis of Hantash et al. (212,214) that this mode of resurfacing produces improvements in the skin signs of photoaging (improvement moderate-to-severe rhytides, dyschromia and skin mottling, and other texture abnormalities) analogous to that only previously achievable with full-ablative resurfacing.

Specifically, several prior reports have confirmed the efficacy of AFR in the treatment of moderate to severe acne scarring and moderate to severe photoaging (deep rhytides, dyschromia, and texture abnormalities) (216,217,220,221). In addition, several split-face studies have confirmed that the degree of improvement with ablative fractionated resurfacing significantly surpasses that of the original prototype nonablative fractionated devices, with only slightly longer downtimes and similar low side-effect profiles.

Similar to those reported in white-skinned patients (103,204,223,224), studies on the NAFR and AFR techniques based on the concept of FP have demonstrated its safety and efficacy in dark-skinned individuals (Fig. 13.22) (101,206,216,225,226). However, PIH remained the most common adverse effects following NAFR and AFR in Asian individuals (216,217,225). Graber et al. retrospectively studied 961 treatments with the 1550-nm erbium-doped fiber laser and found that PIH occurred more frequently in darker skin types (incidence of 2.6%, 11.6%, and 33% for skin types III, IV, and V, respectively), appeared later posttreatment and lasted longer than other complications (227). However, we noted that PIH after NAFR and AFR was much less severe than that after traditional ablative laser resurfacing and mostly cleared within 2–3 months (Fig. 13.23).

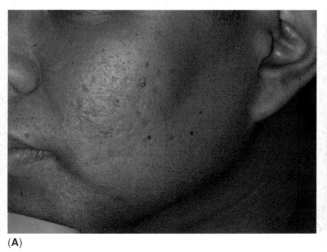

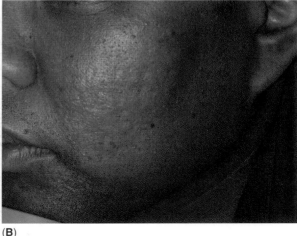

(A)   (B)

Figure 13.22 (**A**) Atrophic acne scars in a Thai man with skin phototype IV at baseline and (**B**) six months after three treatments. There was a marked improvement of boxcar scars. Pulse energy settings of 90 mJ/MTZ and MTZ density of 49/cm² were used. *Abbreviation*: MTZ, microthermal zone. *Source*: From Ref. 216.

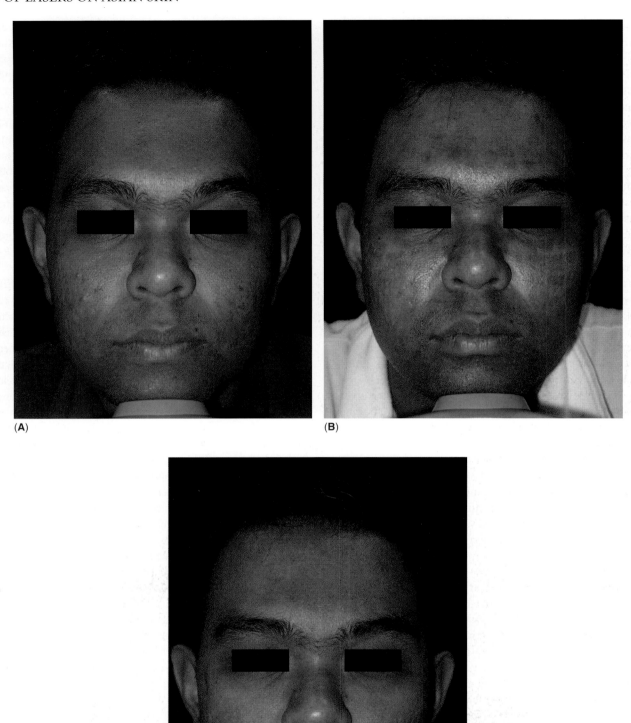

(A)

(B)

(C)

Figure 13.23 Resolution process of moderate PIH of patient in Figure 13.22. (**A**) Patient at baseline, (**B**) three weeks posttreatment with pulse energy of 90 mJ/MTZ and MTZ density of 49/cm², and (**C**) complete clearing of PIH 8 weeks after irradiation with treatment of topical hydroquinone 4% cream. *Abbreviations*: MTZ, microthermal zone; PIH, postinflammatory hyperpigmentation. *Source*: From Ref. 216.

Previous studies investigating the use of NAFR (225,228) and AFR (229) indicated that treatment density, rather than energy, was a stronger determining factor in the development of PIH in predisposed patients. Therefore, to reduce the risk of PIH associated with NAFR and AFR when treating Asian patients, the total treatment density (MTZ/cm^2) should be reduced. However, on the other hand, the total number of treatment sessions should be increased in order to maintain the clinical efficacy.

LASER HAIR REMOVAL

The use of laser and pulsed light sources for hair removal is increasing because the treatment is relatively safe and effective in removing large areas of unwanted hair. Although it has been well documented that the ideal patients for this procedure are individuals with dark hair and fair skin, unwanted or excessive hair is also a cosmetic concern for the Asian population.

Most of the available laser and light source systems with wavelengths in the red and near-infrared regions have been designed to cause selective photothermal damage to pigmented hair follicles. Improved efficacy is accomplished by the high specificity and selectivity contributed by the accurate selection of an appropriate wavelength and pulse duration to maximize follicular damage and minimize unwanted injury to the epidermis. To target the follicle, these lasers and light sources either count on endogenous melanin within the follicular epithelium or hair shaft.

When using light to target these endogenous chromophores, there is also risk of epidermal injury when laser light penetrates the target. Melanin-containing structures, including melanocytes, melanosome-containing keratinocytes, or nevus cells may also be thermally injured when irradiated by red and near-infrared lasers. Consequently, epidermal injury due to the absorption of laser energy by epidermal melanin may occur to a certain degree during the laser impacts.

Most clinical studies on the efficacy of laser and IPL systems in removing unwanted hair have been performed in fair-skinned individuals because it was theoretically postulated that a larger amount of epidermal melanin in Asian and non-white individuals may result in a decrease in clinical efficacy and cause an increase in the incidence of adverse effects, especially pigmentary and textural changes, and scarring. Currently, several reports on these light-assisted hair removal systems performed on darker-skinned persons have shown comparable results to those of fair-skinned persons with a slightly increased risk of complications (230–238). In addition, laser and pulsed light hair-removal systems have been proven to be safe and effective in treating some follicular-related disorders in dark-skinned patients, including pseudofolliculitis barbae (239) and trichostasis spinulosa (240,241).

It is difficult to compare the efficacy and side effects of light-assisted hair removal systems because of the variability in the treated anatomic sites and in the types, pulse widths, spot sizes, and repetition rates of the light sources used, as well as differences in the treatment regimens. All laser and IPL systems have been shown to temporarily remove hair. Reduction of hair growth occurs for all hair colors and at all fluences. Blonde, red-, or white-haired individuals are unlikely to experience permanent hair reduction, but hair loss in these persons can be sustained by treatment at approximately 3-month intervals (168). We note a similar response rate when treating Asian and black patients. Studies have demonstrated that in the ideal patients with fair skin and dark hair, the possibility for long-term hair reduction after a single treatment is approximately 80% (242,243).

A critical threshold fluence is needed to obtain efficacy. This fluence is determined as the lowest fluence that can produce perifollicular swelling and erythema appearing a few minutes after laser irradiation. When treating individuals with skin types IV–VI, we carefully select the endpoint that produces slight perifollicular swelling and erythema. If there is a sign of acute epidermal injury, including whitening, blistering, or Nikolsky's sign (forced epidermal separation), the fluence should be reduced. Generally, the treatment fluence should be at 75% of the Nikolsky's threshold fluence (244). A 2-year follow-up study on the efficacy of normal-mode ruby laser hair removal notes that sites treated with highest fluence (60 J/cm^2) obtained the greatest hair reduction (64.3%) (245).

Epidermal injury is an anticipated consequence when treating a darker complexioned patient. Whereas the goal of light-assisted hair removal is permanent follicular destruction, there is also a risk of epidermal damage during hair removal, especially in nonwhite individuals whose epidermis contains larger amounts of melanin. When treating this group of patients, in order to be able to use the highest tolerable fluence to achieve better hair reduction while minimizing epidermal damage, three important considerations, including wavelength and pulse duration of the light sources, and epidermal cooling methods, should be taken into account.

The first important determinant is wavelength of the light source. The ideal laser wavelength for hair removal is a wavelength that is preferentially absorbed by melanin but not by surrounding tissue. Lasers emitting longer wavelengths have the advantage of being able to penetrate deeper into the dermis, minimizing the possibility of absorptive interference by epidermal melanin (242,244). Color contrast between epidermis and the hair shaft (and bulb) are crucial in determining the optimal wavelength. For high contrast (dark hair, light skin), the low range of the wavelength (650–700 nm) can be employed without risking serious injury to the epidermis (and subsequent hypo- and hyperpigmentation). For lighter hair and darker skin, the longer wavelength (800 nm and greater) should be applied (246).

Studies in patients with skin phototypes III–V have shown that temporary hair reduction after treatment with normal-mode ruby (694 nm) laser (237,247), LP ruby (694 nm) laser (248,249), LP alexandrite (755 nm) laser (233,250), diode (810 and 940 nm) laser (236,251,252), long-pulsed Nd:YAG (1064 nm) laser (231,252), and IPL (253,254) hair-removal systems was comparable in skin phototypes I–II. However, the incidence of undesirable side effects occurred more often compared with those noted in fair-skinned patients. Although most of these side effects, including treatment pain, erythema, edema, blistering, crusting, erosion, purpura, folliculitis, and pigmentary changes (hypopigmentation and hyperpigmentation), were transient and self-limited, pigmentary alterations usually required longer to resolve (more than 3 months). In addition, these side effects often occurred on tanned skin, in patients with skin phototype III and higher, or on sites treated with excessively high-energy fluences.

In our experience, when treating subjects with dark skin, the ruby laser system is associated with higher risk of adverse effects, especially transient hyper- and hypopigmentation. This results from the melanin interface of the 694-nm light pulse of the ruby lasers. However, the alexandrite, diode, and LP 1064-nm Nd:YAG lasers; and the IPL source operating at longer wavelength and longer pulse widths have been used to treat these patients safely when combined with cooling devices. Permanent pigmentary alterations (Fig. 13.24) and scarring were rare except in cases of overaggressive treatment or post-operative infection.

A retrospective study of the side effects of laser-assisted hair removal treatment in skin phototypes I–V found that the QS Nd:YAG laser resulted in the fewest side effects, whereas the LP ruby and the LP alexandrite lasers produced equivalent adverse effects but greater efficacy than that of QS 1064-nm Nd:YAG laser (249). Long-term adverse sequelae and scarring were not observed with any of the laser systems under study. Although it caused the fewest side effects, the 1064-nm QS Nd:YAG system does not typically produce long-term hair reduction because of its very low absorption by melanin and the use of low treatment energy fluences (255).

As anticipated, lasers with longer wavelengths produce fewer adverse effects. A hair removal study comparing the efficacy and complications of diode and LP 1064-nm Nd:YAG lasers in Chinese patients with skin phototypes IV or V noted no pigmentary or textural changes after treatment, even in skin phototype V patients (231). However, the disadvantage of the LP Nd:YAG hair removal system is that the absorption of this laser light by melanin is decreased compared with that of the ruby laser, such that absorption by the completing chromophore, oxyhemoglobin, is substantially increased.

Pulse duration of hair removal light sources is the second important parameter for effective hair removal without epidermal injury (256). A pulse duration of approximately 10–50 ms will damage hair follicles with less epidermal injury. However, caution should be exercised when using very long pulse widths to treat dense hair areas because of thermal conduction between closely adjacent hair follicles.

The last important factor to be considered is epidermal cooling. Integrating surface cooling into the delivery configuration is one way to protect the epidermis and consequently prevent or minimize the adverse sequelae of the procedure. Presently, five types of cooling are used in conjunction with lasers and IPL systems: (*i*) passive cooling with a chilled aqueous gel; (*ii*) active cooling with water encased in a glass housing; (*iii*) active conductive cooling with water encased in a sapphire window; (*iv*) dynamic active cooling with a cryogenic spray; and (*v*) air cooling with a refrigerated air stream. These cooling configurations can provide epidermal preservation compared with no surface cooling (242,246).

Paradoxical hypertrichosis is a rare but significant side effect of photoepilation that has received more attention in the literature (257–259). Initially reported with IPL therapy (260), this adverse effect has now been seen after long-pulse alexandrite (257) and diode laser (261) treatment and is likely to be common to all current laser and light hair removal devices (258,259,262). The most common location of terminal hair growth, which has been noted in several studies, is on the lower face in women although reports on the backs of men have also been described. The majority of patients developing hair induction had dark skin types (III or IV).

The etiology of this "paradoxical effect" of increased hair growth in response to laser and light photoepilation remains unclear but some have speculated that it is lower-range fluences of laser and light in individuals with darker skin types, which paradoxically stimulates hair growth. Therapy for paradoxical hypertrichosis is based on two facets: treatment of the already present induced hair and the prevention of hair induction. Several researchers suggest the continuation of treatments by using higher fluences and inclusion of the new hairy areas in the treatment areas, because induced hair responds to treatment in the same manner as other hair follicles.

In conclusion, in Asian patients, laser- and pulsed light hair removal systems provide comparable clinical efficacy to that of white-skinned patients. Treatment parameters must be individualized for each patient and with each device. When performing this procedure in darker skin individuals, a range of test fluences should be performed in an inconspicuous area prior to performing complete treatment. A delay of at least 1 hour should elapse prior to evaluation of test spots. In our practice, darker skin tones can be safely and effectively treated using a light source with a longer wavelength than that of a ruby laser (>694 nm) with a pulse duration of 10–50 ms and an adequate cooling device. Although laser hair removal treatments are generally effective, clinical challenges still exist. An optimal fluence setting needs to be found that is not low enough to stimulate hair growth and not high enough to cause burning, erythema, and other unwanted side effects.

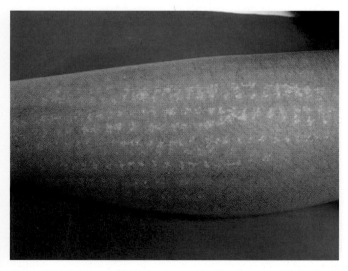

Figure 13.24 A 24-year-old Thai woman with skin phototype IV developed persistent postinflammatory hypopigmentation 8 months after one treatment with an 800-nm diode laser hair removal with a sapphire contact-cooling tip using a fluence of 30 J/cm² with a 30-ms pulse duration.

PREVENTION AND MANAGEMENT OF COMPLICATIONS

Various attempts have been made to reduce the occurrence of side effects of laser treatment in Asian skin. These include sun avoidance, the use of preoperative and postoperative treatment regimens and proper techniques for epidermal cooling.

Sun Avoidance

UV exposure prior to laser treatment has been shown to interfere with laser treatment by increasing epidermal melanin pigmentation and epidermal thickness leading to a change in the optical property of the skin (183). UV exposure may also interfere with the posttreatment healing process (263,264), altering the treatment outcome, and occurrence of side effects. Moreover, laser exposure may influence the carcinogenic potential of UV radiation, which serves as a complete carcinogen, as both tumor initiation and promotion are induced by UV (265). Nonetheless, results from an experimental study conclude that CO_2 laser treatment does not have a carcinogenic potential in itself nor does CO_2 laser treatment influence UV-induced carcinogenesis (266).

In our practice, several recommendations to minimize the effects of UV light have been suggested. From a practical standpoint, it is not easy to avoid sun exposure when living in tropical countries. Most laser treatments are elective surgeries. Thus, surgery may be postponed during summer months. Topical sunscreens protecting against both UVA and UVB, usually zinc oxide based, should be applied regularly at least 6 weeks prior to the treatment to obtain the optimal outcome (188). Patients should not visit tanning booths or go sunbathing, although the influence of acquired pigmentation compared with constitutional pigmentation for the development of adverse effects remains unidentified.

Preoperative and Postoperative

Treatment Regimen

Although the advantage of preoperative treatment regimens with various topical bleaching agents remains controversial (169,267), in current practice we regularly pretreat our patients with a minimal 2-week course of topical retinoic acid (268,269) each night, combined with any of the following topical preparations, including hydroquinone (270), kojic acid (271), azelaic acid (272), arbutin (273), licorice (274), or vitamin C (275). On the postoperative visit, these topical preparations are started as soon as possible (2–4 weeks), depending on the individual healing response. However, we often observe that PIH occurred even with careful preoperative treatment, and

this complication resolved spontaneously without using any topical preparations other than a broad-spectrum sunscreen and sun avoidance.

Epidermal Cooling

Selective epidermal cooling during laser surgery provides great benefits, allowing the use of higher fluences, permitting treatment of darker skin tones and decreasing procedure discomfort. For treating pathology that is situated beneath either the epidermis or superficial dermis, it may often be necessary to use higher fluences to deliver sufficient photons to the intended target. This applies especially to laser surgery for Asian patients, in whom higher epidermal levels of melanin effectively decrease the number of photons reaching the dermis.

Because scarring is related to the generation of excessive heat, which is greatest at or near the skin surface, methods that cool the superficial compartment of the skin should permit the safe use of higher fluences when necessary and minimize epidermal injury when it occurs (Fig. 13.25). When the epidermis and/or superficial dermis are selectively cooled either immediately before or during laser exposure, the peak temperature reached at these sites is insufficient to cause irreversible thermal damage. However, targets that are situated more deeply and that are, therefore, not cooled are able to reach the thermal threshold necessary for successful treatment.

Lowering the temperature of the skin's surfaces is therefore a method for selectively controlling the depth at which heat is produced in the skin by lasers or light sources. The effect of epidermal cooling has been shown to enhance clinical efficacy and minimize epidermal damage caused by the laser treatment process (276–280). The increased efficacy is a consequence of an increase in the depth of penetration (200) and an allowance of higher energy fluence used (281,282).

When not using a dynamic cooling device, the depth to which skin cooling protects the skin from excessive superficial heat injury is largely determined by the temperature and contact time of the handpiece or cryogen with the skin. An appropriate cooling time and technique permit heat extraction from the epidermis before, during, and after each laser pulse. Thus epidermal damage/heating can be minimized. In contrast, an

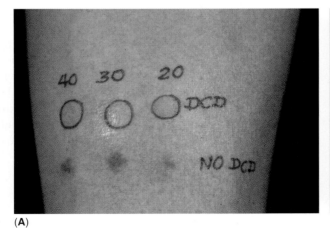

(A)

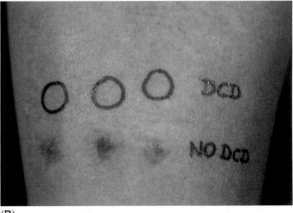

(B)

Figure 13.25 (**A**) Immediate reaction after a 595-nm pulse dye laser irradiation on a skin type IV subject at a fluence of 10 J/cm² and pulse duration of 20, 30, and 40 ms, with and without epidermal cooling using DCD. The epidermis was well protected when cooled; (**B**) 24 hours after laser irradiation. *Abbreviation:* DCD, dynamic cooling device.

overcooled epidermis may cool down the dermal target and result in a decrease in the desired clinical response. The commercial cooling methods/devices include passive cooling with aqueous gel, active cooling with water or refrigerated air, and dynamic active cooling with cryogen spray. Most of these cooling devices have been used in conjunction with vascular lasers, IPL systems, and laser hair removal.

In a less technically sophisticated manner, we find that precooling and postcooling the skin with an ice pack or ice cube can also be performed. This method, like water cooling at 0°C with a glass window, will decrease the dermoepidermal junction temperature, depending on application time. However, because it is done manually, the efficacy of this method may be unpredictable. Studies comparing cooling systems suggest that cryogen spray cooling (CSC) and contact cooling with water encased in a sapphire window provide the most effective/efficient epidermal preservation followed by cold air, water encased in a glass housing, and finally cold gel or ice (246,280).

CONCLUSIONS

The majority of laser and pulsed light treatments on Asian skin can be performed safely and effectively. However, treatments must be approached with caution. Epidermal pigmentation is perhaps the most fundamental limitation because it diminishes laser light reaching the dermis and causes unwanted thermal damage to the epidermis. Thorough patient counseling regarding the risks of cutaneous laser treatment remains an essential part of therapy.

Careful preoperative and postoperative treatment programs should be used as well as a prudent selection of types of lasers and light source suited to a patient's treatment purposes. Treatment parameters (wavelength, pulse duration, and fluence) can be tailored for specific cutaneous applications to effect maximal target destruction with minimal collateral thermal damage. Epidermal cooling is a useful method to minimize undesired epidermal damage. Finally, when treating an Asian individual with any laser, a conservative approach is the best.

REFERENCES

1. United Nations DoEaSA, Population Division. World population prospects: the 2010 revision. [Available from: http://esa.un.org/wpp/Excel-Data/population.htm] [11 July 2012].
2. Berardesca E, Maibach H. Ethnic skin: overview of structure and function. J Am Acad Dermatol 2003; 48: S139–42.
3. Berardesca E, Maibach HI. Racial differences in skin pathophysiology. J Am Acad Dermatol 1996; 34: 667–72.
4. Richards GM, Oresajo CO, Halder RM. Structure and function of ethnic skin and hair. Dermatol Clin 2003; 21: 595–600.
5. Chan HH, Alam M, Kono T, et al. Clinical application of lasers in Asians. Dermatol Surg 2002; 28: 556–63.
6. Ho SG, Chan HH. The Asian dermatologic patient: review of common pigmentary disorders and cutaneous diseases. Am J Clin Dermatol 2009; 10: 153–68.
7. Chung JH. Photoaging in Asians. Photodermatol Photoimmunol Photomed 2003; 19: 109–21.
8. Alaluf S, Atkins D, Barrett K, et al. Ethnic variation in melanin content and composition in photoexposed and photoprotected human skin. Pigment Cell Res 2002; 15: 112–18.
9. Taylor SC. Skin of color: biology, structure, function, and implications for dermatologic disease. J Am Acad Dermatol 2002; 46: S41–62.
10. Sykes JM. Management of the aging face in the Asian patient. Facial Plast Surg Clin North Am 2007; 15: 353–60; vi–vii.
11. Davis EC, Callender VD. Aesthetic dermatology for aging ethnic skin. Dermatol Surg 2011; 37: 901–17.
12. Astner S, Anderson RR. Skin phototypes 2003. J Invest Dermatol 2004; 122: xxx–xxxi.
13. Lancer HA. Lancer Ethnicity Scale (LES) [letter]. Lasers Surg Med 1998; 22: 9.
14. Wolbarsht ML, Urbach F. The Lancer Ethnicity Scale [letter]. Lasers Surg Med 1999; 25: 105–6.
15. Goldman MP. Universal classification of skin type. Cosmet Dermatol 2002; 15: 53–7.
16. Battle EF Jr, Soden CE Jr. The use of lasers in darker skin types. Semin Cutan Med Surg 2009; 28: 130–40.
17. Tanzi EL, Lupton JR, Alster TS. Lasers in dermatology: four decades of progress. J Am Acad Dermatol 2003; 49: 1–31; quiz 31–4.
18. Anderson RR, Parrish JA. The optics of human skin. J Invest Dermatol 1981; 77: 13–19.
19. Ashinoff R, Geronemus RG. Treatment of a port-wine stain in a black patient with the pulsed dye laser. J Dermatol Surg Oncol 1992; 18: 147–8.
20. Tan OT, Kerschmann R, Parrish JA. The effect of epidermal pigmentation on selective vascular effects of pulsed laser. Lasers Surg Med 1986; 4: 365–74.
21. Tong AKF, Tan OT, Boll J, et al. Ultrastructure: effect of melanin pigment on target specificity using a pulsed dye laser (577 nm). J Invest Dermatol 1987; 88: 747–52.
22. Fitzpatrick RE, Lowe NJ, Goldman MP, et al. Flashlamp-pumped pulsed dye laser treatment of port-wine stains. J Dermatol Surg Oncol 1994; 20: 743–8.
23. Haedersdal M, Gniadecka M, Efsen J, et al. Side effects from the pulsed dye laser: the importance of skin pigmentation and skin redness. Acta Derm Venereol 1998; 78: 445–50.
24. Haedersdal M, Wulf HC. Pigmentation-dependent side effects to copper vapor laser and argon laser treatment. Lasers Surg Med 1995; 16: 351–8.
25. Haedersdal M, Wulf HC. Risk assessment of side effects from copper vapor and argon laser treatment: the importance of skin pigmentation. Lasers Surg Med 1997; 20: 84–9.
26. Haedersdal M, Wulf HC. Pigmentation dependent, short time skin reactions to copper vapour laser and argon laser treatment. Burns 1994; 20: 195–9.
27. Chan HH, Chan E, Kono T, et al. The use of variable pulse width frequency doubled Nd:YAG 532 nm laser in the treatment of port-wine stain in Chinese patients. Dermatol Surg 2000; 26: 657–61.
28. Ho WS, Chan HH, Ying SY, et al. Laser treatment of congenital facial port-wine stains: long-term efficacy and complication in Chinese patients. Lasers Surg Med 2002; 30: 44–7.
29. Kono T, Sakurai H, Takeuchi M, et al. Treatment of resistant port-wine stains with a variable-pulse pulsed dye laser. Dermatol Surg 2007; 33: 951–6.
30. Sommer S, Sheehan-Dare RA. Pulsed dye laser treatment of port-wine stains in pigmented skin. J Am Acad Dermatol 2000; 42: 667–71.
31. Dong X, Yu Q, Ding J, et al. Treatment of facial port-wine stains with a new intense pulsed light source in Chinese patients. J Cosmet Laser Ther 2010; 12: 183–7.
32. Ho WS, Ying SY, Chan PC, et al. Treatment of port wine stains with intense pulsed light: a prospective study. Dermatol Surg 2004; 30: 887–91.
33. Chang CJ, Kelly KM, Van Gemert MJ, et al. Comparing the effectiveness of 585-nm vs 595-nm wavelength pulsed dye laser treatment of port wine stains in conjunction with cryogen spray cooling. Lasers Surg Med 2002; 31: 352–8.
34. Greve B, Raulin C. Prospective study of port wine stain treatment with dye laser: comparison of two wavelengths (585 nm vs. 595 nm) and two pulse durations (0.5 milliseconds vs. 20 milliseconds). Lasers Surg Med 2004; 34: 168–73.
35. Chang CJ, Nelson JS. Cryogen spray cooling and higher fluence pulsed dye laser treatment improve port-wine stain clearance while minimizing epidermal damage. Dermatol Surg 1999; 25: 767–72.
36. Chiu CH, Chan HH, Ho WS, et al. Prospective study of pulsed dye laser in conjunction with cryogen spray cooling for treatment of port wine stains in Chinese patients. Dermatol Surg 2003; 29: 909–15; discussion 15.
37. Alster TS, Tanzi EL. Combined 595-nm and 1,064-nm laser irradiation of recalcitrant and hypertrophic port-wine stains in children and adults. Dermatol Surg 2009; 35: 914–18; discussion 18–19.
38. Li G, Sun J, Shao X, et al. The Effects of 595- and 1,064-nm Lasers on Rooster Comb Blood Vessels Using Dual-Wavelength and Multipulse Techniques. Dermatol Surg 2011; 37: 1473–9.

39. Alster TS, Williams CM. Treatment of keloid sternotomy scars with 585 nm flashlamp-pumped pulsed-dye laser. Lancet 1995; 345: 1198–200.

40. Goldman MP, Fitzpatrick RE. Laser treatment of scars. Dermatol Surg 1995; 21: 685–7.

41. Wittenberg GP, Fabian BG, Bogomilsky JL, et al. Prospective, single-blind, randomized, controlled study to assess the efficacy of the 585-nm flashlamp-pumped pulsed-dye laser and silicone gel sheeting in hypertrophic scar treatment. Arch Dermatol 1999; 135: 1049–55.

42. Manuskiatti W, Fitzpatrick RE, Goldman MP. Energy density and numbers of treatment affect response of keloidal and hypertrophic sternotomy scars to the 585-nm flashlamp-pumped pulsed-dye laser. J Am Acad Dermatol 2001; 45: 557–65.

43. Chan HH, Wong DS, Ho WS, et al. The use of pulsed dye laser for the prevention and treatment of hypertrophic scars in Chinese persons. Dermatol Surg 2004; 30: 987–94; discussion 94.

44. Manuskiatti W, Wanitphakdeedecha R, Fitzpatrick RE. Effect of pulse width of a 595-nm flashlamp-pumped pulsed dye laser on the treatment response of keloidal and hypertrophic sternotomy scars. Dermatol Surg 2007; 33: 152–61.

45. Ash K, Kauver A, Lord J, et al. Long term results of treatment of stretch marks with the 585 nm flashlamp-pumped pulsed dye laser, a follow-up study. Lasers Surg Med 1998; 10(Suppl): 41.

46. McDaniel DH, Ash K, Zukowski M. Treatment of stretch marks with the 585-nm flashlamp-pumped pulsed dye laser. Dermatol Surg 1996; 22: 332–7.

47. Nehal KS, Levine VJ, Ashinoff R. Treatment of mature striae with the pulsed dye laser. Lasers Surg Med 1998; 10(Suppl): 41.

48. Nouri K, Romagosa R, Chartier T, et al. Comparison of the 585 nm pulse dye laser and the short pulsed CO$_2$ laser in the treatment of striae distensae in skin types IV and VI. Dermatol Surg 1999; 25: 368–70.

49. Kim BJ, Lee DH, Kim MN, et al. Fractional photothermolysis for the treatment of striae distensae in Asian skin. Am J Clin Dermatol 2008; 9: 33–7.

50. Lee SE, Kim JH, Lee SJ, et al. Treatment of striae distensae using an ablative 10,600-nm carbon dioxide fractional laser: a retrospective review of 27 participants. Dermatol Surg 2010; 36: 1683–90.

51. Manuskiatti W, Boonthaweeyuwat E, Varothai S. Treatment of striae distensae with a TriPollar radiofrequency device: a pilot study. J Dermatolog Treat 2009; 20: 359–64.

52. Anderson RR, Margolis RJ, Watanabe S, et al. Selective photothermolysis of cutaneous pigmentation by Q-switched Nd:YAG laser pulsed at 1064, 532, and 355 nm. J Invest Dermatol 1989; 93: 28–32.

53. Polla LL, Margolis RJ, Dover JS, et al. Melanosomes are a primary target of Q-switched ruby laser irradiation in guinea pig skin. J Invest Dermatol 1987; 89: 281–6.

54. Ohshiro T, Maruyama Y. The ruby and argon lasers in the treatment of naevi. Ann Acad Med Singapore 1983; 12: 388–95.

55. Alster TS, Williams CM. Cafe-au-lait macule in type V skin: successful treatment with a 510 nm pulsed dye laser. J Am Acad Dermatol 1995; 33: 1042–3.

56. Kunachak S, Kulapraditharom B, Kunachakr S, et al. Copper vapor laser treatment of cafe-au-lait macules. Br J Dermatol 1996; 135: 964–8.

57. Li YT, Yang KC. Comparison of the frequency-doubled Q-switched Nd:YAG laser and 35% trichloroacetic acid for the treatment of face lentigines. Dermatol Surg 1999; 25: 202–4.

58. Suh DH, Han KH, Chung JH. The use of Q-switched Nd:YAG laser in the treatment of superficial pigmented lesions in Koreans. J Dermatolog Treat 2001; 12: 91–6.

59. Murphy MJ, Huang MY. Q-switched ruby laser treatment of benign pigmented lesions in Chinese skin. Ann Acad Med Singapore 1994; 23: 60–6.

60. Sadighha A, Saatee S, Muhaghegh-Zahed G. Efficacy and adverse effects of Q-switched ruby laser on solar lentigines: a prospective study of 91 patients with Fitzpatrick skin type II, III, and IV. Dermatol Surg 2008; 34: 1465–8.

61. Shimbashi T, Kamide R, Hashimoto T. Long-term follow-up in treatment of solar lentigo and cafe-au-lait macules with Q-switched ruby laser. Aesthetic Plast Surg 1997; 21: 445–8.

62. Jang KA, Chung EC, Choi JH, et al. Successful removal of freckles in Asian skin with a Q-switched alexandrite laser. Dermatol Surg 2000; 26: 231–4.

63. Xi Z, Hui Q, Zhong L. Q-switched alexandrite laser treatment of oral labial lentigines in Chinese subjects with Peutz-Jeghers syndrome. Dermatol Surg 2009; 35: 1084–8.

64. Dover JS, Smoller BR, Stern RS, et al. Low-fluence carbon dioxide laser irradiation of lentigines. Arch Dermatol 1988; 124: 1219–24.

65. Huang YL, Liao YL, Lee SH, et al. Intense pulsed light for the treatment of facial freckles in Asian skin. Dermatol Surg 2002; 28: 1007–12; discussion 12.

66. Wang CC, Sue YM, Yang CH, et al. A comparison of Q-switched alexandrite laser and intense pulsed light for the treatment of freckles and lentigines in Asian persons: a randomized, physician-blinded, split-face comparative trial. J Am Acad Dermatol 2006; 54: 804–10.

67. Kilmer SL, Goldman MP, Fitzpatrick RE. Treatment of Benign Pigmented Cutaneous Lesions, 2nd edn. St. Louis: Mosby, 1999.

68. Hruza GJ, Dover JS, Flotte TJ, et al. Q-switched ruby laser irradiation of normal human skin. Histologic and ultrastructural findings. Arch Dermatol 1991; 127: 1799–805.

69. Chan HH, Fung WK, Ying SY, et al. An in vivo trial comparing the use of different types of 532 nm Nd:YAG lasers in the treatment of facial lentigines in Oriental patients. Dermatol Surg 2000; 26: 743–9.

70. Ho SG, Yeung CK, Chan NP, et al. A comparison of Q-switched and long-pulsed alexandrite laser for the treatment of freckles and lentigines in oriental patients. Lasers Surg Med 2011; 43: 108–13.

71. Ara G, Anderson RR, Mandel KG, et al. Irradiation of pigmented melanoma cells with high intensity pulsed radiation generates acoustic waves and kills cells. Lasers Surg Med 1990; 10: 52–9.

72. Negishi K, Wakamatsu S, Kushikata N, et al. Full-face photorejuvenation of photodamaged skin by intense pulsed light with integrated contact cooling: initial experiences in Asian patients. Lasers Surg Med 2002; 30: 298–305.

73. Grossman MC, Anderson RR, Farinelli WA, et al. Treatment of cafe au lait macules with lasers: a clinicopathlogic correlation. Arch Dermatol 1995; 131: 1416–20.

74. Taylor CR, Anderson RR. Treatment of benign pigmented epidermal lesions by Q-switched ruby laser. Int J Dermatol 1993; 32: 908–12.

75. Kagami S, Asahina A, Watanabe R, et al. Treatment of 153 Japanese patients with Q-switched alexandrite laser. Lasers Med Sci 2007; 22: 159–63.

76. Chan HH, Ying SY, Ho WS, et al. An in vivo trial comparing the clinical efficacy and complications of Q-switched 755 nm alexandrite and Q-switched 1064 nm Nd:YAG lasers in the treatment of nevus of Ota. Dermatol Surg 2000; 26: 919–22.

77. Rashid T, Hussain I, Haider M, et al. Laser therapy of freckles and lentigines with quasi-continuous, frequency-doubled, Nd:YAG (532 nm) laser in Fitzpatrick skin type IV: a 24-month follow-up. J Cosmet Laser Ther 2002; 4: 81–5.

78. Trelles MA, Verkruysse W, Pickering JW, et al. Monoline argon laser (514 nm) treatment of benign pigmented lesions with long pulse lengths. J Photochem Photobiol B 1992; 16: 357–65.

79. Anderson RR, Parrish JA. Selective photothermolysis: precise microsurgery by selective absorption of pulsed radiation. Science 1983; 220: 524–7.

80. Kono T, Manstein D, Chan HH, et al. Q-switched ruby versus long-pulsed dye laser delivered with compression for treatment of facial lentigines in Asians. Lasers Surg Med 2006; 38: 94–7.

81. Grekin RC, Shelton RM, Geisse JK, et al. 510-nm pigmented lesion dye laser. Its characteristics and clinical uses. J Dermatol Surg Oncol 1993; 19: 380–7.

82. Rendon M, Berneburg M, Arellano I, et al. Treatment of melasma. J Am Acad Dermatol 2006; 54: S272–81.

83. Taylor CR, Anderson RR. Ineffective treatment of refractory melasma and postinflammatory hyperpigmentation by Q-switched ruby laser [see comments]. J Dermatol Surg Oncol 1994; 20: 592–7.

84. Gupta AK, Gover MD, Nouri K, et al. The treatment of melasma: a review of clinical trials. J Am Acad Dermatol 2006; 55: 1048–65.

85. Li YH, Chen JZ, Wei HC, et al. Efficacy and safety of intense pulsed light in treatment of melasma in Chinese patients. Dermatol Surg 2008; 34: 693–700; discussion 00–1.

86. Negishi K, Kushikata N, Tezuka Y, et al. Study of the incidence and nature of "very subtle epidermal melasma" in relation to intense pulsed light treatment. Dermatol Surg 2004; 30: 881–6; discussion 86.

87. Choi M, Choi JW, Lee SY, et al. Low-dose 1064-nm Q-switched Nd:YAG laser for the treatment of melasma. J Dermatolog Treat 2010; 21: 224–8.

88. Jeong SY, Shin JB, Yeo UC, et al. Low-fluence Q-switched neodymium-doped yttrium aluminum garnet laser for melasma with pre- or post-treatment triple combination cream. Dermatol Surg 2010; 36: 909–18.

89. Wattanakrai P, Mornchan R, Eimpunth S. Low-fluence Q-switched neodymium-doped yttrium aluminum garnet (1,064 nm) laser for the treatment of facial melasma in Asians. Dermatol Surg 2010; 36: 76–87.

90. Cho SB, Kim JS, Kim MJ. Melasma treatment in Korean women using a 1064-nm Q-switched Nd:YAG laser with low pulse energy. Clin Exp Dermatol 2009; 34: e847–50.

91. Chan NP, Ho SG, Shek SY, et al. A case series of facial depigmentation associated with low fluence Q-switched 1,064 nm Nd:YAG laser for skin rejuvenation and melasma. Lasers Surg Med 2010; 42: 712–19.

92. Kim MJ, Kim JS, Cho SB. Punctate leucoderma after melasma treatment using 1064-nm Q-switched Nd:YAG laser with low pulse energy. J Eur Acad Dermatol Venereol 2009; 23: 960–2.

93. Manaloto RMP, Alster T. Laser resurfacing for refractory melasma. Dermatol Surg 1999; 25: 121–3.

94. Polnikorn N, Goldberg DJ, Suwanchinda A, et al. Erbium:YAG laser resurfacing in Asians. Dermatol Surg 1998; 24: 1303–7.

95. Angsuwarangsee S, Polnikorn N. Combined ultrapulse CO_2 laser and Q-switched alexandrite laser compared with Q-switched alexandrite laser alone for refractory melasma: split-face design. Dermatol Surg 2003; 29: 59–64.

96. Nouri K, Bowes L, Chartier T, et al. Combination treatment of melasma with pulsed CO_2 laser followed by Q-switched alexandrite laser: a pilot study. Dermatol Surg 1999; 25: 494–7.

97. Minwalla L, Zhao Y, Le Poole IC, et al. Keratinocytes play a role in regulating distribution patterns of recipient melanosomes in vitro. J Invest Dermatol 2001; 117: 341–7.

98. Seiberg M. Keratinocyte-melanocyte interactions during melanosome transfer. Pigment Cell Res 2001; 14: 236–42.

99. Wanitphakdeedecha R, Manuskiatti W, Siriphukpong S, et al. Treatment of melasma using variable square pulse Er:YAG laser resurfacing. Dermatol Surg 2009; 35: 475–81; discussion 81–2.

100. Katz TM, Glaich AS, Goldberg LH, et al. Treatment of melasma using fractional photothermolysis: a report of eight cases with long-term follow-up. Dermatol Surg 2010; 36: 1273–80.

101. Lee HS, Won CH, Lee DH, et al. Treatment of melasma in Asian skin using a fractional 1,550-nm laser: an open clinical study. Dermatol Surg 2009; 35: 1499–504.

102. Rokhsar CK, Fitzpatrick RE. The treatment of melasma with fractional photothermolysis: a pilot study. Dermatol Surg 2005; 31: 1645–50.

103. Sherling M, Friedman PM, Adrian R, et al. Consensus recommendations on the use of an erbium-doped 1,550-nm fractionated laser and its applications in dermatologic laser surgery. Dermatol Surg 2010; 36: 461–9.

104. Hantash BM, Bedi VP, Sudireddy V, et al. Laser-induced transepidermal elimination of dermal content by fractional photothermolysis. J Biomed Opt 2006; 11: 041115.

105. Naito SK. Fractional photothermolysis treatment for resistant melasma in Chinese females. J Cosmet Laser Ther 2007; 9: 161–3.

106. Wind BS, Kroon MW, Meesters AA, et al. Non-ablative 1,550 nm fractional laser therapy versus triple topical therapy for the treatment of melasma: a randomized controlled split-face study. Lasers Surg Med 2010; 42: 607–12.

107. Karsai S, Fischer T, Pohl L, et al. Is non-ablative 1550-nm fractional photothermolysis an effective modality to treat melasma? Results from a prospective controlled single-blinded trial in 51 patients. J Eur Acad Dermatol Venereol 2012; 26: 470–6.

108. Hidano A, Kajima H, Ikedea S, et al. Natural history of nevus of Ota. Arch Dermatol 1967; 95: 187–95.

109. Halasa A. Malignant melanoma in a case of bilateral nevus of Ota. Arch Ophthalmol 1970; 84: 176–8.

110. Sang DN, Albert SM, Sober AJ. Nevus of Ota with contralateral cerebral melanoma. Arch Ophthalmol 1977; 95: 1820–4.

111. Geronemus RG. Q-switched ruby laser therapy of nevus of Ota. Arch Dermatol 1992; 128: 1618–22.

112. Taylor CR, Flotte TJ, Gange RW, et al. Treatment of nevus of Ota by Q-switched ruby laser. J Am Acad Dermatol 1994; 30: 743–51.

113. Watanabe S, Takahashi H. Treatment of nevus of Ota with the Q-switched ruby laser. N Engl J Med 1994; 331: 1745–50.

114. Alster TS, Williams CM. Treatment of nevus of Ota by the Q-switched alexandrite laser. Dermatol Surg 1995; 21: 592–6.

115. Kang W, Lee E, Choi GS. Treatment of Ota's nevus by Q-switched alexandrite laser: therapeutic outcome in relation to clinical and histopathological findings. Eur J Dermatol 1999; 9: 639–43.

116. Suh DH, Hwang JH, Lee HS, et al. Clinical features of Ota's naevus in Koreans and its treatment with Q-switched alexandrite laser. Clin Exp Dermatol 2000; 25: 269–73.

117. Wang HW, Liu YH, Zhang GK, et al. Analysis of 602 Chinese cases of nevus of Ota and the treatment results treated by Q-switched alexandrite laser. Dermatol Surg 2007; 33: 455–60.

118. Chan HH, King WW, Chan ES, et al. In vivo trial comparing patients' tolerance of Q-switched Alexandrite (QS Alex) and Q-switched neodymium:yttrium-aluminum-garnet (QS Nd:YAG) lasers in the treatment of nevus of Ota. Lasers Surg Med 1999; 24: 24–8.

119. Ueda S, Isoda M, Imayama S. Response of naevus of Ota to Q-switched ruby laser treatment according to lesion colour. Br J Dermatol 2000; 142: 77–83.

120. Kono T, Nozaki M, Chan HH, et al. A retrospective study looking at the long-term complications of Q-switched ruby laser in the treatment of nevus of Ota. Lasers Surg Med 2001; 29: 156–9.

121. Kono T, Chan HH, Ercocen AR, et al. Use of Q-switched ruby laser in the treatment of nevus of Ota in different age groups. Lasers Surg Med 2003; 32: 391–5.

122. Teekhasaenee C, Ritch R, Rutnin U, et al. Glaucoma in oculodermal melanocytosis. Ophthalmology 1990; 97: 562–70.

123. Sun CC, Lu YC, Lee EF, et al. Naevus fusco-caeruleus zygomaticus. Br J Dermatol 1987; 117: 545–53.

124. Manuskiatti W, Eimpunth S, Wanitphakdeedecha R. Effect of cold air cooling on the incidence of postinflammatory hyperpigmentation after Q-switched Nd:YAG laser treatment of acquired bilateral nevus of Ota like macules. Arch Dermatol 2007; 143: 1139–43.

125. Kunachak S, Leelaudomlipi P, Sirikulchayanonta V. Q-Switched ruby laser therapy of acquired bilateral nevus of Ota-like macules. Dermatol Surg 1999; 25: 938–41.

126. Manuskiatti W, Sivayathorn A, Leelaudomlipi P, et al. Treatment of acquired bilateral nevus of Ota-like macules (Hori's nevus) using a combination of scanned carbon dioxide laser followed by Q-switched ruby laser. J Am Acad Dermatol 2003; 48: 584–91.

127. Lam AY, Wong DS, Lam LK, et al. A retrospective study on the efficacy and complications of Q-switched alexandrite laser in the treatment of acquired bilateral nevus of Ota-like macules. Dermatol Surg 2001; 27: 937–41; discussion 41–2.

128. Kunachak S, Leelaudomlipi P. Q-switched Nd:YAG laser treatment for acquired bilateral nevus of Ota-like maculae: a long-term follow-up. Lasers Surg Med 2000; 26: 376–9.

129. Polnikorn N, Tanrattanakorn S, Goldberg DJ. Treatment of Hori's nevus with the Q-switched Nd:YAG laser. Dermatol Surg 2000; 26: 477–80.

130. Suh DH, Han KH, Chung JH. Clinical use of the Q-switched Nd:YAG laser for the treatment of acquired bilateral nevus of Ota-like macules (ABNOMs) in Koreans. J Dermatolog Treat 2001; 12: 163–6.

131. Ee HL, Goh CL, Khoo LS, et al. Treatment of acquired bilateral nevus of ota-like macules (Hori's nevus) with a combination of the 532 nm Q-Switched Nd:YAG laser followed by the 1,064 nm Q-switched Nd:YAG is more effective: prospective study. Dermatol Surg 2006; 32: 34–40.

132. Kopera D, Hohenleutner U, Landthaler M. Quality-switched ruby laser treatment of solar lentigines and Becker's nevus: a histopathological and immunohistochemical study. Dermatology 1997; 194: 338–43.

133. Grevelink JM, Gonzalez S, Bonoan R, et al. Treatment of nevus spilus with the Q-switched ruby laser. Dermatol Surg 1997; 23: 365–9; discussion 69–70.

134. Milgraum SS, Cohen ME, Auletta MJ. Treatment of blue nevi with the Q-switched ruby laser. J Am Acad Dermatol 1995; 32: 307–10.

135. Duke D, Byers HR, Sober AJ, et al. Treatment of benign and atypical nevi with the normal-mode ruby laser and the Q-switched ruby laser: clinical improvement but failure to completely eliminate nevomelanocytes. Arch Dermatol 1999; 135: 290–6.

136. Grevelink JM, van Leeuwen RL, Anderson RR, et al. Clinical and histological responses of congenital melanocytic nevi after single treatment with Q-switched lasers. Arch Dermatol 1997; 133: 349–53.

137. Nelson JS, Kelly KM. Q-Switched ruby laser treatment of a congenital melanocytic nevus. Dermatol Surg 1999; 25: 274–6.

138. Vibhagool C, Byers HR, Grevelink JM. Treatment of small nevomelanocytic nevi with a Q-switched ruby laser. J Am Acad Dermatol 1997; 36: 738–41.

139. Imayama S, Ueda S. Long- and short-term histological observations of congenital nevi treated with the normal-mode ruby laser. Arch Dermatol 1999; 135: 1211–18.

140. Nanni CA, Alster TS. Treatment of a Becker's nevus using a 694-nm long-pulsed ruby laser. Dermatol Surg 1998; 24: 1032–4.

141. Ueda S, Imayama S. Normal-mode ruby laser for treating congenital nevi. Arch Dermatol 1997; 133: 355–9.

142. Gold MH, Foster TD, Bell MW. Nevus spilus successfully treated with an intense pulsed light source. Dermatol Surg 1999; 25: 254–5.

143. Manuskiatti W, Fitzpatrick RE, Goldman MP. Treatment of facial skin using combinations of CO_2, Q-switched alexandrite, flashlamp-pumped pulsed dye, and Er:YAG lasers in the same treatment session. Dermatol Surg 2000; 26: 114–20.

144. Park SH, Koo SH, Choi EO. Combined laser therapy for difficult dermal pigmentation: resurfacing and selective photothermolysis. Ann Plast Surg 2001; 47: 31–6.

145. Momosawa A, Yoshimura K, Uchida G, et al. Combined therapy using Q-switched ruby laser and bleaching treatment with tretinoin and hydroquinone for acquired dermal melanocytosis. Dermatol Surg 2003; 29: 1001–7.

146. Kono T, Ercocen AR, Chan HH, et al. Effectiveness of the normal-mode ruby laser and the combined (normal-mode plus q-switched) ruby laser in the treatment of congenital melanocytic nevi: a comparative study. Ann Plast Surg 2002; 49: 476–85.

147. Kono T, Ercocen AR, Kikuchi Y, et al. A giant melanocytic nevus treated with combined use of normal mode ruby laser and Q-switched alexandrite laser. J Dermatol 2003; 30: 538–42.

148. Kono T, Nozaki M, Chan HH, et al. Combined use of normal mode and Q-switched ruby lasers in the treatment of congenital melanocytic naevi. Br J Plast Surg 2001; 54: 640–3.

149. Alster TS. Q-switched alexandrite laser treatment (755 nm) of professional and amateur tattoos. J Am Acad Dermatol 1995; 33: 69–73.

150. Fitzpatrick RE, Goldman MP. Tattoo removal using the alexandrite laser. Arch Dermatol 1994; 130: 1508–14.

151. Kilmer SL, Anderson RR. Clinical use of the Q-switched ruby and the Q-switched Nd:YAG (1064 nm and 532 nm) lasers for treatment of tattoos. J Dermatol Surg Oncol 1993; 19: 330–8.

152. Zelickson BD, Mehregan DA, Zarrin AA, et al. Clinical, histologic, and ultrastructural evaluation of tattoos treated with three laser systems. Lasers Surg Med 1994; 15: 364–72.

153. Chang SE, Choi JH, Moon KC, et al. Successful removal of traumatic tattoos in Asian skin with a Q-switched alexandrite laser. Dermatol Surg 1998; 24: 1308–11.

154. Grevelink JM, Duke D, van Leeuwen RL, et al. Laser treatment of tattoos in darkly pigmented patients: efficacy and side effects. J Am Acad Dermatol 1996; 34: 653–6.

155. Jones A, Roddey P, Orengo I, et al. The Q-switched ND:YAG laser effectively treats tattoos in darkly pigmented skin. Dermatol Surg 1996; 22: 999–1001.

156. Kilmer SL, Lee MS, Grevelink JM, et al. The Q-switched Nd:YAG laser effectively treats tattoos. Arch Dermatol 1993; 129: 971–8.

157. Lim Y, Choi H, Myung K. Effects of treatment according to tattoo color, site and duration with the Q-switched alexandrite laser. Kor J Dermatol 1998; 36: 844–9.

158. Suzuki H. Treatment of traumatic tattoos with the Q-switched neodymium:YAG laser. Arch Dermatol 1996; 132: 1226–9.

159. Taylor CR, Gange RW, Dover JS, et al. Treatment of tattoos by Q-switched ruby laser. Arch Dermatol 1990; 126: 893–399.

160. Al-Mutairi N, Manchanda Y, Almutairi L. Tattooing in the Gulf region: a review of tattoo practices and response to treatment with the Q-switched ruby laser. J Cosmet Laser Ther 2010; 12: 132–7.

161. Moreno-Arias GA, Casals-Andreu M, Camps-Fresneda A. Use of Q-switched alexandrite laser (755 nm, 100 nsec) for removal of traumatic tattoo of different origins. Lasers Surg Med 1999; 25: 445–50.

162. Sherwood KA, Murray S, Kurban AK, et al. Effect of wavelength on cutaneous pigment using pulsed irradiation. J Invest Dermatol 1989; 92: 717–20.

163. Anderson RR. Laser-Tissue Interactions, 2nd edn. St. Louis: Mosby, 1999.

164. Bernstein LJ, Kauvar ANB, Grossman MC, et al. The short- and long-term side effects of carbon dioxide laser resurfacing. Dermatol Surg 1997; 23: 519–25.

165. Manuskiatti W, Fitzpatrick RE, Goldman MP. Long-term effectiveness and side effects of carbon dioxide laser resurfacing for photoaged facial skin. J Am Acad Dermatol 1999; 40: 401–11.

166. Nanni CA, Alster TS. Complications of carbon dioxide laser resurfacing. An evaluation of 500 patients. Dermatol Surg 1998; 24: 315–20.

167. Ruiz-Esparza J, Barba Gomez JM, Gomez de la Torre OL, et al. Ultra-Pulse laser skin resurfacing in Hispanic patients. A prospective study of 36 individuals. Dermatol Surg 1998; 24: 59–62.

168. Sriprachya-anunt S, Marchell NL, Fitzpatrick RE, et al. Facial resurfacing in patients with Fitzpatrick skin type IV. Lasers Surg Med 2002; 30: 86–92.

169. West TB, Alster TS. Effect of pretreatment on the incidence of hyperpigmentation following cutaneous CO_2 laser resurfacing. Dermatol Surg 1999; 25: 15–17.

170. Haedersdal M, Bech-Thomsen N, Poulsen T, et al. Ultraviolet exposure influences laser-induced wounds, scars, and hyperpigmentation: a murine study. Plast Reconstr Surg 1998; 101: 1315–22.

171. Alexiades-Armenakas MR, Dover JS, Arndt KA. The spectrum of laser skin resurfacing: nonablative, fractional, and ablative laser resurfacing. J Am Acad Dermatol 2008; 58: 719–37; quiz 38–40.

172. Alster TS. Cutaneous resurfacing with Er: YAG lasers. Dermatol Surg 2000; 26: 73–5.

173. Ratner D, Tse Y, Marchell N, et al. Cutaneous laser resurfacing. J Am Acad Dermatol 1999; 41: 365–89; quiz 90–2.

174. Khatri KA, Ross V, Grevelink JM, et al. Comparison of erbium: YAG and carbon dioxide lasers in resurfacing of facial rhytides. Arch Dermatol 1999; 135: 391–7.

175. Goldman MP, Manuskiatti W. Combined laser resurfacing with the 950-Msec pulsed CO_2 + Er:YAG lasers. Dermatol Surg 1999; 25: 160–3.

176. Cho SI, Kim YC. Treatment of facial wrinkles with char-free carbon dioxide laser and erbium: YAG laser. Kor J Dermatol 1999; 37: 177–84.

177. Alster T, Hirsch R. Single-pass CO_2 laser skin resurfacing of light and dark skin: extended experience with 52 patients. J Cosmet Laser Ther 2003; 5: 39–42.

178. Avram DK, Goldman MP. The safety and effectiveness of single-pass erbium:YAG laser in the treatment of mild to moderate photodamage. Dermatol Surg 2004; 30: 1073–6.

179. Ruiz-Esparza J, Barba Gomez JM. Long-term effects of one general pass laser resurfacing. A look at dermal tightening and skin quality. Dermatol Surg 1999; 25: 169–73; discussion 74.

180. Kunzi-Rapp K, Dierickx CC, Cambier B, et al. Minimally invasive skin rejuvenation with Erbium: YAG laser used in thermal mode. Lasers Surg Med 2006; 38: 899–907.

181. Manuskiatti W, Siriphukpong S, Varothai S, et al. Effect of pulse width of a variable square pulse (VSP) erbium:YAG laser on the treatment outcome of periorbital wrinkles in Asians. Int J Dermatol 2010; 49: 200–6.

182. Tanzi EL, Alster TS. Treatment of atrophic facial acne scars with a dual-mode Er:YAG laser. Dermatol Surg 2002; 28: 551–5.

183. Wanitphakdeedecha R, Manuskiatti W, Siriphukpong S, et al. Treatment of punched-out atrophic and rolling acne scars in skin phototypes III, IV, and V with variable square pulse erbium:yttrium-aluminum-garnet laser resurfacing. Dermatol Surg 2009; 35: 1376–83.

184. Ho C, Nguyen Q, Lowe NJ, et al. Laser resurfacing in pigmented skin. Dermatol Surg 1995; 21: 1035–7.

185. Kim JW, Lee JO. Skin resurfacing with laser in Asians. Aesthetic Plast Surg 1997; 21: 115–17.

186. Song MG, Park KB, Lee ES. Resurfacing of facial angiofibromas in tuberous sclerosis patients using CO_2 laser with flashscanner. Dermatol Surg 1999; 25: 970–3.

187. Jeong JT, Kye YC. Resurfacing of pitted facial acne scars with a long-pulsed Er:YAG laser. Dermatol Surg 2001; 27: 107–10.

188. Kye YC. Resurfacing of pitted facial scars with a pulsed Er:YAG laser. Dermatol Surg 1997; 23: 880–3.

189. Cho SI, Kim YC. Treatment of atrophic facial scars with combined use of high-energy pulsed CO_2 laser and Er: YAG laser: a practical guide of laser techniques for the Er: YAG laser. Dermatol Surg 1999; 25: 959–64.

190. Fitzpatrick RE. Maximizing benefits and minimizing risk with CO_2 laser resurfacing. Dermatol Clin 2002; 20: 77–86.

191. Lowe NJ, Lask G, Griffin ME. Laser skin resurfacing: pre- and posttreatment guidelines. Dermatol Surg 1995; 21: 1017–19.

192. Trau H, Orenstein A, Schewach-Miller M, et al. Pseudomelanoma following laser therapy for congenital nevus. J Dermatol Surg Oncol 1986; 12: 984–6.

193. Alam M, Hsu TS, Dover JS, et al. Nonablative laser and light treatments: histology and tissue effects–a review. Lasers Surg Med 2003; 33: 30–9.

194. Ang P, Barlow RJ. Nonablative laser resurfacing: a systematic review of the literature. Clin Exp Dermatol 2002; 27: 630–5.

195. Goldberg DJ. Nonablative dermal remodeling: does it really work? Arch Dermatol 2002; 138: 1366–8.

196. Sadick NS. Update on non-ablative light therapy for rejuvenation: a review. Lasers Surg Med 2003; 32: 120–8.

197. Chan HH, Lam LK, Wong DS, et al. Use of 1,320 nm Nd:YAG laser for wrinkle reduction and the treatment of atrophic acne scarring in Asians. Lasers Surg Med 2004; 34: 98–103.

198. Negishi K, Kushikata N, Takeuchi K, et al. Photorejuvenation by intense pulsed light with objective measurement of skin color in Japanese patients. Dermatol Surg 2006; 32: 1380–7.

199. Negishi K, Tezuka Y, Kushikata N, et al. Photorejuvenation for Asian skin by intense pulsed light. Dermatol Surg 2001; 27: 627–31; discussion 32.

200. Anderson RR. Fire and ice. Arch Dermatol 2003; 139: 787–8.

201. Kelly KM, Svaasand LO, Nelson JS. Optimization of laser treatment safety in conjunction with cryogen spray cooling. Arch Dermatol 2003; 139: 1372–3.

202. Manstein D, Herron GS, Sink RK, et al. Fractional photothermolysis: a new concept for cutaneous remodeling using microscopic patterns of thermal injury. Lasers Surg Med 2004; 34: 426–38.

203. Jih MH, Kimyai-Asadi A. Fractional photothermolysis: a review and update. Semin Cutan Med Surg 2008; 27: 63–71.

204. Tierney EP, Kouba DJ, Hanke CW. Review of fractional photothermolysis: treatment indications and efficacy. Dermatol Surg 2009; 35: 1445–61.

205. Rerknimitr P, Pongprutthipan M, Sindhuphak W. Fractional photothermolysis for the treatment of facial wrinkle in Asians. J Med Assoc Thai 2010; 93(Suppl 7): S35–40.

206. Lee H, Yoon JS, Lee SY. Fractional laser photothermolysis for treatment of facial wrinkles in Asians. Korean J Ophthalmol 2009; 23: 235–9.

207. Cohen SR, Henssler C, Johnston J. Fractional photothermolysis for skin rejuvenation. Plast Reconstr Surg 2009; 124: 281–90.

208. Cho SB, Lee SJ, Cho S, et al. Non-ablative 1550-nm erbium-glass and ablative 10 600-nm carbon dioxide fractional lasers for acne scars: a randomized split-face study with blinded response evaluation. J Eur Acad Dermatol Venereol 2010; 24: 921–5.

209. Geronemus RG. Fractional photothermolysis: current and future applications. Lasers Surg Med 2006; 38: 169–76.

210. Glaich AS, Rahman Z, Goldberg LH, et al. Fractional resurfacing for the treatment of hypopigmented scars: a pilot study. Dermatol Surg 2007; 33: 289–94; discussion 93–4.

211. Rahman Z, Alam M, Dover JS. Fractional Laser treatment for pigmentation and texture improvement. Skin Therapy Lett 2006; 11: 7–11.

212. Hantash BM, Bedi VP, Chan KF, et al. Ex vivo histological characterization of a novel ablative fractional resurfacing device. Lasers Surg Med 2007; 39: 87–95.

213. Hantash BM, Mahmood MB. Fractional photothermolysis: a novel aesthetic laser surgery modality. Dermatol Surg 2007; 33: 525–34.

214. Hantash BM, Bedi VP, Kapadia B, et al. In vivo histological evaluation of a novel ablative fractional resurfacing device. Lasers Surg Med 2007; 39: 96–107.

215. Xu XG, Luo YJ, Wu Y, et al. Immunohistological evaluation of skin responses after treatment using a fractional ultrapulse carbon dioxide laser on back skin. Dermatol Surg 2011; 37: 1141–9.

216. Manuskiatti W, Triwongwaranat D, Varothai S, et al. Efficacy and safety of a carbon-dioxide ablative fractional resurfacing device for treatment of atrophic acne scars in Asians. J Am Acad Dermatol 2010; 63: 274–83.

217. Chan NP, Ho SG, Yeung CK, et al. Fractional ablative carbon dioxide laser resurfacing for skin rejuvenation and acne scars in Asians. Lasers Surg Med 2010; 42: 615–23.

218. Tierney EP, Eisen RF, Hanke CW. Fractionated CO_2 laser skin rejuvenation. Dermatol Ther 2011; 24: 41–53.

219. Hu S, Hsiao WC, Chen MC, et al. Ablative fractional erbium-doped yttrium aluminum garnet laser with coagulation mode for the treatment of atrophic acne scars in Asian skin. Dermatol Surg 2011; 37: 939–44.

220. Lapidoth M, Yagima Odo ME, Odo LM. Novel use of erbium:YAG (2,940-nm) laser for fractional ablative photothermolysis in the treatment of photodamaged facial skin: a pilot study. Dermatol Surg 2008; 34: 1048–53.

221. Dierickx CC, Khatri KA, Tannous ZS, et al. Micro-fractional ablative skin resurfacing with two novel erbium laser systems. Lasers Surg Med 2008; 40: 113–23.

222. Ciocon DH, Hussain M, Goldberg DJ. High-Fluence and High-Density Treatment of Perioral Rhytides Using a New, Fractionated 2,790-nm Ablative Erbium-Doped Yttrium Scandium Gallium Garnet Laser. Dermatol Surg 2011; 37: 776–81.

223. Shamsaldeen O, Peterson JD, Goldman MP. The adverse events of deep fractional CO(2): a retrospective study of 490 treatments in 374 patients. Lasers Surg Med 2011; 43: 453–6.

224. Metelitsa AI, Alster TS. Fractionated laser skin resurfacing treatment complications: a review. Dermatol Surg 2010; 36: 299–306.

225. Chan HH, Manstein D, Yu CS, et al. The prevalence and risk factors of post-inflammatory hyperpigmentation after fractional resurfacing in Asians. Lasers Surg Med 2007; 39: 381–5.

226. Mahmoud BH, Srivastava D, Janiga JJ, et al. Safety and efficacy of erbium-doped yttrium aluminum garnet fractionated laser for treatment of acne scars in type IV to VI skin. Dermatol Surg 2010; 36: 602–9.

227. Graber EM, Tanzi EL, Alster TS. Side effects and complications of fractional laser photothermolysis: experience with 961 treatments. Dermatol Surg 2008; 34: 301–5; discussion 05–7.

228. Kono T, Chan HH, Groff WF, et al. Prospective direct comparison study of fractional resurfacing using different fluences and densities for skin rejuvenation in Asians. Lasers Surg Med 2007; 39: 311–14.

229. Chapas AM, Brightman L, Sukal S, et al. Successful treatment of acneiform scarring with CO_2 ablative fractional resurfacing. Lasers Surg Med 2008; 40: 381–6.

230. Alster TS, Bryan H, Williams CM. Long-pulsed Nd:YAG laser-assisted hair removal in pigmented skin: a clinical and histological evaluation. Arch Dermatol 2001; 137: 885–9.

231. Chan HH, Ying SY, Ho WS, et al. An in vivo study comparing the efficacy and complications of diode laser and long-pulsed Nd:YAG laser in hair removal in Chinese patients. Dermatol Surg 2001; 27: 950–4.

232. Galadari I. Comparative evaluation of different hair removal lasers in skin types IV, V, and VI. Int J Dermatol 2003; 42: 68–70.

233. Garcia C, Alamoudi H, Nakib M, et al. Alexandrite laser hair removal is safe for Fitzpatrick skin types IV-VI. Dermatol Surg 2000; 26: 130–4.

234. Goh CL. Comparative study on a single treatment response to long pulse Nd:YAG lasers and intense pulse light therapy for hair removal on skin type IV to VI--is longer wavelengths lasers preferred over shorter wavelengths lights for assisted hair removal. J Dermatolog Treat 2003; 14: 243–7.

235. Hussain M, Polnikorn N, Goldberg DJ. Laser-assisted hair removal in Asian skin: efficacy, complications, and the effect of single versus multiple treatments. Dermatol Surg 2003; 29: 249–54.

236. Hussain M, Suwanchinda A, Charuwichtratana S, et al. A new long pulsed 940 nm diode laser used for hair removal in Asian skin types. J Cosmet Laser Ther 2003; 5: 97–100.

237. Liew SH, Grobbelaar A, Gault D, et al. Hair removal using the ruby laser: clinical efficacy in Fitzpatrick skin types I-V and histological changes in epidermal melanocytes. Br J Dermatol 1999; 140: 1105–9.

238. Yeung CK, Shek SY, Chan HH. Hair removal with neodymium-doped yttrium aluminum garnet laser and pneumatic skin flattening in Asians. Dermatol Surg 2010; 36: 1664–70.

239. Leheta TM. Comparative evaluation of long pulse Alexandrite laser and intense pulsed light systems for pseudofolliculitis barbae treatment with one year of follow up. Indian J Dermatol 2009; 54: 364–8.

240. Manuskiatti W, Tantikun N. Treatment of trichostasis spinulosa in skin phototypes III, IV, and V with an 800-nm pulsed diode laser. Dermatol Surg 2003; 29: 85–8.

241. Toosi S, Ehsani AH, Noormohammadpoor P, et al. Treatment of trichostasis spinulosa with a 755-nm long-pulsed alexandrite laser. J Eur Acad Dermatol Venereol 2010; 24: 470–3.

242. Dierickx CC. Hair removal by lasers and intense pulsed light sources. Dermatol Clin 2002; 20: 135–46.

243. Haedersdal M, Gotzsche PC. Laser and photoepilation for unwanted hair growth. Cochrane Database Syst Rev 2006; CD004684.

244. Dierickx CC, Alora MB, Dover JS. A clinical overview of hair removal using lasers and light sources. Dermatol Clin 1999; 17: 357–66.

245. Dierickx CC, Grossman MC, Farinelli WA, et al. Permanent hair removal by normal-mode ruby laser. Arch Dermatol 1998; 134: 837–42.

246. Ross EV, Ladin Z, Kreindel M, et al. Theoretical considerations in laser hair removal. Dermatol Clin 1999; 17: 333–55.

247. Haedersdal M, Egekvist H, Efsen J, et al. Skin pigmentation and texture changes after hair removal with the normal-mode ruby laser. Acta Derm Venereol 1999; 79: 465–8.

248. Campos VB, Dierickx CC, Farinelli WA, et al. Ruby laser hair removal: evaluation of long-term efficacy and side effects. Lasers Surg Med 2000; 26: 177–85.

249. Nanni CA, Alster TS. Laser-assisted hair removal: side effects of Q-switched Nd:YAG, long-pulsed ruby, and alexandrite lasers. J Am Acad Dermatol 1999; 41: 165–71.

250. Cho S, Kim Y, Baek R. Removal of unwanted hair using the long pulse alexandrite laser. J Kor Soc Laser Med 1999; 3: 8–10.

251. Campos VB, Dierickx CC, Farinelli WA, et al. Hair removal with an 800-nm pulsed diode laser. J Am Acad Dermatol 2000; 43: 442–7.

252. Wanitphakdeedecha R, Thanomkitti K, Sethabutra P, et al. A split axilla comparison study of axillary hair removal with low fluence high repetition rate 810 nm diode laser vs. high fluence low repetition rate 1064 nm Nd:YAG laser. J Eur Acad Dermatol Venereol 2011; doi: 10.1111/j.1468-3083.2011.04231.x; Epub ahead of print.

253. Haak CS, Nymann P, Pedersen AT, et al. Hair removal in hirsute women with normal testosterone levels: a randomized controlled trial of long-pulsed diode laser vs. intense pulsed light. Br J Dermatol 2010; 163: 1007–13.

254. Manuskiatti W, Fitzpatrick RE, Goldman MP, et al. Effects of long pulse duration and short interval retreatment on the efficacy of hair removal using broad-band, intense pulsed light system. Dermatol Cosmet 2000; 10: 67–75.

255. Nanni CA, Alster TS. Optimizing treatment parameters for hair removal using a topical carbon-based solution and 1064-nm Q-switched neodymium:YAG laser energy. Arch Dermatol 1997; 133: 1546–9.

256. Grossman MC, Dierickx C, Farinelli W, et al. Damage to hair follicles by normal-mode ruby laser pulses. J Am Acad Dermatol 1996; 35: 889–94.

257. Alajlan A, Shapiro J, Rivers JK, et al. Paradoxical hypertrichosis after laser epilation. J Am Acad Dermatol 2005; 53: 85–8.

258. Desai S, Mahmoud BH, Bhatia AC, et al. Paradoxical hypertrichosis after laser therapy: a review. Dermatol Surg 2010; 36: 291–8.

259. Tierney EP, Goldberg DJ. Laser hair removal pearls. J Cosmet Laser Ther 2008; 10: 17–23.

260. Moreno-Arias G, Castelo-Branco C, Ferrando J. Paradoxical effect after IPL photoepilation. Dermatol Surg 2002; 28: 1013–16; discussion 16.

261. Bernstein EF. Hair growth induced by diode laser treatment. Dermatol Surg 2005; 31: 584–6.

262. Lolis MS, Marmur ES. Paradoxical effects of hair removal systems: a review. J Cosmet Dermatol 2006; 5: 274–6.

263. Kaiser MR, Davis SC, Mertz PM. Effect of ultraviolet radiation-induced inflammation on epidermal wound healing. Wound Rep Peg 1995; 3: 331–51.

264. Nordback I, Kulmala R, Jarvinen M. Effect of ultraviolet therapy on rat skin wound healing. J Surg Res 1990; 48: 68–71.

265. Baadgaard O. In vivo ultraviolet irradiation of human skin results in profound perturbation of the immune system. Arch Dermatol 1991; 127: 99–109.

266. Hedelund L, Haedersdal M, Egekvist H, et al. CO_2 laser resurfacing and photocarcinogenesis: an experimental study. Lasers Surg Med 2004; 35: 58–61.

267. Kato H, Araki J, Eto H, et al. A prospective randomized controlled study of oral tranexamic acid for preventing postinflammatory hyperpigmentation after Q-switched ruby laser. Dermatol Surg 2011; 37: 605–10.

268. Kligman AM, Grove GL, Hirose R, et al. Topical tretinoin for photoaged skin. J Am Acad Dermatol 1986; 15: 836–59.

269. Pathak MA, Fitzpatrick TB, Kraus EW. Usefulness of retinoic acid in the treatment of melasma. J Am Acad Dermatol 1986; 15: 894–9.

270. Jimbow K, Obata H, Pathak MA, et al. Mechanism of depigmentation by hydroquinone. J Invest Dermatol 1974; 62: 436–49.

271. Grimes PE. Management of hyperpigmentation in darker racial ethnic groups. Semin Cutan Med Surg 2009; 28: 77–85.

272. Pathak MA, Ciganek ER, Wick M, et al. An evaluation of the effectiveness of azelaic acid as a depigmenting and chemotherapeutic agent. J Invest Dermatol 1985; 85: 222–8.

273. Chakraborty AK, Funasaka Y, Komoto M, et al. Effect of arbutin on melanogenic proteins in human melanocytes. Pigment Cell Res 1998; 11: 206–12.

274. Yokota T, Nishio H, Kubota Y, et al. The inhibitory effect of glabridin from licorice extracts on melanogenesis and inflammation. Pigment Cell Res 1998; 11: 355–61.

275. Kameyama K, Sakai C, Kondoh S, et al. Inhibitory effect of magnesium L-ascorbyl-2-phosphate (VC-PMG) on melanogenesis in vitro and in vivo. J Am Acad Dermatol 1996; 34: 29–33.

276. Chan HH. Special considerations for darker-skinned patients. Curr Probl Dermatol 2011; 42: 153–9.

277. Milanic M, Jia W, Nelson JS, et al. Numerical optimization of sequential cryogen spray cooling and laser irradiation for improved therapy of port wine stain. Lasers Surg Med 2011; 43: 164–75.

278. Nelson JS, Majaron B, Kelly KM. Active skin cooling in conjunction with laser dermatologic surgery. Semin Cutan Med Surg 2000; 19: 253–66.

279. Raulin C, Greve B, Hammes S. Cold air in laser therapy: first experiences with a new cooling system. Lasers Surg Med 2000; 27: 404–10.

280. Zenzie HH, Altshuler GB, Smirnov MZ, et al. Evaluation of cooling methods for laser dermatology. Lasers Surg Med 2000; 26: 130–44.

281. Nelson JS, Milner TE, Anvari B, et al. Dynamic epidermal cooling in conjunction with laser-induced photothermolysis of port wine stain blood vessels. Lasers Surg Med 1996; 19: 224–9.

282. Sturesson C, Andersson-Engels S. Mathematical modelling of dynamic cooling and pre-heating, used to increase the depth of selective damage to blood vessels in laser treatment of port wine stains. Phys Med Biol 1996; 41: 413–28.

283. Manuskiatti W. Laser treatment of pigmented lesions. In: Manuskiatti W, ed. Skin Laser Therapy in Clinical Practice, 1st edn. Bangkok: Morchaobann, 2009: 53–76.

284. Manuskiatti W. Laser treatment of tattoos. In: Manuskiatti W, ed. Skin Laser Therapy in Clinical Practice, 1st edn. Bangkok: Morchaobann, 2009: 77–84.

14 Laser lipolysis

Melanie D. Palm, Ane B.M. Niwa Massaki,
Sabrina G. Fabi, and Mitchel P. Goldman

BACKGROUND

Liposuction is one of the most popular cosmetic procedures. During the past several decades, liposculpting has evolved dramatically with many changes that have substantially improved efficacy and safety (1). The advent of tumescent anesthesia by Klein has greatly improved the safety of liposuction by eliminating the need for general anesthesia and hospital stays and decreasing the risks of bleeding complications (2,3).

Several adjunctive techniques to routine liposuction have been developed such as ultrasound-assisted liposuction (internal and external), power-assisted liposuction, and laser-assisted liposuction (1,4).

Laser lipolysis (LAL), also known as laser lipoplasty, was piloted first in Europe and Latin America before gaining acceptance (and FDA approval) in the USA as well as in Japan (5). The earliest description of laser-assisted liposuction was by Dressel in 1990 (6). Shortly thereafter, Apfelberg with colleagues reported on the use of a 1064-nm light source in 51 liposuction patients. The lack of statistically significant improvements or minimization of adverse effects on the laser-treated areas compared with traditional liposuction halted the application for FDA approval of this device (6,7).

Blugerman, Schavelzon, and Goldman used a 1064-nm neodymium:yttrium-aluminum-garnet (Nd:YAG) system for LAL and were the first group to demonstrate the effect of this laser energy on fat, surrounding dermis, vasculature, apocrine, and eccrine glands (8–11). In 2002, Badin and colleagues reported histologic changes after thermal damage by the laser, including rupture of fat cell membranes, coagulation of small vessels, and collagen remodeling (12). The authors found that LAL was less traumatic than conventional liposuction methods due to smaller cannula diameter (1 mm) and the effects of the laser–tissue interaction.

After FDA approval of a 1064-nm Nd:YAG laser (manufactured by DEKA and distributed by Cynosure Inc., Westford, Massachusetts, USA) in 2006, additional systems employing a variety of wavelengths were introduced to the market and LAL found its place as a potential adjunct and an alternative to traditional tumescent liposuction (13).

INDICATIONS FOR LASER LIPOLYSIS

Like liposculpture, the main indication for LAL is body contouring (14). Beyond this function, the addition of laser energy creates other biological effects that result in additional indications for this procedure. Photothermal energy from LAL melts fat (15,16), making LAL ideal for some traditionally challenging cases in liposculpture: (*i*) fibrous areas such as the male breasts, abdomen, and flanks (15); (*ii*) revisional surgery where tissue is difficult to penetrate or suffers from irregularities (12,17); (*iii*) small areas of adiposity that may be inadequately removed (e.g., periumbilical fat) (12,18); and (*iv*) large volume liposuction in highly vascularized areas such as the scapula, waist, and flanks (12).

In addition to its ability to melt fat, the neocollagenesis afforded by LAL lends itself to areas that require skin tightening. The neck, arm, and abdomen are areas well suited for this indication (12,14–16,19).

Stebbins and colleagues reported that LAL alone or in conjunction with suction can be a highly effective and a minimally invasive method for removing large lipomas (>10 cm), particularly fibrous lesions, resulting in excellent cosmetic outcome (20).

ADVANTAGES

The most commonly mentioned advantages of LAL relate to the ease of recovery (14,15,21,22). Compared with traditional liposuction, LAL may diminish postoperative pain and decrease the extent of edema and bruising after the procedure (12,14,15,22–24). Laser-induced thrombosis of blood vessels and closure of lymphatic channels may explain the reduction in the severity of bruising and swelling following LAL (21). Laser-operated liposculpture allows for reduced trauma to the tissue during fat removal, allowing improved wound healing (25). As a result, patients have a more rapid return to daily activities (14,25). All in all, the safety of body contouring using LAL may be increased when compared with traditional liposuction (22).

Operator as well as patient safety is increased with the procedure. The process of fat emulsification allows for efficient fat extraction and less operator fatigue (7,17,21). The frequency of touch-up procedures may be decreased compared with traditional tumescent liposuction performed by experienced surgeons (16).

Two specific clinical goals make LAL a superior choice to liposuction. When the primary goal of a surgical intervention is to treat skin laxity rather than body contouring, LAL is the appropriate choice for inducing collagen production and subsequent skin contraction (14,18,21,22,26). In larger-volume cases of body contouring, LAL may facilitate volume debulking by liquefying the fat prior to aspiration as well as decreasing blood loss during the procedure (7,12,21).

DISADVANTAGES

Several drawbacks exist in performing LAL. For large areas, LAL alone may be insufficient for proper correction; therefore, although LAL has been used successfully as a sole procedure for body contouring, some physicians assert that LAL is not a substitute for conventional liposuction but a complement to it (12,18). Undercorrection following LAL may result from inadequate cumulative energies used, as many studies do not calculate this parameter (12,21). As with any new technology, there is a significant learning curve associated with LAL (12), although the slope is relatively steep in experienced hands (18). For this reason, results following LAL vary, with some studies demonstrating no improvement over traditional liposuction (22). In addition, thermal injury is a possible complication, since there is a relatively narrow therapeutic window between heat accumulation that stimulates collagen contraction and thermal injury resulting in dermal–epidermal burns and potential scarring (27).

As earlier generation and most contemporary LAL devices require two steps—first for the tissue to be treated with the laser and second a separate aspiration step—procedure time is increased (12,22). The innovation of dual functioning cannulas, allowing simultaneous laser firing and suction, resolves this issue (28). Finally, the cost of additional laser equipment is a barrier to entry for some practitioners (18).

MECHANISM OF ACTION

Two properties must be considered in determining the efficacy of LAL given a particular device—the wavelength employed and the energy delivered (14). Unique chromophores are more selectively targeted depending on the wavelength, and the energy used will determine the thermal effect on tissues.

Different wavelengths have been selected for LAL in an attempt to specifically target fat, collagen (water), and blood vessels. According to the theory of selective photothermolysis, these chromophores will preferentially absorb laser energy according to their absorption coefficients at specific wavelengths. Various wavelengths, including 924, 968, 975, 980, 1064, 1319, 1320, 1344, and 1440 nm, alone or in combinations have been evaluated for interactions within the subcutaneous compartment. Some wavelengths have unique advantages. The 924-nm wavelength has the highest selectivity for fat melting (22) but may not be as effective for skin tightening unless combined with another wavelength. The 1064 nm targets oxyhemoglobin providing vessel coagulation (24) has superior heat distribution and therefore skin tightening effect (27), whereas the 1320 nm has greater fat absorption with less tissue penetration and scatter, decreasing the chance for collateral tissue damage (22). The 1440 nm has demonstrated to be preferentially absorbed by subcutaneous fat compared with other wavelengths previously utilized. This implies that the laser beam will be absorbed in a very small primary tissue volume, potentially inducing high temperatures (29).

Photoacoustic (17), photomechanical, photostimulatory, and photothermal effects are theorized mechanisms of action in LAL (14,30). Most of these hypothesized actions are either secondary to or have been replaced by the idea that heat-generated effects on tissue are the primary mode of action in LAL. For example, Khoury et al. asserted that photoacoustic ablation lends to thermal damage (31) although photoacoustic damage is difficult to evaluate histologically. Likewise, photostimulatory effects on tissue are secondary to photothermal effects (14).

Thus, the favored mechanism of action in LAL is a purely thermal effect (17,24,32,33), which is coined as "photohyperthermia" (17). Thermal effects following LAL include the following: coagulation of collagen fibers, thrombosis of vessels, damage to nerve endings, and reversible (tumefaction) and irreversible damage (lysis) to adipocytes depending on the energy employed (5,17,25). At low laser energy, intra- and extracellular sodium and potassium balance is altered, resulting in adipocyte tumefaction (5,25). Eventually, heat generated in the tissue from laser energy results in cellular membrane degradation (adipolysis) secondary to protein denaturation (25). Some authors believe a thermomechanical effect also plays a role in LAL, as laser treatment on fat tissue results in adipocyte rupture (5,34).

A mathematical model of LAL using two systems—one with a 980-nm wavelength and the other 1064 nm—demonstrated skin contraction due to a heating effect. Mordon and coworkers demonstrated that bioheat transfer initiated from laser light resulted in collagen remodeling (34). In other words, laser light energy is converted into heat energy within the adipose layer. This diffuses to the dermis and eventually to the skin surface. According to the mathematical model, temperatures of 48–50°C must be reached within the dermis to induce collagen contraction and resultant skin tightening (22,26,34). Depending on the study, a dermal temperature between approximately 50°C and 70°C translates to a skin surface temperature of approximately 40–41°C (22,26,34).

Damage is energy dependent (5,18). Compared with an area treated by lower energy (1000 J), 3000 J of energy resulted in significant irreversible damage (25). The dose-dependent relationship between laser energy and thermal damage has been duplicated by other histologic studies (5,26,31).

Increasing energy creates not only adipocyte changes but also tissue fibrosis (24). Collagen damage from thermal damage promotes collagen remodeling, leading to increases in skin tone and texture. These effects continue to improve for 3–6 months following the procedure (12,26).

HISTOLOGIC FINDINGS

The histologic findings from human tissue models support the photothermal effect of LAL, regardless of laser wavelength. In 2002, Badin and colleagues found the immediate cellular changes following laser treatment of subcutaneous tissue to include ballooning and rupture of fat cells with reduced bleeding due to vessel coagulation (12). At 3 months following treatment, histologic studies demonstrated new collagen formation and remodeling (12).

Additional histologic studies using and comparing wavelengths of 980, 1064, and 1320 nm all provided similar evidence for the dose-dependent nature of cellular changes following LAL (5,25,26,31,35). Cadaveric studies as well as ex vivo and in vivo studies first showed reversible cellular damage seen as cellular ballooning (tumefaction). Further energy delivery resulted in cell membrane destruction and irreversible cell lysis. Laser treatment also caused thermal damage to collagen fibers, vessel thrombosis, and reduced areas of bleeding compared with liposuction-treated areas (5,25,35).

Liquefaction of adipocytes, carbonization of tissues, and finally epidermal injury were observed only at the highest energy settings (5,26,31,35).

A histologic evaluation of LAL comparing different wavelengths and continuous wave (CW) versus pulsed lasers in an *in vivo* pig model was conducted by Levi and colleagues (36). Three CW lasers (980, 1370, and 1470 nm) and three pulsed lasers (1064, 1320, and 1440 nm) were used followed by histopathologic evaluations at 1 day, 1 week, and 1 month after exposure. The authors found that skin damage occurred at temperatures exceeding 46°C regardless of wavelength. Tissue treated with the CW laser at 1470 nm demonstrated a greater hemorrhage and denser histiocytic infiltration than tissue treated with the 1440-nm pulsed laser. Overall, there was more collagen deposition with increased power levels. Furthermore, increasing numbers of histiocytes (a marker of fat necrosis) occurred with increasing power and energy levels at 1 month after laser exposure. Lasers with a low coefficient of absorption (980, 1064, and 1320 nm) achieved similar degrees of collagen deposition as high-absorption lasers (1370 and 1470 nm) by using higher power, lower speed, or both. However, due to higher power and lower speed being used for this low-absorption group, total energy delivered under the skin was much higher and resulted in a much higher temperature increase on the skin surface. Therefore, the authors concluded that pulsed lasers with high peak power provided better hemostatic effect than CW lasers likely due to quick coagulation of blood vessels from the pulsed laser at high peak power. Considering skin safety and efficacy, a high-absorption wavelength (e.g., 1440 nm) with low power (6–12 W) would be a better choice for promoting controlled collagen deposition in the subdermal tissue and reticular dermis. Further clinical studies comparing different wavelengths are still required to confirm that histologic findings correlate with clinical results.

INVASIVE LASER LIPOLYSIS TECHNOLOGY

Devices of six wavelengths have been FDA approved for use in the USA for LAL: 924/975, 980 (CW), 1064, 1320, and 1444 nm (14). All devices described for use in LAL in the medical literature are discussed in the next sections (Table 14.1).

Carbon Dioxide Laser

Carbon dioxide laser (wavelength 10,600 nm) was used briefly during the early development of LAL (37). The ablative laser was used during neck and jowl liposuction to create platysmal tightening, dermal remodeling, and fat vaporization. Although the clinical results in terms of skin tightening were impressive, the large submental incision necessary for introduction of the laser to the subcutaneous layer was a major drawback of the procedure.

Diode Laser

The 924/975-nm Multiplex System

This dual wavelength diode laser system was cleared by the FDA for LAL and appears to independently target lipid and water-based tissues (SlimLipo, Palomar Medical Technologies, Inc., Burlington, Massachusetts, USA). The 924-nm wavelength has a peak in the adipose tissue absorption spectrum to provide sufficient penetration and heating for the release of intracellular lipids, while the 975 nm has a peak in the water absorption spectrum to target collagen and promote tissue retraction (38). The laser system consists of three different-sized laser fibers measuring 0.8, 1.0, and 1.5 mm and a continuous wattage output power of up to 30 W. Weiss and Beasley treated 19 subjects in the submental area, abdomen, thighs, and flanks and observed good-to-excellent improvement across all patients after 3 months (Fig. 14.1) (38). Aspiration was performed with 3- or 4-mm diameter cannulas. Seventy-two percent of subjects felt their skin was smoother and tighter. In addition, the authors also observed reduced operator fatigue, uniformity of treatment, and a significantly reduced recovery time. Specifically, in terms of tumescent fluid drainage, the authors observed that drainage following suction-assisted lipectomy occurred post-procedure for 48–72 hours, compared with 12–24 hours with laser-assisted lipectomy alone. Side effects were generally mild and resolved by 2 weeks after treatment.

The 980-nm Device

A study by Reynaud et al. reported on the effects of a 980-nm diode device (Pharaon, OSYRIS, Hellemmes, France) for use in LAL (21). The laser system consists of a 600-μm optical fiber contained within a rounded 1-mm microcannula. The laser is fired in a continuous mode at energy settings from 6 to 15 W depending on the treatment area. Fat lysate may be removed by aspiration or manual massage following laser treatment. Five hundred thirty-four procedures were performed in 334 patients over various locations. Mean cumulative energies ranged from a minimum of 2200 J (knee) to a maximum of 51,000 J (abdomen). Patient satisfaction was high, with 58% of patients very satisfied and 22% reporting they were satisfied with the procedure. Patients were able to return to normal daily activities within 24 hours. Adverse events included mild pain reported in 17% of cases at 1 week, ecchymoses in most of patients that resolved within 1 week, three cases of paresthesias at 3 months, and one report of skin necrosis at a prior surgical site. Ultrasound imaging showed a thermal effect, which results in the melting and rupturing of collagenous and subdermal bands. Physicians observed a reduction of contour irregularities and immediate skin retraction during the procedure.

Diode lasers such as the 980-nm LAL device may offer an advantage of increased power and efficiency (by approximately 30%) compared with other wavelengths (5). This is particularly interesting given that the coefficient of fat absorption of both the 980-nm and 1064-nm wavelengths were found to be very similar (5). However, with higher energy and continuous pulsing comes an increased risk of tissue damage and subsequent scarring. Carbonization of adipose tissue has been documented with use of the 980-nm device (14).

The only FDA-approved 980-nm device for LAL is Lipotherme™ (MedSurge Advances, Dallas, Texas, USA).

Nd:YAG Laser Devices

The 1064-nm Device

The 1064-nm wavelength targets oxyhemoglobin, allowing for efficient vessel coagulation (24). Dermal collagen-bound water and fat also absorb the laser wavelength but less efficiently than the longer 1320-nm wavelength, especially at increasing tissue depths (22,33). The thermal energy spread is diffuse, causing bulk heating of the treated tissues (26).

Table 14.1 Devices Used in LAL

Trade Name (Manufacturer)	FDA Approval Date	Wavelength (nm)	Laser Type	Fiber Size (μm)	Power (W)	Pulse Duration (μs)	Repetition Rate (Hz)	Pulse Energy (mJ)
SlimLipo (Palomar, Burlington, Massachusetts, USA)	April 2008	924, 975	Diode	1500	30	Continuous	Continuous	N/A
Lipotherme (Osyris/Med Surge Advances, Dallas, Texas, USA)	Not FDA approved	980	Diode	600	25	Continuous	Continuous	N/A
SmartLipo (Cynosure, Westford, Massachusetts, USA)	October 2006	1064	Nd:YAG	300, 600	18	100	40	150
LipoLite (Syneron, Yokneam, Israel)	May 2008	1064	Nd:YAG	550	20	100–800	50	<250–800
SmartLipo MPX (Cynosure, USA)	October 2006	1064 1320	Nd:YAG	600	20 12	150	40	500 300
CoolLipo (CoolTouch, Roseville, California, USA)	January 2008	1320	Nd:YAG	200, 320, 500	20, 25	100	20–50	
ProLipo (Sciton, Palo Alto, California, USA)	July 2007	1064	Nd:YAG	600–1000	20 (25 outside USA)	10–100	50	800
ProLipo Plus (Sciton USA)	December 2008 March 2009 (higher energy system with 1319 nm)	1064 1319	Nd:YAG	600–1000	30–40 (1064 nm) 20–40 (1319 nm)	10–250	60	800
AccuSculpt (Lutronic, Inc., San Jose, California, USA)	February 2009	1444	Nd:YAG	600	12	Not specified	5–40	300
SmartLipo Triplex (Cynosure,USA)		1064 1320 1440	Nd:YAG		40 24 15	500 1000 1000	40 40 25	

Abbreviations: LAL, laser lipolysis; N/A, not applicable.

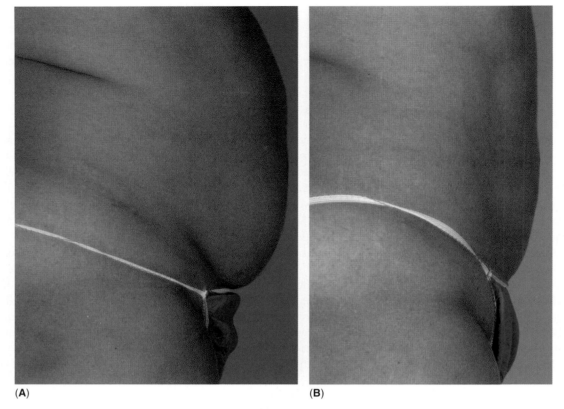

(A)   **(B)**

Figure 14.1 (**A**) Preoperative and (**B**) 3-month postoperative view of the abdomen treated with laser lipolysis using the dual 924/975-nm device. The 46-year-old woman was treated with a total of 60 kJ using a 1.5-mm quartz rod for energy delivery. The first pass was treated with 20 W at 924 nm and 10 W at 975 nm. Second and third passes were completed at 20 W using the 924-nm wavelength only. Two lipoaspiration passes were completed; the first pass after the first laser pass and the second pass following second laser pass. Total volume of aspirated fat was 820 cc.

Apfelberg and colleagues reported in 1994 on the first 1064-nm laser device for use in LAL. In a clinical trial intended for a new device application to the FDA, this study consisted of 51 patients treated with a 1064-nm Nd:YAG laser (Heraeus Lasersonics, acquired by Laserscope Inc., San Jose, California, USA) during liposuction. Fifteen of these patients had split area treatment with LAL and conventional liposuction (7). The system incorporated a 600-µm fiber contained within a 4- or 6-mm cannula. A chilled saline infusion was required to flow through the cannula chamber to cool the tip during the procedure. No clear benefit for LAL was demonstrated in terms of clinical improvement or patient discomfort (7). Furthermore, no statistically significant difference was found in postoperative edema or ecchymosis between either treatment side, although there was a trend toward superior results on the LAL-treated side (6). Although the device may have reduced surgeon fatigue during the procedure, the five participating physicians commented the system was cumbersome to utilize (7). Given the lack of benefit of LAL using this YAG laser, the FDA approval of this device was not pursued.

In October 2006, the SmartLipo™ device (Cynosure Inc.; DEKA, Calenzano, Italy) gained FDA approval for the "surgical incision, excision, vaporization, ablation, and coagulation of soft tissues" as well as for LAL (14,15). The 1064-nm Nd:YAG SmartLipo device currently delivers a maximum energy of 18 W, increased from the original 6-W output. The optical fiber has been increased from 300 to 600 µm, and treatment is usually administered at 150 mJ/pulse, 40 Hz, with a 100-ms pulse width (14).

As the SmartLipo device has been on the market the longest, the largest body of published literature accompanies this laser wavelength. Two studies have observed high patient satisfaction following treatment with this 1064-nm Nd:YAG platform. Dudelzak performed LAL on the arms of 20 patients with a 10-W, 300-µm fiber encased in 1-mm microcannula (39). The liquefied fat was removed via standard liposuction aspiration in 50% of patients. All patients were "very satisfied" with their results despite modest arm circumference reductions that did not differ from traditional liposculpture. Treatment with and without post-LAL suction aspiration produced similar results. Lack (40), in a comparative cohort study of 46 patients, found patients had higher treatment satisfaction scores with the 1064-nm device compared with tumescent liposuction, and another study demonstrated a 37% subject-rated improvement 3 months following LAL (18).

Several other studies have examined the safety and efficacy of LAL using the 1064-nm wavelength. In a noncomparative study of 245 patients undergoing LAL, Badin and colleagues found less trauma, bleeding, and swelling after LAL compared with their personal experience with liposuction (12). Both Sun et al. and Kim and Geronemus reported no serious adverse effects following case studies of LAL in 35 and 29 patients, respectively (18,24). Kim and Geronemus used MRI to evaluate the volume of fat reduction in 10 patients treated with LAL, using the pulsed Nd:YAG laser and found 17% fat volume reduction. In addition, patients noted a 37% improvement at 3 months, quick recovery times and visible skin retraction (18). Smaller baseline volume areas, such as the submentum, showed better results, suggesting a dose–response relationship.

Nonetheless, Prado and colleagues conducted a prospective randomized, double-blind controlled clinical trial comparing LAL with conventional suction lipoplasty in 25 patients and found no major clinical differences between conventional suction lipoplasty and laser-assisted liposuction (41). They used the SmartLipo System and applied 500 J for each area equivalent to the size of the patient's "palm" of the hand on one side followed by aspiration with a 3-mm cannula. The contralateral side was also infiltrated with tumescent fluid and aspirated with a 3-mm cannula. There was no difference in cosmetic results, ecchymosis, edema, and retraction between the two groups. There was less pain in the LAL side; however, surgical time was longer for the LAL side (median 60 minutes; range 45–80 minutes) compared with the suction-assisted lipoplasty side (median 45 minutes; range 40–80 minutes).

Goldman and colleagues have examined the effect of the 1064-nm LAL platform in several treatment areas. In one study, 82 subjects with submental lipodystrophy were treated using a 1064-nm Nd:YAG laser, with 6-W power, 40-Hz frequency, 150-mJ energy, and 100-μs pulse width parameters (SmartLipo, Cynosure) (17). Histology was performed on fatty tissue samples. Some patients received liposuction immediately following LAL. The histologic studies revealed coagulation of small blood vessels, rupture of adipocytes, reorganization of the reticular dermis, coagulation of collagen, and the appearance of channels produced by the laser action. However, the final results obtained with LAL were similar to the results utilizing traditional liposuction. In a separate study by Goldman and colleagues (19), laser liposuction using the 1064-nm SmartLipo device was compared with liposuction alone in 28 female patients with skin flaccidity and lipodystrophy of the arms. One arm in each patient was treated with laser liposuction followed by traditional liposuction. The contralateral arm was treated with pretunneling of the SmartLipo device with no optical fiber, followed by traditional liposuction. Treatment end points 3 months postprocedure included blinded, clinical photographic comparisons and arm circumference measurements. Arm circumference reduction was superior in the laser-treated group compared with liposuction alone ($P = 0.001$). Skin retraction in the laser-treated group versus liposuction alone-treated group was 11.4% ± 3.17% versus 8.70% ± 2.40%, respectively. These results complemented higher photographic clinical outcome ratings in the laser- versus liposuction alone-treated groups.

Another 1064-nm pulsed Nd-YAG device became available for LAL in the US market in May 2008. Lipolite™ (Syneron, Yokneam, Israel) consists of a variable pulse system (pulse width of 100–800 ms) with a maximum power of 12 W, maximum pulse energy of 800 mJ/pulse, and a repetition rate up to 50 Hz. Energy is delivered with a 550-μm fiber ensheathed within a 1.2-mm microcannula. Like the SmartLipo system, aspiration must be performed in a separate step following LAL.

Therefore, LAL using an Nd:YAG laser has been shown to be effective and safe in previous studies, with apparent advantages over traditional liposuction such as fast patient recovery and a possible skin tightening effect. A longer operative time is also a minor relative drawback, which needs to be measured against the possible advantages. Some authors defend that

early reports regarding the lack of efficacy of skin tightening were related to the steep learning curve of the procedure, inadequate energy delivery, or insufficient heat application (42). However, further studies are still needed to standardize methods that will optimize results, safety, and efficacy.

The 1320-nm Device

This wavelength is efficiently absorbed by fat and water (22,26) and targets mostly dermal and subcutaneous collagen, water-containing adipocytes, and collagen-bound water (33). The 1320-nm device may provide less collateral tissue damage, as energy deposition to tissues is concentrated around the laser tip (22,26). Because of its preferential targeting of water, the 1320-nm laser device may allow for greater tissue tightening (22).

The 1320-nm device was FDA approved in January 2008 and marketed as CoolLipo (CoolTouch, Roseville, California, USA). CoolLipo delivers a maximum of 25 W through 200-, 320-, and 500-μm fibers. The pulsed firing is delivered with a 100-ms pulse width at 20–50 Hz (14). A dual-port microcannula allows both LAL and aspiration to occur simultaneously (Figs. 14.2–14.6).

One study has examined the clinical effects of the 1320-nm device to the 1064-nm and multiplex (1064 + 1320 nm) devices (28). Mild-to-moderate improvement in skin laxity was noted in 10 patients undergoing LAL of the arms, abdomen, flanks, or thighs with the 1320-nm device at 10 W, 40–50 Hz, followed by aspiration. However, there was not a control of liposuction only to determine whether the improvement in skin laxity was much greater than liposuction alone.

Multiplex Devices

The 1064/1320-nm multiplex device (SmartLipo MPX, Cynosure, Inc.) incorporates sequential firing of the dual wavelengths although either wavelength can be fired alone (14). The newer platform also includes a handpiece with motion-sensing feedback, termed "SmartSense," allowing an automatic shut-off mechanism when maximum temperatures are reached. The platform is capable of firing a maximum of 20 W at 1064 nm and 12 W at 1320 nm through a 600-μm fiber contained within a 1.0- to 1.5-mm microcannula (14).

The scientific premise for combining the 1064- and 1320-nm wavelengths is to exploit their individual properties and allow for them to act synergistically, particularly in regard to hemostasis. The 1320-nm wavelength converts hemoglobin to methemoglobin (22). The 1064 nm not only targets oxygenated hemoglobin but also has a great affinity to methemoglobin, thereby enhancing the effects of the 1320-nm firing (22).

McBean and Katz evaluated the safety and efficacy of the 1064/1320-nm (SmartLipo MPX™, Cynosure, Inc.) system for lipolysis of localized fat and skin tightening in 20 patients (27). Five of the subjects had 4 × 4 cm temporary India ink tattoos placed at treatment sites and the tattooed areas were measured at baseline and 1-month and 3-month intervals. Suction aspiration followed laser treatment to remove the liquefied adipose tissue. Independent observers found reduction in localized fat in all patients (76–100% improvement in 85% of subjects and 51–75% improvement in 15% of subjects) with no adverse events. India ink tattoo maps demonstrated an 18% decrease in surface area indicating a significant skin tightening effect.

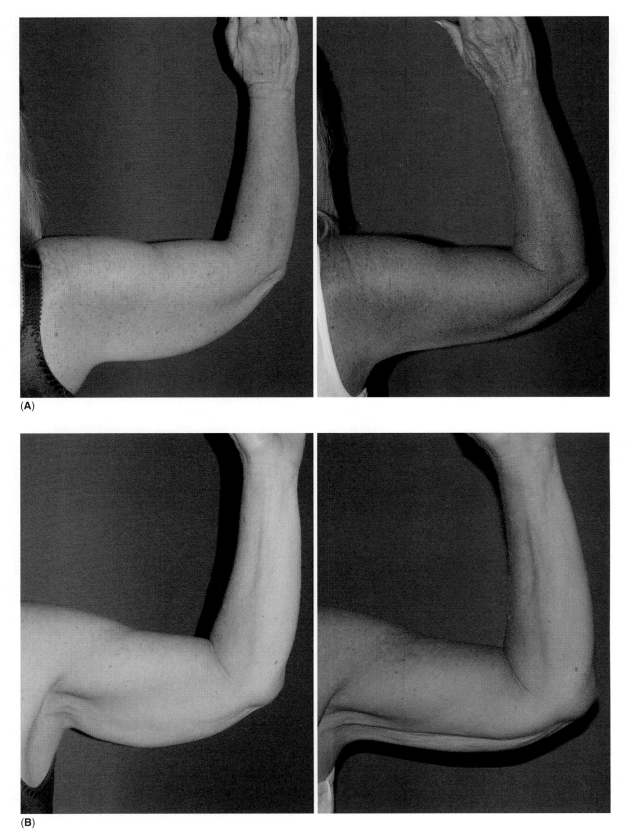

Figure 14.2 (**A**) Preoperative views of the arms of a 58-year-old woman and (**B**) 6-month postoperative views following laser lipolysis with the CoolLipo system (1320 nm) at 17 W, 50 Hz, and 7466 J.

Histology by hematoxylin and eosin, methylene blue stains, and electron microscopy showed new collagen and myofibroblast formation compared with baseline. One limitation of the study was that no patients were treated with liposuction alone.

A three-arm treatment study was conducted by Woodhall and coworkers comparing the SmartLipo MPX device, to either wavelength alone for LAL of various body areas (28). In the first study, both arms were treated with tumescent liposculpture with one arm randomized to treatment with a subcutaneous 10-W, 1064-nm Nd:YAG laser. The second study treated multiple sites with half of the area randomized to receive 10-W, 1064-nm versus 10-W, 1320-nm system followed by aspiration

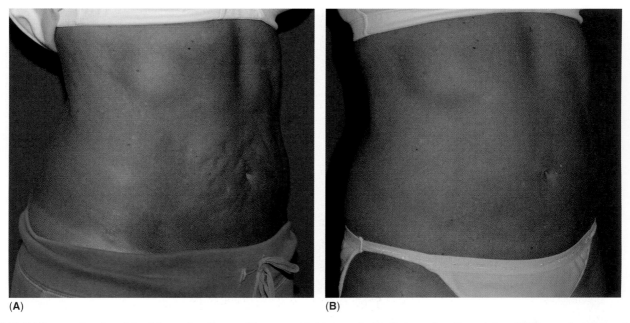

Figure 14.3 (**A**) Preoperative view of the abdomen in a 62-year-old woman with skin irregularities from previous liposculpture. (**B**) Six-month postoperative view of the treatment area demonstrating improved skin irregularities and decreased skin flaccidity. CoolLipo system (1320 nm) was used at 15 W, 50 Hz, and 8602 J.

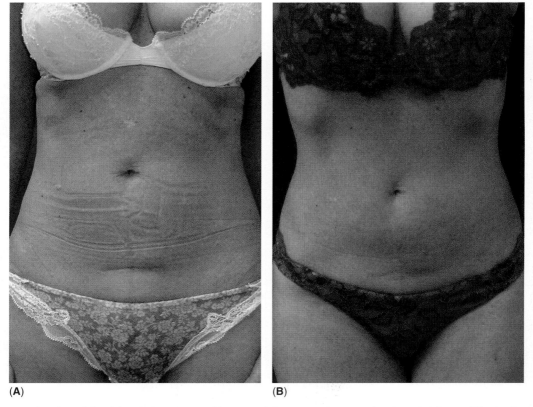

Figure 14.4 (**A**) Preoperative view of the abdomen in a 48-year-old woman. (**B**) One-year postoperative view of abdomen following laser lipolysis with the CoolLipo system (1320 nm) at 10 W and 50 Hz. Improvement is also noted on the scar on the lower abdomen.

at equal power. The third study used the combined 1064/1320-nm multiplex laser system at multiple sites. The end point of laser treatment was determined by reaching an external skin surface temperature of 40°C. In the first study, no significant improvement over tumescent liposculpture alone was noted using the 1064-nm laser. The second study showed no difference using the 1320- versus the 1064-nm LAL system. The authors believe that the results found in the first two studies were likely secondary to suboptimal energies. Finally, the multiplex 1064/1320-nm system appeared to show better clinical improvement in skin laxity and fat reduction, possibly due to higher energies produced with the multiplex than either the 1064- or the 1320-nm 10-W system alone. Two of the 20 patients receiving treatment with the multiplex device sustained thermal burns and in both cases intraoperative skin surface temperatures exceeded 40°C.

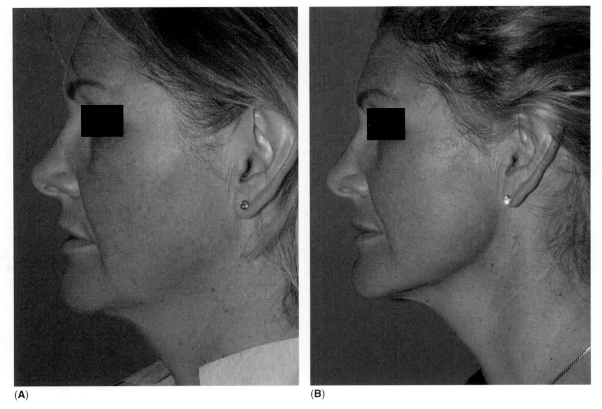

Figure 14.5 (**A**) Preoperative view of the neck/submental area of a 50-year-old woman and (**B**) 4-month postoperative view following laser lipolysis with the CoolLipo system (1320 nm) at 15 W and 50 Hz. Significant improvement in submental fat and skin tightening can be observed.

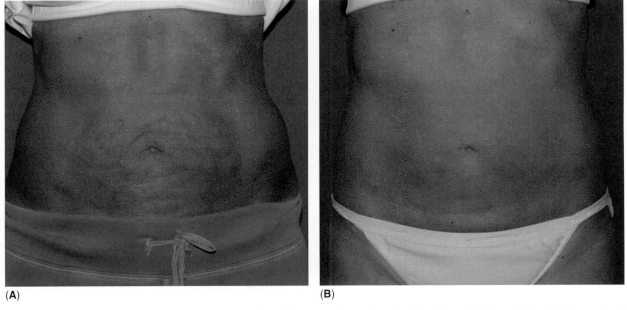

Figure 14.6 (**A**) A 62-year-old woman 2 years after aggressively performed liposuction by another physician with marked irregularities. (**B**) Six months after liposuction with the 1320-nm CoolLipo system without aspiration of fat. Note the smoother appearance and tighter skin. Treatment parameters were 15 W, thermal mode, and 8602 J, beginning skin temperature 23.2°C with a final skin temperature of 34.2°C.

In 2010, Dibernardo conducted a randomized blinded split abdomen study to evaluate skin shrinkage and skin tightening in laser-assisted liposuction (SmartLipo MPX, Cynosure, Inc.) versus liposuction control in 10 patients (43). Skin shrinkage was quantified by measuring temporary ink markings and then calculating the changes in surface area by region. Skin tightening was quantified by changes in the skin stiffness index measured with an elasticity device in the treated regions. The author found significantly higher mean shrinkage ratios on the laser-treated side than on the suction side both at the 1- and 3-month evaluations. The skin stiffness and skin tightening were significantly higher on the laser-treated site at 3 months posttreatment.

A second multiplex device is also available from Sciton (Palo Alto, California, USA) as ProLipo™, incorporating the

1064- and 1319-nm wavelengths. The ProLipo 1064-nm platform has been approved since July 2007. The 1319-nm component was initially FDA approved on December 1, 2008, with a higher energy system gaining FDA approval on March 6, 2009. The newest platform is capable of delivering a maximum energy of 40 W for both the 1064- and the 1319-nm wavelengths. The 1064-nm wavelength was selected in this multiplex system for its affinity for oxyhemoglobin, while the 1319 nm for its high absorption of water. In addition, the company reports that the energy produced from the 1319-nm wavelength concentrates around the fiber tip and targets fibrous septae by damaging associated collagen. The multiplex system may use differential blending of wavelengths to exert more vascular effects with the 1064-nm predominance or more skin tightening effects by favoring the 1319-nm wavelength.

Alexiades-Armenakas conducted a study of the 1064/1319-nm multiplex LAL device for 12 patients with lipodystrophy and skin laxity of the submentum and neck (44). Three treatment arms (1064 nm only, 1319 nm only, and 1064/1319-nm multiplex) of the study showed similar degrees of skin tightening. This study is notable for its use of in situ tissue monitoring to a target tissue temperature of 45–48°C. No thermal injuries were reported.

A multiplex LAL device (Cynosure's Triplex Workstation, Cynosure, Inc.) utilizes three wavelengths: 1064, 1320, and 1440 nm. These wavelengths can be used independently or can be blended (1064 and 1320 nm or 1064 and 1440 nm) with the objective of enhancing the efficacy of lipolysis and improving skin tightening. This device also includes a subcutaneous temperature monitoring system and motion sensing devices to minimize overtreatment and thermal injuries.

The 1444-nm Device

In 2009 the FDA gave clearance for the surgical incision, excision, vaporization, ablation, and coagulation of soft tissue by the 1444-nm device called AccuSculpt™ (Lutronic Inc., San Jose, California, USA). The laser system is a neodymium-doped laser operating on a micropulsed mode (100 μs) through a 600-μm silica fiber.

The selection of this wavelength is based on the fact that both the fat and the water absorption spectra have pronounced peaks near 1444 nm. Theoretically, this may allow for more selective, focused destruction of adipocytes in the treatment area with less thermal diffusion to adjacent tissues (45). A Korean study conducted by Tark and Song found greater lipolytic effect with the 1444-nm Nd:YAG laser compared with the 1064-nm Nd:YAG laser in an in vivo mini pig and in vitro human fat experiments (46). However, considering the association between powerful lipolytic effect and thermal damage, there were theoretical concerns of complications of thermal burns and oil collection from the 1444-nm laser. A 2012 follow-up porcine study by Youn and Holcomb compared fat ablation crater depth, tissue mass loss, and thermal temperature monitoring on ex vivo samples (45). While measuring fat ablation depth and tissue mass loss, the 1444-nm laser treatment demonstrated the greatest effect, followed by the 1320-nm laser and then the 1064-nm fiber. In terms of temperature changes, laser irradiation by the 1444 nm demonstrated the least amount absolute temperature elevation and slowest rate (slope) of temperature elevation, indicating the 1444 nm

created less thermal diffusion compared with the other two wavelengths. The 1064-nm wavelength had intermediate temperature elevation and rate of temperature increase, while the 1320-nm wavelength created the highest temperature diffusivity. These findings would suggest that the 1444-nm wavelength compared with 1064 nm and 1320 nm has the highest degree of thermal confinement to the area treated. These studies indicate that 1444 nm may be a more efficient wavelength for fat destruction. This may decrease work required for fat lipolysis; however, there is likely less collateral tissue damage. This effect is desirable when considering a need to protect nearby vital structures such as nerves and vasculature. However, if thermal diffusivity creates collateral thermal destruction and subsequent collagen production and tissue tightening, this may be a potential limitation of the 1444-nm wavelength. Further studies are still required to establish safety and efficacy guidelines comparing all of the FDA-approved wavelengths utilized for LAL.

TECHNIQUE

Patient workup and preparation are similar to that of the tumescent liposuction technique. Patients are marked in a standing position. Patients are prepped in a sterile fashion and typically given a light sedative medication by the oral, intramuscular, or intravenous route. Less commonly, some physicians will perform LAL under spinal or general anesthesia (14).

LAL may be performed independently or in combination with traditional liposuction. In the majority of cases, tumescent anesthetic fluid similar to the Klein formulation is infiltrated in the area to be treated. Once the infiltration is complete, a baseline temperature is taken with an infrared temperature sensor and small adit sites are created by a direct puncture technique using a #11 surgical steel blade. The microcannula housing the laser fiber is inserted under the skin into the fat compartment. With currently used devices, the laser fiber tip must be advanced outside the cannula tip, usually by 2–3 mm (12).

Some practitioners begin LAL in the deep fat compartment first and then move more superficially within the adipose layer in a fan-like motion. A red aiming beam (HeNe) is visible under the surface of skin, with the intensity increasing as the laser light becomes more superficial. Protective eyewear should be used by all individuals in the operating room through the entirety of the procedure. The cannula is moved in a to-and-fro manner in a fanning pattern at a velocity of approximately 100 mm/s. Some authors stress the need for slow movement of the cannula through the tissue, to maximize laser–tissue interaction (12). The operator's dominant hand is used to propel the cannula back and forth within the treatment area, while the nondominant hand is placed on the skin surface for tactile feedback on the skin surface temperature.

Typical starting temperatures at the skin surface are 26–28°C. Serial temperature readings are taken during the procedure, and treatment discontinued in a given area when the skin surface temperature registers 38–40°C or there is a complete loss of resistance, signaling emulsification of the fat, whichever end point is reached first. At this clinical end point, the skin feels moderately warm to touch (21). Areas with a thinner dermal and adipose layer (e.g., submental area) will reach the target temperature more quickly, and special care must be taken in treating such areas (26). Some of the available technology now takes thermal readings at the cannula tip as well as provides skin surface temperature readings through an infrared thermal monitor screen (SmartLipo MPX). Total energies utilized for the laser range from 5000 to 60,000 J/cm². Size of the treatment location, the total amount of fat, the number of strokes, distance of cannula placement from the skin and depth within the fat layer, number of repeated cycle passes, and individual surgical techniques prevent recommending an absolute number of kilojoules for each region. Reynaud has published guidelines using a 980-nm diode laser (21). His average totals for each area are listed here: 24,600 J for abdomen, 21,900 J for back, 14,600 J for hip, 13,100 J for buttock, 8100 J for knee, and 10,400 J for inner thigh. The cumulative total for the submandibular region seems a bit high, since we typically use about 50% of the total of 11,700 J reported.

After LAL is complete, the emulsified fat may be removed by aspiration with traditional liposuction or extrusion through incision sites by gentle physician massage (24). One system (CoolLipo) has integrated cannulas that allow for LAL and aspiration simultaneously. Aspiration continues until the appropriate body contour is reached. A pinch test is used at the conclusion of the procedure to test for any contour irregularities.

Entry sites are left open for drainage and wound dressings applied in a fashion similar to traditional tumescent liposuction. Patients wear compression bandages and/or garments between 3 and 30 days depending on the area treated (12). Patients may resume daily activities as tolerated, usually within 24 hours. Pain management usually requires only acetaminophen and, occasionally, a codeine-containing medication. Patients can usually resume vigorous physical activity within 7 days. Postoperative physiotherapeutic treatments or lymphatic drainage massage is used by some to accelerate patient recovery and enhance the clinical result (14,30).

COMPLICATIONS, ADVERSE EFFECTS, AND PRECAUTIONS

The complication rate following LAL is extremely low in well-trained hands, estimated at 0.93% according to a prospective trial in 537 patients (16). A second large study by Chia and Theodorou of 1000 consecutive cases of suction-assisted and laser-assisted lipectomy under local anesthesia confirms these findings (47). Ecchymoses, edema, and pain are the most commonly experienced adverse events (18,30), similar to those expected following liposuction and usually mild in severity. Paresthesias and hyperpigmentation have also been reported (14,18). Rare side effects similar to liposuction-related complications are also possible including seroma, infection, neuropathy, and minor contour irregularities. Touch-up rates following laser-assisted liposuction are low, reported as 7.3% in one study of laser-assisted and suction-assisted liposuction (47). Adverse events can largely be avoided. Inappropriately high laser settings resulting in high radiant energy, overly aggressive tissue treatment with concentration in a single treatment area for long periods of time all increase the risk of tissue hyperthermia and a risk of irreversible tissue injury (45).

Some of the most common adverse effects related to LAL are often secondary to the heat produced by the laser fiber, resulting in residual tissue damage (45). If the laser energy is inappropriately high, or the local temperature rises above 47°C, the

likelihood of a thermal burn increases (14). In this same study of 537 patients using a 1064-nm Nd:YAG laser, four skin burns occurred (16).

Although the majority of reports on LAL indicate decreased bruising as a distinct advantage over traditional liposuction, one author has disputed this advantage with a case series and a retrospective review (40,48). Three of 44 patients in one series experienced severe ecchymoses, with tenderness lasting beyond the resolution of bruising following LAL with an Nd:YAG system (48). Lack also found a higher degree of edema, ecchymosis, skin sensitivity, and pain in LAL patients compared with those undergoing traditional liposuction, although no statistical analysis was performed (40).

Blistering of the skin is a direct result of superficial thermal damage. Superficial treatment more readily leads to epidermal injury (26). Epidermal injury is typical when the skin surface temperature reaches 47°C, with blistering at temperatures of 58°C or greater (26). However, in clinical practice, we have witnessed epidermal blistering when surface temperatures are far below 58°C. For this reason, continuous thermal monitoring is necessary and the temperature end point should not exceed 40°C.

In addition, the accumulated energy could be employed as a surgical end point; however, few studies have tried to quantify energy levels by treatment area. In addition, there is a wide range of energy levels reported in the literature due to lack of knowledge in early studies. In 2009, Reynaud and colleagues reported their experience with 534 LAL procedures using a 980-nm diode laser (21). Data recorded during the 534 procedures allowed for a calculation of the mean cumulative energy applied for each location: 8100 J for the knee, 14,600 J for the hip, 10,400 J for the inner thigh, 11,700 J for the chin, 12,800 J for the arm, 13,100 J for the buttock line, 21,900 J for the back, and 24,600 J for the abdomen. However, wide ranges of energies were identified when the mean energy levels were calculated, with accumulated energies between 6000 and 51,000 J while treating the abdomen. Other factors such as the treatment area, the depth of cannula placement, and individual techniques will also interfere with the final accumulated energy. Therefore, other clinical end points, such as palpation, use of a handheld infrared temperature gauge, and integrated internal sensing devices, should be used to avoid thermal injury.

The presence of tumescent fluid may provide some epidermal protection. According to Mordon et al., cooled tumescent fluid infiltration decreases skin surface temperature greatly (34). The large volume of tumescent fluid used for anesthesia serves as a large reservoir for heat transfer. Just as cooled tumescent fluid lowers the skin surface temperature, tumescent fluid heated by laser light from bioheat transfer could produce epidermal heating, with increasing temperatures occurring beyond the treatment time. For this reason, we advocate close monitoring of skin surface temperatures with an infrared temperature sensor or similar technology. We often discontinue LAL in an area once a temperature of 38–40°C has been reached, knowing that the maximum temperature may reach 41°C several minutes later. If this does occur, we quench the area quickly with an ice bath.

A theoretical concern of LAL is its effects on serum lipid levels. Laser-induced adipocyte rupture causes the release of intracellular lipid contents, and how this is metabolized by the body is unclear. Studies on lipid levels following LAL indicate no change in serum lipid levels following the procedure (11,34). Mordon et al. followed serial lipid panels in four patients for 30 days following LAL and found no deviation from baseline levels (34). Goldman and coworkers conducted LAL with a 1064-nm device and observed no increase in cholesterol or triglyceride levels following the procedure (11). Woodhall et al. also found no change in triglycerides in 39 patients undergoing LAL with the 1064 nm, 1320 nm, or multiplex (1064 + 1320 nm) device (28). Given the lack of serum lipid level elevation following LAL, there appears to be no lipid-related renal or hepatotoxicity risk. Lipid metabolism following LAL has not been studied although mechanisms of action have been postulated. Lipid metabolism may occur slowly, avoiding changes in serum lipid levels or alternatively, lipids may be cleared through a phagocytic route via macrophage digestion (34).

NONINVASIVE LASER LIPOLYSIS TECHNOLOGY
Several technologies have appeared in the medical literature as possible noninvasive laser alternatives for adipocyte destruction. The advantage of such technology, if effective, would be the nonsurgical delivery of therapy. However, the relative paucity of available studies as well as the lack of reproducibility from one of the studies casts doubts on the true effects and efficacy of these light sources.

The first noninvasive laser light source reported to produce fat liquefaction was a 635-nm, low-level energy laser source (49). Low-level laser therapy (LLLT) requires that the delivery of laser energy does not result in a temperature increase in the treated tissue. A similar light source has been used in a variety of applications in the fields of physical therapy and anti-inflammatory research (50) and is FDA approved for pain alleviation and for use with lipoplasty (51). Other applications include promotion of wound healing and edema reduction (49). The clinical effects may be partially explained by the multitude of effects on the skin from the action spectra produced within the wavelengths of 630–640 nm. These include fibroblast and keratinocyte proliferation, microcirculatory stimulation, and scar diminution (49).

In an effort to exploit the biomodulatory effects of low-level 635-nm laser light (Erchonia Laser PL3000™, Majes-Tec Innovations, Inc., Mesa, Arizona, USA), Neira and coworkers subjected 12 human post-lipectomy adipose tissue samples to treatment for increasing time periods (49). The device consists of a single diode, variable hertz, red light source. Neira et al. reported 80% adipocyte membrane disruption after 4 minutes of exposure to laser light and 99% disruption after 6 minutes. An electron microscopic examination revealed transitory pores within cell membranes, deflation of adipocytes, and emptying of cellular contents (49).

The favorable results reported by Neira et al. in 2002 failed to be reproduced by an independent study in 2004 by Brown and coworkers (51). Using both porcine and human models, no cellular changes were observed following low-level 635-nm laser treatment. Despite lengthy exposure times of up to 60 minutes, no change in adipocyte structure or morphology was demonstrated, casting doubt in the belief that this diode laser source produces adipocyte liquefaction (51). In addition, a study by Elm and colleagues evaluated the efficacy of LLLT (Zerona System™, Santa Barbara Medical Innovations, Dallas, Texas, USA) for body contouring, independent of body suction (52). Five patients received six treatments over a 2-week period on one side of the body and were evaluated by three blinded dermatologists 7 days and 1 month after last treatment. The authors found that circumference measurements revealed no statistically significant reduction in fat layer thickness, a finding confirmed also by ultrasound evaluation. Evaluation by three blinded dermatologists resulted in average correct photo identification of 51.1%, reflecting little clinical difference between posttreatment and baseline images. Therefore, the authors conclude that more studies are required to show clinical improvement in body contouring before LLLT can be recommended.

A second noninvasive laser light source has been used to target adipocytes. Wanner et al. used a 1210-nm, CW semiconductor diode laser to treat 24 patients (53). A 3-second exposure with precooling was used at increasing fluences to treat the abdominal area. The treatment was painful, necessitating the use of local anesthesia. Erythema persisted after treatment in some cases for several days. Histologic evidence of fat necrosis was noted, but dermal damage was also present with increasing energy. The authors concluded that this laser light source may preferentially target adipocytes but within a narrow therapeutic window. Further refinement in pain management, epidermal cooling, and energy delivery is necessary before this laser light source is a safe and reliable device for targeting fat.

DEVELOPMENTS AND FUTURE APPLICATIONS
Appropriate uses for LAL will continue to develop as this technology matures. It has been suggested that LAL may be a suitable treatment for axillary hyperhidrosis (15), for revising flaps (14), facial sculpting, and periorbital adipose tissue and skin tightening (42). A study utilized LAL with a 980-nm diode device to successfully treat a series of 28 male patients with gynecomastia (54). Twenty-two patients (78.6%) had very good results, and no complications were reported.

There is a particular interest in utilizing LAL for the treatment of cellulite, a condition that affects approximately 85% of postpubertal women (55). Cellulite continues to be a frustrating esthetic problem for many women without treatment modalities that offer dramatic improvement. In fact, traditional liposuction affords only minimal improvement of cellulite and may even worsen its appearance (30).

Combination treatment of LAL with autologous fat transfer was used in a small case series of 52 female patients (30). A 1064-nm Nd:YAG system (SmartLipo) was combined with subsequent fat transfer to treat Curri grades III–IV cellulite of the hips, buttocks, thighs, and abdomen. Patients were very pleased with the clinical outcome, with 84.6% of patients rating their results as good to excellent, but the effect of the laser alone was unknown (30).

We conducted our own study to answer this question. Nine patients and 11 sites were treated in a comparative study of LAL (CoolLipo) to mechanical disruption with a liposuction microcannula (Palm, Goldman, presented at the ASDS National Meeting, Oct 4, 2009, Phoenix, Arizona, USA). There was no difference between treatment groups in regard to cellulite grading following treatment, with both LAL and mechanical disruption improving one point on a 4-point scale. Patient-scored improvement did not differ between treatment sides, but physician scoring indicated increased improvement on the LAL-treated side. Future, large-scale studies are necessary to determine whether LAL is a viable treatment option for cellulite.

In situ temperature feedback has been reported using the 1064/1319-nm multiplex laser liposuction device (44). Employing a target tissue temperature of 45–48°C, the study of 12 subjects treated for submental lipodystrophy demonstrated no dermal injury, thermal burns, or postoperative complications.

Finally, the 1444-nm wavelength has been used as an alternative means of facial contouring. In a study of 478 patients who underwent "laser-assisted facial contouring," Holcomb et al. (56) treated mid and lower face localized adiposity with a wide breadth of outcomes from minimal improvement to marked changes in facial contour. Treatment complications were 13%, but over 60% of complications were undercorrection of the perceived defect.

CONCLUSION

LAL development has occurred rapidly over the last decade with the advancement of device platforms, usable wavelengths, surgical techniques, and new indications. Six wavelengths have been FDA approved for use with LAL: 924/975, 980, 1064, 1320, and 1444 nm. To date, the 1064-nm wavelength has the largest body of cumulative clinical studies regarding its use in LAL (57).

LAL is a safe technique in experienced hands and proper monitoring. Although LAL theoretically may have distinct advantages to traditional liposuction, well-constructed clinical studies are needed to definitively demonstrate possible advantages, as some experts still debate the utility of this technology (58). More precise laser and light devices, improved technology, and a reduced side effect profile will be introduced into the market. Future studies may better characterize treatment parameters and the optimal technology for use in LAL.

ACKNOWLEDGMENTS

This chapter derives material from the chapter on laser lipolysis by Melanie Palm and Mitchel Goldman in *Seminars in Cutaneous Medicine and Surgery* 2009; 28(4): 212–19.

REFERENCES

1. Heymans O, Castus P, Grandjean FX, et al. Liposuction: review of the techniques, innovations, and applications. Acta Chir Belg 2006; 106: 647–53.
2. Klein JA. Anesthesia for liposuction in dermatologic surgery. J Dermatol Surg Oncol 1988; 14: 1124–32.
3. Klein JA. Tumescent technique for local anesthesia improves safety in large-volume liposuction. Plast Reconstr Surg 1993; 92: 1085–98.
4. Mann MW, Palm MD, Sengelmann RD. New advances in liposuction technology. Semin Cutan Med Surg 2008; 27: 72–82.
5. Mordon S, Eymard-Maurin AF, Wassmer B, Ringot J. Histologic evaluation of laser lipolysis: pulsed 1064-nm Nd:YAG laser versus CW 980-nm diode laser. Aesth Surg J 2007; 27: 263–8.
6. Apfelberg DB. Results of multicenter study of laser-assisted liposuction. Clin Plast Surg 1996; 23: 713–19.
7. Apfelberg DB, Rosenthal S, Hunstad JP, Achauer B, Fodor PB. Progress report on multicenter study of laser-assisted liposuction. Aesth Plast Surg 1994; 18: 259–64.
8. Blugerman GB. Laser lipolysis for the treatment of localized adiposity and "cellulite". Abstracts of World Congress on Liposuction Surgery. Dearborn, Michigan, 2000.
9. Schavelzon DS, Blugerman G, Goldman A, et al. Laser lipolysis. Abstracts of the 10th International Symposium on Cosmetic Laser Surgery. Las Vegas, Nevada, 2001.
10. Goldman AG, Schavelzon D, Blugerman G. Liposuction using neodymium:yttrium-aluminium-garnet laser. Abstr Plast Reconstr Surg 2003; 111: 2497.
11. Goldman A, Schavelzon DE, Blugerman GS. Laserlipolysis: Liposuction using Nd:YAG laser. Rev Soc Bras Cir Plast 2002; 17: 17–26.
12. Badin AZD, Moraes LM, Gondek L, Chiaratti MG, Canta L. Laser lipolysis: flaccidity under control. Aesth Plast Surg 2002; 26: 335–9.
13. Uebelhoer NS, Ross EV. Introduction: update on lasers. Semin Cutan Med Surg 2008; 27: 221–6.
14. Goldman A, Gotkin RH. Laser-assisted liposuction. Clin Plast Surg 2009; 36: 241–53.
15. Katz B, McBean J. The new laser liposuction for men. Dermatol Ther 2007; 20: 448–51.
16. Katz B, McBean J. Laser-assisted lipolysis: a report on complications. J Cosmet Laser Ther 2008; 10: 231–3.
17. Goldman A. Submental Nd:YAG laser-assisted liposuction. Lasers Surg Med 2006; 38: 181–4.
18. Kim KH, Geronemus RG. Laser lipolysis using a novel 1064 nm Nd:YAG laser. Dermatol Surg 2006; 32: 241–8.
19. Goldman A, Wollina U, de Mundstock EC. Evaluation of tissue tightening by the subdermal Nd:YAG laser-assisted liposuction versus liposuction alone. J Cutan Aesthet Surg 2011; 4: 122–8.
20. Stebbins WG, Hanke CW, Petersen J. Novel method of minimally invasive removal of large lipoma after laser lipolysis with 980 nm diode laser. Dermatol Ther 2011; 24: 125–30.
21. Reynaud JP, Skibinski M, Wassmer B, Rochon P, Mordon S. Lipolysis using a 980-nm diode laser: a retrospective analysis of 534 procedures. Aesth Plast Surg 2009; 33: 28–36.
22. Parlette EC, Kaminer ME. Laser-assisted liposuction: here's the skinny. Semin Cutan Med Surg 2008; 27: 259–63.
23. Mordon SR, Wassmer B, Reynaud JP, Zemmouri J. Mathematical modeling of laser lipolysis. Biomed Eng Online 2008; 7: 10–24.
24. Sun Y, Wu SF, Yan S, et al. Laser lipolysis used to treat localized adiposis: a preliminary report on experience with Asian patients. Aesth Plast Surg 2009; 33: 701–5.
25. Badin AZED, Gondek LBE, Garcia MJ, et al. Analysis of laser lipolysis effects on human tissue samples obtained from liposuction. Aesth Plast Surg 2005; 29: 281–6.
26. DiBernardo BE, Reyes J, Chen B. Evaluation of tissue thermal effects from 1064/1320-nm laser-assisted lipolysis and its clinical implications. J Cosmet Laser Ther 2009; 11: 62–9.
27. McBean JC, Katz B. A pilot study of the efficacy of a 1064 nm and 1320 nm sequentially firing Nd:YAG laser device for lipolysis and skin tightening. Lasers Surg Med 2009; 41: 779–84.
28. Woodhall KE, Saluja R, Khoury J, Goldman MP. A comparison of three separate clinical studies evaluating the safety and efficacy of laser-assisted lipolysis using 1,064, 1,320 nm, and a combined 1,064/1,320 nm multiplex device. Lasers Surg Med 2009; 41: 774–8.
29. Wassmer B, Zemmouri J, Rochon P, Mordon S. Comparative study of wavelengths for laser lipolysis. Photomed Laser Surg 2010; 28: 185–8.
30. Goldman A, Gotkin RH, Sarnoff DS, Prati C, Rossato F. Cellulite: a new treatment approach combining subdermal Nd:YAG laser lipolysis and autologous fat transplantation. Aesth Surg J 2008; 28: 656–62.
31. Khoury JG, Saluja R, Keel D, Detwiler S, Goldman MP. Histologic evaluation of interstitial lipolysis comparing a 1064, 1320, and 2100 nm laser in an ex vivo model. Lasers Surg Med 2008; 40: 402–6.
32. Mordon S, Blanchemaison Ph. Letter to the editor: "Histologic evaluation of interstitial lipolysis comparing a 1064, 1320 and 2100 nm laser in an ex vivo model". Lasers Surg Med 2008; 40: 519.
33. Reszko AE, Magro CM, Diktaban T, Sadick N. Histological comparison of 1064 nm Nd:YAG and 1320 nm Nd:YAG laser lipolysis using an ex vivo model. J Drugs Dermatol 2009; 8: 377–82.
34. Mordon S, Wassmer B, Rochon P, et al. Serum lipid changes following laser lipolysis. J Cosmet Laser Ther 2009; 11: 74–7.
35. Ichikawa K, Miyasaka M, Tanaka R, et al. Histologic evaluation of the pulsed Nd:YAG laser for laser lipolysis. Lasers Surg Med 2005; 36: 43–6.

36. Levi JR, Veerappan A, Chen B, et al. Histologic evaluation of laser lipolysis comparing continuous wave vs pulsed lasers in an in vivo pig model. Arch Facial Plast Surg 2011; 13: 41–50.

37. Cook WR. Laser neck and jowl liposculpture including platysma laser resurfacing, dermal laser resurfacing, and vaporization of subcutaneous fat. Dermatol Surg 1997; 23: 1143–8.

38. Weiss RA, Beasley K. Laser-assisted liposuction using a novel blend of lipid-and water-selective wavelengths. Lasers Surg Med 2009; 41: 760–6.

39. Dudelzak J, Hussain M, Goldberg DJ. Laser lipolysis of the arm, with and without suction aspiration: clinical and histologic changes. J Cosmet Laser Ther 2009; 11: 70–3.

40. Lack EB. A retrospective analysis of the postoperative course of patients receiving suction-assisted liposuction versus laser lipolysis. Am J Cosmet Surg 2009; 26: 82–6.

41. Prado A, Andrades P, Danilla S, et al. A prospective, randomized, double-blind, controlled clinical trial comparing laser-assisted lipoplasty with suction-assisted lipoplasty. Plast Reconstr Surg 2006; 118: 1032.

42. McBean JC, Katz BE. Laser lipolysis: an update. J Clin Aesthet Dermatol 2011; 4: 25–34.

43. DiBernardo BE. Randomized, blinded split abdomen study evaluating skin shrinkage and skin tightening in laser-assisted liposuction versus liposuction control. Aesthet Surg J 2010; 30: 593–602.

44. Alexiades-Armenakas M. Combination laser-assisted liposuction and minimally invasive skin tightening with temperature feedback for treatment of the submentum and neck. Dermatol Surg 2012; 38: 871–81.

45. Youn JI, Holcomb JD. Ablation efficiency and relative thermal confinement measurements using wavelengths 1,064, 1,320, and 1,444 nm for laser-assisted lipolysis. Lasers Med Sci 2012; electronic version ahead of print.

46. Tark KC, Jung JE, Song SY. Superior lipolytic effect of the 1444 nm Nd:YAG laser comparison with the 1064 nm Nd:YAG laser. Lasers Surg Med 2009; 41: 721–7.

47. Chia CT, Theodorou SJ. 1,000 consecutive cases of laser-assisted liposuction and suction-assisted lipectomy managed with local anesthesia. Aesth Plast Surg 2012; 36: 767–79.

48. Lack EB. Three cases of severe ecchymoses following laser lipolysis. Am J Cosmet Ther 2009; 26: 101–4.

49. Neira R, Arroyave J, Ramirez H, et al. Fat liquefaction: effect of low-level laser energy on adipose tissue. Plast Reconstr Surg 2002; 110: 912–22.

50. King PR. Low level laser therapy: a review. Lasers Med Sci 1989; 4: 141.

51. Brown SA, Rohrich RJ, Kenkel J, et al. Effect of low-level laser therapy on abdominal adipocytes before lipoplasty procedures. Plast Reconstr Surg 2004; 113: 1796–804.

52. Elm CM, Wallander ID, Endrizzi B, Zelickson BD. Efficacy of a multiple diode laser system for body contouring. Lasers Surg Med 2011; 43: 114–21.

53. Wanner M, Avram M, Gagnon D, et al. Effects of noninvasive, 1,210 nm laser exposure on adipose tissue: results of a human pilot study. Lasers Surg Med 2009; 41: 401–7.

54. Trelles MA, Mordon SR, Bonanad E, et al. Laser-assisted lipolysis in the treatment of gynecomastia: a prospective study in 28 patients. Lasers Med Sci 2012; 14: 59–66.

55. Goldman MP, Hexsel D. Cellulite: Pathophysiology and Treatment, 2nd edn. London and New York: Informa Healthcare, 2010.

56. Holcomb JD, Turk J, Baek SJ, Rousso DE. Laser-assisted facial contouring using a thermally confined 1444-nm Nd-YAG laser: a new paradigm for facial sculpting and rejuvenation. Facial Plast Surg 2011; 27: 315–30.

57. Fakhouri TM, El Tal AK, Abrou AE, Mehregan DA, Barone F. Laser-assisted lipolysis: a review. Dermatol Surg 2012; 38: 155–69.

58. Coleman WP. Lasers for liposuction: no benefit over tumescent liposuction. Dermatol Surg 2012; 38: 170.

15 Laser, light, and energy devices for cellulite and lipodystrophy

Mitchel P. Goldman, Jennifer D. Peterson, and Sabrina G. Fabi

BACKGROUND

Historically a sign of beauty and wealth, the presence of cellulite is now considered esthetically objectionable. The term "cellulite" is used in modern times to describe the dimpled or puckered skin of the posterior and lateral thighs and buttocks seen in many trim and overweight women. The appearance is often described to resemble the surface of an orange peel or that of cottage cheese. It affects all races and is estimated that 85% of women over 20 years of age have some degree of cellulite (1). Cellulite is known medically as liposclerosis, gynoid dystrophy, edematofibrosclerosis, or dermopanniculitis (2). The condition is best described by Goldman as a normal physiologic state in postadolescent women, which maximizes adipose retention to ensure adequate caloric availability for pregnancy and lactation (3). Adipose tissue is also essential for nutrition, energy, support, protection, and thermal insulation (4).

Many of the currently accepted cellulite therapies target deficiencies in lymphatic drainage and microvascular circulation. Devices utilizing either exclusively or in combination are radiofrequency (RF)-, laser-, and light-based energies; many coupled with tissue manipulation are available for the improvement of cellulite. Laser-assisted liposuction with and without autologous fat transfer for the improvement of the appearance of cellulite has also been utilized. Although improvement using these devices is temporary, they may last for several months. Thus, patients who wish to have smoother skin with less visible cellulite can have a series of treatments and then return for additional treatments as necessary.

Predisposing Factors

There are many predisposing factors that contribute to cellulite development. These include the following:

1. Gender—Due to the underlying structure of fat and connective tissue described below, women are more likely to develop cellulite.
2. Heredity—The degree and presence of cellulite, as with body habitus, are often similar between females within the same family.
3. Race—Cellulite is more common in Caucasian women than in Asian or African-American women (5).
4. Increased subcutaneous fat—Due to the unique histology of cellulite-affected skin, more adipose tissue in the subcutaneous layer enhances the appearance of cellulite on the skin surface (6).
5. Age—Post puberty, women begin to develop cellulite as part of normal anatomic and physiologic development. With advancing age, cellulite increases in severity as a reflection of thinning of the epidermis.

Unfortunately, these predisposing factors are difficult if not impossible to alter and thus cellulite prevention is currently not attainable.

Histology

At the histologic level, cellulite is the result of localized adipose deposits and edema within the subcutaneous tissue. In women, fascial bands of connective tissue are oriented longitudinally and extend from the dermis to the deep fascia. These bands form fibrous septa, which segregate fat into channels resembling a down quilt or mattress, and the subcutaneous fat is projected superficially into the reticular and papillary dermis. As the fat layer expands, the perpendicular connective tissue remains fixed and anchored to the underlying tissue, creating a superficial puckered appearance of the skin (4,7,8). Ultrasonic studies of cellulite have shown the striking feature of herniation of the subcutaneous fat into the reticular and papillary dermis (Fig. 15.1) (9).

Fatty acids are believed to be modified through peroxidation by free radicals. These events are hypothesized to contribute to the worsening of local microcirculation by disrupting venous and lymphatic drainage. This skin phenomenon is rarely found in men as the connective tissue in males is not normally arranged vertically, but rather in a crisscross pattern that is gender-typical for the skin of the thighs and buttocks (Fig. 15.2) (4,7).

Pathophysiologic Mechanisms of Cellulite

The pathophysiology of cellulite is multifactorial. Adipose tissue is vascular, leading to the theory that cellulite may worsen in predisposed areas where circulation and lymphatic drainage have been decreased, possibly due to local injury or inflammation. Under normal conditions, fat cells are embedded in a network of reticular fibers. In cellulite, interstitial edema results from an increased permeability in the local microvasculature. As a result, a chronic inflammatory process ensues around the reticular fiber network. Subsequently, the reticular fibers increase in number (hyperplasia) and thickness (hypertrophy), worsening the compromised microcirculation (3). This is evident clinically as the classic "orange peel" appearance of overlying skin and in reduced blood perfusion.

The formation of cellulite is also under a hormonal influence. Estrogen is known to stimulate lipogenesis and inhibit lipolysis, resulting in adipocyte hypertrophy. This may explain the onset of cellulite at puberty, the condition being more prevalent in females, and the exacerbation of cellulite with

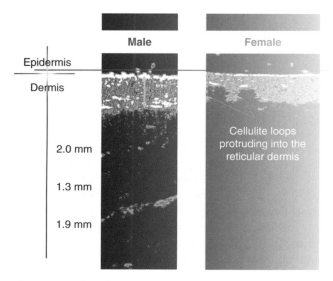

Figure 15.1 High-resolution ultrasound images of male and female subcutaneous fat. Note the fat herniations into the dermis for the female, which are absent in the male. *Source*: Courtesy of Dr. Agustina Vila Echague and Dr. Mathew Avram, from Dr. Avram's chapter in Goldman MP, Hexsel D, eds. *Cellulite: Pathophysiology and Treatment*, 2nd edn. New York, NY: Informa Healthcare, 2010.

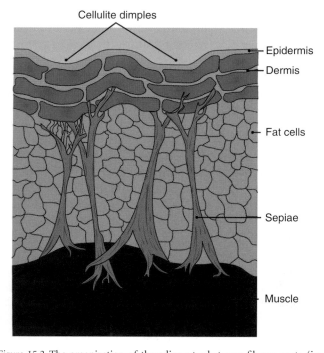

Figure 15.2 The organization of the adipocytes between fibrous septa (in a crisscross pattern) results in the dimpling of the skin characteristic of cellulite. *Source*: Courtesy of Dr. Zoe Draelos, from her chapter in Goldman MP, Hexsel D, eds. *Cellulite: Pathophysiology and Treatment*, 2nd edn. New York, NY: Informa Healthcare, 2010.

pregnancy, nursing, menstruation, and estrogen therapy (oral contraceptive use and hormone replacement) (10). The opposite seems true for men. Although there are a limited number of studies involving men, it is hypothesized that the combination of gender-specific soft tissue histology at the cellulite-prone anatomic sites, with a relatively lower circulating estrogen level, may be responsible for the lower incidence of cellulite in men (3,4). Although not proved, it is possible that

Table 15.1 Nurnberger–Muller Cellulite Classification Scale

Grade I	No or minimal cellulite based on observation when standing, the pinch test, or gluteal muscle contraction.
Grade II	Irregular skin topography upon observation. Cellulite is enhanced by pinching or gluteal contraction. Subjects may have skin pallor or decreased temperature and sensation.
Grade III	Skin exhibits the classic orange peel dimpling, "peau d'orange," at rest. Small subcutaneous nodularities may be palpated.
Grade IV	In addition to the characteristics described above, there is more severe puckering and palpable nodules.

circulating androgens may have an inhibitory effect on cellulite development by contributing to a different pattern of adipose tissue storage (i.e., more truncal than on the buttocks and thighs).

Classification

Nurnberger and Muller developed a classification system for grading cellulite severity. For this method, the physician accentuates cellulite dimpling by gently pinching an area of tissue between the fingers and the thumb. For larger areas, the skin of the thigh can be compressed between two hands. This technique is referred to as the "mattress phenomenon" as the dimpled pinched skin resembles a bed mattress. Cellulite may be graded for severity on a scale of I–IV (Table 15.1) (3,5,6).

ENERGY-BASED TREATMENT OVERVIEW

Many of the currently accepted cellulite therapies target deficiencies in lymphatic drainage and microvascular circulation. Based on our understanding of the etiology and nature of this condition, several treatment modalities have been developed and can be divided into five main categories: attenuation of aggravating factors, physical and mechanical methods, pharmacologic agents, RF energy, and laser energy (5). Treatments such as topical creams and lotions, ultrasound, electrolipolysis, iontophoresis, and mesotherapy have all been tried; while effective for temporary, mild improvement (11), none of these have proved to provide long-term resolution of cellulite (2). The below sections describe the developments of multiple devices utilizing either exclusively or in combination: RF-, laser-, and light-based energies, many coupled with tissue manipulation for the improvement of cellulite. Laser-assisted liposuction for the improvement of cellulite is also reviewed below.

Mechanical Devices
Tri-Active

Tri-Active (Cynosure, Inc., Westford, Massachusetts, USA) has the capability to treat cellulite and postliposuction fibrosis using a trifold treatment approach with diode laser delivery, contact cooling, and massage, to work synergistically to restore the body's normal homeostatic environment. It is cleared as an over-the-counter laser cellulite treatment, for temporary cellulite reduction. The Tri-Active laser energy is emitted through six 808-nm diode lasers to target the endothelial cells in order to enhance arterial, venous, and lymphatic flow and promote neovascularization. The contact cooling system can manually be adjusted from 10°C to 25°C and aids in decreasing edema by causing an initial vasoconstriction followed by a compensatory vasodilatation allowing for pooled fluid to remobilize. The rhythmic massage, which can either be selected as either single or dual phase, counteracts circulatory stasis, thereby mobilizing fluids by stimulating lymphatic drainage. In addition, the massage stretches the connective tissue smoothing the interface between the dermis and the epidermis.

The parameters of the Tri-Active system can be manipulated to optimize patient results. The depth and intensity of the rhythmic massage can be controlled by the frequency (0.1–5 Hz) and duty cycle (20–80%). The frequency (Hz) measures the number of aspirations per second. At higher frequencies, a superficial mechanical action is achieved, whereas lower repetition rates stimulate deeper tissue. The duty cycle is the percentage of time the aspiration is active between one aspiration and the next. For example, a duty cycle of 70% indicates that the aspiration is active 70% of the time between the two aspirations. The higher the value, the stronger the action. Thus by manipulating the duty cycle and frequency, one can increase or decrease the intensity and depth of the message.

For Fitzpatrick skin types I–III, it is recommend to start at 30 W and adjusting for patient discomfort and erythema. The frequency should initially be set at 3 Hz with duty cycle of 60%, and the operator may increase it to 4 or 5 Hz but would need to decrease the duty cycle to 50%. The dual mode is advised for the massage setting. When treating darker skin types, Fitzpatrick skin types IV–VI, the energy should be adjusted down to an initial fluence of 20 W. The fluence should be adjusted based on patient discomfort and the level of erythema. The same repetition rates (Hz) and duty cycles as listed above for skin types I–III can be utilized. No matter which skin type, the contact cooling function should be on and set at coolest level (10°C) and can be adjusted during the treatment.

A seal of the applicator should be always chambered to the skin—if the air is heard to be sucked into the chamber, this indicates that the applicator is not positioned properly for ideal vacuum suction on the skin. Five minutes should be spent on each major surface, that is, posterior thigh, outer thigh and hip, inner thigh, anterior thigh, and buttocks. Each treatment should last approximately for 30 minutes, and each zone should be treated with three to five passes, with the end point being significant erythema and warmth radiating from the treated skin. The Tri-Active device has also been used before, during, and after other surgical procedures, including liposuction and abdominoplasty. We have noted a marked improvement in irregularities when Tri-Active is performed after liposculpture. This improvement may be due to the redistribution of dystrophic adipose cells (12).

The experimental studies in Europe regarding the efficacy of Tri-Active were conducted by Nicola Zerbinati, MD, assistant professor of dermatology, University of Insubria, Milan, Italy. Ten patients were enrolled and each treated with 20-minute sessions three times a week. To evaluate the efficacy of the technique, all patients were requested not to change habits such as diet, physical activity, and lifestyle in general. Clinical observation, circumference of the thighs and hips, plicometry, skin elasticity, and thermography were recorded. All patients noted an increase in skin tone and a reduction in the circumference of the areas treated (13).

A similar study to those presented above to evaluate the efficacy of the Tri-Active without the lymphatic drainage protocol confirmed the importance of lymphatic drainage. Thirteen healthy females from 19- to 51-year old group with a mean age of 36.6 years and a mean body mass index of 22.26 kg/m² (19.2–29.3 kg/m²) were included in the study. The mean starting body fat percentage of the subjects was 22.18% (16.46–31.02%). Subjects underwent biweekly treatments for 6 weeks for a total of 12 treatments. Treatments were administered locally only on the hips and thighs. Efficacy was measured via waist, hip, and thigh circumference, elasticity, and thermography. Analysis of results included a subjective evaluation of pre- and posttreatment photos by five blinded evaluators. An overall improvement of 21% was noted among the treated patients. The most notable improvement was in the appearance of cellulite (23%), skin texture (16%), size (15%), and skin tone (14%). The results of thermography evaluated in this study show neither changes of mean temperature nor variations in uniformity of temperature distribution in the treated areas. The results revealed a trend toward modest but steady improvements in hip and thigh circumferences. A comparison with the pretreatment photos also suggests modest improvements in the appearance of cellulite and overall appearance, with those subjects starting with the least symptoms showing the greatest degree of improvement. Comparing these results with those of the previous studies suggests the importance of considering the entire system and method as a whole concept to be diligently performed for maximizing results (14).

Gold evaluated the Tri-Active on 10 females with cellulite treated with 15 biweekly sessions. Nine of the 10 subjects completed the study and the 1-month follow-up period. There were no significant changes in the subject's weight. An approximate 50% improvement in the visual grading scale was noted in 80% of the subjects (15).

Nootheti and Goldman performed the first comparative study to determine the relative efficacy of treatment of cellulite using two novel modalities, Tri-Active versus VelaSmooth. The VelaSmooth is based on a combination of two different ranges of electromagnetic energy, which produce heat: infrared (IR) light (700–2000 nm) and bipolar RF combined with mechanical manipulation of the skin and has also been demonstrated to improve the appearance of cellulite (see below). Patients were treated twice a week for 6 weeks with the randomization of Tri-Active on one side and VelaSmooth on the other side. There were a total of 12 treatments per leg. Cellulite grading was determined utilizing the four-stage Nurnberger–Muller scale; measurements of thigh circumference were taken before treatment and after the final treatment. Visual inspection and photographic grading were quantified and statistically examined.

In comparing efficacy between VelaSmooth treatment and Tri-Active treatment, they calculated a 28% versus a 30% improvement, respectively, in the upper thigh circumference measurements, whereas a 56% versus a 37% improvement was observed, respectively, in lower thigh circumference measurements. These differences in treatment efficacy, using the thigh circumference measurements, were not found to be significant ($p > 0.05$). Based on before and after blinded photographic evaluations, we found 25% (5 of 19) of the subjects showed improvement in cellulite appearance for both Tri-Active and VelaSmooth. The average percent improvement based on random photography grading from a scale of 1–5 (1 = no improvement, 5 = most improvement) for the VelaSmooth versus Tri-Active was 7% and 25%, respectively. This difference was also found not to be significant ($p = 0.091$). Perceived change grade was also calculated based on random side-by-side comparisons of before and after photographs. Seventy-five percent (15 of 19) subjects showed improvement in the VelaSmooth leg, whereas 55% (11 of 19) subjects showed improvement in the Tri-Active leg. The average mean percent improvement was roughly the same for both treatments (22% and 20%, respectively) and showed no statistically significant difference ($p > 0.05$).

Incidence of bruising was reported in 60% of the subjects. Bruising incidence and intensity were 30% higher in the VelaSmooth leg than in the Tri-Active leg. Seven of 20 subjects reported bruising with VelaSmooth, 1 subject reported bruising with Tri-Active, and 3 reported bruising with both VelaSmooth and Tri-Active. The extent of bruising ranged from minor purpura to larger and diffused bruises, which lasted for an average of a week with no intervention. This study revealed that both machines effectively reduced the appearance of cellulite; however, when using a P value of 0.05, there was no statistically significant difference between using either the Tri-Active or the VelaSmooth in the reduction of cellulite. The Tri-Active provides low-energy diode laser, contact cooling, suction, and massage, whereas the VelaSmooth provides a combination of two different ranges of electromagnetic energy: IR light and RF combined with mechanical manipulation of the skin. After twice weekly treatment for 6 weeks, there was no statistical significance between the two units in upper or lower thigh circumference measurements, randomized photographic evaluations, or perceived change in before and after photographic evaluations. Incidence and extent of bruising were higher for VelaSmooth than for Tri-Active (16).

SmoothShapes

SmoothShapes (Cynosure, Inc., Westford, Massachusetts, USA) is a Food and Drug Administration (FDA)-cleared device for the temporary improvement in the appearance of cellulite, which employs the application of dual wavelengths of laser energy (650 and 915 nm) along with vacuum and massage.

Neira et al., investigated the effects of low-level laser energy on adipose tissue. This group demonstrated when adipocyte cells were exposed to a 635-nm wavelength, a transitory pore was produced within the adipocyte membrane releasing fat into the intracellular space (17). Pore formation in the adipocyte membrane was repeated in another controlled study (18). As a result, the 650-nm wavelength was chosen for its action in enhancing adipocytes' membrane permeability and fat emulsification. Of note, the 650-nm wavelength has minimal absorption in the epidermis and dermis, which allows for enhanced penetration into the subcutaneous tissue. The

915-nm wavelength shows less scattering than 650 nm and is preferentially absorbed by the lipids in fat cells. A temperature rise within the adipocytes results in fat liquefaction. Both wavelengths are reported to stimulate neocollagenesis and improve blood and lymphatic circulation. Tissue manipulation, using vacuum and massage, enhances the transference of the liquefied fat within adipocytes into the intracellular spaces along with improving circulation of blood and lymphatic fluid.

The most current SmoothShapes treatment head (also known as the Photomology™ module) consists of two rollers, a vacuum chamber, four 650-nm light-emitting diodes (LEDs) (1 W), and eight 915-nm laser diodes (15 W) in a 90 mm × 90 mm dimension. Prior models delivered maximum energies of 1 W from the 650-nm LED and 10 W from the 915-nm diodes. Subcutaneous tissue up to 10 mm in depth is heated via the dual laser energy with surface temperatures remaining below 40°C.

Ecchymoses, erythema, edema, pain, burn, abrasions, scaling, infection, dyspigmentation, and scarring are adverse effects from SmoothShapes.

The suction level is recommended not to exceed 500 mbar (375 mmHg). When initiating treatment, the treatment head is placed on the skin surface and then moved across the treatment area. Each treatment area (e.g., posterior thigh, lateral thigh, anterior thigh) is approximately 8.5 in. × 11 in. The time of each treatment area can be selected with a maximum treatment time of 30 minutes and a default time of 10 minutes (SmoothShapes XV User Manual, 2010).

To date, the majority of SmoothShapes clinical trials have investigated the volumetric effects of SmoothShapes in patients with cellulite, as graded by circumferential reduction and magnetic resonance imaging (MRI), but not the improvement in the appearance of cellulite itself (19–21). In the study by Lach et al., 88.9% of subjects who completed the study reported that they were "somewhat" or "definitely" pleased with the results of their treatment (19). In a study by Fournier et al. (abstract presented at the 2009 ASLMS annual meeting), they performed 8–12 biweekly treatments using the 915-nm (10 W) and 650-nm (1 W) SmoothShapes device to evaluate the effects on cellulite. Thirty female patients, Fitzpatrick skin types I–V, with mild-to-moderate cellulite of the thighs were enrolled in this split-leg study, utilizing the untreated leg as the control. The group reported a high level of patient satisfaction was achieved (22).

The SmoothShapes was performed on 20 women, skin types II–VI, with mild-to-moderate lateral thigh cellulite in a study by Kulick. Patients received biweekly treatments for 4 weeks with the application of the Photomology™ treatment head for 15 minutes per lateral thigh. Energy was delivered at the maximum settings (1 W 650 nm, 10 W 915 nm). Photographic evaluations were performed with standard digital photography and three-dimensional (3D) digital photography at baseline and at 1, 3, and 6 months after the final treatment. Textural images for all patients were developed from the 3D digital photography computer database (23).

The author reported improved resolution of textural changes with the 3D digital photography system. Physician-rated improvement was seen in 82% of subjects at 1 month and 76% at both 3 and 6 months posttreatment. Seventeen patients completed the study, and no adverse events were reported. Textural images showed elevations of depressed areas and reduction of surface bulges. Computer-generated volumetric analysis demonstrated a decrease in thigh volume. At 6 months after the final treatment, 94% of subjects reported sustained improvement in the appearance of cellulite. Percentile improvements based on quartile scales or a similar grading system was not performed (23). Further studies evaluating the clinical appearance of cellulite are necessitated.

RF Energy Devices

VelaSmooth

VelaSmooth (Syneron Medical Ltd., Yokneam Illit, Israel) is based on a combination of two different ranges of electromagnetic energy, which produce heat: IR light and RF, known as ELOS.

VelaSmooth was the first energy-based medical device to be approved by the FDA for reducing the appearance of cellulite. It is a device that combines controlled IR light (700–2000 nm, in the most current model) and conducted bipolar RF energies with mechanical manipulation of the skin to improve the appearance of cellulite (24–26). In the most current model, the VelaSmooth peak optical energy is 35 W and peak RF energy is 60 W. Prior models had a peak optical energy of 12.5–20 W and a peak RF energy of 20–50 W.

By combining RF energy with optical energy, the required amount of optical energy may be reduced. As a result, the majority of skin types can be successfully treated as RF does not target melanin and therefore the epidermal heating is reduced. Manipulation is provided via vacuum suction and mechanical rollers in a 40 mm × 40 mm applicator head.

Before initiating treatment, the skin should be cleaned. Conductive lotion is applied to the treatment area and gel should never be used. Once rehydrated, the skin does not need constant reapplication of conductive lotion even if it appears dry; the electrode rollers will remain coupled to the skin as long as proper pressure and contact are made by the operator. However, additional lotion should be applied during treatment if the applicator becomes difficult to move across the treatment area. Proper applicator seal to the skin surface is indicated by a lack of air being heard sucked into the chamber in addition to a nonflashing light indicator on the applicator. For the effective and safe delivery of RF energy, ensure the RF rollers maintain equal compression and contact with the skin surface.

Each treatment area (i.e., posterior thigh, anterior thigh, inner thigh, outer thigh/hip, buttocks) should be treated for 5 minutes with three to six passes of the VelaSmooth applicator. The targeted end point is significant erythema and warmth (40–42°C, which is maintained for 5–10 minutes) of the treatment area. The time for each treatment session is approximately 20–30 minutes per side of the body. With the most current model of VelaSmooth, the manufacturer recommends treatments once a week for 4–6 weeks; however, the majority of studies have been performed using earlier, less powerful models, using biweekly treatments for 4 weeks (24–27).

All three parameters on this device can be independently adjusted to tailor treatment to each patient's needs. The treatment levels on all three components range from 1 to 3. To maximize the effectiveness of the device for the treatment of cellulite, areas should be treated with the highest levels of light and RF (as tolerated by the patient) with a vacuum level of 1–2, except in the following situations. All treatment levels

should never be simultaneously set at maximum parameters. In skin types IV–VI or tanned skin, the light should be set to 1–2. If the patient does not experience lasting erythema or excessive heat, the level may be increased to 2–3 and the skin response reevaluated. To increase the degree of patient comfort in sensitive areas, such as the inner thighs and abdomen, the vacuum can be adjusted to a level 1 or 2. Adverse events include erythema, pain, edema, bullae formation, scabbing, ecchymoses, postinflammatory hyperpigmentation, and scarring (24,25,27,28).

Thirty-five female patients with cellulite of the thighs and/or buttocks were treated in a two-arm, multicenter study by Sadick and Mulholland. The first group (n = 20) received biweekly treatments for 4 weeks, whereas the second group (n = 15) received biweekly treatments for 8 weeks. All patients were treated with maximum tolerance parameters for all energies (RF maximum energy 20 W and optical maximum energy of 20 W). Two patients developed crusting, which resolved within 3 days. All patients were evaluated on a quartile scale for percent improvement from baseline to 3–4 weeks after the last treatment session. All patients demonstrated some improvement in the appearance of cellulite. However, patients treated with 16 treatments achieved higher levels of physician-graded improvement, corresponding to a 50–75% or 75–100% improvement (25).

Alster and Tanzi investigated 20 patients with moderate thigh and buttock cellulite using biweekly VelaSmooth (20-W RF, 20-W IR) treatments for 4 weeks. This study was conducted in a randomized, split-leg manner with the untreated leg serving as the control. Physician-graded improvement was based on a quartile scale, similar to Sadick et al. Ten percent of patients experienced ecchymoses. Ninety percent of subjects experienced improvement in the appearance of cellulite on the treated leg, with a mean improvement of nearly 50% at 1 month after the last treatment. All but one of these subjects was interested in receiving treatments to the control leg. Of note, at 3 and 6 months after the last treatment, the physician-graded improvement scale decreased to approximately 35% and 25%, respectively (24).

Sixteen patients were treated with biweekly treatments for thigh cellulite for 4 weeks in a study by Kulick. All patients were treated with maximal machine parameters using an RF energy of 20 W and optical energy of 12.5 W. All patients were followed for 6 months after their last treatment. Transient erythema occurred posttreatment in all patients. Bruising occurred in 32.25% of subjects but resolved within a week. A single patient sustained a second-degree burn. At 3 and 6 months after the last treatment, the mean investigator-graded improvement scores were 62% and 50%, respectively. At both time points, all patients graded their cellulite to be improved over 25% (27).

In a study by Boey, 17 women received VelaSmooth (using the earlier, low-energy model) treatments for mild-to-moderate cellulite on thighs, buttocks, and abdomen. The mean investigator-graded improvement from baseline was 32.9%, whereas the mean subject-graded improvement from baseline was 30.6%. Follow-up times and a description of the treatment regimen were not provided. Bruising was reported in 58.8% of patients but no crusting. The majority of patients experienced temporary erythema and edema (28).

Twenty patients with thigh and buttock cellulite were randomized to receive 12 biweekly VelaSmooth treatments in a split-leg fashion. Of the 16 patients who completed the study, 31.25% experienced bruising at some point during the study. At 4 and 8 weeks after the last treatment, 50% (at both time points) of subjects had over 25% improvement in the appearance of cellulite in the treated leg, as graded by the investigator's quartile-based scale. At 4 and 8 weeks after the last treatment, 50% and 68.75%, respectively, of subjects had over 25% improvement in the appearance of cellulite in the treated leg, as graded by an independent investigator-evaluated, quartile-based scale. At 8 weeks of follow-up, 31.25% of patients had greater than 51% improvement in the appearance of cellulite in the treated leg as graded by the independent investigator (26).

Similar, split-anatomic controlled studies with the 20-W RF and 20-W IR VelaSmooth have continued to show improvement in the appearance of cellulite as rated by investigator-based (29,30) and subject-based (29) grading scales. Many authors have recommended monthly maintenance treatments to help sustain the clinical improvements (24,29).

VelaShape

VelaShape (Syneron Medical Ltd., Yokneam Illit, Israel) is an FDA class II-cleared device for the noninvasive temporary circumferential reduction in thigh size and temporary cellulite reduction, based on the same combination of bipolar RF, IR light (700–2000 nm), vacuum, and mechanical tissue manipulation as the original VelaSmooth device. The VelaShape platform combines the previous VelaSmooth treatment head along with a smaller (30 mm × 30 mm) treatment head, the VelaContour.

VelaShape II is a newer version of the original VelaShape, with 20% more power allowing for shorter treatment sessions, as well as an improved interface terminal to optimize treatments and facilitate device maintenance. The applicator heads have different energy and vacuum parameters. On the VelaShape II platform, the VelaContour is able to achieve up to 440 mbar of negative pressure, 20-W peak IR energy, and 23-W peak RF energy, whereas the VelaSmooth is able to achieve up to 380 mbar of negative pressure, 35-W IR energy, and 60-W RF energy. Instructions for the use of the VelaSmooth are identical to that listed above in the previous section. Additional instructions for VelaShape are as follows: large areas (such as the waist, hips, and thighs) are treated with the VelaSmooth applicator for the majority of the treatment session. In curved, small areas such as the lower abdomen and the periumbilical area, and/or over local fatty deposits, the VelaContour applicator is used instead. For the VelaContour, treatment is identical to the VelaSmooth; however, a 20% overlap is recommended with the VelaContour. With the new higher energy VelaShape II, treatments are delivered at weekly intervals (VelaShape II User Manual, 2009). Clinical studies with these newer devices are presently underway. In our office, we see a significant improvement over the VelaSmooth.

Accent

The Accent XL platform (Alma Lasers Ltd., Caesarea, Israel) consists of two treatment heads, one employing unipolar RF and the other bipolar RF, which is FDA-cleared for the treatment of wrinkles and rhytides. As compared with bipolar RF, unipolar RF is able to affect deeper structures (up to 15–20 mm) (31–33). The Accent XL UniPolar treatment head emits electromagnetic radiation, and heat production is generated through high-frequency (40.68 MHz) oscillations within water molecules. Heat is then subsequently transferred into neighboring tissues (32,33). Due to the increased depth of penetration, the unipolar treatment head has been investigated for the improvement of the appearance of cellulite (31,32).

Due to the lack of melanin absorption by RF energy, all skin types can be successfully treated (33). The Accent XL UniPolar treatment head has an integrated cooled treatment tip to increase patient comfort. The unipolar RF energy is delivered up to 200 W. Prior to initiation of treatment, mineral oil is applied to the treatment area. The operator moves the handpiece across the treatment (6 in. × 10 in. gridded) area in 30-second passes in a circular fashion. Consecutive passes are applied to the gridded area until the treatment end point (40–43°C, measured via IR thermometer) is achieved (34).

Treatment sessions are performed every other week for up to 3 to 4 months (34). Transient erythema is common and expected. Crusting, blistering, scarring, dyspigmentation, pain, and ecchymoses are potential adverse events associated with unipolar RF treatment (31–33).

Alexiades-Armenakas and colleagues assessed 10 female patients with cellulite distributed over the thighs using a novel cellulite grading scale (0–4), which reflected the appearance of contours and dimple depth, density, and distribution. In a randomized, split-leg manner, all patients received a mean of 4.22 (range, 3–6) treatments (administered every other week) to the investigational limb with the untreated leg serving as a control. Unipolar RF energy was emitted at 150–200 W per 30-second pass. Two blinded physicians assessed photographs at each treatment and 1 and 3 months after the last treatment. Three months after the final treatment, dimple density, distribution, and depth improved by 11.25%, 10.75%, and 1.75–2.5%, respectively. Overall, an average 7.83% improvement in the appearance of cellulite was discovered on the treated leg; however, statistical significance was not obtained. While the majority of patients demonstrated transient erythema, no episodes of scarring, crusting, or dyspigmentation developed (31).

Thirty patients with moderate-to-severe thigh cellulite were treated every other week for 3 months with 150–170 W of unipolar RF. All areas were treated with three passes and 30 seconds per pass. Patients were evaluated 6 months after the final treatment via photography, MRI, plasma lipids, and skin biopsy. No changes in plasma lipids or occurrence of blistering, dyspigmentation, or scarring were observed. MRI evaluations at the conclusion of the study failed to reveal a change in the subcutaneous tissue. Fibroplasia of the dermis was noted on histologic examination at 6 months after the final treatment. No changes were present in the subcutaneous tissue on histology. Using standardized digital photography, performed at baseline and 6 months after the final treatment, the mean cellulite improvement was 2.9 (as graded on a 4-point scale). The authors concluded the longevity of results seen in this study was due to the induction of dermal fibroplasias (32). Although studies have revealed a good safety profile with unipolar RF, there is a general lack of consensus regarding the efficacy in the improvement of the clinical appearance of cellulite (31,32).

Thermage

Thermage (Solta Medical, Inc., Hayward, California, USA) delivers monopolar RF through a cooled epidermis and superficial dermis to the deeper dermis, creating thermal damage. It is proposed that the remodeling of deep dermal collagen (fibrous septa) allows modeling of contours and improvement of cellulite appearance in a single treatment. Thermage has FDA clearance for the noninvasive treatment of wrinkles and rhytides, as well as temporary improvement in the appearance of cellulite when used with vibration. The new Comfort Pulsed Technology (CPT) enables energy delivery in short, rapid pulses at varying energy levels, which patients find tolerable. The depth of penetration of the RF, the depth of damage, and hence remodeling depend on the type of tip used in the machine and the energy delivered by the machine through the tip.

The device has three main components: a generator, a cryogen unit, and a hand piece with a treatment tip. The generator supplies the RF and monitors through a display unit the output current, output energy, number of treatments, duration of treatment, and impedance (35,38). The Thermage Cellulite Tip 3.0 (CL) is utilized for cellulite treatments (36). Prior to initiation of treatment, a return pad is applied to the patient, allowing the generator to supply the monopolar RF in a closed circuit between the device and the patient. A temporary marking grid is applied so that the operator can place the treatment tip accurately for each pulse. Coupling lubricant is then applied. Before beginning the treatment, the patient's individual impedance is automatically measured by the system (35,38). Treatment levels typically employed range from 372.5 to 374. The operator delivers two staggered consecutive passes to the full treatment area, and the remaining treatment passes are used at the providers' discretion on vectors needing greater skin contouring. In general, energy levels between 27 and 44 J/cm² are used with an average of 900 pulses when the area above the knee or small thigh areas are treated bilaterally. Larger thigh areas and upper thigh and buttocks may need two to three staggered passes plus vectors, requiring up to 1800 total pulses between two sides. It is estimated that the device heats tissue to 65–75°C, the critical temperature at which collagen denaturation occurs (36–38). The device has a feedback mechanism to alert the user if maximum temperatures have been reached in a particular area, so that the area is avoided. It also features a feedback system to notify the user if there is insufficient contact with the skin. The lateral aspects of the abdomen, inner thighs, and under arms are sensitive sites (35,38).

No further treatments are advisable within 6 months. Treatment may be repeated yearly. In addition to the adverse events associated with unipolar RF treatments, mentioned above, inconsistent results, blistering, scarring, development of temporary nodules and swellings, and contour irregularities have been reported with the older machines, particularly over the temporal or cheek regions, where there possibly has been fat atrophy because of the elevated energy levels and single-pass protocols once used.

No studies have been published on the use of the older Thermacool Thermage system or CPT system for the treatment of cellulite and/or subcutaneous tissues of the buttocks and thighs.

Exilis

Exilis (BTL Industries, Inc., Prague, Czech Republic), a device combines monopolar RF and ultrasonic energy, was introduced to the market with FDA clearance for the noninvasive treatment of wrinkles and rhytides in 2009. Animal studies in porcine tissue have demonstrated that a penetration depth of 30 mm is safely obtainable. The Exilis body treatment head has a cooling tip, constant temperature monitoring of the skin surface via an integrated IR thermometer, and adjustable RF (W) energy control. Peak monopolar RF energy and ultrasonic energy are 120 W and 3 W/cm², respectively. The integrated "Energy Flow Control System" eliminates peaks of RF energy. A unique feature of this device, as compared with other RF devices, is the sensor monitors for constant contact between the skin surface and the applicator. If the treatment head is removed from the skin surface during treatment, arcing, pain, blistering, or a burn will not result (39).

Anecdotally, this device has been used off-label for improvement in the appearance of cellulite; however, randomized clinical trials are lacking. For the treatment of cellulite, the treatment area is divided into 20 cm × 10 cm sections. The grounding electrode is placed adjacent to the zone of treatment and mineral oil is applied to the skin surface within the gridded area. The cooling tip is adjusted to 10°C and the treatment head is moved continuously in a circular array within the 200 cm² grid. Fifty watts is the recommended starting RF energy and should be increased over 1 minute until a surface temperature of 40–41°C is reached. Once attainment of the targeted temperature end point, treatment is continued for an additional 3 minutes to maintain the skin surface at 40–41°C while the RF energy is simultaneously decreased. The average treatment time per grid is 6 minutes, with a total treatment time of 30 minutes per session. Treatments are administered weekly for 3–4 weeks. For the following 48 hours after treatment, the patient is encouraged to increase their fluid intake, which enhances treatment efficacy by allowing degraded adipose tissue by products to be eliminated (Exilis User Manual, 2009). Further studies are necessitated to investigate the effects of Exilis on the appearance of cellulite.

TriPollar

TriPollar (Pollogen Ltd., Tel Aviv, Israel) combined three RF electrodes to deliver low-level (5–30 W) RF energy into the dermis and subcutaneous tissues at a depth of up to 20 mm to produce volumetric heating for immediate collagen contraction and neocollagenesis. The depth of heating is roughly equivalent to the mean difference between the spacing of the RF electrodes. The polarity of the three electrodes is in constant, alternating rotation between all electrodes (i.e., all electrodes have the capability to act as positive or negative, although one is always positive and two are negative), to avoid overheating of the positive electrode. Cutaneous cooling is not required with this device (40). Of note, this product has not received FDA clearance for usage on the body at the time of this writing (January 2013).

Prior to treatment, the skin surface is cleansed and dried. Glycerin oil is applied to the treatment area and then the treatment head is glided across the skin surface in either circular or linear strokes. Erythema and warmth during treatment is expected. Skin temperature should be monitored with an IR thermometer to prevent surface temperatures rising above 40–42°C; once the target temperature is obtained (40), treatment is continued for an additional 2 minutes (41). Treatments are administered weekly for 6–8 weeks, and monthly maintenance treatments are encouraged. Adverse events include erythema (although expected and transient), burn, bruising, and mild discomfort during treatment (40).

The only study on cellulite was performed by Manuskiatti on 39 patients with mild-to-severe cellulite involving the arms, abdomen, buttocks, or thighs. Treatments were administered weekly for eight treatments using 20–28.5 W total per treatment. Thirty-seven patients (81 anatomic sites) completed the study. One month after the final treatment session, nearly a 50% mean improvement in the clinical appearance of cellulite, as graded by a blinded investigator, was discovered (41).

In a study using classic and high-frequency ultrasound to evaluate the effectiveness of another tripolar RF device, the T1 Tripolar RF Beauty Machine (Beauty Light Science and Technology Co., Ltd., Beijing, China) for anticellulite treatment, cellulite was reduced in 89.27% of the 28 women who underwent treatment (42). Eight treatments were administered weekly. Ultrasound images were taken before initiating therapy and 4 weeks after the last treatment. The following structures were evaluated using high-frequency ultrasound: epidermal thickness, dermal thickness, dermal echogenicity, the length of the subcutaneous tissue bands growing into the dermis, and the presence/absence of edema. When compared with the placebo group ($n = 17$), there was statistically significant reduction in both epidermal and dermal thickness in the RF-treated group ($p = 0.006$). There was also a statistically significant increase in dermal echogenicity, decrease in the length of the subcutaneous tissue bands growing into the dermis, and decrease in the presence/absence of edema, as well as decrease in the stage of cellulite as measured by Nurnberger–Muller scale ($p \leq 0.001$). The placebo group showed no statistically significant changes in the above parameters. This device is not FDA approved for use in the USA.

Laser Energy Devices
Cellulaze
Cellulaze (CelluLaze, Cynosure, Inc., Westford, Massachusetts, USA) is a pulsed laser that delivers 1440-nm energy internally to the dermal–hypodermal interface via a fiber. Energy is delivered to the subdermal tissue through a 600-μm "side-firing" fiber (SideLight 3D, Cynosure, Inc.) enclosed in a 1-mm cannula and extending 1–2 mm beyond the distal end of the cannula. The side-firing fiber delivers approximately half its laser energy perpendicular to the fiber axis as the other half moves forward along the axis. The transient bubble on the distal tip creates an air–glass interface in the tissue and deflects the beam. A thermal camera ThermaCAM E45, FLIR, Niceville, Florida, USA) is used to monitor skin surface temperature. This makes it possible to thermally subscise hypodermal septa, thermally denature adipocytes protruding into the dermis, stimulate neocollagenesis at the dermal–hypodermal junction, resulting in thickened and tightened skin, and selectively melt hypodermal adipocytes in the risen areas of the skin (43). Of note, this product has not received FDA clearance at the time of this writing (September 2011).

Prior to treatment the skin is marked with the patient standing. The target area is divided into square sectors (5 cm × 5 cm) and each sector is treated individually. The treatment area is anesthetized with tumescent lidocaine solution. The laser cannula is inserted via an incision made with a trocar or blade close to the target area. A red aiming beam from an He:Ne laser source allows one to visualize the tip of the fiber during treatment. The cannula is gently positioned below the skin surface and the procedure is then divided into three steps, with the fiber in the *down*, *horizontal*, and *up* positions. The fiber is first placed in the *down* position (1–2 cm beneath the skin), once in place the cannula-fiber unit is moved back and forth in a fan-like pattern until the delivered energy totals 300–600 J. When all selected raised sectors are treated, the fiber position is changed to *horizontal* direction, with the side-firing energy parallel to the skin surface (rather than perpendicular). In this step, energy is delivered only to areas premarked as dimples, with the horizontal fiber moving in a fan-like pattern and in the same plane. The end point in this second step is loss of resistance as the cannula passes through the tissue, indicating that the septa no longer connect the dermal and muscle layers. The fiber is then set at *up* and positioned 2–3 mm below the skin surface, just under the dermal–hypodermal interface. All sectors are then uniformly treated. Total treatment time (including pretreatment and posttreatment care) is approximately 90 minutes, depending on the area treated. Once the laser treatment is complete, the liquefied adipocytes are removed by gently squeezing the incision point tissue. Standard pressure dressings are applied to the treated areas, and patients are instructed to wear a compression garment for 2 to 3 weeks. Results from treatment can persist for up to 1 year (43). Adverse events include mild discomfort, bruising, swelling, and numbness, which typically resolve after 3 months (43).

In a study on 10 healthy women with moderate-to-severe cellulite involving their thighs (lateral, posterior, or both), participants received a single treatment with the CelluLaze system to one thigh, while the other served as a control, using power settings at 8–10 W and pulse frequency at 40 Hz (43,44). Surface temperatures reached 40°C and 42°C during treatment. Delivered energy ranged from 300 J for raised areas and dimples measuring 3 cm × 3 cm to 600 J for raised areas and dimples measuring 5 cm × 5 cm. An average subdermal temperature below 47°C was monitored and maintained by a temperature-sensing cannula (ThermaGuide, Cynosure, Inc.) attached to the laser cannula. To ensure uniform delivery of energy during treatment, an accelerometer (SmartSense A, Cynosure, Inc.) is attached to the laser hand piece, which causes the energy level to decrease (if the motion of the hand piece is slowed) or increase (if the hand piece is moved more rapidly); if the hand piece stops moving, energy delivery ceases within 0.2 seconds. Mean skin thickness (as shown by ultrasound) and skin elasticity were shown by objective measurements to increase significantly at 1, 3, 6, and 12 months. Subjective physician and subject evaluations on cellulite reduction, skin texture, and satisfaction at 1 year were roughly equal to those, if not greater, than at 3 and 6 months.

Laser-Assisted Lipolysis for the Treatment of Cellulite

Laser-assisted lipolysis (LAL) is indicated for body contouring (45). While some physicians use exclusively LAL without liposuction, others feel that it is best served as an adjunct to liposuction (46,47). With traditional liposuction, the improvement in appearance of cellulite is modest to say the least and in certain instances may exacerbate cellulite (48). Due to the simultaneous capabilities of LAL to emulsify fat and stimulate neocollagenesis, resulting in skin shrinkage and tightening (45,46,49–51), it was extrapolated that this technology may have a role in the treatment of cellulite.

Goldman and colleagues investigated a combination approach of laser lipolysis using a pulsed 1064-nm neodymium-doped:yttrium-aluminum-garnet (SmartLipo, Deka, Calenzo, Italy) and autologous fat transplantation in 52 females with moderate-to-severe cellulite of the hips, buttocks, thighs, flanks, and/or abdomen. Fat was manually harvested via syringe aspiration from a site distant to the areas treated with LAL. An average volume of 240 mL of centrifuged adipose tissue was then transferred to the depressed areas with a 10–15% overcorrection. Ecchymoses and edema were common, but no burns or infections occurred. At 1 year postoperatively, patient evaluation of improvement was greater than 75% in 30.8% of patients and 51–75% in 53.8% of patients. Although patient satisfaction was high, the isolated effect of the laser was unknown (48).

In a small study by Palm and Goldman, nine patients (11 sites) received treatment with either LAL (CoolLipo, CoolTouch, Inc., Roseville, California, USA) or mechanical disruption with a liposuction microcannula. At the conclusion of the study, there was no difference in the efficacy between the two treatment regimens with both groups improving by 1 point on a 4-point investigator-evaluated scale. Patient evaluated improvement did not differ between the two regimens (52). Furthermore, larger studies will be needed to investigate the effects of LAL alone in the management of cellulite.

Radiofrequency-Assisted Lipolysis for the Treatment of Cellulite

BodyTite (Invasix, Inc., Yokneam, Israel) uses a bipolar RF device with one electrode on the skin and one RF electrode under the skin immediately in the subdermal and hypodermal area. The internal cannula is coated with dielectric material and has a conductive tip that emits RF energy into the adipose tissue toward the skin surface, while the external electrode moves along the surface of the skin delivering RF energy (53). Areas to be contoured are divided into 10 cm × 15 cm sections and up to 50 W of RF power is applied between the two electrodes. The RF energy coagulates the adipose, connective, and vascular tissues in the vicinity of the internal cannula tip and gently heats the dermis below the external electrode. The internal electrode also serves as an internal suction cannula, aspirating the coagulated adipose, vascular, and fibrous tissues. Real-time epidermal temperatures are continuously provided by a builtin thermal sensor in the external electrode. Target temperatures are set at 38–42°C, and maintained for 1–3 minutes (53,54). FDA clearance is presently pending on the device and is only available in the USA through investigational studies. The RF CelluTite applicator (Invasix, Inc., Yokneam, Israel) is specifically designed to target cellulite by treating in the immediate hypodermal space, which results in an enhanced collagen barrier in the deep hypodermis, improving the appearance of cellulite, both clinically and histologically (55). Presently only anecdotal reports exist, and randomized clinical trials are lacking (55).

The incidence of thermal injury reported with the Invasix internal and external device is less than 1%; however, the technique is very user sensitive (55).

CONCLUSION

In short, cellulite is a normal female sexual characteristic that cannot be "cured." It has only been brought to the attention of the female population as a condition to be treated by the mass media. However, as cosmetic dermatologists, we have developed a variety of methods to improve the appearance of cellulite. While this improvement is temporary, it may last for several months. Thus, patients who wish to have smoother skin with less visible cellulite can have a series of treatments and then return for additional treatments as necessary. Future research will try and extend both treatment efficacy and duration. The extent of research will be stimulated by the public's demand for treatment.

REFERENCES

1. Draelos ZD, Marenus KD. Cellulite—etiology and purported treatment. Dermatol Surg 1997; 23: 1177–81.
2. Avram MM. Cellulite: a review of its physiology and treatment. J Cosmet Laser Ther 2004; 6: 181–5.
3. Goldman MP. Cellulite: a review of current treatments. Cosmet Dermatol 2002; 15: 17–20.
4. Querleux B, Cornillon C, Jolivet O, et al. Anatomy and physiology of subcutaneous adipose tissue by in vivo magnetic resonance imaging and spectroscopy: relationships with sex and presence of cellulite. Skin Res Technol 2002; 8: 118–24.
5. Rossi ABR, Vergnanini AL. Cellulite: a review. J Eur Acad Dermatol Venerol 2000; 14: 251–62.
6. Nurnberger F, Muller G. So-called cellulite: an invented disease. J Dermatol Surg Oncol 1978; 4: 221–9.
7. Pierard GE, Nizet JL, Pierard-Franchimont C. Cellulite: from standing fat herniation to hypodermal stretch marks. Am J Dermatopathol 2000; 22: 34–47.
8. Pellicier F, Andre P, Schnebert S. The adipocyte in the history of slimming agents. Pathol Biol 2003; 51: 244–7.
9. Salter DC, Hanley M, Tynan A, et al. In-vivo high-definition ultrasound studies of subdermal fat lobules associated with cellulite. J Invest Dermatol 1990; 29: 272–4.
10. Sainio EL, Rantanen T, Kanerva L. Ingredients and safety of cellulite creams. Eur J Dermatol 2000; 10: 596–603.
11. Rao J, Goldman MP. A double-blinded randomized trial testing the tolerability and efficacy of a novel topical agent with and without occlusion for the treatment of cellulite: A study and review of the literature. J Drugs Dermatol 2004; 3: 417–27.
12. Goldman MP. The use of Tri-Active in the treatment of cellulite. In: Goldman MP, Hexsel D, eds. Cellulite: Pathophysiology and Treatment, 2nd edn. New York, NY: Informa Healthcare, 2010: 99.
13. Zerbinati N, Vergani R, Beltrami B, et al. The TriActive system; a simple and effective way of combating cellulite. Internal study conducted by Deka 2002.
14. Boyce S, Pabby A, Chuchaltkaren P, et al. Clinical evaluation of a device for the treatment of cellulite: triactive. Am J Cosmetic Surg 2005; 22: 233–7.
15. Gold M. The use of rhythmic suction massage, low level laser irradiation, and superficial cooling to effect changes in adipose tissue/cellulite. Laser Surg Med (Sup) 2006; 18: 65.

16. Nootheti PK, Magpantay A, Yosowitz G, et al. A single center, randomized, comparative, prospective clinical study to determine the efficacy of the VelaSmooth system versus the Triactive system for the treatment of cellulite. Lasers Surg Med 2006; 38: 908–12.

17. Quatresooz P, Xhauflaire-Uhoda E, Piérard-Franchimont C, et al. Cellulite histopathology and related mechanobiology. Int J Cosmet Sci 2006; 28: 207–10.

18. Smalls LK, Hicks M, Passeretti D, et al. Effect of weight loss on cellulite: gynoid lypodystrophy. Plast Reconstr Surg 2006; 118: 510.

19. Lach E. Reduction of subcutaneous fat and improvement in cellulite appearance by dual-wavelength, low-level laser energy combined with vacuum and massage. J Cosmet Laser Ther 2008; 10: 202–9.

20. Pankratov MM, Morton S. SmoothShapes treatment of cellulite and thigh circumference reduction: when less is more. In: Goldman MP, Hexsel D, eds. Cellulite: Pathophysiology and Treatment, 2nd edn. New York, NY: Informa Healthcare, 2010: 126.

21. Gold MH, Khatri KA, Hails K, Weiss RA, Fournier N. Reduction in thigh circumference and improvement in the appearance of cellulite with dual-wavelength, low-level laser energy and massage. J Cosmet Laser Ther 2011; 13: 13–20.

22. Fournier N, Pankratov M, Aubree AS, et al. Cellulite treatment with photomology technology. American Society for Laser Medicine and Surgery Meeting, 2009.

23. Kulick MI. Evaluation of a noninvasive, dual-wavelength laser-suction and massage device for the regional treatment of cellulite. Plast Reconstr Surg 2010; 125: 1788–96.

24. Alster TS, Tanzi EL. Cellulite treatment using a novel combination radiofrequency, infrared light, and mechanical tissue manipulation device. J Cosmet Laser Ther 2005; 7: 81–5.

25. Sadick NS, Mulholland RSA. Prospective clinical study to evaluate the efficacy and safety of cellulite treatment using the combination of optical and RF energies for subcutaneous tissue heating. J Cosmet Laser Ther 2004; 6: 187–90.

26. Sadick N, Magro C. A study evaluating the safety and efficacy of the VelaSmooth system in the treatment of cellulite. J Cosmet Laser Ther 2007; 9: 15–20.

27. Kulick M. Evaluation of the combination of radio frequency, infrared energy, and mechanical rollers with suction to improve skin surface irregularities (cellulite) in a limited treatment area. J Cosmet Laser Ther 2006; 8: 185–90.

28. Boey G. Cellulite treatment with a radiofrequency, infrared light, and tissue manipulation device. The American Society of Dermatologic Surgery Annual Meeting, 2006.

29. Romero C, Caballero N, Herrero M, et al. Effects of cellulite treatment with RF, IR light, mechanical massage and suction treating one buttock with the contralateral as a control. J Cosmet Laser Ther 2008; 10: 193–201.

30. Wanitphakdeedecha R, Manuskiatti W. Treatment of cellulite with a bipolar radiofrequency, infrared heat, and pulsatile suction device: a pilot study. J Cosmet Dermatol 2006; 5: 284–8.

31. Alexiades-Armenakas M, Dover JS, Arndt KA. Unipolar radiofrequency treatment to improve the appearance of cellulite. J Cosmet Laser Ther 2008; 10: 148–53.

32. Goldberg DJ, Fazeli A, Berlin AL. Clinical, laboratory, and MRI analysis of cellulite treatment with a unipolar radiofrequency device. Dermatol Surg 2008; 34: 204–9.

33. Del Pino ME, Rosado RH, Azulea A, et al. Effect of controlled volumetric tissue heating with radiofrequency on cellulite and the subcutaneous tissue of the buttocks and thighs. J Drugs Dermatol 2006; 5: 709–17.

34. Unaeze J, Goldberg DJ. Accent unipolar radiofrequency. In: Goldman MP, Hexsel D, eds. Cellulite: Pathophysiology and Treatment, 2nd edn. New York, NY: Informa Healthcare, 2010: 115.

35. Hodgkinson DJ. Clinical applications of radiofrequency: nonsurgical skin tightening (Thermage). Clin Plast Surg 2009; 36: 261–8; viii.

36. Arnoczky SP, Aksan A. Thermal modification of connective tissues: basic science considerations and clinical implications. J Am Acad Orthop Surg 2000; 8: 305–13.

37. Sukal SA, Geronemus RG. Thermage: the nonablative radiofrequency for rejuvenation. Clin Dermatol 2008; 26: 602–7.

38. Polder KD, Bruce S. Radiofrequency: thermage. Facial Plast Surg Clin North Am 2011; 19: 347–59.

39. Simotova P, Berankova B. Evaluation of non-invasive body sculpting method based on novel efficient application of high-frequency energy administered to human adipose tissue. Journal of Czecho-Slovak Association of Anti-Aging Medicine; 2009; 2: 21–4.

40. Manuskiatti W. TriPollar radiofrequency. In: Goldman MP, Hexsel D, eds. Cellulite: Pathophysiology and Treatment, 2nd edn. New York, NY: Informa Healthcare, 2010: 158.

41. Manuskiatti W, Wachirakaphan C, Lektrakul N, et al. Circumference reduction and cellulite treatment with a TriPollar radiofrequency device: a pilot study. J Eur Acad Dermatol Venereol 2009; 23: 820–7.

42. Mlosek RK, Woźniak W, Malinowska S, Lewandowski M, Nowicki A. The effectiveness of anticellulite treatment using tripolar radiofrequency monitored by classic and high-frequency ultrasound. J Eur Acad Dermatol Venereol 2012; 26: 696–703.

43. DiBernardo BE. Treatment of cellulite using a 1440-nm pulsed laser with one-year follow-up. Aesthet Surg J 2011; 31: 328–41.

44. Burns AJ. Commentary on: Treatment of cellulite using a 1440-nm pulsed laser with one-year follow-up: preliminary report. Aesthet Surg J 2011; 31: 342–3.

45. Goldman A, Gotkin RH. Laser-assisted liposuction. Clin Plast Surg 2009; 36: 241–53.

46. Badin AZD, Moraes LM, Gondek L, Chiaratti MG, Canta L. Laser lipolysis: flaccidity under control. Aesthet Plast Surg 2002; 26: 335–9.

47. Kim KH, Geronemus RG. Laser lipolysis using a novel 1064 nm Nd:YAG laser. Dermatol Surg 2006; 32: 241–8.

48. Goldman A, Gotkin RH, Sarnoff DS, Prati C, Rossato F. Cellulite: a new treatment approach combining subdermal Nd:YAG laser lipolysis and autologous fat transplantation. Aesthet Surg J 2008; 28: 656–62.

49. Katz B, McBean J. The new laser liposuction for men. Dermatol Ther 2007; 20: 448–51.

50. Katz B, McBean J. Laser-assisted lipolysis: a report on complications. J Cosmet Laser Ther 2008; 10: 231–3.

51. DiBernardo BE. Randomized, blinded split abdomen study evaluating skin shrinkage and skin tightening in laser-assisted liposuction versus liposuction control. Aesthet Surg J 2010; 30: 593–602.

52. Palm MD, Goldman MP. Presented at the American Society of Dermatologic Surgery National Meeting, 2009.

53. Paul MD, Mulholland RS. A new approach for adipose tissue treatment and body contouring using radiofrequency-assisted liposuction. Aesthetic Plast Surg 2009; 33: 687–94.

54. Paul M, Blugerman G, Kreindel M, Mulholland RS. Three-dimensional radiofrequency tissue tightening: a proposed mechanism and applications for body contouring. Aesthet Plast Surg 2011; 35: 87–95.

55. Mulholland RS, Paul MD, Chalfoun C. Noninvasive body contouring with radiofrequency, ultrasound, cryolipolysis, and low-level laser therapy. Clin Plast Surg 2011; 38: 503–20.

16 Anesthesia for cutaneous laser surgery

Mitchel P. Goldman, Sabrina G. Fabi, and Jennifer G. Wojtczak

CHILDREN

Laser surgery can be uncomfortable, both for adults and for children. Some laser treatments can be accomplished without anesthesia, depending on the location, extent of the lesion, and age and cooperation of the patient. Certain treatments are limited because of the pain experienced by the patient. This phenomenon is particularly evident in the treatment of vascular malformations in children, particularly port-wine stains (PWS) and especially with large surface areas. Both children and adults often complain of increased perception of pain with each subsequent treatment. The reason for this increased pain perception remains to be elucidated; however, several potential explanations exist.

PWS have been shown to be derived from a progressive ectasia of the superficial vascular plexus. One hypothesis on the etiology of PWS stresses the importance of a near absence of sympathetic innervation, which modulates blood flow, possibly leading to defective maturation of the cutaneous sympathetic component and forming the basis for this progressive vascular ectasia (1,2). One would assume that as the lesion lightens (losing its target vascularity), less laser energy would be absorbed, leading to less pain. However, as previously noted, patients often note that, as lesions lighten, successive treatments actually result in a slight increase in their perception of pain. This increased pain perception may occur because treating PWS reestablishes a normal vessel growth pattern leading to normalization of vessel innervation. Regardless of the exact reason for this phenomenon, treating vascular malformations with minimal pain in children is an important dilemma facing laser surgeons.

Nonetheless, the use of anesthetics in children undergoing cutaneous laser surgery remains a controversial issue, and its use is left to the discretion of the treating physician (3–9). Painful laser treatments are made more tolerable by the use of different anesthetic techniques. Anesthesia may be delivered simply by precooling the lesion, applying a topical anesthetic or administering intralesional/block anesthesia using 1% lidocaine with or without epinephrine. Larger lesions in young children may be more effectively managed with the aid of general anesthesia or sedation. These anesthetic modalities along with their advantages and disadvantages are detailed below.

The surgeon must balance the advantages and disadvantages when deciding to use anesthesia. If the treating physician decides to use anesthesia, he or she must then decide which anesthetic modality to use. The list of criteria below will help discern physicians which anesthetic type would be most appropriate (3,8):

1. patient's age
2. patient's medical history
3. patient and family preference
4. duration of procedure
5. skill and experience of anesthesiologist in different technique options
6. availability of appropriate monitoring equipment, medications, emergency equipment, and personnel prevention of ignition by limiting ambient oxygen concentration near the laser.
7. prevention of ignition by limiting ambient oxygen concentration near the laser

The advantages of anesthesia in laser cutaneous surgery in children include less long-term emotional trauma because fewer details of treatments will be remembered, more treatment compliance, and more thorough treatments in each session (thereby decreasing the number of treatments required). In addition, it is particularly crucial that children are comfortable during a laser treatment, as erratic patient movement can result in excessive overlapping and double pulsing of laser impacts leading to possible adverse results. Furthermore, anesthesia serves to maintain a friendly rapport among the laser center staff, physician, patient, and family by making the patient feel comfortable. This is especially important in performing cosmetic procedures paid for entirely by the patient where the treating physician would like to see the patient in the future for additional treatments.

Nonetheless, there are several disadvantages of anesthesia that must be considered. An exhaustive list of each complication of every anesthetic technique is beyond the scope of this chapter. However, the most significant complications from various anesthetic techniques include hypoxia from airway obstruction, bronchospasm, aspiration, hypoventilation, pulmonary edema, and laryngospasm. Allergic reactions to the anesthetic agent may also occur, with the rare possibility of malignant hyperthermia from inhalational anesthetic agents. Dysphoric and dystonic reactions, including emergence delirium, hallucinations, and flashbacks, may also occur with certain anesthetic agents (e.g., ketamine hydrochloride). In particular, with general anesthesia, children (especially those under 2 years of age) are at greater risk for hypoxia for various reasons. These reasons include the propensity for airway obstruction from their relatively large tongue, a small functional residual lung capacity, high oxygen consumption, possibility of undiagnosed arterial cardiac shunts, possible patency of foramen ovale, and frequent upper respiratory tract infections, which result in prolonged hyperreactivity of airways.

HYPNOSIS "TALKATHESIA"

All patients may benefit from soothing verbal and tactile reinforcement from both their doctors and their families. This method uses hypnosis as an aid to improving a patient's tolerance level. The physician should coach the patient in a calm, monotone voice to relax and modify his or her own state of consciousness. Relaxing background music is also helpful. One useful method is to have the patient concentrate on breathing. This simple maneuver is performed by having the patient take a slow, steady breath in to the count of "one-two-three" and a slow, steady breath out to the count of "one-two-three." Timing the laser impact to a point in expiration appears to be less traumatic. Holding the patient's hand, with or without gentle stroking, is also a calming procedure. Adults sometimes wish to squeeze a nurse's hand. If this occurs, to prevent a "workman's compensation" injury, substituting a rubber object for the nurse's hand seems prudent. A complete discussion on formal hypnotic techniques is beyond the scope of this chapter. The reader is referred to an excellent text on this subject (10).

When additional anesthesia is required, one can use a variety of physical techniques, which stimulate neurologic pathways to counteract sensory input from pain fibers. This is commonly referred to as the gate theory (11,12). Commonly used techniques are cooling, pressure, and vibration. Additional methods to minimize pain include topical anesthetic agents, local injected anesthetics or systemic antianxiolytics, and narcotics. This chapter reviews the safety and efficacy of these procedures or techniques.

TOPICAL CRYOTHESIA

Pretreatment application of ice bags and/or cryogen spray minimizes treatment pain and posttreatment tenderness. However, cooling the vessels to be treated will result in the need for a higher fluence to achieve effective treatment (see chaps. 1 and 2). For this reason, pretreatment ice application should be limited to a few seconds and repeated immediately after treatment. In addition, the ice bag is then moved over previously treated areas during the course of the treatment. A decreased efficacy with this form of laser has not been reported.

Cooling the skin can be accomplished through a variety of techniques. The simplest is using water ice directly applied as an ice cube to minimize melting water, which may interfere with the procedure, by enclosing the ice within a plastic and/or cloth covering. The advantage here is simplicity and low cost. The disadvantage is the inability to regulate the extent of epidermal cooling as well as to cool the skin during the laser impact. However, decreasing epidermal temperature will lead to its protection for nonspecific heating from the laser or other energy source. As detailed later, epidermal cooling allows for the use of higher laser and/or energy settings to better target the heat below the epidermal–dermal layer.

Cold, clear, water-based gels also provide pain relief. Although a gel may not get to the freezing temperature of ice, it is a more efficient heat sink, absorbing epidermal heat and also increases the transmission of light into the skin. The gel can be kept cold on the skin by using cold air as described later. The use of cold, clear gel was pioneered during the development of the intense pulsed light (IPL) device and actually was one of the major developments that allowed its safe use.

The first cold air delivery system was developed by Zimmer Elektromedizin GmbH (Neu-Ulm, Germany). The advantage of using continuous cold air is that cooling can be delivered before, during, and after the laser or other energy delivery without interfering with the laser beam. With these devices, room air is filtered and cooled to −30°C. A variety of air speeds can be used to increase epidermal cooling. The extent of epidermal cooling can be measured through infrared temperature to prevent excessive cooling if necessary. Studies have demonstrated a two- to threefold decrease in pain by cooling the skin to 20°C and 17°C, respectively (13–15).

Disadvantages to cold air cooling are (*i*) the inability to precisely regulate epidermal cooling and (*ii*) when used during ablative procedures, blowing the plume of vaporized skin away from the smoke evacuator with the potential risks of laser plume inhalation by the surgeon and others in the laser room. In addition, its effect on cutaneous blood flow may be disadvantageous during photodynamic therapy activation since blood flow and oxygenation are a key component in activating the photosensitizing agent to produce superoxides. Whether this adverse effect affecting patient outcome is presently under investigation (16,17).

Cryothesia can also be administered by spraying a cryogen onto the skin before, during, or after a laser pulse. This has been patented and termed "dynamic cooling device" (DCD) (18–20). The CoolTouch™ lasers (New Star Lasers, Inc., Rosemont, California, USA) and almost all Candela lasers (Syneron/Candela, Wayland, Massachusetts, USA) have utilized this device in potentiating the effect of their lasers. The DCD cryogen spurt is controlled through an electronically controlled solenoid valve. This allows the laser surgeon to vary the timing and output of the cryogen with the laser pulse. Typically laser fluence can be raised 10–20% through the use of the DCD without any increase in pain. Postoperative purpura from pulsed dye lasers is also less pronounced and resolves more quickly. Finally, use of the cryogen spurt after the laser pulse has been termed "thermal quenching" as it cools the epidermis from diffusion of thermal effects in the deeper dermal target tissue (blood vessel, hair follicle, etc.) to the epidermis.

Care must be taken when performing cryoanesthesia to hold the cryogen spray nozzle perpendicular to the skin and not to overcool the skin. Failure to do so can produce hyper- or hypopigmentation (Figs. 16.1 and 16.2).

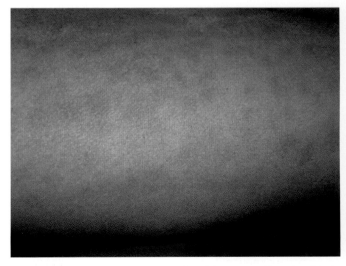

Figure 16.1 Hyperpigmentation induced by overcooling the skin in cryoanesthesia.

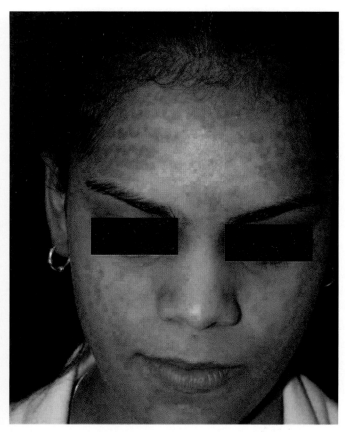

Figure 16.2 Hyperpigmentation developed after the use of alexandrite laser hair removal with cryogen spray; this lasted over 2 years.

PNEUMATIC SKIN FLATTENING

Pain can be reduced by applying a vacuum to the treated skin area under the laser. The associated vacuum provides a decrease in pain through various mechanisms. The skin compression stimulates tactile and pressure neural receptors in the skin to inhibit afferent pain transmission in the dorsal horn (gate theory) (11,12). According to the gate theory, nerve impulses from nociceptors (pain) and their sensory fibers, which are slower and thinner, arrive at synapses in the spinal cord on their way to the brain. The myelinated sensory neurons – of larger diameter and thus faster – carry pressure and tactile sensation from the surrounding skin, thereby activating secondary neurons, which secrete endogenous opioids into the pain synapse, thus suppressing the pain sensation.

Pneumatic skin flattening (PSF) was first demonstrated to reduce pain from IPL treatment, which was given through a PSF vacuum chamber Inolase (Netanya, Israel), Candela/Syneron (Wayland, Massachusetts and Irvine, California) (21). In this study, three different IPL devices were tested and a significant pain reduction was seen with all the treatments (21). An additional PSF study was performed on hair removal using the Lightshear 800-nm diode laser (Lumenis, Santa Clara, California, USA) (22). This study also demonstrated a reduction in pain. Regarding hair removal, an additional benefit suggested was the blood expelled from the skin being sucked up into the chamber, which eliminates a secondary target that would further reduce nonspecific absorption of laser light. The authors recognized that efficacy was preserved despite a 5% decrease in attenuation by the sapphire window. This concept of using the gate theory through vacuum to minimize pain with the addition of

minimizing absorption of laser energy through expulsion of blood led to further enhancement in developing the Lightshear High Speed Duet hair removal laser (Lumenis). Here, there is no sapphire window to attenuate the energy; instead, the vacuum draws the targeted hair-bearing skin into a chamber surrounded by six diode laser arrays, which stretches epidermal melanocytes and melanin particles to further decrease the epidermal absorption targets (melanin) so that the laser energy can more selectively penetrate into the melanin-containing follicular hair, allowing the use of decreased fluence while maintaining efficacy. Ross and Kilmer have confirmed both significant pain reduction and enhanced treatment efficacy in laser hair removal using this novel "pain-reducing" treatment technique (23).

TOPICAL ANESTHETICS
Lidocaine/Prilocaine (EMLA)
EMLA cream (Astra Pharmaceutical Products, Inc., Westborough, Massachusetts, USA) is a 5% eutectic mixture of two local anesthetics, lidocaine (107 mmol/L = 25 mg/L) and prilocaine (113 mmol/L = 25 mg/L), with Arlatone 289 (emulgent), Carbopol 934 (thickener), and distilled water in 1 mL cream. The pH is adjusted to 9.4 with sodium hydroxide. One gram of cream is applied to a 10-cm^2 area.

EMLA cream has been found to be nontoxic, with plasma levels in the circulation measured at 100 times lower than those associated with toxicity (24,25). In 22 infants, ranging in age from 3 to 12 months, 2 mL of EMLA was applied to 15 cm^2 of skin surface for 4 hours. In each case, the plasma concentration of lidocaine and prilocaine was below toxic levels (24).

The only adverse sequelae reported in the literature include mild local reactions, such as pallor, erythema, or edema, observed in treated skin areas (24,26–32). Cutaneous blanching is thought to be secondary to vasoconstriction, which raises the possibility of decreasing the efficacy of laser treatment. Decreased efficacy was not found in one clinical study (33), nor have we noted a decreased efficacy in our patients treated with EMLA.

EMLA is recommended to be applied thickly under occlusion with a polyurethane dressing (Tegaderm) for 60 minutes (Fig. 16.3). A maximum of 10 g should not be exceeded at any time in any patient. Below the age of 1 year, the maximum application quantity is 2 g. A prospective double-blind randomized study assessing pain during laser treatment of PWS skin occluded with either EMLA or placebo showed that pain scores for EMLA-treated sites were significantly lower ($p < 0.0001$) (34).

A study with the argon laser compared injectable lidocaine hydrochloride with EMLA cream. Experimental subjects were adults with normal skin. The argon laser was used at a duration of 200 ms, beam diameter of 3 mm, and maximal intensity of 2.4 W. Interestingly, after 60 minutes of EMLA application, pain blockade was obtained in 9 of 12 subjects, with total sensory blockade in the remaining three subjects. In addition, after a 60-minute application of EMLA, analgesia did not immediately occur after removal of the cream, but reached a maximum extent of 15 minutes after cream removal. The analgesic efficiency of EMLA cream increased with longer application time (60–120 minutes), approaching an analgesic state similar to conventional lidocaine infiltration. Lack of anesthetic effect of the EMLA returned to baseline 90 minutes after removal of the cream (35).

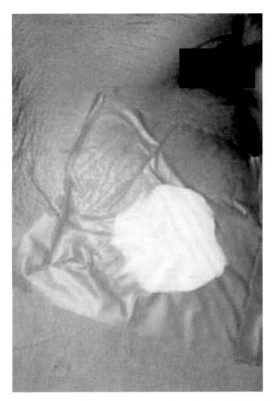

Figure 16.3 Appearance of EMLA under Tegaderm dressing. The level of anesthesia has not been reported to be proportional to the thickness of anesthetic cream applied.

Unfortunately, there has been some indication that experience with EMLA cream may be variable. Anecdotal evidence indicated that some patients will have excellent anesthetic results with an almost imperceptible reaction to laser pulses, whereas on another day the same patient may have absolutely no response to the cream. Therefore, it has been recommended by some to use EMLA for small lesions, but that it may not be useful for total, predictable anesthesia.

Lidocaine/Tetracaine (LaserCaine)

Another topical anesthetic agent available for physician use within the office is LaserCaine (Unit Dose Pharmacy and Packaging, Phoenix, Arizona, USA). LaserCaine Compound contains 1% lidocaine and 3% or 4% tetracaine in a proprietary formulation. It is available in 2- and 3-oz sizes in two strengths, Classic, 3% tetracaine, and Forte, 4% tetracaine. It is intended for use on intact skin.

Preliminary observations indicate that LaserCaine has a 30–50% faster onset than EMLA, produces little to minimal skin changes, and does not require the use of an occlusive dressing. It appears to have minimal toxicity. LaserCaine is rapidly metabolized in tissue through hydrolysis by serum cholinesterase. The half-life in serum is 1½ to 2½ minutes with a toxic blood level of 8 mg/mL, which is higher than the toxic level of lidocaine, 5 mg/mL. In addition, only 5% of tetracaine is present in the nonionized or active form at physiologic pH. However, patients with atypical plasma cholinesterase enzyme may be at increased risk for developing excessive plasma concentrations of local ester anesthetics because of absent or minimal hydrolysis. There have been reports of anaphylaxis with the use of tetracaine-containing topical anesthetics.

The efficacy of topical anesthetic creams may be affected by a variety of conditions. A decrease in penetration of the cream can occur if the skin contains makeup moisturizing creams and/or sunscreens. In addition, some topical compounds, such as benzoyl peroxide, may affect the anesthetic efficacy. One study demonstrated a 75% increased perception of pain when 5% benzoyl peroxide was applied prior to application of 6% benzocaine cream (36). Benzoyl peroxide reacts with tetracaine, procaine, pramoxine, prilocaine, and lidocaine. Thus, since benzoyl peroxide is one of the most commonly used topical antiacne creams, one should make sure that the skin where topical anesthetics are applied is totally devoid of any previous treatment with benzoyl peroxide.

Iontophoresis of Lidocaine

Iontophoresis describes the process of transporting charged ions across a membrane by means of an electric current. This technique can be used to deliver a large amount of medication into the skin, including local anesthetics (37). Anesthesia induced by iontophoretic delivery of lidocaine is most effective when treating lesions within the epidermis and upper dermis (4). The procedure entails adding 1.5 mL lidocaine hydrochloride 4% with epinephrine 1:50,000 to the polymer gel medication delivery electrode. Anesthesia is achieved with a minimum current delivered over 20 minutes. The duration of anesthetic effect with this mixture lasts between 60 and 90 minutes (38,39). Two studies evaluating three (40) and eleven (41) patients, respectively, with PWS were conducted to test the efficacy of iontophoresis. Patients demonstrated significant decreases in discomfort of pulsed dye laser impulses with this iontophoretic mixture. In addition, no detrimental effect on flashlamp-pumped pulsed dye laser (FLPDL) ablation of PWS occurred despite significant decreases in perfusion, as measured by laser–Doppler velocimetry of the PWS receiving iontophoresis with the lidocaine/epinephrine mixture (41).

The average time of iontophoresis is approximately 12 minutes. This usually yields a 30-minute anesthetic effect. The most common side effects to this treatment are prolonged erythema under the dispersive electrode and a burning sensation to underlying skin. A metallic taste has been noted by patients during some procedures when the electrode was placed on the face (40,41). In a cooperative patient with a limited lesion, this modality may be useful (Fig. 16.4).

General Anesthesia

Use of general anesthesia is highly regulated by the Federal and State governments and can only be administered in approved surgical centers that are meticulously monitored. Each surgical center must have specified updated equipment, including anesthesia machines with appropriate vaporizers, intraoperative and postoperative monitoring systems, and resuscitation equipment (defibrillator, oxygen delivery, intubation equipment, various intravenous (IV) drugs, etc.). A strict record-keeping system of the monitoring environment and procedures, as prescribed by the US Occupational Safety and Health Administration (OSHA), is also mandatory. Finally, specifically trained personnel are required. The physician is referred to the American Academy of Pediatrics (AAP) guidelines for the use of conscious sedation, deep sedation, and general anesthesia in pediatric patients for further information on this subject (41).

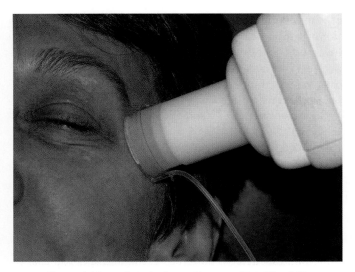

Figure 16.4 Iontophoresis. *Source:* Courtesy of Jaggi Rao, MD.

A complete discussion regarding these requirements is beyond the scope of this chapter.

Gaseous Anesthesia

Nitrous oxide (N_2O) is a sweet-smelling, nonexplosive gas with low anesthetic potency. It is administered with at least 30% oxygen (O_2) to prevent hypoxia. N_2O also has good analgesic properties and thus is useful as the sole analgesic agent for brief procedures. Its safety and efficacy have been well documented in numerous studies (42,43,102–105).

Anesthesia is usually given initially at a flow rate of 6 L/min N_2O and 6 L/min O_2. After approximately 1 minute, the O_2 and N_2O flows are reduced to 3 L/min. Patients usually experience some lightheadedness and relaxation after approximately 2–3 minutes. Patients usually report a tingling sensation of the toes or fingers. We typically use "talkathesia" during N_2O use to facilitate the anesthetic state. N_2O sedation is a helpful method for calming both children and adults and has been extremely safe in approximately 3000 pediatric procedures (43).

N_2O is 35 times more soluble in blood than nitrogen. Therefore, at the end of the procedure, it is important to wash out all alveolar N_2O. To avoid diffusion hypoxia, we discontinue the N_2O flow and ventilate the patient for 1 minute with 100% O_2 after the procedure has concluded.

Complications from N_2O anesthesia use are limited. The most common adverse effect is postoperative nausea and vomiting occurring in up to 15% of patients (44). A more serious complication from N_2O use is fire. Gauze is capable of igniting when the FLPDL is used at 7 J/cm² in the presence of 100% O_2 (6). Hair has also been reported to ignite in room air when struck repeatedly at this laser energy or in the setting of 100% O_2 (6). Anecdotal report indicates one episode of ignition of a patient's eyebrow hair by the FLPDL during the use of nitrous oxide/oxygen. Therefore, it is recommended to wet hair and gauze with saline and apply saline-soaked gauze to cover the exit ports of the nose inhalation piece.

INTRAVENOUS SEDATION

Preoperative Preparation

A history and physical examination is recommended for each patient. The anesthetic plan should be discussed with parent(s) or guardian, and informed consent should be obtained. Families should be alerted to the possibility of unpleasant dreams and emergence phenomena for the patient. Such occurrences should be reported to modify future anesthesia (45–50).

Routine laboratory tests are usually not required. Patients should be fasting overnight prior to the administration of the anesthetic, with the exception of clear liquids, which are allowed 2 hours before the procedure. This regimen can probably be liberalized further based on certain studies (51). In patients with acute, resolving, or recent respiratory infections, the procedure should be postponed until symptoms, especially nasal secretions and cough, resolve (52).

Premedication

Typically, no premedication is given for the first treatment. Subsequently, families are given the option of administering oral diazepam (Valium, 0.1–0.2 mg/kg) preoperatively.

Induction/Maintenance/Emergence

The treatment room is prepared as follows. Oxygen E cylinder is checked and linked to a resuscitation bag. Suction equipment is assembled and kept ready with both a Yankauer suction and a soft suction tip. An IV solution of lactated Ringer's solution with or without 5% glucose with microdrip system is prepared. Endotracheal tube (ET) and laryngoscope are kept ready. Medications are prepared, including ketamine, midazolam, fentanyl citrate hydrochloride, glycopyrrolate, atropine, succinylcholine chloride, droperidol, epinephrine, lidocaine, diphenhydramine hydrochloride, and others, as needed. Monitors include precordial stethoscope, temperature monitor, Criticare #506 [contains noninvasive blood pressure measurement, pulse oximetry, electrocardiography (ECG)], and backup manual blood pressure cuff with sphygmomanometer. Ohmeda 9000 continuous/bolus infusion pump is kept ready with diluted ketamine solution, usually with milligrams of ketamine three to six times patient weight in kilograms in a final volume of 20 mL (Fig. 16.5).

The patient and at least one family member are brought to the treatment room. Most patients allow IV placement with parental presence. Some patients are given an initial intramuscular (IM) dose of ketamine, 3–5 mg/kg IM of body weight with or without atropine, 0.02 mg/kg, as sedation for placing the IV catheter.

Once the IV 22-gauge catheter is secured, IV sedation is started. Initially, 0.01 mg/kg of glycopyrrolate (Robinul) is given, followed by small increments of midazolam (Versed) to induce amnesia and anxiolysis and prevent unpleasant dreaming and emergence phenomena from ketamine. Doses of midazolam vary with age, weight, and level of anxiety, for example, 0.25 mg for a 1-year-old versus 11 mg for a 10-year-old child. Ketamine is started, usually with a small bolus followed by an infusion. The typical initial bolus is usually up to about 1–2 mg/kg, sometimes in increments. This is followed by ketamine infusion titrated to effect. The dose range for infusion is typically between 20 and 200 mcg/kg/min, using higher rates initially and lower rates as the procedure progresses. The infusion is stopped shortly before or at the conclusion of the procedure. The level of sedation varies among patients, with most patients calm and quiet on this regimen.

Some patients talk and move during the procedure. If patients move excessively or begin to cry, the rate of ketamine

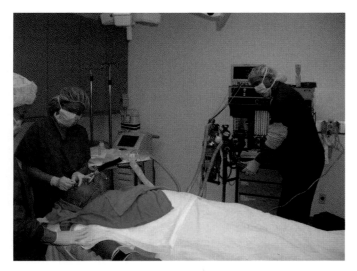

Figure 16.5 Typical laser operatory with monitoring, anesthesia, if desired and emergency equipment readily available.

infusion is increased or supplemented with other IV agents (usually, small doses of midazolam or fentanyl). Ondansetron (Zofran) is a serotonin (5HT3) receptor antagonist that is frequently used for the prevention and treatment of PONV. The recommended dose is 4mg IV in adults and 0.1 mg/kg in children, best given within 30 minutes of conclusion of the procedure. It has minimal associated side effects and is generally considered safe. Patients with a history of emesis during the procedure can be given prophylactic droperidol (Inapsine), 0.625–1.25 mg IV. Some patients also receive IV diphenhydramine at the beginning of the procedure to help limit erythematous flaring around the lesion, which at times obscures the margins for treatment.

At the conclusion of the procedure, the patient is closely observed and monitored until consciousness resumes. In particular, the patient is monitored for any problems with emergence, such as vomiting, delirium, and coughing. Most patients do very well with the above regimen; they maintain stable vital signs, tolerate the procedure well, and awake calmly. As with any technique, some problems are encountered, as follows:

- coughing during procedure
- coughing on emergence
- hiccups during procedure
- emesis during procedure
- emesis on emergence
- excitement on emergence
- irregular or decreased respiratory rate.

Each of these events occurs infrequently (less than 4% of procedures), and most of them are mild. Coughing responses are the most worrisome reactions because of the concern for potential laryngospasm (53,54). Occasional respiratory rate irregularity or slowing is extremely mild and responds well to adjustment of ketamine infusion and avoidance of other IV agents. Emesis is usually mild; vomitus is gently suctioned if necessary and droperidol occasionally given. Hiccups rarely occur secondary to midazolam or possibly ketamine use (49,53,55).

The use of ketamine in small boluses and infusion usually permits adequate spontaneous ventilation so that supplemental

O_2 is not routinely required (although O_2 must always be available in case needed, and oximetry is critical). This lack of necessity of oxygen is desirable in laser procedures where ignition is always a risk and also allows for avoidance of masks, which could restrict the field of the laser treatment for facial lesions. The continuous infusion of ketamine helps limit the total dose of the drug and allows flexible and delicate titration during the procedure. The recommended dosage range is well documented (56–62). Glycopyrrolate prevents the excessive secretions that ketamine typically causes, and midazolam promotes tranquility and amnesia.

Furthermore, the disadvantages of IV sedation should be considered. Although ketamine usually permits adequate or even increased ventilation, hypoventilation can occur (50,54,63–66). Coughing and laryngospasm, although rare, may also occur (49,53,54). Excessive salivation with ketamine, although usually blocked with a drying agent, may predispose to coughing and laryngospasm (49). Emergence phenomena can be a problem with ketamine, but midazolam seems to control this problem adequately (45,46,50,66). Midazolam itself can cause hypoventilation, hiccups, excessive sedation, emesis, and emergence delirium; careful dosing and vigilance are critical (49).

Propofol Anesthesia

Propofol (Diprivan) is an IV sedative-hypnotic agent that can be used for sedation, induction, and maintenance of general anesthesia. It is slightly soluble in water and is formulated as an emulsion containing the active agent 2,6 diisopropylphenol (10 mg/mL) along with soybean oil, egg lecithin, and glycerol. Propofol may be used as a single agent or in combination with other sedatives, narcotics, or inhaled anesthetics. Induction of anesthesia with propofol is smooth and rapid. Intermittent bolus injections or a continuous infusion can be used to maintain anesthesia.

Propofol may offer advantages over the other sedative-hypnotics because of its short duration of effect, rapid recovery, and minimal side effects (67). Propofol is highly lipid soluble, so after an induction dose, rapid blood–brain equilibration occurs, resulting in rapid loss of consciousness. After a single bolus, blood concentrations fall rapidly because of extensive tissue redistribution and rapid elimination. Metabolic clearance is the highest of any IV hypnotic, even with impairment of renal and hepatic function. Propofol blood concentration and depth of sedation may be maintained by intermittent bolus or continuous infusion.

Numerous dosage guidelines for propofol are provided in the literature (68–72). A dosage range of 2–3 mg/kg for induction followed by an initial infusion of 25–300 mcg/kg/min is common, depending on whether IV sedation or general anesthesia is being performed. If the infusion rate is titrated to match the level of anesthesia to the level of surgical stimulation, excessive drug level and prolonged recovery may be avoided. Dosage requirements decrease with age and debility, as well as with adjuvant opiates and premedication. Maintenance of anesthesia should be administered by continuous infusion rather than intermittent boluses, which may result in undesirable oscillations of the propofol blood concentrations and will vary the anesthetic depth. The infusion rate should be titrated to the level of desired central nervous system depression and to the duration of the procedure (68).

The major hemodynamic effect of propofol is arterial hypotension (up to 30%) with minimal change in heart rate. Both decreased systemic vascular resistance and direct myocardial depression have been implicated as important factors in producing hypotension after large bolus doses of propofol (67). The cardiovascular effects are accentuated and may be significant in the presence of hypovolemia (excessive nothing-by-mouth status) and preexisting cardiovascular disease and in elderly patients. Most investigators seem to agree that the clinical significance of these changes in young, healthy, normovolemic patients is negligible (73). Once again, dosage should be titrated for the individual patient and surgical procedure.

Propofol has a profound respiratory depressive effect, including a decrease in tidal volume, minute ventilation, and a depressed ventilatory response to hypoxemia (74) and hypercarbia. Apnea (20–30 seconds) may occur after a large bolus, stressing the importance of infusion rate titration to allow spontaneous ventilation without supplemental oxygen. The expertise and equipment necessary to monitor and maintain the airway, including supplemental oxygen and ventilatory support, are implicit in the use of this drug (75).

Several minor disadvantages accompany this technique. IV access must be established in small children with each treatment. With an uncooperative or very frightened child, low-dose IM ketamine, 2–3 mg/kg, with atropine, 0.02 mg/kg, is used as a preinduction sedative to facilitate establishment of IV access. Pain on injection of propofol into a vein in the dorsum of the hand is common (30–45%). The incidence of pain can be decreased (6–12%) if injection is made into a large vein of the forearm or antecubital fossa (71,75). The incidence of injection pain can be decreased with a dose of IV lidocaine, modified Bier block (76), or addition of 1 mg/mL lidocaine to the propofol emulsion will significantly reduce the incidence of injection pain.

Nonetheless, the aforementioned emulsion formulation is capable of supporting rapid growth of bacteria if contaminated. Therefore, strict aseptic techniques must be maintained when handling propofol. In addition, it is recommended that unused drug be discarded at the end of the procedure or at 6 hours, whichever occurs sooner.

Overall, propofol is a desirable sedative agent because of its rapid induction, rapid redistribution, rapid recovery with clear emergence, and a low incidence of nausea and vomiting (67). Studies also suggest that propofol can be used safely in malignant hyperthermia-susceptible patients (77–79). For these reasons, propofol anesthesia is popular among children and their parents.

Inhalation Anesthesia

When general anesthesia has been selected as the anesthetic technique, no single approach will be effective for all children in all situations. Inhalation induction of anesthesia may be preferred for small infants and children with abnormal airways. Nausea and vomiting may occur, but recovery is usually uneventful. Anesthetic agents such as isoflurane sevoflurane, and desflurane have a longer induction period and produce a higher incidence of coughing and breath holding (80). Both appear to have significant advantages over present agents (81). A detailed discussion is beyond the scope of this chapter.

SUMMARY

A variety of anesthetic modalities can be employed when treating children with laser surgery depending on the need and preferences of the physicians, the patient, and the families. The choice of agents and technique should be based on the needs of the individual child (82) and the surgical requirements while balancing the risks and benefits of the various techniques.

Adults

As with children, many laser treatments in adults can be painful and uncomfortable, although some treatments can be accomplished without anesthesia or with limited application of topical agents. Nonetheless, more painful procedures may require more invasive anesthetic techniques (83,84). For example, facial laser resurfacing is a highly stimulating and often painful procedure requiring a combination of anesthetic modalities. Furthermore, the anesthetic goal during surgery is to render the patient insensitive to pain over the treated area, motionless during the procedure, and amnestic for the time spent in the operating suite. Specific pharmacologic agents are selected to meet these clinical objectives. Anxiolytics, hypnotics, dissociative agents, narcotics, and nonsteroidal antiinflammatory drugs (NSAIDs), as well as inhaled anesthetics, all may play a role in meeting anesthetic goals. The advantages and disadvantages of various techniques are discussed below.

General Anesthesia

General anesthesia with ET intubation may be administered quickly and is usually safe when proper monitoring occurs. General anesthesia ensures airway control and allows the administration of adequate narcotic analgesia without concern for respiratory depression. However, not all facilities are equipped to provide general anesthesia, and because of potential complications while the patient is unconscious, the patient or physician may be reluctant to use this technique.

Intravenous Anesthesia

Advances in anesthetic airway management, specifically the development of the laryngeal mask airway (LMA), have allowed for increased flexibility in office-based practice. For example, LMA allows facial laser resurfacing to be safely performed using IV and/or inhaled agents while maintaining spontaneous ventilation and airway control. If necessary, the technique of IV anesthesia combined with the use of an LMA can provide safe and effective anesthesia for laser facial resurfacing without the need for an anesthesia machine.

Although some surgeons have utilized a combination of local and regional anesthetic techniques, total IV anesthesia offers several advantages since infiltration of local anesthetics may often distort facial anatomy and increase postoperative discomfort. In addition, any movement of the patient may alter the surgical result and increase the risk of complications. Given these risks, total IV anesthesia provides a cost-effective method to provide anesthesia with minimal risk to patients undergoing laser facial resurfacing. Sore throats, however, related to LMA use, are common (85). Despite this minimal risk, proper patient monitoring and availability of airway management equipment, emergency airway and cardiac medications, and a defibrillator should be ensured. A potential IV anesthesia regimen is discussed below.

Oftentimes in laser resurfacing, propofol (Diprivan) is the primary IV sedative agent used because it provides rapid induction, easy maintenance, and quick termination. Analgesia is provided by fentanyl (Sublimaze) supplemented intermittently with ketamine (Ketalar). To counteract the potentially troublesome side effects of ketamine, as well as to provide sedation and amnesia, all patients receive midazolam (Versed) on initiation of IV access and the total dose of ketamine is limited to 1 mg/kg. This regimen decreases the risk of "bad dreams" and adverse psychic experiences. In addition, Glycopyrrolate (Robinul) can be used as a drying agent to help keep the airway free of excess secretions.

After IV access has been secured, sedation is generally achieved with midazolam at a dose of 0.05–0.1 mg/kg. Glycopyrrolate, 0.2 mg, and fentanyl, 1–2 mcg/kg, are given, followed by an initial dose of propofol, 1–2 mg/kg, to facilitate the placement of the LMA. With the LMA in proper position and the patient breathing spontaneously, propofol is administered in a continuous infusion using an IV infusion pump in a dose of 100–300 mcg/kg/min. Supplemental oxygen may be supplied from the circle system of an anesthetic machine or through tubing from an oxygen cylinder at 2–4 L/min. If an anesthetic machine is being used, N_2O and anesthetic gases may also be used; however, their addition may lead to an increased incidence of postoperative nausea and vomiting. IV analgesia is provided as needed with small doses of ketamine, 10–20 mg, and/or fentanyl, 25–50 mcg. Continuous ECG, pulse oximetry, blood pressure at 5-minute intervals, and continuous end-tidal CO_2 volume are used to monitor the patient. At the conclusion of the laser resurfacing, the propofol infusion is discontinued, and the patient rapidly awakens. The LMA is removed when the patient is able to follow commands, usually within about 5 minutes.

The aforementioned anesthetic technique requires an ECG machine, blood pressure monitor, functional suction apparatus, pulse oximeter, supplemental oxygen source, LMA, and IV infusion pump. Capnography, although only optional for anything other than minimal sedation, is desirable to monitor the adequacy of ventilation. Any facility administering narcotics or sedatives must have appropriately trained medical personnel, a fully stocked resuscitation cart, intubation equipment (laryngoscope, blades, ET tubes), a method for delivering positive-pressure ventilation (Ambubag or Jackson–Rees circuit), and a charged and functional defibrillator. In addition, a recovery area staffed with qualified nursing personnel should have the capacity to monitor ECG, blood pressure, and pulse oximetry.

Even in a properly monitored environment, there has been some concern over the safety of using lasers in close proximity to oxygen. The use of opioids may require the use of oxygen to maintain the pulse oximetry above 90%. Although modern inhaled anesthetics are nonflammable, CO_2 and N_2O are combustible. Therefore, it is imperative that flammable liquids and prep solutions not be used in the facial preparation. The LMA and its pilot tube used to inflate the pharyngeal cuff are both very resistant to damage from inadvertent laser strikes, but green O_2 tubing is easily damaged by a few laser pulses. However, the oxygen flowing through the tube will not ignite. ET and LMA tubes can be fully protected by wrapping them with saline-soaked gauze or towels. With proper technique and caution preventing combustible liquids near operative areas, laser resurfacing in the presence of oxygen and an anesthetic delivery system, such as an ET or LMA, can be very safe.

Conscious Sedation

Conscious sedation is defined as a depressed level of consciousness during which a patient retains control over his protective reflexes and can respond to commands. This type of anesthesia is being used more frequently for outpatient dermatologic and cosmetic surgery and is particularly relevant in laser rejuvenation. Sedation renders a patient less mobile than simply injecting a local anesthetic or using topically applied cream, thereby decreasing the risks of complications from the surgical procedure. A combination of propofol, a nonbarbiturate anesthetic, and fentanyl, an opioid agonist, is often used. The nonbarbiturate anesthetic provides amnesia as well as mental detachment from the procedure.

In a study, 20 patients received conscious sedation for procedures, including dermabrasions, blepharoplasties, facelifts, CO_2 laser resurfacing, and liposuction. First, each patient was given 1 mg/kg IV of fentanyl. Then, the patient received an initial bolus of propofol of 0.5 mg/kg followed by a infusion rate at 150 mg/kg/min to achieve sedation. A total of 95% of the patients reported a lack of pain from the procedure; only two experienced nausea after the procedure. Other analgesic choices include ketorolac (up to a total of 30 mg IV or 60 mg IM), phenoperidine, and pentazocine. Midazolam (up to a maximum of 20 mg) has also been used as a short-acting powerful sedative. Although this technique is designed to maintain protective reflexes, it should be avoided in patients who are at high risk for airway incompetence during sedation. Basic monitoring should occur throughout the procedure, including pulse oximetry, blood pressure, and ECG. Emergency drugs and equipment must be available. Pulse oximetry should be continued for about 20 minutes after the conclusion of the procedure. Generally, the patient can then be discharged after an hour with a responsible adult. Potential problems with conscious sedation include oversedation, undersedation, and drug reactions (86,87).

Propofol–Ketamine Technique with Opioid Avoidance

Opioid use has been associated with an 8.3% incidence of postoperative nausea and vomiting when used with droperidol and ondansetron prophylaxis. A retrospective study using propofol–ketamine anesthetic technique with opioid avoidance, room air, and spontaneous ventilation indicates that this combination may be an excellent anesthetic alternative for full-face laser resurfacing. Patients in this study were given glycopyrrolate 0.2 mg at the onset. Some patients then received 2 or 4 mg of midazolam to reduce propofol requirements. Propofol was administered as a dilute (5 mg/mL) solution in a 50-mL bag connected via a 60 drops/mL IV set piggybacked into the most proximal main IV port. The patients were titrated to a loss of lid reflex and verbal response and then given a 50 mg IV bolus of ketamine. Within 2 minutes, injection of local anesthetic could begin. The main branches of the trigeminal nerve were blocked with 2–5 mL of 2% lidocaine with 1:100,000 epinephrine (Fig. 16.6). One milliliter of this solution was also injected into the zygomaticotemporal and zygomaticofacial branches. Then, a field block of 1% lidocaine with 1:100,000 epinephrine was injected along the entire perimeter of the face, and

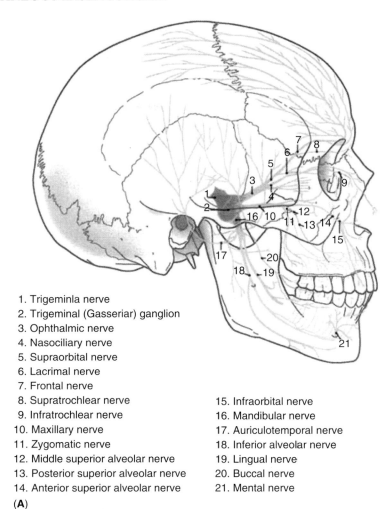

1. Trigeminla nerve
2. Trigeminal (Gasseriar) ganglion
3. Ophthalmic nerve
4. Nasociliary nerve
5. Supraorbital nerve
6. Lacrimal nerve
7. Frontal nerve
8. Supratrochlear nerve
9. Infratrochlear nerve
10. Maxillary nerve
11. Zygomatic nerve
12. Middle superior alveolar nerve
13. Posterior superior alveolar nerve
14. Anterior superior alveolar nerve

15. Infraorbital nerve
16. Mandibular nerve
17. Auriculotemporal nerve
18. Inferior alveolar nerve
19. Lingual nerve
20. Buccal nerve
21. Mental nerve

(A)

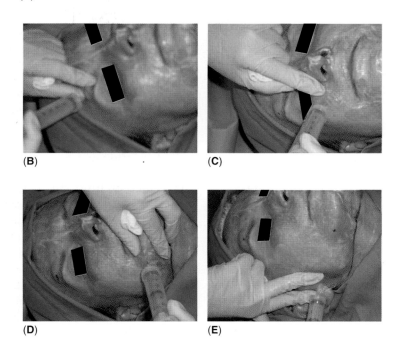

(B) (C)

(D) (E)

Figure 16.6 (**A**) Nerve blocks required for facial analgesia (Redrawn after Scott DB. Techniques of regional anaesthesia, East Norwalk, Connecticut, USA: Appleton & Lange; 1989). (**B**) Supraorbital injection. (**C**) Maxillary nerve injection. (**D**) Mandibular nerve injection. (**E**) Auriculotemporal nerve injection.

sometimes this was followed by a fan injection in the cheek area with the 1% solution. A retrospective chart review of 95 consenting adults receiving this anesthesia regimen in an office-based setting indicates no evidence of hallucinations, postoperative nausea and vomiting, and no cardiovascular instability or seizures (signs of lidocaine toxicity). In addition, this technique allowed for an immobile, unconscious patient with adequate local anesthesia, without the increased equipment requirements and complication risk associated with general anesthesia (88).

Iontophoresis

Iontophoresis, the introduction of various ions into the skin through the use of electricity, has been increasingly used by dermatologists to provide pain relief in outpatient procedures. Iontophoresis uses an electric current to overcome some of the barriers of the skin and assist the penetration through the movement of ions into the skin via sweat glands, hair follicles, and sebaceous glands. Generally, a constant direct current is used, although pulsed currents have also been shown to be effective. Constant direct current is generally limited to 10–15 minutes and 1 mA/cm^2 secondary to burns that can result from generated hydrogen and hydroxide ions. Ultimately, iontophoresis can be used to deliver chemicals to both superficial and deeper layers of the skin. The advantages of this technique are multifold: (*i*) it avoids the pain associated with injection and IV modalities; (*ii*) it prevents the variation in absorption seen with oral medications; (*iii*) it bypasses first-pass elimination; (*iv*) drugs with short half-lives can be delivered directly to tissues; and (*v*) rapid termination can occur. Disadvantages to this technique include discomfort and erythema at the site of iontophoresis secondary to pH changes. There is also the potential for skin irritation and burns; however, these risks can be minimized by thoroughly cleansing the skin, using well-saturated pads for electrodes, and ensuring even skin contact (89).

Iontophoresis of lidocaine diluted in distilled water has allowed for anesthesia to the depth of at least several millimeters. This mechanism allows for minimal systemic absorption of the drug and direct delivery of the drug to the tissues. The addition of epinephrine assists in penetration and increases the duration of anesthesia. According to the "bottleneck theory," which states that there are a threshold number of molecules able to penetrate the skin via iontophoresis, the duration of current flow and the amount of applied current predominantly determine drug penetration. Recent research has shown that iontophoresis of 4% lidocaine with epinephrine (1:50,000) using a mean total current of 3.4 mA for an average of 8 minutes caused an 80–100% relief of pain from injections, dermabrasions, superficial laser surgery, and electrosurgery. Approximately 25% of patients experienced adverse effects, including erythema, mild tingling, stinging, burning, and a transient metallic taste. Furthermore, a study conducted by Greenbaum and Bernstein comparing the efficacy of iontophoresis of a lidocaine solution for 30 minutes with topical EMLA applied for 30–60 minutes. Iontophoresis of lidocaine was found to be more anesthetizing to pinprick. Overall, it seems that iontophoresis may be very useful in superficial ablative procedures with lasers, electrosurgery, dermabrasion, scalpel, or scissors. For deeper procedures, this technique can allow for enough anesthesia to allow for painless infiltration with lidocaine (89).

Topical Anesthesia

In addition to the aforementioned techniques, topical anesthesia continues to be used with laser and surgical techniques. Recently, the movement toward less aggressive laser resurfacing techniques (such as single-pass CO_2 laser ablation and nonablative laser remodeling) has increased the demand for adequate topical anesthetics to replace IV sedation. Generally, topical anesthetics function by inhibiting sodium channels, leading to a block of nerve impulse conduction.

As mentioned previously, EMLA cream is a 5% eutectic mixture of lidocaine and prilocaine and remains the most widely used topical anesthetic. Several studies have indicated that EMLA is effective in reducing or eliminating pain associated with pulsed dye laser treatments after a 60-minute application period. EMLA has been shown to be effective on the face and thighs after 25 minutes. Potential side effects that must be considered include methemoglobinemia (rare), blanching, redness, pruritus, burning, and purpura. Caution must be exercised when EMLA is used near the eyes as it may cause chemical eye injuries, including but not limited to corneal abrasions and ulcerations.

LMX is another topical anesthetic consisting of 4% or 5% lidocaine in a liposomal delivery system. After a 60-minute application period under occlusion, 5% liposomal lidocaine was shown to be effective in producing anesthesia to laser-induced pain stimuli. Its efficacy seems to be comparable with EMLA but superior to Betacaine-LA and tetracaine (see below). Its liposomal delivery system enhances its effects by facilitating penetration of the anesthetic into the skin and providing sustained release. A study evaluated the efficacy and onset of action of EMLA versus LMX using a high-energy pulsed light source. Results of the study indicated that a maximum anesthetic effect was achieved 20 minutes after application of LMX, and that a similar maximum effect was achieved after 1.5 hours of EMLA under occlusion. Nonetheless, lidocaine toxicity may occur when LMX is used over large areas for more than 2 hours (90–92). We use LMX routinely with or without nerve blocks to perform one- or two-pass erbium:yttrium-aluminum-garnet (Er:YAG) laser resurfacing of the face (Fig. 16.7). We have found that a 20-minute application of LMX provides adequate anesthesia for the 20–40 mm ablative effects of the Er:YAG laser at 1–2 J/cm^2.

Betacaine-LA is another topical anesthetic consisting of lidocaine, prilocaine, and a vasoconstrictor. Some preliminary anecdotal reports indicate that this anesthetic may be more effective than EMLA; however, more controlled research is necessary. Betacaine-LA is not approved by the FDA. In addition, Amethocaine 4.0% gel, which contains 4% tetracaine, has been used extensively in Europe. Studies have indicated that tetracaine may be significantly effective in reducing pain associated with pulsed dye laser treatment. Potential side effects include local erythema, pruritus, and edema. Tetracaine gel is a compounded anesthetic containing 4% tetracaine in lecithin-gel base. This gel has not yet received FDA approval; however, it may be beneficial. Another topical anesthetic agent is Topicaine, consisting of 4% lidocaine in gel microemulsion. Studies indicate that Topicaine has a very rapid onset of action with a long duration of effect. Topicaine is FDA approved with a recommended application time of 30–60 minutes with occlusion and is gaining popularity in laser hair removal. Side effects include erythema, blanching, and edema (90).

S-Caine Patch

The S-Caine local anesthetic patch (ZARS, Inc., Salt Lake City, Utah), which utilizes a disposable, oxygen-activated heating element to assist in dermal penetration, contains a eutectic 1:1 mixture of lidocaine base and tetracaine base. After it dries, this peel becomes a flexible membrane that provides inherent occlusion and is readily removed (Fig. 16.8). Studies have indicated that the S-Caine local patch has been effective in alleviating pain associated with shave biopsies, venipuncture, and vascular access procedures.

This peel is currently in FDA Phase III clinical trials, and its use for laser and surgical procedures is still being investigated. A randomized, double-blind, placebo-controlled trial with

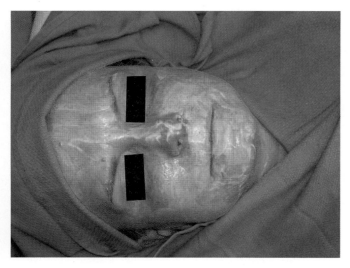

Figure 16.7 Application of LMX to full face prior to a one- or two-pass erbium:yttrium-aluminum-garnet laser resurfacing.

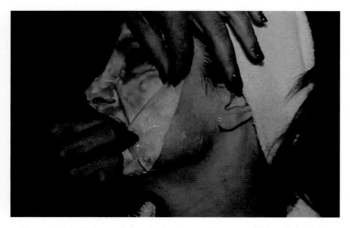

Figure 16.8 S-Caine peel anesthesia. *Source*: Courtesy of Tina Alster, MD.

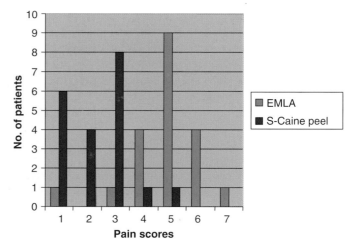

Figure 16.9 EMLA versus S-Caine peel. *Source*: From Ref. (99).

the S-Caine peel for anesthesia prior to pulsed dye laser treatments indicates that a 60-minute application of the peel is more effective than placebo in pain relief for these procedures.

Alster has evaluated the efficacy of the S-Caine peel versus EMLA cream in providing anesthesia prior to cutaneous laser resurfacing (91). Twenty patients were enrolled in a double-blind institutional review board-approved study in which a 4-cm × 4-cm patch of each cheek was randomized to receive either EMLA cream or S-Caine peel. The creams were applied for 30 minutes (previous studies indicate that the optimal application time for the S-Caine peel is 30 minutes) with EMLA cream being occluded under plastic. After removal of the creams, the area was evaluated for erythema, edema, and skin blanching. The patients then underwent single-pass CO_2 laser resurfacing to each area using the UltraPulse 5000C with an 8 mm^2 computer pattern generator scan at a density of 5. The laser has a pulse energy of 300 mJ, pulse power of 60 W, and pulse duration of 950 ms. After each area, patients evaluated their discomfort, pain relief, and side effects. The blinded investigator and independent assessor also evaluated the patients' level of discomfort. Results indicated that the pain scores were significantly lower using the S-Caine peel and side effects were limited to mild transient erythema and skin blanching (Fig. 16.9). In addition, 95% of patients reported

adequate pain relief for the laser procedure on the side that had the S-Caine, compared with only 20% on the side with the EMLA cream. The investigator and independent observer had similar results regarding observed patient discomfort. The same study also makes reference to successful use of the S-Caine peel as a sole anesthetic in full-face ablative laser skin surgery (although some patients may require an additional local or nerve block in certain areas).

Others have also analyzed the efficacy of this peel as a topical anesthetic prior to pulsed dye laser treatment for vascular lesions of the face (92–94). Results indicate that patients experienced significant pain reduction using peel and that an application time of 20 or 30 minutes was as effective as 60 minutes. Another clinical trial evaluated the efficacy of the S-Caine peel for the induction of anesthesia after a 30-minute application period and found that it provided effective dermal anesthesia for nonablative laser treatment with the 1450-nm diode laser (95). In this study, 20 patients received concurrent 30-minute applications of the S-Caine peel and a placebo cream to either side of their face. After one pass of the 1450-nm diode laser, pain levels of patients were evaluated using a visual analog scale and through investigator and independent observer evaluation. The results indicated a statistically significant decrease ($p < 0.001$) in pain perception between the active and placebo sites. Also, a painless procedure was noted in 50% and 65% of the active sites by the independent observer and investigator, respectively, whereas at the placebo sites a painless procedure was noted in 0% and 5%, respectively. A study on pain relief with Q-switched laser tattoo demonstrated adequate pain relief in 50% of patients who applied the S-Caine peel versus 7% with placebo (96). This study also showed that 70% of patients had less pain with the S-Caine peel versus 10% with placebo cream. However, when the S-Caine was used as anesthesia in minor dermatologic procedures, such as shave biopsy or superficial excision, there was no statistically significant difference compared with placebo (97). Therefore, the depth of anesthetic effects of the S-Caine peel is fairly superficial.

The treatment of leg veins with the long-pulsed 1064-nm Nd:YAG laser can be quite painful (see ch. 11). Topical application of S-Caine for 60–90 minutes has been shown to reduce pain associated with laser treatment of leg veins (98,99). Ninety-minute application was demonstrated to be no better than a 60-minute application in both of these studies. Table 16.1 compares various topical anesthetics.

Table 16.1 Topical Anesthetics

Anesthetic	Ingredients	Vehicle	Application dose	Occlusion required	FDA approved	Advantages	Disadvantages	Maximum dose/patient
Betacaine-LA	Lidocaine, prilocaine, dibucaine[a]	Vaseline ointment	60–90	No	No	Anecdotal reports of rapid onset	More clinical and safety trials needed	300 cm²—adults
LMX	4% Lidocaine	Liposomal	60	No	Yes	Liposomal delivery, long duration of action	Postapplication residue	100 cm²—children 600 cm² > 10 kg—adults + children
LMX 5	5% Lidocaine	Liposomal	30	No	Yes	Rapid onset of action	More clinical trials needed	100 cm²—children 600 cm² > 10 kg—adults + children
EMLA	2.5% Lidocaine, 2.5% prilocaine	Oil in water	60	Yes	Yes	Proven efficacy and safety profile	Long application, occlusion required	20 g/200 cm²—adults and children older than 7 years and >20 kg
Tetracaine gel	4% Tetracaine gel[a]	Lecithin gel	60–90	Yes	No	Anecdotal reports of rapid onset	More clinical and safety trials needed	None reported
Amethocaine	4% Tetracaine		40–60	Yes	No	Rapid onset, prolonged effect	Ester anesthetic, avoid mucosal surfaces	50 mg—adults
Topicaine[a]	4% Lidocaine	Microemulsion	30–60	Yes	Yes	Rapid onset, cost-effective	More clinical trials needed	600 cm²—adults (children > 10 kg)
S-Caine	2.5% Lidocaine, 2.5% tetracaine	Oil in water	30–60	No	Phase III clinical trails	Unique delivery system	Contains an ester anesthetic	To be determined

[a]Over-the-counter product. *Source:* From Ref. 90.

FULL-FACE LASER RESURFACING AND SUPPLEMENTED TOPICAL ANESTHESIA

Traditionally, full-face laser resurfacing, which removes the epidermis and upper portions of the dermis, has required general anesthesia or regional nerve blocks (with or without IV sedation and regional infiltration). The complications associated with general anesthesia were previously discussed. Regional nerve blocks often leave areas that are still sensitive to pain and require needle injections that increase patient discomfort. Research indicates that EMLA in a supplemented topical anesthesia protocol for full-face CO_2 laser resurfacing is safe, tolerable, and effective (100). This protocol is as follows: After washing the face, hot compresses are placed for 10 minutes. Then, 30 g of EMLA cream is applied to the face under occlusion. An hour-and-a-half later, the patient is given one to two tablets of 5 mg hydrocodone/500 mg acetaminophen PO, 5–10 mg of diazepam PO, and/or 30–60 mg ketolac IM. Then, an additional 30 g of EMLA is applied under occlusion (anatomic areas are covered with individual pieces of plastic wrap). Approximately 1 hour later, laser resurfacing is performed by removing the plastic wrap from one area and wiping the area clean with a dry gauze. If possible, repeat passes are performed on the same area before moving to the next quadrant. This protocol was applied to 200 patients requiring full-face CO_2 laser resurfacing procedures. The procedure was tolerated with minimal pain, and only 5% required adjuvant anesthesia (nerve blocks or local infiltration). No adverse effects were seen in the study with topical EMLA. Patients generally reepithelialized by day 7. One year later, only one patient had hypopigmentation and scarring. In addition, EMLA-treated skin and skin without EMLA treatment revealed similar depths of thermal damage as indicated through histologic examination. It has been hypothesized that because CO_2 lasers target water, the hydrating effects of EMLA may contribute to the low rate of hypopigmentation and scarring seen in this study. In addition, research indicates that there is potential to use EMLA as a single agent since it has been shown to penetrate up to 5 mm 2.5 hours after application (the minimum required depth of anesthesia is general 100 mm) (100).

Fractionated ablative lasers also require significant anesthesia. We have used a similar technique where patients are medicated with either IM Demerol and Phenergan or IV midazolam and fentanyl along with topical anesthetic. Newer topical anesthetics that do not require hours of occlusion may be used such as 7% lidocaine and 7% tetracaine. Pretreatment of the treatment area with microdermabrasion may facilitate penetration of the topical anesthetic. However, patients should be monitored to prevent lidocaine toxicity.

LASERS AND PENETRATION OF TOPICAL ANESTHETICS

The skin forms a barrier to the penetration of topically applied anesthetics. Therefore, traditionally lidocaine has been administered via subcutaneous injection (which is often painful), iontophoresis-aided delivery (which may cause irritation and burning), topical application after repeated tape stripping of the skin (which is inconvenient and uncomfortable), or topical application with occlusion (which is time consuming). The Er:YAG laser is used in superficial skin resurfacing and is readily absorbed by the epidermis. Research indicates that a single pass of the Er:YAG (wavelength 2940 nm) laser enhanced the absorption and penetration of lidocaine, by disrupting the stratum corneum (101). With this method, anesthesia can be induced in just 5 minutes compared with the 60 minutes required if lidocaine was applied under occlusion. Data from clinical trials evaluating pain associated with hypodermic needle insertion indicate that there is a 62% pain reduction with laser pretreatment plus lidocaine compared with laser pretreatment plus placebo and a 61% pain reduction with laser pretreatment plus lidocaine compared with lidocaine alone. Although this technique may not be adequate for invasive procedures, it may minimize pain and discomfort for more superficial cutaneous procedures, such as hypodermic needle insertion.

Despite these advances in safety in the office-based setting, patients with severe medical problems, such as poorly controlled hypertension, congestive heart failure, severe/easily triggered asthma, orthopnea, morbid obesity, and other significant conditions, are better treated in a hospital or outpatient surgery center setting. Nonetheless, with proper preoperative screening, appropriate patient selection, and careful monitoring, the anesthetic techniques described can readily be adapted to meet the specific needs of practitioners and patients in a variety of clinical settings.

REFERENCES

1. Rosen S, Smoller BR. Port-wine stains: a new hypothesis. J Am Acad Dermatol 1987; 17: 164.
2. Smoller BR, Rosen S. Port-wine stains: a disease of altered neural modulation of blood vessels? Arch Dermatol 1986; 132: 177.
3. Lowe NJ, Burgess P, Borden H. Flash pump dye laser fire during general anesthesia oxygenation: case report. J Clin Laser Med Surg 1990; 8: 39.
4. Garden JM, Polla LL, Tan OT. The treatment of port-wine stains by the pulsed dye laser. Arch Dermatol 1988; 124: 889.
5. Tan OT, Sherwood K, Gilchrest BA. Treatment of children with port-wine stains using the flashlamp-pulsed tunable dye laser. N Engl J Med 1989; 320: 416.
6. Tan OT, Stafford TJ. Treatment of port-wine stains at 577 nm: clinical results. Med Instru 1987; 21: 218.
7. Garden JM, Burton CS, Geronemus R. Dye-laser treatment of children with port-wine stains. N Engl J Med 1989; 321: 901; letter.
8. Epstein RH, Brummett RR, Lask GP. Incendiary potential of the flash-lamp pumped 585 nm tunable dye laser. Anesth Analg 1990; 71: 171.
9. Rabinowitz LG, Esterly NB. Anesthesia and/or sedation for pulsed dye laser therapy: special symposium. Pediatr Dermatol 1992; 9: 132.
10. Spiegel H, Spiegel D. Trance and treatment clinical uses of hypnosis. New York: Basic Books, 1978.
11. Melzack R, Wall PD. On the nature of cutaneous sensory mechanisms. Brain 1962; 85: 331–56.
12. Melzack R, Wall PD. Pain mechanisms: a new theory. Science 1965; 150: 171–9; 2007; 9: 210-212.
13. Hammes S, Raulin C. Evaluation of different temperatures in cold air cooling with pulsed dye laser. Lasers Surg Med 2005; 36: 136–40.
14. Greve B, Hammes S, Raulin C. The effect of cold air on 585-nm pulsed dye laser treatment of port-wine stains. Dermatol Surg 2001; 27: 633–6.
15. Pagliaro J, Elliott T, Bulsara M, King C, Vinciullo C. Cold air analgesia in photodynamic therapy of basal cell carcinoma and Bowen's disease: an effective addition to treatments: a pilot study. Dermatol Surg 2004; 30: 63–6.
16. Baseradi M, Fabi SG, Goldman MP. Evaluating the efficacy of cold air cooling in improving patient comfort during photodynamic therapy as well as its effect on therapeutic outcomes. Lasers Surg Med 2012 (submitted).
17. Tyrrell J, Campbell SM, Curnow A. The effect of air cooling pain relief on protoporphyrin IX photobleaching and clinical efficacy during dermatological photodynamic therapy. J Photochem Photobiol B 2011; 103: 1–7

18. Sturesson C, Anderson-Engels S. Mathematical modeling of dynamic cooling and pre-heating used to increase the depth of selective damage to blood vessels in laser treatment of port wine stains. Phys Med Biol 1996; 41: 413–28.

19. Waldorf HA, Alster TS, McMillan K, et al. Effect of dynamic cooling on 585-nm pulsed dye laser treatment of port wine stain birthmarks. Dermatol Surg 1997; 23: 657–62.

20. Nelson JS, Milner TF, Anvert B, et al. Dynamic epidermal cooling in conjunction with laser-induced photothermolysis of port wine stain blood vessels. Lasers Surg Med 1996; 19: 234–29.

21. Fournier N, Elman M. Reduction of pain and side effects in the treatment of solar lentigines with pneumatic skin flattening (PSF). J Cosmet Laser Ther 2007; 9: 167–72.

22. Ke M. Pain inhibition with pneumatic skin flattening (PSF) in permanent diode laser hair removal. J Cosmet Laser Ther 2007; 9: 210–12.

23. Xia Y, Moore R, Cho S, Ross EV. Evaluation of vacuum-assisted handpiece compared with the sapphire-cooled handpiece of the 800-nm laser system for the use of hair removal and reduction. J Cosmet Laser Ther 2010; 12: 264.

24. Juhlin L, Hagglund G, Evers H. Absorption of lidocaine and prilocaine after application of a eutectic mixture of local anesthetics (EMLA) on normal and diseased skin. Acta Derm Venerol 1989; 69: 18.

25. Engberg G, Danielson K, Henneberg S, et al. Plasma concentrations of prilocaine and lidocaine and methaemoglobin formation of infants after epicutaneous application of a 5% lidocaine-prilocaine (EMLA). Acta Anaesthesiol Scand 1987; 31: 624.

26. Hallen B, Olsson GL, Uppfeldt A. Pain-free venipuncture: effect of timing of application of local anaesthetic cream. Anaesthesia 1984; 39: 969.

27. Moller C. A lidocaine-prilocaine cream reduces venipuncture pain. Upps J Med Sci 1985; 90: 293.

28. Ohlsen L, Englesson S, Evers H. An anaesthetic lidocaine/prilocaine cream (EMLA) for epicutaneous application tested for cutting split skin grafts. Scand J Plast Reconstr Surg 1985; 19: 201.

29. Rosdahl I, Edmar B, Gisslen H, et al. Curettage of molluscum contagiosum in children: analgesia by topical application of a lidocaine/prilocaine cream (EMLA). Acta Derm Venerol 1988; 68: 149.

30. Ehrenstrom-Reiz GM, Reiz SL. EMLA—a eutectic mixture of local anaesthetics for topical anaesthesia. Acta Anaesthesiol Scand 1982; 26: 596.

31. Ehrenstrom-Reiz G, Reiz S, Stockmar O. Topical anaesthesia with EMLA, a new lidocaine-prilocaine cream and the Cresum technique for detection of minimal application time. Acta Anaesthesiol Scand 1983; 27: 510.

32. Evers H, von Dardel O, Juhlim L, et al. Dermal effects of composition based on the eutectic mixture of lidocaine and prilocaine (EMLA): studies in volunteers. Br J Anaesth 1985; 57: 997.

33. Ashinoff R, Geronemus RG. Effect of the topical anesthetic EMLA on the efficacy of pulsed dye laser treatment of port-wine stains. J Dermatol Surg Oncol 1990; 16: 1008.

34. Tan OT, Stafford TJ. EMLA for laser treatment of port-wine stains in children. Lasers Surg Med 1992; 12: 543.

35. Arendt-Nielsen L, Bjerring P. Laser-induced pain for evaluation of local analgesia: a comparison of topical application (EMLA) and local injection (lidocaine). Anesth Analg 1988; 67: 115.

36. Burkhardt CG, Burkhart CN. Decreased efficacy of topical anesthetic creams in the presence of benzoyl peroxide. Dermatol Surg 2005; 31: 1479–80.

37. Gangarosa LP, Park NH, Fong BC, et al. Conductivity of the drugs used by iontophoresis. J Pharm Sci 1978; 67: 1439.

38. Bezzant JL, Stephen RL, Petelenz TJ. Painless cauterization of spider veins with the use of iontophoretic local anesthesia. J Am Acad Dermatol 1988; 19: 869.

39. Kennard CD, Whitaker DC. Iontophoresis of lidocaine for anesthesia during pulsed dye laser treatment of port-wine stains. J Dermatol Surg Oncol 1992; 18: 287.

40. Maloney JM, Bezzant JL, Stephen RL, et al. Iontophoretic administration of lidocaine anesthesia in office practice: an appraisal. J Dermatol Surg Oncol 1992; 18: 937.

41. Committee on Drugs, Section on Anesthesiology, American Academy of Pediatrics. Guidelines for elective use of conscious sedation, deep sedation, and general anesthesia in pediatric patients. Pediatrics 1985; 75: 317.

42. Ruben H. Nitrous oxide analgesia in dentistry: its use during 15 years in Denmark. Br Dent J 1982; 132: 195.

43. Griffin GC, Campbell VD, Jones R. Nitrous oxide–oxygen sedation for minor surgery. JAMA 1981; 245: 2411.

44. American Medical Association. AMA Drug Evaluations: Nitrous Oxide. Chicago: AMA, 1983.

45. Mattila MAK, Larni HM, Nummi SE, et al. Effect of diazepam on emergence from ketamine anaesthesia. Anaesthesia 1979; 28: 20.

46. Cartwright PD, Pingel SM. Midazolam and diazepam in ketamine anaesthesia. Anaesthesia 1984; 39: 439.

47. Miller RD, ed. Anesthesia, 2nd edn. New York: Churchill Livingstone, 1986.

48. Gregory GA, Levine J, Miaskowski C, et al. Pediatric Anesthesia. New York: Churchill Livingstone, 1983.

49. Physicians' Desk Reference, 47th edn. Montvale, NJ: Medical Economics, 1993.

50. Brown TCK, Cole WHJ, Murray GH. Ketamine: a new anaesthetic agent. Aust NZ Surg 1970; 39: 305.

51. Schreiner MS, Triebwasser A, Keon TP. Ingestion of liquids compared with preoperative fasting in pediatric outpatients. Anesthesiology 1990; 72: 593.

52. Cohen MM, Cameron CB. Should you cancel the operation when a child has an upper respiratory tract infection? Anesth Analg 1991; 72: 282.

53. Dundee JW, Wyatt GM. Dissociative anaesthesia. In: Dundee JW, ed. Intravenous Anaesthesia. Boston, MA: Little Brown, 1964.

54. Coppel DL, Dundee JW. Ketamine anaesthesia for cardiac catheterization. Anaesthesia 1972; 27: 25.

55. Bailey PL, Pace NL, Ashburn MA, et al. Frequent hypoxemia and apnea after sedation with midazolam and fentanyl. Anesthesiology 1990; 73: 826.

56. Scarborough DA, Bisaccia E, Swensen RD. Anesthesia for outpatient dermatologic cosmetic surgery: midazolam-low-dosage ketamine anesthesia. J Dermatol Surg Oncol 1989; 15: 658.

57. Pandit SK, Kothary SP, Kumar SM. Low dose intravenous infusion technique with ketamine. Anaesthesia 1980; 35: 669.

58. Lilburn JK, Dundee JW, Moore J. Ketamine infusions. Anaesthesia 1978; 33: 315.

59. Sher MH. Slow dose ketamine – a new technique. Anaesth Intens Care 1980; 8: 359.

60. White PF. Use of continuous infusion versus intermittent bolus administration of fentanyl or ketamine during outpatient anesthesia. Anesthesiology 1983; 59: 294.

61. Jastak JT, Goretta C. Ketamine HCl as a continuous-drip anesthetic for outpatients. Anesth Analg 1983; 52: 341.

62. Ackerly JA. Ketamine anesthesia in burn patients. In: Anesthesiology Forum. vol IV Ketamine anesthesia in open heart and burn patients. Presented in part at the Ketalar Roundtable, New Orleans, 13 October 1984. Morris Plains, NJ: Parke-Davis, 1984.

63. Virtue RW, Alanis JM, Mori M, et al. An anesthetic agent: 2 orthochlorophenyl, 2-methylamino cyclohexanone HCl (CI 581). Anesthesiology 1967; 28: 823.

64. Wilson RD, Traber DL, McCoy NR. Cardiopulmonary effects of CI-581: the new dissociative anesthetic. South Med J 1968; 61: 692.

65. Kelly RW, Wilson RD, Traber DL, et al. Effects of two new dissociative anesthetic agents, ketamine and CL-1848C, on the respiratory response to carbon dioxide. Anesth Analg 1971; 50: 262.

66. Corssen G, Domino EF. Dissociative anesthesia: further pharmacologic studies and first clinical experience with the phencyclidine derivative CI-581. Anesth Analg 1966; 45: 29.

67. Van Hemelrijck J, Gonzales JM, White PF. Pharmacology of intravenous anesthetic agents. In: Rogers MC, et al. ed. Principles and Practice of Anesthesiology. St Louis: Mosby, 1993.

68. Stanski DR, Shafer SL. New intravenous anesthetics (no. 274). Presented at 41st Annual Refresher Course Lectures and Clinical Update Program, Park Ridge, IL, 1990. Park Ridge: ASA Inc., 1990.

69. Fragen RJ, ed. Drug infusions in anesthesiology. New York: Raven, 1991.

70. Bloomfield EL, Masaryk TJ, Caplan A, et al. Intravenous sedatives for MR imaging of the brain and spine in children: pentobarbital versus propofol. Radiology 1993; 186: 93.

71. Cauldwell CB, Fisher DM. Sedating pediatric patients: is propofol a panacea? Radiology 1993; 186: 9.

72. Patel DK, Keeling PA, Newman BG. Induction dose of propofol in children. Anaesthesia 1988; 43: 949.

73. Apfelbaum JL. Outpatient anesthesia for adult patients (no. 412). Presented at 43rd Annual Refresher Course Lectures, Park Ridge, IL, 1992. Park Ridge: ASA Inc., 1992.

74. Blouin RT, Seifert HA, Babenco HD, et al. Propofol depresses the hypoxic ventilatory response during conscious sedation and isohypercapnia. Anesthesiology. 1993; 79: 1177–82.

75. Valtonen M, Iisalo E, Kanto J, et al. Propofol as an induction agent in children: pain on injection and pharmacokinetics. Acta Anaesthesiol Scand 1989; 33: 152.

76. Mangar D, Holak E.Tourniquet at 50 mm Hg followed by intravenous lidocaine diminishes hand pain associated with propofol injection. Anesth Analg. 1992; 74: 250–2.

77. Raff M, Harrison GG. The screening of propofol in MHS swine. Anesth Analg 1989; 68: 750.

78. Denborough M, Hopkinson KC. Propofol and malignant hyperpyrexia. Lancet 1988; 1: 191.

79. Verburg MP, DeGrood PMRM. Safety of propofol in malignant hyperthermia: preliminary results. Anaesthesia 1988; 43(Suppl): 121.

80. Steward DJ. Anesthesia for pediatric outpatients. In: White PF, ed. Outpatient Anesthesia. New York: Churchill Livingstone, 1990.

81. Eger EI. New inhalational anesthetic agents (no. 245). Presented at 43rd Annual Refresher Course Lectures, Park Ridge, IL, 1992. Park Ridge: ASA Inc., 1992.

82. Hannallah RS. Anesthesia for pediatric outpatients (no. 133). Presented at 43rd Annual Refresher Course Lectures, Park Ridge, IL, 1992. Park Ridge: ASA Inc., 1992.

83. Stafford TJ, Crocker D. Role of anesthesia in laser therapy. In: Tan OT, ed. Management and Treatment of Benign Cutaneous Vascular Lesions. Philadelphia: Lea & Febiger, 1992.

84. Anesthesia Patient Safety Foundation Newsletter 5: 4, 1990–1991.

85. Trytko R, Werschler W. Total intravenous anesthesia for office-based laser facial resurfacing. Lasers Surg Med 1999; 25: 126–30.

86. Balance J. Sedational anaesthesia for laser skin therapy. J Cutan Laser Ther 1999; 1: 57–9.

87. Friedberg BL. Facial resurfacing with the propofol–ketamine technique: room air, spontaneous ventilation anesthesia. Dermatol Surg 1999; 25: 569–72.

88. Abeles G, Sequeira M, Swensen R, et al. The combined use of propofol and fentanyl for outpatient intravenous conscious sedation. Dermatol Surg 1999; 25: 559–62.

89. Greenbaum SS. Iontophoresis as a tool for anesthesia in dermatologic surgery: an overview. Dermatol Surg 2001; 27: 1027–30.

90. Friedman PM, Mafong E, Friedman E, et al. Topical anesthetics update: EMLA and beyond. Dermatol Surg 2001; 27: 1019–26.

91. Alster T, Lupton J. Evaluation of a novel topical anesthetic agent for cutaneous laser resurfacing: a randomized comparison study. Dermatol Surg 2002; 28: 1004–6.

92. Wahlgren CF, Quiding H. Depth of cutaneous analgesia after application of a eutectic mixture of the local anesthetics lidocaine and prilocaine (EMLA cream). J Am Acad Dermatol 2000; 42: 584–8.

93. Altman D, Gildenberg S. High-energy pulsed light source hair removal device used to evaluate the onset of action of a new topical anesthetic. Dermatol Surg 1999; 25: 816–18.

94. Bryan H, Alster T. The S-Caine peel: a novel topical anesthetic for cutaneous laser surgery. Dermatol Surg 2002; 28: 999–1003.

95. Doshi S, Friedman P, Marquez D, et al. Thirty-minute application of the S-Caine peel prior to nonablative laser treatment. Dermatol Surg 2003; 29: 1008–11.

96. Chen ZSJ, Jacobson LG, Bakus AD, et al. Evaluation of the S-Caine peel for induction of local anesthesia for laser-assisted tattoo removal: Randomized, double-blind, placebo-controlled, multicenter study. Dermatol Surg 2005; 31: 281–6.

97. Schecter AK, Pariser DM, Pariser RJ, et al. Randomized, double-blind, placebo-controlled study evaluating the lidocaine/tetracaine patch for induction of local anesthesia prior to minor dermatologic procedures in geriatric patients. Dermatol Surg 2005; 31: 287–91.

98. Jih MH, Friedman PM, Sadick N, et al. 60-minute application of S-Caine peel prior to 1,064 nm long-pulsed Nd:YAG laser treatment of leg veins. Lasers Surg Med 2004; 34: 446–50.

99. Chen JZS, Alexiades-Armenakas MR, Bernstein LJ, et al. Two randomized, double-blind, placebo-controlled studies evaluating the S-Caine peel for induction of local anesthesia before long-pulsed Nd:YAG laser therapy for leg veins. Dermatol Surg 2003; 29: 1012–18.

100. Kilmer S, Chotzen V, Zelickson B, et al. Full-face laser resurfacing using a supplemental topical anesthesia protocol. Arch Dermatol 2003; 139: 1279–83.

101. Baron E, Harris L, Redpath WS, et al. Laser-assisted penetration of topical anesthetic in adults. Arch Dermatol 2003; 139: 1288–90.

17 Laser safety: Risk assessment and quality management

Penny J. Smalley

Laser safety is much more than wearing safety goggles and posting a sign on the treatment room door. Audit results from around the country have revealed a number of misconceptions, areas of noncompliance with standards, and potential unsafe practices, as well as potential medicolegal problems should an accident or incident occur, and safe practice has to be defended.

A laser is safe or hazardous depending on how a user handles it; the user's knowledge and skill define how well and safely a clinical practice operates. Healthcare lasers are the same, with the same risks and hazards, regardless of where they are used. Therefore, standards and guidelines for safety are the same for all practice settings, including hospitals, clinics, or private office facilities.

Of all hazards, "complacency" is the most dangerous, and it is imperative to develop a risk management perspective on laser safety. Proper safety management requires a fourfold approach including: knowledge of standards, identification of hazards and risks, implementation of appropriate control measures, and consistent program audit and management.

RISK MANAGEMENT STEP 1: KNOWLEDGE OF STANDARDS, REGULATIONS, AND PRACTICE GUIDELINES

Standards are generally nonregulatory, but serve as consensus documents for best practice. As such, they are often considered as the usual and customary practice in a given area, and are the basis for medicolegal decisions in cases of patient or staff injury, incident, accident, or unanticipated occurrence. Because standards provide this foundation, laser clinicians should acknowledge them as the key to individual laser safety practices.

There are a number of levels of governance in the USA, ranging from best practice at the professional level to mandatory compliance with law.

American National Standards

National safety requirements are based on the American National Standards Institute (ANSI) Z136.3, Guide to the Safe Use of Lasers in Healthcare. This document is a benchmark standard, for safe practice in the USA. Though not regulatory, and without legal enforcement, this document is evidence based and is considered best practice, and as such, is the foundation for state laws, Occupational Safety and Health Administration (OSHA) guidance, the Joint Commission (TJC) surveys, and professional recommended practices. It applies to all healthcare laser systems (HCLS), and all practice settings, including non-hospital environments, mobile laser units, and private practices.

Every 5 years, ANSI requires published standards to undergo a review by a committee of experts, and if necessary, a revision to ensure that they accurately reflect the current state of practice. The Z136.3 has just been revised extensively and is now available to the medical community. Guidance in this chapter is based on the newly revised edition of the standard, Z136.3-2011, and has been available as of January 1, 2012.

An ever-evolving universe of laser safety guidance documents, laws, regulations, rules, standards, and recommended practices exists in varying forms from state to state. States may have regulations that mandate a range of requirements, from registration of equipment, to verification of staff qualifications. Unfortunately, there is no national guidance for either the content or enforcement of state laws regarding medical lasers, and so they vary a great deal. It is essential that all users investigate their own state laws and incorporate compliance with those laws into their laser safety programs.

Because these laws are inconsistent and may change, it is imperative to access the state's website and locate the agency that governs the laser use. This may be the Department of Health, The Bureau of Radiation Safety, The Department of Nuclear Safety, the Department of Emergency Management, or other state bureaus. Keywords to use in searching current and pending legislation may include non-ionizing radiation, medical laser regulation, or medical laser safety.

Healthcare laser users must understand their responsibilities relative to the standards, regardless of practice setting. These responsibilities and requirements are clearly provided in the ANSI Z136.3. The document contains engineering controls required by the Food & Drug Administration and the Center for Devices and Radiological Health, administrative controls, and procedural controls, and provides guidance for development and implementation of hazard-based and operational policies and procedures.

Material in the standard is either informative (appendices, narrative text related to clinical application, and references), or normative (containing the mandatory requirements). The terms "should" and "shall" are found throughout the normative part of the standard.

The term "should" means that a material is strongly recommended but not necessarily mandatory if the user has a rationale for opting for noncompliance. Because it is best practice compliance is strongly recommended, but remains at the discretion of the laser safety officer (LSO) to implement.

The term "shall" means that material is mandatory for compliance. Only normative material found up to but not including tables and appendices contains "shalls."

Where there is a "NOTE:" following a normative statement, the material is intended as further explanation or support, but it cannot contain "shalls."

Though ANSI standards have no office of compliance, nor enforcement capabilities, its contents parallel the requirements found in OSHA regulations for workplace safety. Further, the fact that the USA has a national standard defining the risks and hazards of HCLS, it is appropriate to classify these known hazards as workplace safety issues, and therefore, OSHA law can be used as the basis for mandatory compliance with ANSI.

OSHA applies the General Duty Clause as the mechanism for citing facilities for noncompliance. The General Duty Clause places a duty of care on both employee and employer. The law requires employers to provide their employees with a workplace free of known hazards, to ensure appropriate education and training relative to workplace hazards, and to mandate the use of personnel protective equipment and work practices that mitigate exposure to those hazards.

OSHA requires the elimination or control of exposure to known hazards in the workplace. In terms of laser safety, these known hazards may include but are not limited to possible ocular exposure and injury, flammability and reflectivity hazards, exposure to airborne contaminants in surgical plume, inadvertent exposure to the beam, and electrical hazards.

OSHA and TJC both use the ANSI standards as the basis for their regulations and guidance, so ensuring compliance with these regulations depends on knowledge of the ANSI standards.

The reason for OSHA to use the ANSI Standard comes from its definition of standard:

- 1910.2(f): "Standard" requires conditions, or the adoption or use of one or more practices, means, methods, operations, or processes, reasonably necessary or appropriate to provide safe or healthful employment and places of employment.
- 1910.2(g) "National consensus standard" means any standard or modification thereof, which (1) has been adopted and promulgated by a nationally recognized standards-developing organization under procedures whereby it can be determined by the Secretary of Labor or by the Assistant Secretary of Labor that persons interested and affected by the scope or provisions of the standard have reached substantial agreement on its adoption, (2) was formulated in a manner which afforded an opportunity for diverse views to be considered.

Both OSHA and ANSI require these:

1. Education and training for all personnel.
   a) Education is noncommercial, didactic knowledge, presented at a professional level, and is validated by exam or other mechanism for measurement of acquired knowledge. Training is competency based, validated by physical demonstration of proficiency. Both of these are needed to prepare users, operators, and all ancillary persons that may be present in the laser treatment room, to work safely with HCLS.

2. Equipment maintenance
   a) The user is responsible for ensuring that all equipment is kept in proper working order; can produce documentation that validates a history of service and maintenance; and meets all federal, state, and local registrations and regulations.

3. A safety program is to be implemented and enforced.
   a) A laser safety program contains requirements for management and employee involvement, compliance with all standards and regulations, education, audit, and quality assurance. The laser safety plan can be incorporated into a facility safety plan, but it must contain the specific hazards and control measures associated with HCLS.

If a laser safety program investigation is conducted by OH&S, the focus will be on reviewing administrative control measures, documentation, and interviewing personnel to assess their level of knowledge. By looking at the process of safety management, a compliance officer can assess whether or not a facility has demonstrated that they have done the following:

1. Established written safety policies and procedures.
2. Identified criteria for selection of protective equipment.
3. Implemented adequate education and training programs for all employees who may be exposed to the hazards.
4. Performed and documented periodic safety audits.

OH&S should be viewed as an advocate for safe practice, and can offer education, assistance, advice, and resources to help the individual practice comply with standards and regulations. It is to everyone's benefit, especially the patient's, for laser users to take advantage of these resources during the early phases of program planning, and well ahead of treating the first patient, or making the decision to purchase or rent laser equipment.

Many healthcare facilities, including ambulatory surgery centers and private practices, are accredited by, or have applied to be accredited by one of the national accreditation organizations such as TJC or the Accreditation Association for Ambulatory Health Care. This credential is given when a healthcare organization undergoes rigorous preparation, and then passes an extensive on-site survey based on demonstrating compliance with its standards, as applied to its physical plant, administration, and clinical practices. Accreditation enables the institution to prove a level of excellence in every aspect of its services to the community.

Evidence of the requirement for establishing a formal laser safety plan, can be found in TJC standards, Environment of Care 02.02.01: The hospital manages risks related to hazardous materials and waste (3). The hospital minimizes risks associated with selecting, and using hazardous energy sources... including but not limited to ionizing and non-ionizing radiation equipment and lasers. Surveyors will require the facility to demonstrate compliance through audit reports, and appropriate documentation of administrative controls.

Standards should be kept in every use site for easy reference by users and operators during laser use; knowledge of the guidance in the ANSI standards should be included in all education and training programs.

RISK MANAGEMENT STEP 2: IDENTIFICATION OF HAZARDS AND RISKS

In order to assess the presence of potential hazards, risk of exposure to those hazards, and what appropriate control measures are required to prevent that risk, it is necessary for all personnel (nurses, technicians, physician assistants, private scrubs, and physicians) in a laser practice to have a thorough understanding of laser science.

So how does laser science education relate to safety standards? Follow this simple formula for the rationale behind the requirement for comprehensive education and training for all—beyond the basics of vendor-taught operational inservice.

- Tissue interaction depends on the knowledge of the wavelength (absorption, selective photothermolysis, etc.).
- Wavelength depends on knowing what the medium is [neodymium (Nd):YAG, CO_2, erbium (Er):YAG, holmium (Ho):YAG, etc.].
- Medium determines the delivery system (fiber, handpiece, scanner, etc.).
- Delivery system affects application (open surgical, endoscopic, cutaneous, etc.).
- Application indicates risks/hazards (fire, ocular, plume, etc.).
- Risks and hazards determine the control measures (policies and procedures for each hazard identified).
- Control measures are found in ANSI standards!

It is impossible to provide a safe laser environment without understanding the science. Therefore, everyone who may work within a laser treatment room must have that knowledge. Safety is only ensured when everyone has equal training, responsibility, and understanding of what occurs when a laser is switched on. And since not all lasers have the same hazards, this understanding must be specific to the user's equipment and the practice in which it is used.

Laser science includes the following:

1. Properties of laser light that make it different from ambient or white light
2. Characteristics of each laser wavelength
3. Absorbing chromophores of each wavelength
4. Dosimetry (power, pulse parameters, fluence, energy density, etc.)
5. Spot size and delivery systems
6. Application techniques

Once these properties are well understood, the clinician can anticipate potential hazards. Hazards are all of those potentially dangerous conditions that are associated with an unanticipated interaction or exposure of tissues or materials, to laser energy. These include both direct beam hazards such as tissue burns, eye damage, endotracheal tube fire, drape fire, and explosion of gases, or indirect non-beam hazards (those that are secondary to the actual beam interaction) such as laser-generated airborne contaminants, electrical damage, toxic dyes, and system failures.

Each wavelength, system, delivery device, and application must be assessed for associated hazards, since they are all different and will require different management and procedures.

Once the hazards are identified, risk must be assessed. Risk is often defined as the level of potential for exposure to, or injury resulting from, identified hazards. Risk levels may differ for each member of the laser team and for each person involved with the laser equipment. The level of risk may also vary with clinical applications of a system, depending on the delivery device, power parameters, and target tissues.

While all in the laser treatment room have the risk of eye exposure and damage if they are unprotected, there are going to be varied risks for physician, assistant, nurse practitioner, patient, patient support person, technician, office manager, LSO, scrub nurse, sales representative, biomedical engineer, and manager. Therefore, the LSO must understand each person's level of interaction with the system and their job responsibilities, before developing appropriate policies and procedures.

For example, a photothermal laser such as a 1064-nm Nd:YAG creates enough heat to cause flammability hazards. Users of such a laser will need to follow procedures to prevent fire, including eliminating dry materials or alcohol-containing solutions from the target zone, correctly placing an appropriate fire extinguisher, having an open container of water available, preventing specular reflections, observing the path of the beam for interference of any kind, and removing sources of oxygen or other flammable gases.

Should a laser, based on its science, be assessed to have minimal hazards, the user may modify standards and procedures to reflect that individual level of hazard. This is the reason it is so important for users to write their own facility policies and procedures, and not simply adopt generic documents obtained from manufacturers, course materials, or other institutions. An example of how the same laser used in two different practice settings may require different safety measures as follows.

- Setting A: A suite on the top floor of an office building overlooking a park land sets up a green diode laser, emitting at 532 nm. Window barriers do not have to be installed to cover the windows on the outside facing wall, because the laser beam, even if transmitted accidentally through the window, cannot strike anything that could be harmed.
- Setting B: A suite on the ground floor of a busy professional building, with a window facing directly across from another window in the adjacent suite, sets up the same laser. In this case, appropriate window coverings must be installed to prevent accidental transmission of the beam through to the adjacent suite. The specifications for appropriate window coverings will be addressed further on in this text.

Clinically relevant risk assessment provides safety in a sensible and appropriate manner often at lower cost to the user, and always, at greater levels of protection for all concerned.

RISK MANAGEMENT STEP 3: IMPLEMENTATION OF CONTROL MEASURES

Establishing Control Measures

Control measures are the actions taken by healthcare personnel, to prevent injury or exposure to identified hazards. Once hazard-based risks are identified, and the potential of exposure to those risks assessed, the user can develop and implement control measures. These measures translate into policies and procedures, which have clear statements of scope (Who does the policy affect?), rationale (Why is it necessary?), who is responsible for implementation and enforcement, and how it should be monitored.

Each policy should be updated on an annual basis, when new systems, accessories, or clinical applications are introduced, and whenever a new regulation or standard is published. It is the responsibility of the LSO to enforce compliance with all control measures.

Once control measures are written and approved by the facility, inservice should be offered to all employees. Copies of all policies and procedures should be distributed, so that everyone can read them. Some facilities require each person to sign a checklist stating that they have received and read the procedure manual, as a supplement to the documentation of safety training.

There are three kinds of control measures:

1. Engineering controls: These are inbuilt safety features supplied by the manufacturer in compliance with International Electrotechnical Commission (IEC) standards. These include guarded footswitch, audible and visible emission indicators, stand-by control, emergency off control, housing interlocks, and beam attenuators.
2. Procedural controls: standard operating procedures, or SOPs, in standards, and policies and procedures in hospitals. These are operational activities, specific to equipment and practice, and include ocular protection, flammability hazard prevention, controlled access, management of plume, control of electrical hazards, and control of the delivery system and beam emissions.
3. Administrative controls: These constitute the infrastructure of the laser safety program. These must be in place before the laser can be used, and include appointment of an LSO, organization of a laser safety committee, development of documentation tools, education and training of all personnel, compliance with Occupational Health and Safety rules, development of a formal audit and technical management plan.

A written safety plan should be completed and kept in a book at the laser use site. This should include all policies and procedures, verification of education and training of all personnel, samples of documentation forms, and audit reports. Everyone involved should become familiar with this book, as it is the medicolegal documentation of safe practices.

The Laser Safety Officer

The LSO is the person who is responsible for the management of risk, and the authority to ensure compliance with all applicable standards and rules. This person should be competent to assess all systems, and validate the knowledge and skills of all personnel involved in the laser practice. The LSO can be a physician, a nurse, a practice manager, or a consultant, biomedical engineer, or other properly qualified person.

The LSO is the contact person and spokesperson for the laser program, should there be an audit, a medicolegal situation, a compliance inspection, or questions from accrediting bodies.

There must be only one LSO but in his or her absence from the facility during any use of the laser, there should be someone designated as a deputy LSO, who has equal levels of authority and knowledge. The duties of the LSO will vary depending on the size and scope of the laser facility; however, standards do require the LSO to be responsible for:

1. advising facility administration;
2. hazard evaluation [determination of the nominal ocular hazard area (NOHA)];
3. implementing appropriate control measures;
4. approving all policies and procedures;
5. approving and maintaining all protective equipment;
6. approval of all signage and labels;
7. authorization of laser technicians and service providers;
8. ensuring that all staff members are properly educated and trained;
9. investigating all accidents and incidents;
10. ensuring that a periodic audit is conducted, documented, and followed-up with remedial actions.

The LSO is often responsible for technology assessment and advising users on potential laser purchases, as well as on compliance with standards and regulations. In some situations, especially in a private practice, the physician who owns and runs the practice or clinic seems to be the likely candidate for LSO. A careful analysis of the duties of the LSO must be made before making this decision, remembering that if the laser is to be used by several clinicians, the LSO must be available during all use, and must be responsible for safety regardless of who is operating the system. This may determine who is selected for the position.

It can often be a better decision to assign a permanent office professional, such as the nurse or physician's assistant, to serve as the LSO, as he or she will be on site all the time and can work with all the laser users in the practice. There are no rules as to who may serve as LSO; only that the person identified be appropriately trained and empowered to establish procedures and to enforce compliance.

Compliance with occupational health and safety (OH&S) is an important component of a laser safety program. There are no specific OH&S guidelines for assessing a facility's level of compliance. Assessments are usually made under a broad, generic, general duty clause, which says in summary that there is a shared duty between an employer and an employee for establishing and maintaining a safe working environment.

The employer has a duty of care to provide the proper safety equipment, appropriate education, and training, and a work environment free of known and potential risks and hazards. The employee has a duty of care to access the training, use the personal protective equipment, and to follow safe work practices at all times.

Though often seen as an adversary, an OH&S officer, can be a strong advocate for safety, if viewed as a professional partner. This resource person can be a member of the team approach, assisting the LSO with audit, compliance, education, and staff motivation, and always resulting in fewer risks of injury for patient and staff, less potential for legal entanglement, and overall lower costs for the program. Remember, even though it may seem that the cost of laser safety training is high, it is always far less than the cost of one injury or lawsuit.

Procedural Control Measures

Controlling hazards in the laser treatment room depends on controlled access to the room and to the equipment, proper use of personal protective devices, monitoring testing and operations of the laser and its delivery systems, appropriate applications, and vigilance on the part of each laser team member.

Controlled Access

Controlled access is based on the identification of the NOHA (a term used in IEC standards), or nominal hazard zone (NHZ—a term used in American National Standards). This is the area within which the level of exposure to laser radiation can exceed the maximum permissible exposure (MPE) levels. The MPE is a mathematical calculation based on variables including wavelength, power, distance, and time of exposure, which results in a length of time (usually milliseconds) an unprotected eye can be exposed to laser radiation, without producing injury. The NOHA/NHZ is a mathematical calculation, resulting in an area around the laser, within which laser hazards may exist, and protective devices are required. These values should be readily available from the laser manufacturer's documentation.

Standards indicate procedures for maintaining a controlled access area. Some of the key points are as follows:

1. Regulation CAUTION (DANGER) signs are posted visibly, on each entry way into the NOHA/NHZ.
2. Appropriate protective eyewear for laser in use, is placed with the signs at each entryway. These are removed only at conclusion of the procedure.
3. Windows are covered with blinds, shades, or other nonflammable barriers that reduce transmission of the beam to acceptable levels below the MPE for laser wavelengths that can penetrate glass (long wavelengths that absorb in water do not need window barrier protection).
4. Everyone within the NOHA is authorized by the LSO.
5. Doors are kept closed, but not locked at all times during laser use.

The measurement that defines the NOHA/NHZ may be obtained from the manufacturer of the laser, by having the LSO perform the calculations, or by designating the entire room as the controlled area. If the entire room is so designated, everyone in the room must follow all safety procedures at all times, including wearing of protective eyewear.

Control of access to equipment is accomplished by two procedures: key storage away from the console and positioning a dedicated operator at the control panel whenever the laser is in use. When an individual is operating (activating the equipment) and using (delivering the energy to the target tissue) the laser without assistants present, he or she is responsible for controlling access to all components of the device.

Protective eyewear, corresponding to the laser in use, should be placed with each door sign posted at NOHA/NHZ entryways, to be used by anyone who has to enter the laser room in an emergency. Signs should only be posted when the laser is in actual use, and removed or covered when the laser is turned off and key removed. These are indicators to others in the facility that there is a potentially hazardous situation in the room, and safety procedures are in effect. If the sign is left up all the time, it loses its meaning, and staff tends to become casual about entering the room. When signs are used properly, there is no need to lock doors or connect lasers to interlocks, which are hazardous and should never be utilized in medical settings (Fig. 17.1).

Windows and doors should be covered with barriers for all wavelengths that transmit through glass. The LSO must assess the facility to determine what type of coverings are required, and the options vary from black barrier curtains, to purpose built window films marked with the actual OD of protection (Fig. 17.2). The criteria for selection of window covers include nonflammability, infection control guidelines, and ability of the material to reduce the laser transmission below the MPE.

The control panel of the laser should never be left activated and unattended. If the operator has to leave the room, the laser should be turned off, and the key removed and either stored or taken with the operator or LSO. If the operator sets up and tests the laser, but then must wait while the patient comes into the room, the laser must be kept on standby. This mode deactivates the shutter and prevents accidental misfiring. The only time the laser should be turned to the ready mode, is when the clinician is aimed at target tissue, and is ready to treat.

State law determines the licensing requirements for who can operate a laser under the supervision of a physician. In an operating theater, a technician operating a laser should be supervised by a licensed medical professional. In private practice, the laser user (clinician) frequently functions as the supervisor. No untrained individual should ever be allowed to operate a laser under any circumstance, without immediate supervision of a competent laser user.

In the case of rental lasers, the renter and the staff must be educated about the laser and its delivery systems, accessory equipment, mechanism of action, all safety measures, and minor troubleshooting. Clinicians should insist on comprehensive staff training for two reasons: one in order to meet standards; two, regardless of what equipment is being used, or who owns the equipment, the professional staff are responsible for patient advocacy, management, and safety.

The footswitch for activating the laser must be given only to the credentialed laser user. Position all other footswitch activated devices away from the laser and clearly indicate to the user, which pedal is for the laser, and which ones are for other devices. Accidental activation of the pedal is one of the most commonly reported accidents.

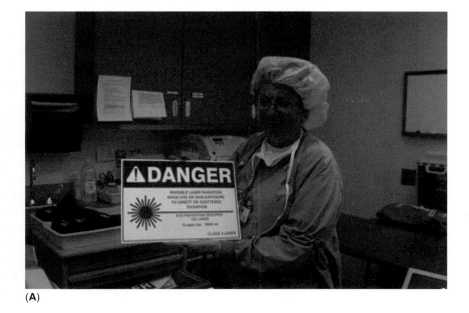

(A)

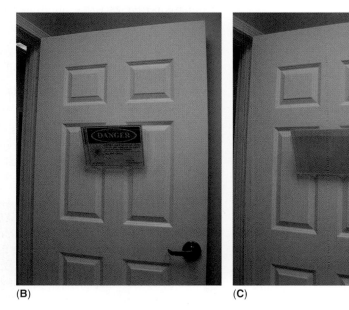

(B) (C)

Figure 17.1 (**A**) Signs and goggles posted properly to establish the NOHA. Signs (**B**) displayed and (**C**) not visibly displayed when laser is not in use. *Source*: Courtesy of Princess Alexandra Hospital, Brisbane, Australia.

Ocular Hazards and Protection

Class 3b and Class 4 lasers, as well as certain uses of other classes (1,2,4) have the potential to damage the eye through both direct and reflected impact, and should NEVER be operated without first assessing the need for proper protective eyewear.

The classification of the laser is based on whether or not the MPE is longer or shorter than the human aversion response. MPE is a calculation that determines how long an unprotected eye can be exposed to a laser beam before injury occurs. The aversion response is the autonomic response (within 0.25 seconds) of the eye moving away from an intense light.

The lower classifications (1,2) have extended MPE measurements and do not require protective eyewear, since the human eye will avert from the bright light long before the beam can injure the unprotected eye.

In the case of a higher classification (5,6) the MPE is shorter than the aversion response, and therefore, protective eyewear must be worn at all times during laser activation.

Safety precautions, including eye protection, flammability, reflection, and administrative control measures, are determined

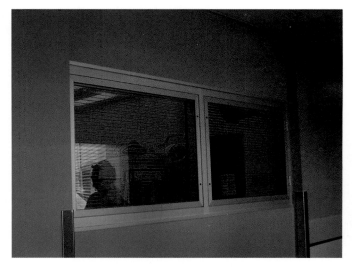

Figure 17.2 Installed permanent window protective covering for argon laser 457–514 nm. *Source*: Courtesy of KenTek Corporation and Princess Alexandra Hospital, Brisbane, Australia.

by the classification of the laser, which must be included by the manufacturer on the device and aperture labels. Current classifications have been adopted by the IEC as follows:

Class 1: safe under every conceivable condition of use

Class 1M: safe for viewing without optical aids, but potentially hazardous with magnification aids (microscopes, loupes, binoculars, etc.)

Class 2: visible wavelengths (400–700 nm) safe if viewed for less than 0.25 seconds

Class 2M: visible wavelengths (400–700 nm) not safe with optical viewing aids

Class 3R: marginally unsafe for intrabeam viewing of beams with diameters >7 mm

Class 3B: unsafe for intrabeam viewing, causing skin and eye injury from direct but not necessarily diffuse energy

Class 4: high power causing skin and eye injury from direct and reflected energy

Low-power lasers (e.g., those used in physiotherapy), are usually of lower classification, and the LSO must determine control measures that are appropriate.

Ocular Hazards

Levels of ocular injury are determined by the interaction with the tissue, and absorption chromophores that are present in the structures that are exposed. Delivery systems, power and energy density, and clinical application techniques also contribute to the type and severity of damage that can occur.

Long wavelengths (CO_2 and Er:YAG) are absorbed by water in the tissues, and therefore, can absorb at the tear layer covering the cornea (Fig. 17.3). As the water is vaporized away, the beam interacts with the tissues of the cornea to cause burns. This is not permanent but can be painful and temporarily disabling or even cause permanent scarring if deep enough. It can be particularly hazardous should it occur intraoperatively, when the staff and patient are at risk of injury should the user lose control of the delivery system due to a "flash blinding" type of injury.

Mid-range infrared (Ho:YAG) can partially absorb, and yet partially transmit through water, and be absorbed at the lens, causing injury to the lens, but not to the retina (Fig. 17.4). This is a permanent injury, similar to cataract damage.

Short wavelengths (near infrared through visible range) penetrate through water and can transmit through all anterior structures of the eye, absorbing in the hemoglobin in the retina, causing permanent damage to central vision (Fig. 17.5). Furthermore, the human lens acts to cause convergence of stray, low-power, reflected or scattered beam emissions, which can increase power density to a significant level.

Standards State

Eye protection devices specifically designated for the wavelength and classification of the laser in use should be worn in addition to other controls that may be in place to ensure that personnel will not be exposed in excess of the MPE level.

This means that everyone in a laser treatment room, within the designated controlled area, must wear appropriate protective eyewear at all times when a laser device is in use. This means all medical lasers, including CO_2 and Er:YAG. The only exception to the rule of wearing safety glasses is when the physician is working through a properly filtered microscope.

There is no such thing as an "eye safe" Class 3b or Class 4 laser!!!

Criteria as follows should be used to select eyewear with emphasis on the fact that all eyewear must be approved by the LSO.

1. Permanent labels stating wavelength in nanometers
2. Permanent label stating the optical density (OD) of >4.5
3. Ruby (694 nm) must have an OD of not <7
4. Side shield protection
5. Adequate visible light transmission
6. Resist shock, scratching, and front surface reflection
7. Have proper fit and be comfortable (no slippage)
8. Be without damage to lenses or frames

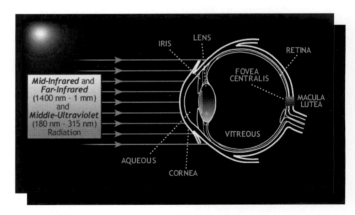

Figure 17.4 Mid-infrared radiation can cause damage to anterior segment, and has the potential for serious injury.

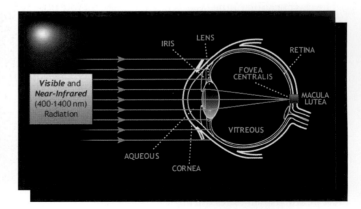

Figure 17.5 Visible and near-infrared (400–1400 nm) radiation can cause damage to the retina and permanent injury.

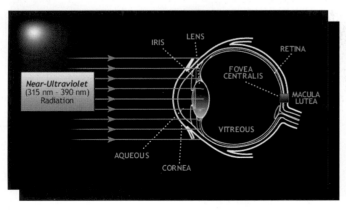

Figure 17.3 Near-ultraviolet and near-infrared radiation (CO_2, Er:YAG, and excimer) penetrate only to the cornea and can cause temporary injury without permanent damage to vision.

This means that personnel should NEVER use splash glasses, prescription eyewear, face shields, tanning booth goggles, contact lenses, or any other gear not specifically designed, tested, and labeled for laser safety use. Infection control goggles do not meet the eyewear selection criteria.

If the LSO has determined the entire treatment room as the NOHA, then everyone in the room must wear eye protection having the same level of optical density, eliminating the use of observer glasses (low OD or marked "for observation only"). It is important that users wear glasses that will allow enough adequate visible light transmission.

Each individual should be responsible for examining their glasses before use, to verify the correct labels, and to assess whether or not the glasses are in proper condition. Look for scratches, cracks, or discoloration in the lenses, as well as loose connections or damage to the frame. If the lenses are discolored as a result of improper cleaning (alcohol degrades optical coatings) or prolonged light exposure (photobleaching), the optical density will be less than expected and the glasses will not provide proper protection.

Regardless of routine safety inspections by the LSO, or assurance by the rental company technician, each individual must ensure that the glasses he or she uses are the right ones and that they are in safe condition, every time they are used.

During fiberoptic procedures, even when the physician is working from the video monitor, he or she should wear the safety glasses. It is a known hazard, as fibers can break or become disconnected, resulting in unanticipated transmission of laser energy in the room. Should that happen, the user may be exposed to laser radiation above the MPE level.

Safety eyewear is the best method of providing patient eye protection (Fig. 17.6). Straps or elastic bands should be in place to keep the goggles from slipping out of place when the patient moves or is repositioned. If unable to wear goggles, due to treatment in the periorbital area, metal corneal eye shields or tightly fitting orbital goggles should be used to prevent damage to the eye. Plastics may not withstand the impact of a laser, and most have not been properly tested for this type of use.

If unsure, request the testing specifications used by the manufacturer, to be sure that the product in question has been tested with the wavelength and within the clinical parameters to be used. If the documentation is not available, do not use the product.

All staff in the room must wear protective eyewear at all times during laser use, with no exceptions. Remember that eye injury is completely preventable if everyone is properly trained and uses proper eye protection.

Flammability and Reflection

The skin and other tissues of all patients and perioperative personnel must be protected from unintended exposure to the laser beam, as well as all personnel in the room.

Flammability is a potential laser hazard associated with most high-power systems, but only rarely in the use of low-power or diffuse beams. Many flammable products are used routinely in clinical procedures, and the LSO as well as everyone on the laser team must continually assess products and devices in use in the laser target site, for compatibility with the beam, and potential hazards. These items may include dry or unwoven fabrics, plastic, rubber, solutions containing alcohol, tape removers, skin degreasers, disposables, and skin preparation solutions.

Solutions that contain iodophors, (Hibiclens, Betadine, etc.) must be thoroughly dry before firing the laser, as heat can cause a chemical burn to the skin if it interacts with wet solution. All of these, as well as many other products, can become a fire hazard when exposed to the heat produced by a high-intensity laser beam as they are flammable.

Some drapes are nonflammable, but melt when heated. These may not cause flame, but can still present a severe hazard by containing heat and in some cases, flames, under the material, and as it melts can cause injury. These unwoven fabrics require smothering to extinguish them. The facilities that use such drapes should have a fire blanket installed in the room.

An open basin of water should be available whenever a laser is used. This serves to extinguish fires caused by ignition of fabric, sponges, etc. on the surgical field. The basin should be positioned near the laser operator.

A standard electrical equipment fire extinguisher should be conveniently installed near every laser room. The device should not be attached to the laser, the supply cart, or the

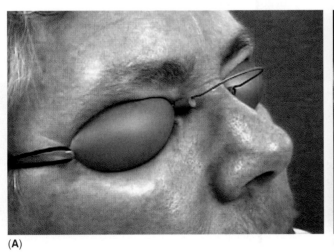
(A)

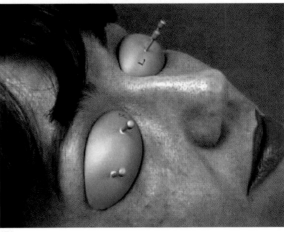
(B)

Figure 17.6 (**A**) Periorbital eye shields protect against all laser wavelengths and fit snugly inside the orbital ridge for procedures on the face. (**B**) Individual eye shields can be used one at a time to protect the non-operative eye during most types of laser procedures. *Source*: Photos courtesy of Oculoplastik, Canada.

plume evacuator. It is best not to keep the fire extinguisher in the laser room, because should the room fill with plume, it may not be possible for the staff to find it (Fig. 17.7). If it is positioned just outside the room, it is quickly available for someone either inside or outside the room. All staff should be inserviced and have current knowledge of how to operate the fire extinguisher.

When patients present for procedures at the hairline, the area must be washed free of any cosmetic preparation (hair spray, gels, mousse, nail polish, etc.) that may contain alcohol. This should be a standard nursing procedure to be completed at the time of pretreatment patient admission and preparation.

All sources of oxygen (nasal cannulas) need to be eliminated from the laser target site. Flammable gases of any kind should not be used in the laser room.

Reflection is a hazard, when exposed reflective or specular materials, instruments, or surfaces are allowed to interfere in the beam path. The beam path extends from the aperture (point of emission from the delivery device) to the target. It is unlikely that a beam can cause a reflection hazard from a wall or cabinet, unless it is directed at that surface. The LSO should assess the potential for hazards from any metal cabinets, wall coverings, or furniture in the laser treatment room, before recommending the costly removal or replacement of such equipment.

Specular surfaces may include speculum blades, retractors, non-anodized black instruments, foil masks, or front surface glass lenses. Surface dulling (sandblasting, anodizing, etching), NOT blackening or ebonizing, will result in diffusion of the incident laser beam and prevent reflection. If anodized instruments are not available, the exposed surfaces should be covered with wet drapes or towels to prevent reflection and unintended burn hazards.

All nonreflective coatings or processes should be tested by the LSO to determine whether or not they are truly effective, before instruments are sent off to be resurfaced or new ones purchased. Some ebonized (blackened) coatings come off quickly during instrument cleaning and sterilization, and some are just as reflective as silver colored finishes. Companies should supply testing materials at no charge.

Plastic or rubber devices (teeth guards, mouth gags, tongue blades, etc.) should not be used in the beam path, unless they are tested for safety by the LSO with the intended laser wavelength, and at surgical levels of power intended to be used. If testing specifications are not available from the manufacturer, the LSO must conduct appropriate tests and verify safety of such devices and instruments.

External, nontargeted tissues in the direct beam path should be draped with wet towels. Metal foil material or any other device that may reflect the beam or heat up upon laser impact should not be used.

Testing and Calibration

It is important to test fire or calibrate a laser prior to use. Infrared lasers with coaxial visible aiming beams must be tested for alignment and for the presence of an appropriate beam mode, whereas fiberoptic lasers must be calibrated for adequate transmission across the fiber, in order to assure accurate and consistent power density delivery to tissue.

Infrared testing consists of firing the beam at a dampened tongue depressor, and watching to see that a burn appears in the same spot where the aiming beam is visible. The test must be done in the delivery system intended for use (handpiece, microscope, etc.) and the delivery system must be held at right angles to the target in order to allow for assessment of the beam mode. No more than 5 W is necessary for this test.

Beam mode must be TEM00 (fundamental mode) indicated by a clean circle without distortion. It is critical to being able to maintain power density.

Testing should be done before the first patient of the day, and then repeated if the laser is moved or if the delivery system is changed (Fig. 17.8 and 17.9). The nurse or operator can test however, should there be a question of suitability; the user must decide whether it can be used on the patient.

Electrical Hazards

Lasers are electrical devices and should be treated with the same caution. This may be overlooked by individual users, especially those using hand-held or small mobile devices. It must be remembered that all electrical safety procedures should be followed, and an occupational health and safety plan for response to fire should be in place and included in staff education programs.

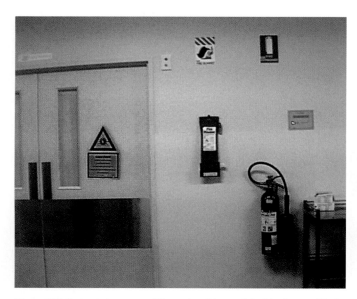

Figure 17.7 Correct placement of fire extinguisher and fire blanket outside the laser procedure room.

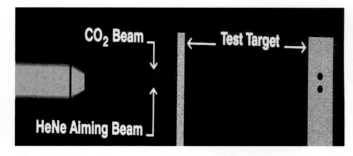

Figure 17.8 Infrared lasers are tested prior to use, to assess whether or not the working beam and the visible aiming beam are properly aligned, and to determine whether or not the beam is in the TEM00 mode.

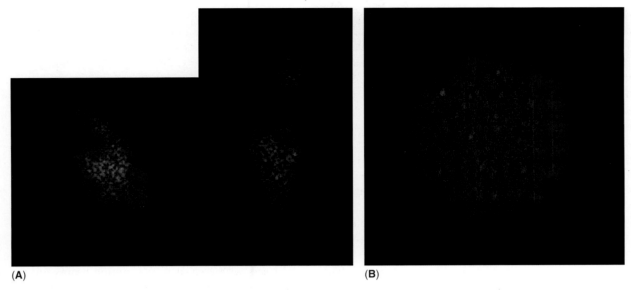

(A)   **(B)**

Figure 17.9 (**A**) Incorrect beam modes, unable to deliver accurate power density due to uneven distribution of energy in the beam spot. (**B**) Correct TEM00 (fundamental) mode beam, which will deliver consistent and accurate power density.

The laser operator should examine the unit while setting up and testing, to be sure that all electrical cords, plugs, and connections are intact and in safe working condition.

Extension cords should not be used on lasers, and in many cases, isolated circuits are necessary to prevent power drains in the laser treatment room.

It is important to check the cord connection to the footswitch, to make sure that there are no damaged or exposed wires. Improper handling of the footswitch can result in this type of damage, and if not repaired properly, it can cause electrical shock upon activation.

Airborne Contaminants

As with all potential hazards, airborne contaminants are associated with only certain wavelengths and applications, and the LSO must evaluate this for each system and use, providing appropriate protection as needed.

This hazard is not present when using low-power lasers; however, it is a hazard associated with many other energy-based devices, such as electrosurgical pencils, harmonic scalpels (ultrasonic devices), plasma generators, argon beam coagulators, and mechanical instruments.

Research has proven that thermal disruption of viable human cells, regardless of the instrument used, results in the release of mutagenic and carcinogenic materials, including carbon particles, virus, bacteria, DNA, aerosolized blood, blood-borne pathogens, and over 41 known hazardous gases such as benzene, formaldehyde, toluene, and acrolein.

Forceful microexplosions of tissue, as in applications of the Q-switched Nd:YAG, or ruby lasers, as well as the tissue splatter associated with the Er:YAG laser, also present airborne contamination hazards, often in excess of that resulting from thermal injury to tissues.

There is a global trend toward eliminating the hazards of plume from our daily lives. The main focus has been on public smoking in confined areas such as airplanes, restaurants, offices, and hotels. The hazards contained in plume are well documented and governments around the world such as America, Canada, the UK, Australia, New Zealand, Germany, and Singapore have taken action.

This same activity has occurred in our healthcare workplaces, as we become more and more aware of the hazards associated with surgical plume (7).

Surgical plume is more than an inconvenience, and must be treated as an occupational hazard with a high level of risk. Effective removal results from both proper filtration equipment, and good work practices, including appropriate capture (device positioned not further than 2 cm from the point of evolution of the plume), systems, closed systems for laparoscopy, in-line filters for wall suction, patient protection during airway procedures, and evacuation systems now known as local exhaust ventilation systems (Fig. 17.10).

Plume evacuation systems should be selected after careful evaluation of needs and options available. Filters must remove particulates to 0.1 μm, which is the mean average diameter of viral particulates found in surgical plume. This requires an ultra low-particulate air filter in order to eliminate the viral hazards, and should be rated to 99.999% efficiency to be effective. Filters should have a filter life monitor, indicating when to change the filters. Units should also be assessed for suction power measured in cubic feet per minute (CFM), (suction should not be <50 CFM), and for the noise factor (should not exceed recommended OH&S decibel levels).

High-efficiency particulate air filters are NOT adequate, filtering only to particle sizes of 0.3 μm (a mean average diameter of bacteria and not an area of greatest concern in medicine).

Masks are not meant to be the first line of protective devices, against plume exposure in the breathing zone. There are no masks on the market today, including N95 masks, which are capable of filtering out all airborne contaminants. Furthermore, high-filtration material works only while dry, so during a lengthy surgical case, the filtration medium stops working when the mask gets damp from breathing, defeating the purpose of the mask. Also a factor is a fit and wearing technique. Masks (particularly N95 masks) must be fit tested for each

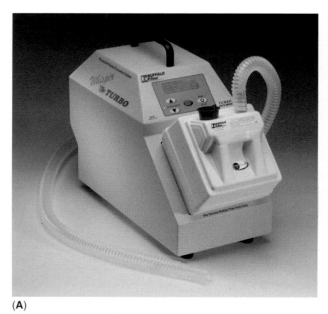

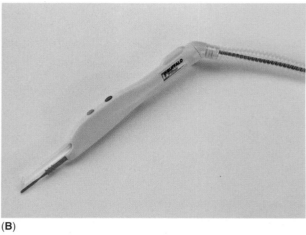

(B)

(A)

Figure 17.10 (**A**) Turbo and (**B**) plume pen: examples of plume evacuation system and capture device for electrosurgery.

employee, to ensure of a tight seal, and must be secured and worn properly at all times if they are to be effective, and in compliance with OSHA regulations on respiratory protection. If a facility is going to follow standard precautions (bloodborne pathogens standard), then high-filtration masks should be worn for all surgical plume producing cases, that is, about 95% of all procedures. This can be a costly and relatively ineffective control measure, and it is recommended that infection control nurses work with facility managers to develop a reasonable policy and procedure for the use of protective face masks.

Wall suction lines should always be protected with in-line filters that are placed between the wall inlet and the floor canister. Though these filters may decrease suction strength, they will prevent the buildup of particulates and debris in suction lines in the wall, which often results in expensive repairs to the central vacuum system.

All materials used to collect and handle surgical plume should be considered as biohazard, and disposed of according to infection control procedures. Staff must wear masks, goggles, and gloves to change and handle filters, and should place all used materials in biohazard bags.

RISK MANAGEMENT STEP 4:
AUDIT FOR SAFETY PROGRAM MONITORING
Safety audits monitor compliance with facility policies and procedures. The LSO will determine the frequency of the audit, which is based on the number of lasers, number of users, case numbers, and number of people involved. The greater the numbers and heavier the use, the more frequent the audit should be. Audit should be done at least once a year.

A laser safety audit, for those that have not done one, is simply an assessment of staff compliance, equipment, supplies, and documents involved in performing laser treatments in a facility. It can be performed by anyone familiar with the systems, but must be supervised by the LSO, who is ultimately responsible. Audits help identify areas of deficit requiring further education and training, purchase of new equipment, or

the need for additional control measures. Audits should always be done when new systems or procedures are initiated.

Audit requires completing each of the following steps:

1. Inventory all equipment and develop a checklist
2. Inspect every item on the checklist, assessing its condition, placement, and handling
3. Interview staff working with the laser systems
4. Observe laser procedures (setup, testing, and intraoperative management)
5. Document results
6. Remedy deficiencies identified
7. Monitor outcomes and follow-up

An inventory/checklist includes laser unit, keys, and storage system; delivery devices, signs, protective eyewear, window barriers, logs, tanks, supply carts, plume evacuation systems, lens filters for microscopes and endoscopes, cleavers and strippers for fibers, operation manuals, adapters, and policy/procedure manuals. Include all lasers and all systems in all areas of the facility, including ophthalmology clinics, hospital owned professional offices, emergency room, day surgery, cardiac cath lab, dental unit, physiotherapy, or any other clinical or research area. If the facility operates a mobile service or satellite centers, all lasers in those areas must be included as well.

Questions to ask during an audit are as follows:

1. Is it where it should be? (stored, covered, cleaned)
2. Does it work properly? (test all delivery systems and controls)
3. Is it being handled and used properly? (observe staff, sign posting, eyewear etc.)
4. Is it safe? (all parts present and correct policies present, etc.)
5. Is it intact?
6. Does it need repair or replacement?
7. Has it been misused or abused?

Results should be documented and reported to the program administrator, for action. The purpose of an audit is to identify potential hazards in equipment or work practices, and to lead to corrective actions. An example might be the discovery that the CO_2 laser arm is not replaced properly, potentially leading to damage and misalignment of the optics. If such an item is noted in the audit report, the resulting action could be to require every staff member to attend an inservice on handling the laser arm, and validate skill by performing a return demonstration for the LSO. Another audit result might be that glasses need to be replaced because they are scratched and have loose frames.

Audits should also include calibration and output testing, which can be delegated to biomedical engineering or the company laser technician. The LSO should keep a copy of audit reports in the laser program files, along with user credentials, equipment history, staff training validation, service agreements, logs, and other documentation.

Should there be an accident, incident, or occurrence, documentation of a current audit will help substantiate that the user maintained both safe systems, and staff compliance, in accordance with the expectations of standards.

Education and Training

Education (didactic knowledge) and training (operational skill) equip clinicians with the foundation information needed to establish a laser-safe environment. This is an individual responsibility without universal criteria, and with varied levels of resources available in different regions of the world. There are no authorities, boards, examinations, agencies, or organizations that can credential or certify anyone in laser use or laser safety, with a very few exceptions. Even if an organization claims to be able to certify, it is still the responsibility of the facilities or practitioners to individually approve that certification, as meeting their own criteria and standards. Course certificates can only verify attendance at a program. Some courses offer written examinations, which validate a certain level of knowledge, but competency and operational skills must be validated with the user's own device in a suitable manner. Education must be an ongoing effort to stay current with the technology through journals, conferences, networking, and professional organizations.

A comprehensive program should include the following topics with ample time for discussion, and relevant questions:

1. Biophysics and Tissue Interactions of all Wavelengths
2. Instrumentation and Delivery Systems
3. Clinical Applications
4. Standards, Regulations, and Professional Recommended Practices
5. Control Measures (Administrative, Engineering, and Procedural)
6. Patient Management
7. Maintenance and Repair (Troubleshooting)
8. Audit and Monitoring
9. Documentation and Reporting

Laser vendors and representatives can provide operational (hands-on) training, but cannot usually provide professional level education, or non–commercially biased information on the science and technology outside their own equipment. All professionals should avail themselves of comprehensive education before taking operational training, so they will have the knowledge base required for safe laser program implementation.

Documentation

Of all "safety" procedures, documentation should become a priority. Logs, operative records, audit reports, policies, repair and maintenance records, and committee minutes all contribute to claims that a clinician established and enforced a laser safe practice. Without proper documentation, there is no factual, objective, or sustainable support for that claim.

Inaccurate, incomplete, and absent documentation is an area of liability for many laser clinicians around the world. More and more emphasis is being placed on compliance with known safety standards, and it is an imperative in today's litigation-conscious environment.

Each facility must develop its own forms and decide on its own requirements for collecting data. Sample forms are found here, to assist in this task, but it must be clearly stated that they should not be copied and used as such, and MUST be formatted to reflect individual practice, and the results of each practice's risk assessment.

Documentation should be included in the formal audit process, with a focus on identifying areas not being completed properly.

Safety is Everyone's Responsibility

Routine audit, troubleshooting, training, policy and procedure development, and compliance enforcement are duties of the LSO, but case by case, day by day, patient by patient, laser safety depends on each and every healthcare professional's commitment and vigilance.

Lasers can offer patients a wonderful range of treatment options, from standard of care to experimental innovation. Laser users are constantly challenged to redefine who they are, what they do, and their scope of practice, with each new laser system or application.

It must be remembered that every new system may demand a new look at safety policies and procedures, and that only through teamwork, communication, and respect for the technology, can we establish the foundation for a truly effective laser safety program.

LASER SAFETY AUDIT PLAN

Audit is essential for any Quality Assurance Program and documents compliance, as well as areas of deficiencies needing improvement. Audit is a means of looking at all aspects of your laser safety program, in a formal and comprehensive manner as follows:

I. Laser Safety Officer

Materials needed: Job Descriptions for LSO
   Written Statement of Authority from Management Points to be evaluated:

1. LSO appointed: statement of authority from administration
2. Training and qualifications documented
3. Time available for related duties
4. Continuing education plan
5. LSO deals appropriately with problems and is available when needed
6. Safety audits and reporting completed

II. Equipment

Materials needed: Lasers and all accessory equipment.
   Points evaluated:

1. Status and condition of equipment (history and documentation)
2. Physical plant (handling and moving, fire extinguishers, storage, etc.)
3. Proper handling, setup, storage by staff

III. Continuing Education

Materials needed: records of all inservice and training programs for nursing and technical staff
   Credentialing criteria, forms, policies for medical staff:
   Points evaluated:

1. Medical staff credentials (policies and forms) in order and current
2. Nursing staff training documented
3. New or additional staff orientation
4. Annual refresher and skills validation
5. Conferences/ workshops attended or planned
6. Learning needs assessment (current and future)

IV. Documentation

Materials needed and points evaluated:

1. Policies/procedures
2. Log sheets (review of current logs and a copy of blank form)

3. Incident/accident report forms and procedures for reporting
4. Problems identified (any QA reports or accidents that have occurred)
5. Knowledge/presence of ANSI standards
6. Equipment inventory (biomed) with service contract information
7. State license or registration (where required)

V. Program Development

No specific materials needed to evaluate the following points:

1. New procedures/instrumentation to be acquired or initiated
2. Clinical research projects—industry partnerships
3. Alternative/ additional practice sites or redesign/ expansion
4. Teaching program involvement (medical and/or nursing)

VI. Use of Third Party Equipment

Laser equipment being rented or borrowed must meet the same standards as owned equipment. Facility is still responsible for all administrative and procedural control measures.
   Materials needed:

Terms of agreement between a facility and rental company
Copies of rental company patient case logs
Rental company policies and procedures
Credentials of technicians running rental lasers
Intake Checklist

Points evaluated:

a. Who is responsible for the intake procedures?
b. Are proper documentation forms being completed?
c. Are facility staff trained in basic operations and equipment handling?
d. Whether surgeons have been credentialed
e. Education and training of rental company staff
f. Do rental company staff comply with ANSI standards and basic OSHA requirements?
g. Appropriate supervision of rental company staff

Audit will be documented in a written report that contains: Identification of areas of noncompliance with standards, needs assessment, recommendations for remedy of deficiencies, and a follow-up plan.
   See further Tables 17.1–17.12.

Table 17.1 Laser Audit Checklist

Item	Yes	No	N/A	Comments on Deficiencies Noted and Action Taken	Date Corrected
1. *Administrative Controls*					
a) Copies of ANSI Z136.3 at the laser use site					
b) Written policies and procedures at use site					
c) Laser log located at laser site and completed properly					
d) All users have read and have knowledge of p/p and standards					
2. *Laser and Accessories*					
a) Keys accessed by authorized persons only					
b) No unauthorized modifications to equipment					
c) Equipment properly cleaned and stored					
d) Laser keys in proper storage location					
3. *Safety Glasses*					
a) Appropriate to the laser in use					
b) Labels intact and clearly readable					
c) Lenses clean and free of defects					
d) Cleaned and stored properly after use					
4. *Electrical Safety*					
a) Electrical components in good repair					
b) Scheduled testing/maintenance up to date and documented					
5. *Fire Safety*					
a) Extinguisher available to every room where laser procedures performed					
b) Fire exits free of obstruction and working properly					
6. *Observation*					
a) Proper staff handling and positioning of laser and accessory equipment					
b) Laser keys removed from laser after use					
c) Only authorized persons allowed in the room during laser use					
d) Patient properly protected					

Comments: _____

_____

Audited by _____ Date _____

Report received by LSO _____ Date _____

Table 17.2 Skills Validation Checklist. Each healthcare facility must develop its own criteria for validating laser operator skills. This sample checklist may be used as a guideline.

Laser Operator Performance Checklist

1. Applicant has read laser policies and procedures   _____
2. Knows applicable standards and rules   _____
3. Has submitted certificate of attendance for an LSO approved course.   _____
4. Has attended an equipment inservice by an instructor approved by the LSO   _____
5. Knows security system for the laser keys   _____
6. Establishes a laser safe treatment room, following all policies and procedures for hazard control   _____
7. Knows how to assemble and position all laser equipment and delivery systems   _____
8. Performs test fire/fiber calibration procedures   _____
9. Operates control panel properly:
                         power setting   _____
                         time exposure   _____
                         standby/ready   _____
                         emergency off   _____
10. Assembles, positions, and checks plume evacuator   _____
11. Completes all documentation forms   _____
12. Knows proper methods for cleaning and storing laser accessories and equipment   _____
13. Demonstrates ability to monitor a laser safe environment   _____
14. Knows proper endotracheal tube protocol   _____

Table 17.3 Procedure for Obtaining Laser Surgery Privileges

Policy: All laser privilege applications will be submitted to the laser committee for review and recommendation. Physicians must have current surgical privileges. Applications must be wavelength and specialty specific.

Procedure:

A. Obtain application forms from the Medical Staff Office
B. Submit proof of current staff privileges
C. Submit documentation of attendance at laser education programs to include course brochure, certificate, and course notes verifying course content.
   1) Course must be no less than 8 hours Category 1 credit
   2) Course may not have been completed more than six months prior to application
   3) Content must include laser physics, tissue interactions, instrumentation and delivery systems, clinical procedures, patient management, alternative treatments, safety and standards, hospital policy and procedure, and laboratory exercises with appropriate tissue models, designed to teach surgical techniques and understanding dosimetry.
D. Residency training must be documented by a letter from the program director, and must verify education equivalent to the course criteria stated in C 3.
E. Five documented cases from another facility may be substituted for the above requirements, provided that they were performed with the same lasers and delivery systems.
F. Under conditional privileges, the applicant will complete three cases under the supervision of a proctor, who will certify safe and appropriate surgical laser use.
G. Applicant will complete an equipment inservice scheduled with the LSO, prior to booking the first case.
H. Privileges will be reviewed every two years, and if the surgeon has not performed a minimum of one case per month, he/she will be required to submit proof of attendance at a refresher course.

Table 17.4 Controlled Access

Purpose: To define the area in which control measures must be applied, and to describe the control measures necessary in order to maintain a laser safe treatment environment.

Policy: Lasers will only be operated in areas where traffic flow can be monitored, and access can be limited by the laser safety officer, in compliance with all safety policies and procedures.

Procedure:

1. Regulation *Danger* signs will be posted at eye level, on all doors that allow access to a room in which a laser will be used.
2. Signs will be removed when the laser is not in use in the room.
3. Safety goggles labeled with the appropriate wavelength and optical density will be placed on each door, adjacent to the sign.
4. Laser keys will be secured and removed only by those authorized to operate the laser.
5. Only those who are authorized by the LSO may enter the laser room (nominal hazard zone) during laser procedures.
6. Doors will remain closed at all times during laser operation.
7. A temporary controlled access area will be established (NOTICE signs posted) during maintenance and/or repair.
8. The laser will be placed in a "STANDBY" mode when the delivery system is not aimed at target tissue.
9. The laser operator will not leave the laser in Ready mode if the control panel is unattended.

Date Approved: Date Reviewed:

Table 17.5 Test Firing the CO_2 Laser

Purpose: To determine the operational and safe functional status, beam alignment (infrared and visible aiming beam), and the beam profile (TEM00), of the CO_2 laser, prior to use.

Policy: CO_2 laser will be test fired each day it is to be used, prior to a scheduled laser procedure. It will also be tested if it is moved from room to room, used for demonstrations, or involved in service or other nonsurgical uses.

Procedure:
1. Set up a room according to controlled access procedures.
2. Drape Mayo stand with wet cloth towels (no exposed metal).
3. Follow all safety policies and procedures.
4. Set up laser with delivery systems to be used in surgery (handpiece, microscope, etc.)
5. Place wet wooden tongue depressor on wet towel surface, at the same angle as the delivery system so beam is emitted at a perpendicular angle.
6. Set laser for 5 W, single pulse, and fire onto the wet target.

Never fire the laser if you do not see the aiming beam
7. Examine the test spot for alignment and beam profile.
8. Repeat the test in all modes (repeat, continuous wave, superpulse, etc.).
9. Turn laser to standby if ready to begin, to off if leaving the room.
10. Document test results in the laser log.
11. For questionable results, request repeat test by the LSO.

Date Approved:	Approved By:

Table 17.6 Flammability Hazards and Fire Safety

Purpose: To prevent the risk of incidents and accidents involving laser ignition of materials, tissues, or other substances.

Policy: All procedures regarding safe application of laser energy will be adhered to during clinical use, demonstrations, service, and all other laser operations.

Procedures:
1. Laser personnel will know the location of the nearest fire extinguisher.
2. Water will be readily available during all laser procedures.
3. Nonreflective instruments and/or devices will be used in the path of the beam and in the operative field.
4. No alcohol-based solutions will be used in the beam path, or on target tissue.
5. Iodophor-based solutions will be allowed to dry thoroughly before the laser is activated.
6. Wet cloth towels will be used to drape the tissues immediately adjacent to the treatment site that may be exposed to direct or diffuse laser energy.
8. The anus will be protected with a wet sponge, during perianal procedures, to prevent ignition of methane gas.
9. No disposable or dry materials will be used near the treatment site or near the path of the laser beam.
10. Nail polish in the treatment area will be removed prior to treatment or covered with wet cloth material throughout the procedure.

Date Approved:	Date Reviewed:

Table 17.7 Handling of Fiber Delivery Systems

Purpose: To promote safe and appropriate handling of laser fiber delivery systems and to limit the potential for fiber breakage, damage, and reduced efficiency during clinical laser procedures.

Policy: Personnel handling laser fibers will assure compliance with all safety procedures, and will consider the fiber an extension of the laser system, governed by all standards and regulations.

Procedures:
1. Examine the fiber for breaks, kinks, or other obvious damage, along the length of the sheath, at the proximal end and at the distal end, prior to attaching to the laser.
2. Insert connector into the laser, taking care not to scratch the optical surface of the proximal end of the cable.
3. Calibrate the fiber according to the manufacturer's directions and chart the results on the laser log.
4. Never fire the laser if you do not observe the aiming beam.
5. Position the fiber on the field and secure safely. Do not use clamps or other instruments to secure the fiber to the operative site.
6. Secure the fiber in the antenna, when it is not in use.
7. Monitor the fiber during use for: distortion of the beam, accumulation of debris on the tip, or decreased power transmission.
8. Never place a hot fiber on the drapes. Wait until the tip is cool, before placing it in contact with potentially flammable materials.
9. When fiber is removed from the unit, the dummy plug must be inserted into the fiber connector port.

Date Approved:	Approved By:

Table 17.8 Laser-Generated Airborne Contaminants (LGAC)

Purpose: To effectively remove the biohazard of plume from the laser energy impact site, in order to reduce the risk of occupational exposure

Policy: A plume evacuation system will be used whenever the potential for the release of gases and/or tissue particulates, associated with the removal of hair or other tissues is anticipated.

Procedures:

1. Position the plume evacuator in the room whenever a laser is set up and plume is anticipated.
2. Check the operation of the unit and document on the log sheet.
3. Check the filter, and if needed, install a clean filter.
4. Hold the distal collection tube not further than 2 cm from the point at the impact site.
6. High-filtration masks will be worn by all personnel in the room, and will be fitted properly, leaving no gaps around the face.
7. Universal precautions will be observed throughout all phases of handling LGAC and evacuation equipment.
8. Biohazard disposal procedures will be followed for all materials involved in collection of LGAC.

Date Approved: Approved By:

Table 17.9 Ocular Safety

Purpose: To prevent injuries to patients receiving laser treatment, or to personnel in the laser treatment room during the use of laser equipment.

Policy: All personnel will adhere to eye protection procedures during all laser operations. Service personnel, technicians, and those involved in demonstrations, labs, or other nonclinical uses of the lasers, will adhere to eyewear policies as stated.

Procedures:

1. The LSO will assure that only properly tested and labeled laser safety eyewear stating the wavelength and an optical density of no less than 4.5 will be used by all personnel in the room during laser procedures.
2. Eyewear will have side protection, and will fit comfortably over prescription eyewear.
3. Each laser team member will be responsible for examining eyewear for defects in the optical coating, or other damage to both lenses and frames, before using them for laser protection. If damaged, eyewear is to be sent to the LSO for replacement or repair, and must NOT be worn.
4. Fluid or splash protectors are not to be worn for laser protection.
5. Patients receiving local or regional anesthesia will wear safety goggles that are secured to the face for the duration of the procedure.
6. Eyewear will be cleaned with only alcohol-free soaps, and returned to the individual storage cases, which are then placed in the laser supply cart, after each use. Responsibility for both staff and patient eyewear lies with designated facility personnel.

Date Approved: Approved By:

Table 17.10 Electrical Safety

Purpose: To prevent electrical accidents involving laser equipment.

Policy: All personnel handling, operating, or providing maintenance service, or demonstration of laser equipment in this facility, will comply will all procedures as stated.

Procedures:

1. Personnel will review hospital policy regarding the use and handling of electrical equipment in a patient care area.
2. All lasers and plume evacuators will be checked for electrical leakage semiannually during routine audit, and whenever brought into the hospital for demonstration, evaluation, or other nonclinical activities, and will be labeled according to biomedical policy.
3. No extension cords will be used on lasers.
4. Daily inspection of the footswitch connectors, circuit breakers, and power cords will be conducted by the laser operator, and charted on the log sheet, prior to use of the equipment.
5. Solutions will not be placed on or near the laser.
6. Defects or damage to electrical components will be properly repaired and documented prior to laser use.

Date Approved: Approved By:

Table 17.11 Criteria for Education of Perioperative Team Members

There are no standards or professional guidelines established for certification or validation of perioperative personnel working with healthcare lasers. The following suggestions are recommendations only.

Three groups of staff requiring education and training include:

1. Personnel who may be exposed incidentally to lasers in the operating room or laser treatment area but who do not have direct responsibility for operating the laser, maintaining the laser safe environment, or caring for the patient, should attend a basic inservice that covers:
   a. Introduction to the types of lasers, accessory equipment, and instrumentation in use in the facility.
   b. Safety hazards and control measures
   c. Relevant national, state, and professional standards
   d. Hospital policies and procedures
2. Personnel who work in a laser room, but do not operate the systems should have the above stated education with additional coverage of:
   a. Appropriate clinical applications for each laser
   b. Mechanisms of action of each wavelength
   c. Organization and administration of the laser safety program
   d. Documentation
   e. Procedures for establishing and maintaining a laser safe environment
3. Personnel who operate the laser equipment should have all of the above with further training including:
   a. Hands-on experience with each laser system, delivery systems, accessory equipment, instrumentation, and safety equipment
   b. Completion of skills validation checklists
   c. Completion of (number) cases with a certified preceptor
   d. Approval and sign-off by the LSO
4. All personnel should be required to participate in an annual continuing education program, with satisfactory completion documented by the LSO. This can be any professional activity if focused on current laser issues or safety issues.

Table 17.12 Laser Safety Officer: Statement of Authority

I. Scope of Authority

The primary responsibility for administering the facility's laser safety program shall be delegated to the Laser Safety Officer (LSO), and in his/her absence, the Deputy LSO. The LSO receives authority directly from the President of the facility, to accomplish all program activities and to intervene, if necessary, in the event of imminent danger or noncompliance with stated policies and procedures.

II. Scope of Responsibility

Specifically, the responsibilities of the LSO include, but may not be limited to:

   a. Management of the Laser Safety Program
   b. Knowledgeable evaluation of hazards
   c. Control of hazards in accordance with organizational policy, regulatory agencies, and consensus standards
   d. Identification of program revisions and enhancements
   e. Establish a formal audit system, and assure its monitoring activity
   f. Communication of audit findings, deficiency, and recommendations, as a result of program audit and management
   g. Provide appropriate education, training, and competency validation, to maintain required registration, licensure, credentialing and certification
   h. Establish facility policies, procedures, and documentation methods
   i. Participate on facility Laser Committee
   j. Provide technical and clinical resources and support as needed

III. Limit of Authority

The LSO is a primary resource to the President, CEO, and all other personnel in support of the organization's goal of providing a safe and effective environment of patient care. The CEO is ultimately responsible for organizational safety through a laser risk management program.

The organization has appointed _____ as the LSO, and _____ as the deputy LSO in his/her absence. The term of appointment is not limited, and will be reviewed periodically by the Administrator.

IV. Authority to Cross Departmental Boundaries

The LSO shall have the authority to cross all departmental boundaries in order to accomplish facility-wide enforcement of approved policies and procedures, and to resolve situations of hazard, imminent danger, and noncompliance. At times, this may require the collaboration of the Administrator On Call.

Signed by Appropriate Facility Administrator

REFERENCES

1. American National Standards Institute, ANSI Z136.3-2011, ISBN #978-0-9122035-69-7.
2. The Joint Commission, Environment of Care Standards EC: 02.02.01.
3. United States Department of Labor, Occupational Safety and Health Administration: 29CFR 1910, OSH Act 1970.
4. Blood Borne Pathogens 29CFR1910.1030.
5. 1910.2(f) "Standard" definitions (basis for using ANSI standards). [Available from: www.OSHA.gov]
6. Canadian Standards Association, Z305-13.09 Plume Scavenging in Surgical, Diagnostic, Therapeutic, and Aesthetic Settings.
7. International Federation of Perioperative Nurses Guideline for Management of Surgical Plume. [Available from: www.IFPN,org.uk]

Index